# THE VITAMINS

*Fundamental Aspects in Nutrition and Health*

*To my Dad,*
*whom I love and admire.*

# THE VITAMINS

*Fundamental Aspects in Nutrition and Health*

GERALD F. COMBS, JR.
*Division of Nutritional Sciences*
*Cornell University*
*Ithaca, New York*

**ACADEMIC PRESS, INC.**
*Harcourt Brace Jovanovich, Publishers*
San Diego  New York  Boston  London  Sydney  Tokyo  Toronto

*Academic Press Rapid Manuscript Reproduction*

Academic Press, Inc.
San Diego, California 92101

*United Kingdom Edition published by*
Academic Press Limited
24–28 Oval Road, London NW1 7DX

Library of Congress Cataloging-in-Publication Data

Combs, Gerald F.
    The vitamins : fundamental aspects in nutrition and health /
  Gerald F. Combs, Jr.
      p.   cm.
    Includes index.
    ISBN 0-12-183490-5
    1. Vitamins.   2. Nutrition.   I. Title.
    [DNLM:   1. Nutrition.   2. Vitamins.   QU 160 C731v]
  QP771.C645   1992
  612.3'99--dc20
  DNLM/DLC
  for Library of Congress                         91-35241
                                                       CIP

PRINTED IN THE UNITED STATES OF AMERICA
91  92  93  94    9  8  7  6  5  4  3  2  1

# CONTENTS

## SECTION I.   PERSPECTIVES ON THE VITAMINS IN NUTRITION

## SECTION II.   CONSIDERING THE INDIVIDUAL VITAMINS

## SECTION III.   USING CURRENT KNOWLEDGE OF THE VITAMINS

## APPENDICES

## INDEX

# PREFACE

I have found it to be true that one learns best what one has to teach. And, because I have had no formal training either in teaching or in the field of education in general, it was not for several years of my own teaching that I began to realize that the good teacher must understand more than the subject matter of his or her course. In my case, that realization developed, over a few years, with the recognition that individuals learn in different ways and that the process of learning itself is as relevant to my teaching as the material I present. This enlightenment has been for me invaluable because it has led me to the field of educational psychology from which I have gained at least some of the insights of the good teacher. In fact, it led me to write this book.

In exploring that field, I came across two books that have influenced me greatly: A Theory of Education[1] by another Cornell professor, Joe Novak, and Learning How to Learn[2] by Prof. Novak and his colleague Bob Gowin. I highly recommend their work to any scientific "expert" in the position of teaching within the area of his or her expertise. From those books and conversations with Prof. Novak, I have come to understand that people think (and, therefore, learn) in terms of *concepts* – not facts. Therefore, for the past few years I have experimented in offering my course at Cornell University, The Vitamins, in ways that are more concept-centered than I (or others, for that matter) have used previously. While I regard this experiment as an ongoing activity, it has already resulted in my shifting away from the traditional lecture format to one based on open classroom discussions aimed at involving the students, each of whom, I have found, brings a valuable personal perspective to discussions. I have found this to be particularly true for discussions concerning the vitamins; while it is certainly possible in modern societies to be misinformed about nutrition, it is virtually impossible to be truly naive. In other words, every person brings to the study of the vitamins some relevant conceptual framework and it is, thus, the task of the teacher to build upon that framework by adding new concepts, establishing new linkages and modifying existing ones where appropriate.

It quickly became clear to me that my own notes, indeed, all other available reference texts on the subject of the vitamins, were insufficient to support a concept-centered approach to the subject. Thus, I undertook to write a new type of textbook on the vitamins, one that would be maximally valuable in this kind of teaching. In so doing, I tried to focus on the key concepts and to make the book itself useful in a practical sense. Because I find myself writing in virtually any book that I really use, I gave this text margins wide enough for the reader to do the same. Because I have found the technical vocabularies of many scientific fields to present formidable barriers to learning, I have listed what I regard as the most important technical terms at the beginning of each chapter and have used each in context. Because I intend this to be an accurate synopsis of present understanding but not a

---

[1] Cornell University Press, Ithaca, N.Y., 1977, 324 pp.

[2] Cambridge University Press, New York, 1984, 199 pp.

definitive reference to the original scientific literature, I have cited only current major reviews that I find useful to the student. Because I have found the discussion of real-world cases to enhance learning of the subject, I have included case reports that can be used as classroom exercises or student assignments. I have designed the text for use as background reading for a one-semester upper-level college course within a nutrition-related curriculum. In fact, I have used draft versions in my course at Cornell as a means of refining it for this purpose.

While The Vitamins was intended primarily for use in teaching, I recognize that it will also be useful as a desk reference for nutritionists, dieticians and many physicians, veterinarians and other health professionals. Indeed, I have been gratified by the comments I have received from colleagues to that effect.

It is my hope that The Vitamins will be read, re-read, written in and thought over. It seems to me that a field as immensely fascinating as the vitamins demands nothing less.

G.F. Combs, Jr.

Ithaca, New York
August, 1991

# HOW TO USE THIS BOOK

**The Vitamins** is intended as a teaching text for an upper-level college course within a nutrition-related curriculum; however, it will also be useful as a desk reference or as a workbook for self-paced study of the vitamins. It has several features that are designed to enhance its usefulness to students as well as instructors.

## *To the student:*

Before reading each chapter, take a few moments to go over the *Anchoring Concepts* and *Learning Objectives* listed on the chapter title page. *Anchoring Concepts* are the ideas fundamental to the subject matter of the chapter; they are the concepts to which the new ones presented in the chapter will be related. The *Anchoring Concepts* identified in the first several chapters should already be very familiar to you; if they are not, then it will be necessary for you to do some background reading or discussion until you feel comfortable in your understanding of these basic ideas. You will find that most chapters are designed to build upon the understanding gained through previous chapters; in most cases, the *Anchoring Concepts* of a chapter relate to the *Learning Objectives* of previous chapters. Pay attention to the *Learning Objectives*; they are the key elements of understanding that the chapter is intended to support. Keeping the *Learning Objectives* in mind as you go through each chapter will help you maintain focus on the key concepts.

Next, read through the *Vocabulary* list and *mark* any terms that are unfamiliar or about which you feel unsure. Then, as you read through the text, look for them; you should be able to get a good feel for their meanings from the contexts of their uses. If this is not sufficient for any particular term, then you should consult a good medical or scientific dictionary.

As you go through the text, note what information the layout is designed to convey. First, note that the major sections of each chapter are indicated with a bold heading above a bar, and that the wide left margin contains key words and phrases that relate to the major topic of the text at that point. These are features that are designed to help you *scan* for particular information. Also note that the footnoted information is largely supplementary but not essential to the understanding of the key concepts presented. Therefore, the text may be read at two levels: at the basic level, one should be able to ignore the footnotes and still get the key concepts; at the more detailed level, one should be able to pick up more of the background information from the footnotes.

Chapters 5-17 are each followed by a *Case Study* comprised of one or more clinical case reports abstracted from the medical literature. For each case, use the associated questions to focus your thinking on the features that relate to vitamin functions. As you do so, try to ignore the obvious connection with the subject of the chapter; put yourself in the position of the attending physician who was called upon to diagnose the problem without prior knowledge that it involved any particular nutrient, much less a certain vitamin.

Take some time and go through the *Study Questions and Exercises* at the end of each chapter. These, too, are designed to direct your thinking back to the key concepts of each chapter and to facilitate integration of those concepts with those you already have. To this end, you are asked in this section of several chapters to prepare a *concept map* of the subject matter. Many people find the *concept map* to be a powerful learning tool; therefore, it you have had no previous experience with this device, then it will be well worth your while to consult Learning How to Learn[1].

At the end of each chapter is a reading list. With the exception of Chapter 2, which lists papers of landmark significance to the discovery of the vitamins, the reading lists consist of key reviews in prominent scientific journals. Thus, while primary research reports are not cited in the text, you should be able to trace research papers on topics of specific interest through the reviews that are listed.

Last, but certainly not least, have *fun* with this fascinating aspect of the field of nutrition!

## To the instructor:

I hope you will find this format and presentation useful in your teaching of the vitamins. To that end, some of my experiences in using **The Vitamins** as a text for my course at Cornell may be of interest to you.

I have found that *every* student comes to the study of the vitamins with *some* background knowledge of the subject, although those backgrounds are generally incomplete, frequently with substantial areas of no information and mis-information. This is true for upper-level nutrition majors and for students from other fields, the difference being largely one of magnitude. This is also true for instructors, most of whom come to the field with specific expertise that relates to only a subset of the subject matter. In addition, I have found that, by virtue of having at least *some* background on the subject and being motivated by any of a number of reasons to learn more, *every* student brings to the study of the vitamins a unique perspective which may not be readily apparent to the instructor. I am convinced that meaningful learning is served when both instructor and students come to understand each others' various perspectives. This has two benefits in teaching the vitamins. First, it is in the instructor's interest to know the students' ideas and levels of understanding concerning issues of vitamin need, vitamin function, etc., such that these can be built upon and modified as may be appropriate. Second, I have found that many upper-level students have interesting experiences (through personal or family histories, their own research, information from other courses, etc.) that can be valuable contributions to classroom discussions, thus, mitigating against the "instructor knows all" notion, which we all know to be false. To identify student perspectives, I have found it useful to assign on the first class period for submission at the second class a written autobiographical sketch. I distribute one I wrote for this purpose and I ask each student to write "as much or as little" as he or she cares to, recognizing that I will distribute copies of whatever is submitted to each

---

[1]Novak, J.D. and D.B. Gowin, 1984, Learning How to Learn, Cambridge University Press, New York, 199 pp.

student in the class. The biographical sketches that I see range from a few sentences that reveal little of personal nature, to longer ones that provide many good insights about their authors; I have found *every one* to help me get to know my students personally and to get a better idea of their understandings of the vitamins and of their expectations of my course. The exercise serves the students in a similar manner, thus, promoting a group dynamic that facilitates classroom discussions.

I have come to use **The Vitamins** in my teaching as the text from which I make regular reading assignments, usually a chapter at a time, as preparation for each class which I generally conduct in an open discussion format. Long ago, I found it difficult, if not impossible, to cover in a traditional lecture format all of the information about the vitamins I deemed important for a nutritionist to know. Thus, I have put that information in this text and have shifted more of the responsibility for learning to the student for gleaning it from reading. I use my class time to assist the student by providing discussions of issues of particular interest or concern. Often, this means that certain points were not clear upon reading or that the reading itself stimulated questions not specifically addressed in the text. Usually, these questions are nicely handled by eliciting the views and understandings of other students and by my giving supplementary information. Therefore, my class preparation involves the collation of research data that will supplement the discussion in the text and the identification of questions that I can use to initiate discussions. In developing my questions, I have found it useful to prepare my own concept maps of the subject matter and to ask rather simple questions about the linkages between concepts, e.g., *"How does the mode of enteric absorption of the tocopherols relate to what we know about its physio-chemical properties?"* If you are unfamiliar with concept mapping, then I strongly recommend your consulting Learning How to Learn[1] and experimenting with the technique to determine whether it can assist you in your teaching.

I have found it useful to give weekly written assignments for which I use the *Study Questions and Exercises* or *Case Studies*. In my experience, regular assignments keep students focused on the topic and prevent them from letting the course slide until exam time. More importantly, I believe there to be learning associated with the thought that necessarily goes into these written assignments. In order to support that learning, I make a point of going over each assignment briefly at the beginning of the class at which it is due, and of returning it by the *next* class with my written comments on *each* paper. You will find that the *Case Studies* I have included are abstracted from actual clinical reports; however, I have presented them without some of the pertinent clinical findings (e.g., responses to treatments) that were originally reported, in order to make of them learning exercises. I have found that students do well on these assignments and that they particularly enjoy the *Case Studies*.

I evaluate student performance on the basis of class participation, weekly written assignments, a review of a recent research paper, and either one or two examinations (i.e., either a final or a final plus a mid-term). In order to allow each student to pursue a topic of specific individual interest, I ask them to review a research paper published within the last year, using the style of Nutrition Reviews. I evaluate each review on its criticalness as well as on the importance of the paper that was selected, which I ask them to discuss. This assignment has also been generally well received. Because many students are inexperienced in research and thus feel uncomfortable in criticizing it, I have found it helpful to conduct in advance of the assignment a discussion dealing with the general principles of experimental design and statistical inference. Because I have adopted a concept-oriented teaching style, I long ago abandoned the use of short-answer questions (e.g., *"Name the species that require dietary sources of vitamin C"*) on examinations. Instead, I use brief case descriptions and actual experimental data and ask for diagnostic strategies, development of hypotheses, design of means of hypothesis testing, interpretation of results, etc. Many students may prefer the more traditional short-answer test; however, I have found that such inertia can be overcome by using examples in class discussions or homework assignments.

**The Vitamins** has been of great value in enhancing my teaching of the course by that name at Cornell. Thus, it is my sincere wish that it will assist you similarly in your teaching. Whatever your experiences with it are, please let me know about them.

G.F. Combs, Jr.

Ithaca, New York
August, 1991

# *SECTION I*

## PERSPECTIVES ON THE VITAMINS IN NUTRITION

# CHAPTER 1  *WHAT IS A VITAMIN?*

*"Imagination is more important than knowledge."*　　　　　A. Einstein

---

## Anchoring Concepts:

| | |
|---|---|
| *i.* | Certain factors, called *nutrients*, are necessary for normal physiological function of animals including man. Some nutrients cannot be synthesized adequately by the host and must, therefore, be obtained from the external chemical environment; these are referred to as *dietary essential nutrients*. |
| *ii.* | *Diseases* involving physiological dysfunction often accompanied by morphological changes can result from insufficient intakes of dietary essential nutrients. |

## Learning Objectives:

| | |
|---|---|
| *i.* | To understand the classical meaning of the term *vitamin* as it is used in the field of nutrition. |
| *ii.* | To understand that the term vitamin describes both a *concept* of fundamental importance in nutrition as well as any member of a rather heterogeneous array of nutrients any one of which may *not* fully satisfy the classical definition. |
| *iii.* | To understand the concepts of a *vitamer* and a *pro-vitamin*. |

## Vocabulary:

vitamin
vitamer
pro-vitamin

## A REVOLUTIONARY CONCEPT

*everyday word or revolutionary idea?*

The term **vitamin**, today a common word in everyday language, was born of a revolution in thinking about the interrelationships of diet and health that occurred at the beginning of the twentieth century.

That revolution involved the growing realization of two phenomena that are now so well understood that they are taken for granted even by the lay person:

> *i.*     Diets are sources of more nutrients than the few then recognized by physiologists, those being *protein*, *fat*, *carbohydrate*, *"ash"* and *water*, which accounted for very nearly 100% of the mass of most foods;
>
> *ii.*    Low intakes of specific nutrients can cause certain diseases.

In today's world, each of these concepts may seem self-evident; but in a world still responding to and greatly influenced by the important discoveries in microbiology of the nineteenth century, each represented a major departure from contemporaneous thinking in the area of health. With this view, it is understandable that, at the turn of the century, experimental findings which now can be seen as indicating the presence of hitherto unrecognized nutrients were interpreted instead as substantiating the presence of natural antidotes to unidentified disease-causing microbes.

Important discoveries in science have ways of directing, even entrapping, one's view of the world - a tendency resistance from which depends upon critical and constantly questioning minds. That such minds were involved in early nutrition research is evidenced by the spirited debates and frequent polemics that ensued over discoveries of apparently beneficial new dietary factors. Still, the systematic development of what emerged as nutritional science depended upon a *new* intellectual construct for interpreting such experimental observations.

*vitamin or vitamine?*

The elucidation of the nature of what was later to be called thiamin occasioned the proposition of such a new construct in physiology[1]. Aware of the impact of what was a departure from prevailing thought, its author, the Polish biochemist **Casimir Funk**, chose to generalize from his findings on the chemical nature of that *"vital amine"* to suggest the term

---

[1]This is a clear example of what T.H. Kuhn has called a "scientific revolution" (The Structure of Scientific Revolutions, 1968), i.e., the discarding of an old paradigm with the invention of a new one.

*vitamine* as a generic descriptor for many such *accessory factors* associated with diets. That the factors soon to be elucidated comprised a somewhat chemically heterogeneous group not all of which were nitrogenous does not diminish the importance of the introduction of what was first pronounced as the *vitamine theory*, later to become a key concept in nutrition: *the vitamin.*

The term *vitamin* has been defined in various ways. While the very concept of a vitamin was crucial to progress in understanding nutrition, the actual definition of a vitamin has evolved in consequence of that understanding.

## AN OPERATING DEFINITION

For the purposes of the study of this aspect of nutrition, a vitamin is defined as follows:

### A vitamin . . .

---

is an *organic compound* distinct from fats, carbohydrates and proteins;

is a *natural component of foods* where it is usually present in minute amounts;

is essential, also usually in minute amounts, for *normal physiological function* (i.e., maintenance, growth, development and/or production);

causes, by its absence or under-utilization, a *specific deficiency syndrome*;

is *not synthesized by the host* in amounts adequate to meet normal physiological needs.

---

This definition will be useful in the study of the vitamins, as it effectively distinguishes this class of nutrients from the others (i.e., proteins and amino acids, essential fatty acids, minerals) and indicates the needs in various normal physiological functions. It also points out the specificity of deficiency syndromes by which the vitamins were discovered. Further, it places the vitamins in that portion of the chemical environment upon which animals (including humans) must depend for survival, thus distinguishing vitamins from hormones.

*some caveats* It will quickly become clear, however, that, for all of its usefulness, this operating definition has serious limitations, notably with respect to the last clause, for many species can indeed synthesize at least some of the vitamins.

Four examples illustrate this point:

*i.*    Most animal species have the ability to synthesize ascorbic acid. Only those few which lack the enzyme l-gulonolactone oxidase (e.g., the guinea pig, humans) cannot; only for them can ascorbic acid properly be called **vitamin C**.

*ii.*   Individuals exposed to modest amounts of sunlight can produce adequate amounts of cholecalciferol which for them functions as a hormone. Only individuals without sufficient exposure to ultraviolet light (e.g., livestock raised in indoor confinement, people spending most of their days indoors) require a dietary source of **vitamin D**.

*iii.*  Most animal species have the metabolic capacity to synthesize choline; however, some (e.g., the chick, the rat) may not be able to employ that capacity if they are fed insufficient amounts of methyl-donor compounds. In addition, some (e.g., the chick) do not develop that capacity fully until several weeks of age. Thus, for the young chick and for individuals of other species fed diets providing limited methyl groups, **choline** is a vitamin.

*iv.*   All animal species can synthesize nicotinic acid mononucleotide (NMN) from the amino acid tryptophan. Only those for which this metabolic conversion is particularly inefficient (e.g., the cat, fishes) and others fed low dietary levels of tryptophan require a dietary source of **niacin**.

With these counter-examples in mind, the definition of a vitamin can be understood as having specific reference to animal species, stage of development, diet or nutritional status, and physical environmental conditions.

Thus, it will be seen that:

**some compounds are vitamins for one species and not another**; and
**some are vitamins only under specific dietary or environmental conditions**.

*the vitamins*    Thirteen substances or groups of substances are now generally recognized as vitamins; others have been proposed[2]. In some cases, the familiar name is actually the *generic descriptor* for a family of chemically related compounds having qualitatively comparable metabolic activities.  For example, the term *"vitamin E"* refers to those analogues of tocol or tocotrienol[3] that are active in preventing such syndromes as fetal resorption in the rat and myopathies in the chick.  In these cases, the members of the same vitamin family are called **vitamers**.  Some carotenoids can be metabolized to yield the metabolically active form of vitamin A; such a precursor of an actual vitamin is called a **pro-vitamin**.

## Study Questions:

i.       What are the key features that define a vitamin?

ii.      What is the fundamental difference between a vitamin and a hormone?

iii.     List the recognized vitamins.

---

[2]These include such factors as inositol, carnitine, bioflavinoids, pangamic acid and laetrile, for some of which there is evidence of vitamin-like activity (*see* Chapter 19).

[3]Tocol is 3,4-dihydro-2-methyl-2-(4,8,12-trimethyltridecyl)-6-chromanol; tocotrienol is the analog with double bonds at the 3',7' and 11' positions on the phytol side chain. See Chapter 7.

## The Vitamins: their *Vitamers*, *Pro-vitamins*[4] and *Functions*

| group | vitamers | pro-vitamins | physiological functions |
|---|---|---|---|
| Vitamin A | retinol<br>retinal<br>retinoic acid | $\beta$-carotene<br>cryptoxanthin | visual pigments<br>epithelial cell differentiation |
| Vitamin D | cholecalciferol ($D_3$)<br>ergocalciferol ($D_2$) | | Ca homeostasis |
| Vitamin E | $\alpha$-tocopherol<br>$\gamma$-tocopherol | | membrane antioxidant |
| Vitamin K | phylloquinones ($K_1$)<br>menaquinones ($K_2$)<br>menadione ($K_3$) | | blood clotting<br>Ca metabolism |
| Vitamin C | ascorbic acid<br>dehydroascorbic acid | | reductant in hydroxylations in the<br>   formation of collagen and carnitine, and<br>   in the metabolism of drugs and steroids |
| Vitamin $B_1$ | thiamin | | coenzyme for decarboxylations of 2-keto<br>   acids (e.g., pyruvate) and<br>   transketolations |
| Vitamin $B_2$ | riboflavin | | coenzymes in redox reactions of fatty<br>   acids and the TCA cycle |
| Niacin | nicotinic acid<br>nicotinamide | | coenzymes for several dehydrogenases |
| Vitamin $B_6$ | pyridoxol<br>pyridoxal<br>pyridoxamine | | coenzymes in amino acid metabolism |
| Folic Acid | folic acid<br>polyglutamyl folacins | | coenzyme in single-carbon metabolism |
| Biotin | biotin | | coenzyme for carboxylations |
| Pantothenic Acid | pantothenic acid | | coenzymes in fatty acid metabolism |
| Vitamin $B_{12}$ | cobalamin | | coenzymes in the metabolism of<br>   propionate, amino acids and single<br>   carbon |

---

[4]Several other carotenoids are also pro-vitamins A; these are discussed in Chapter 5.

# CHAPTER 2  *DISCOVERY OF THE VITAMINS*

*"When science is recognized as a framework of evolving concepts and contingent methods for gaining new knowledge, we see the very human character of science, for it is creative individuals operating from the totality of their experiences who enlarge and modify the conceptual framework of science."*

J. D. Novak

## Anchoring Concepts:

*i.*  A scientific **theory** is a *plausible explanation* for a set of observed phenomena; because theories cannot be tested directly, their acceptance relies upon a preponderance of supporting evidence.

*ii.*  A scientific **hypothesis** is a *tentative supposition* that is assumed for the purposes of argument or testing and is, thus, used in the generation of evidence by which theories can be evaluated.

*iii.*  An **empirical approach** to understanding the world involves the generation of theories strictly by observation, while an **experimental approach** involves the undertaking of operations (experiments) to test the truthfulness of hypotheses.

*iv.*  **Physiology** is that branch of biology dealing with the processes, activities and phenomena of life and living organisms, and that **biochemistry** deals with the molecular bases for such phenomena. The field of **Nutrition**, derived from both of these disciplines, deals with the processes by which animals or plants take in and utilize food substances.

## Learning Objectives:

i.      To understand the nature of the **process of discovery** in the field of nutrition.

ii.     To understand the impact of the **"vitamine theory"**, as an intellectual construct, on that process of discovery.

iii.    To recognize the **major forces** in the emergence of nutrition as a science.

iv.     To understand that the discoveries of the vitamins proceeded along **indirect lines** most often through the seemingly unrelated efforts of many persons.

v.      To know the **key events** in the discovery of each of the vitamins.

vi.     To become familiar with the **basic terminology** of the vitamins and their associated deficiency disorders.

## Vocabulary:

| | |
|---|---|
| accessory factor | pantothenic acid |
| anemia | pellagra |
| animal model | polyneuritis |
| animal protein factor | prothrombin |
| ascorbic acid | purified diet |
| beri-beri | pyridoxine |
| biotin | retinen · |
| black tongue disease | riboflavin |
| $\beta$-carotene | rickets |
| cholecalciferol | scurvy |
| choline | vitamin A |
| dermatitis | vitamin B |
| ergocalciferol | vitamin $B_2$ |
| fat-soluble A | vitamin B complex |
| filtrate factor | vitamin $B_6$ |
| flavin | vitamin $B_{12}$ |
| folic acid | vitamin C |
| hemorrhage | vitamin D |
| lactoflavin | vitamin E |
| niacin | vitamin K |
| night blindness | water-soluble B |
| ovoflavin | xerophthalmia |

## THE EMERGENCE OF NUTRITION AS A SCIENCE

In the span of only five decades commencing at the very end of the nine-teenth century, the vitamins were discovered.  Their discoveries were the result of the activities of hundreds of people that can be viewed retro-spectively as having followed discrete branches of intellectual growth. Those branches radiated from ideas originally derived inductively from observations in the natural world, each starting from the recognition of a relationship between diet and health.  Subsequently, branches were pruned through repeated analysis and deduction, a process that both produced and proceeded from the fundamental approaches used in experimental nutrition today.  Once pruned, the limb of discovery may appear straight to the naive observer.  Scientific discovery, however, does *not* occur that way; rather, it tends to follow a zig-zag course with many participants contributing many branches; the contemporaneous view of each partici-pant may be that of a thicket of tangled hypotheses and facts.  The seemingly straight-forward appearance of the emergent limb of discovery is only an illusion achieved by discarding the dead branches of false starts and unsupported hypotheses, each of which can be instructive about the process of scientific discovery.

With the discovery of the vitamins, therefore, nutrition moved from a largely observational activity to one that relied increasingly upon hypothesis testing through experimentation; it moved from empiricism to science. Both the process of scientific discovery and the course of the development of nutrition as a scientific discipline are perhaps best illustrated by the history of the discovery of the vitamins.

## THE PROCESS OF DISCOVERY IN NUTRITIONAL SCIENCE

*empiricism and experiment*

History shows that the process of scientific discovery starts with the syn-thesis of general ideas about the natural world from observations of particulars in it, i.e., an *empirical phase*.  In the discovery of the vitamins, this initial phase was characterized by the recognition of associations between diet and human diseases, namely, *night blindness*, *scurvy*, *beri-beri*, *rickets* and *pellagra*, each of which was long prevalent in various societies.  The next phase in the process of discovery involves the use of these generalizations to generate hypotheses that can be tested experi-mentally, i.e., the *experimental* phase.  In the discovery of the vitamins, this phase necessitated the development of two key tools of modern experi-mental nutrition:  the **animal model** and the **purified diet**.  The availability of both of these tools proved to be necessary for the discovery of each vitamin; in cases where one was late to be developed (e.g., an animal model for pellagra), the elucidation of the identity of the vitamin was postponed until it was.

## THE EMPIRICAL PHASE OF VITAMIN DISCOVERY

The major barrier to entering the empirical phase of nutritional inquiry proved to be the security provided by pre-scientific attitudes about foods that persisted until the last century. Many societies had observed that human populations in markedly contrasting parts of the world tend to experience similar health standards despite the fact that they subsist on very different diets. These observations were taken by nineteenth century physiologists to indicate that health was not particularly affected by the kinds of foods consumed. Foods were thought important as sources of the only nutrients known at the time: **protein, available energy** and **"ash"**. In the middle part of the century, attention was drawn further from potential relationships of diet and health by the major discoveries of Pasteur, Liebig, Koch and others in microbiology. For the first time, several diseases, first anthrax and then others, could be understood in terms of a microbial etiology. By the end of the century, germ theory, which proved to be of immense value in medicine, directed hypotheses for the etiologies of most diseases. The impact of this understanding as a barrier to entering the inductive phase of nutritional discovery is illustrated by the case of the Dutch physician **Christian Eijkman**, who found a water-soluble factor from rice bran to prevent a beri-beri-like disease in chickens (now known to be the vitamin thiamin) and concluded that he had found a "pharmacological antidote" against the beri-beri "microbe" presumed to be present in rice.

*diseases linked to diet*

Nevertheless, while they appeared to affect little the prevailing views concerning the etiology of human disease, by the late 1800s, several empirical associations had been made between diet and the diseases.

Four diseases empirically associated with diet:

|  |  |
|---|---|
| scurvy | rickets |
| beri-beri | pellagra |

*scurvy*

For several centuries it has been known that scurvy, the disease involving sore gums, painful joints and multiple hemorrhages, could be prevented by including in the diet green vegetables or fruits. Descriptions of cases in such sources as the Eber papyrus (ca. 1150 B.C.) and writings of Hippocrates (ca. 420 B.C.) are often cited to indicate that scurvy was prevalent in those ancient populations. Indeed, signs of the disease are said to have been found in the skeletal remains of primitive man. Scurvy was common in northern Europe during the middle ages where local agriculture provided few sources of vitamin C that were stable to winter storage. It was very highly prevalent among seamen who subsisted for months at a time on dried and salted foods. The Spanish explorer **Vasco da Gama** reported losing more than 60% of his crew of 160 sailors in his voyage around the Cape of Good Hope in 1498. In 1535, the French explorer **Jacques**

**Cartier** reported that signs of scurvy were shown by all but three of his crew of 103 men (25 of whom died) during his second Newfoundland expedition.  In 1593, the British admiral **Richard Hawkins** wrote that, during his career, he had seen some 10,000 seamen die of the disease.

While the link between scurvy and *"preserved"* foods was long evident, the first report of a cure for the disease appears to have been Cartier's description of the rapidly successful treatment of his crew with an infusion of arborvitae prepared by the indigenous people of Newfoundland.  By 1601, the efficacy of regular consumption of citrus fruits or juices was recognized as a means of preventing the disease.  In that year, the English privateer **Sir James Lancaster** introduced regular issues of such foods on the ships of the East India Company.

Against this background, the British physician often called "the founder of modern naval hygiene", **James Lind**, wrote the now-classic <u>Treatise on Scurvy</u> in 1753, which had great impact on medical thought of the time. It detailed past work on the subject, most of which was anecdotal, but also presented the results of his own experiments with British sailors.  Lind's experimental comparisons of putative cures for scurvy are recognized as *the first controlled clinical trials in medical research*.  Their results established clearly the value of fresh fruits in treating the disease.  By 1804, the British Navy had made it a regular practice to issue daily rations of lemon juice to all seaman − a measure that gave rise to the term *"limey"*[1] as a slang expression for a British seaman.  In the early part of the nineteenth century, there remained no doubt of a dietary cause and cure of scurvy; still, it would be more than a century before its etiology and metabolic basis would be elucidated.

*beri-beri*  It is said that signs consistent with beri-beri (e.g., peripheral neuropathy, cardiac enlargement, edema) are described in the ancient Chinese Herbals (ca. 2600 B.C.).  Certainly, beri-beri, too, has been an historic disease prevalent in many Asian populations subsisting on diets in which polished (i.e., "white" or dehulled) rice is the major food.  For example, in the 1860s, the Japanese Navy reported an incidence of the disease that approached one-third of its seamen.  Interesting clinical experiments conducted in the 1870s with sailors by Director General **Takaki** of the Japanese Naval Medical Service showed the association of beri-beri and diet.  Finding that the disease could be very effectively prevented by increasing the daily rations of vegetables, fish, meat and barley in the place of rice, Takaki concluded that it was caused by insufficient dietary protein or by a relative excess of fat and carbohydrate to protein in the diet.  The adoption of Takaki's dietary recommendations by the Japanese navy was most effective, reducing the incidence of beri-beri from nearly 40% in 1869 to 0% in

---

[1] It is a curious fact that the lemon was often called *'lime'*, a source of confusion to many writers on this topic.

1875, despite the fact that his conclusion, reasonable in the light of contemporaneous knowledge, later proved to be incorrect.

*rickets*     The prevalence of rickets, the disease of growing bones, which is manifest as deformations of the long bones (e.g., bowed legs, knock knees, curvatures of the upper and/or lower arms), swollen joints and/or enlarged heads in children, is generally associated with the urbanization and industrialization of human societies.  Its appearance on a wide scale was more recent and more restricted geographically than that of either scurvy or beriberi.  The first written account of the disease is believed to be that of **Daniel Whistler**, who wrote on the subject in his medical thesis at Oxford University in 1645.  A complete description of the disease was published shortly thereafter (in 1650) by the Cambridge professor **Francis Glisson**, so it is clear that by the middle of the seventeenth century rickets had become a public health problem in England.  However, rickets appears not to have affected earlier societies, at least on such a scale.  Studies in the late 1800s by the English physician **T.A. Palm** showed that the mummified remains of Egyptian dead bore no signs of the disease.  By the latter part of the century, the incidence of rickets among children in London exceeded one-third; by the turn of the century, estimates of prevalence were as high as 80% and rickets had become known as *"the English disease"*.  Noting the absence of rickets in southern Europe, Palm in 1890 was the first to point out that rickets was prevalent only where there is relatively little sunlight (e.g., in the northern latitudes).  He suggested that sunlight exposure prevented rickets; but others held that the disease had other causes, e.g., heredity, syphilis.  Through the turn of the century, much of the western medical community remained either unaware or skeptical of a food remedy which had long been popular among the peoples of the Baltic and North Sea coasts and which had been used to treat adult rickets in the Manchester Infirmary by 1848:  cod liver oil.  Not until the 1920s would the confusion over the etiology of rickets become clear.

*pellagra*    Pellagra, the disease characterized by lesions of the skin and mouth and by gastro-intestinal and nervous symptoms, also became prevalent in human societies fairly recently.  There appears to have been no record of the disease, even in folk traditions, prior to the eighteenth century.  Its first documented description, in 1735, was that of the Spanish physician **Gaspar Casal**, whose observations were disseminated by the French physician **François Thieri**, whom he met some years later after having been appointed as physician to the court of King Philip V.  In 1755, Thiery published a brief account of Casal's observations in *Journal de Vandermonde*; this became the first published report on the disease.  Casal's own description was included in his book on the epidemic and endemic diseases of northern Spain, *Historia natural y medic de el Principado de Asturias*, which was published in 1762, i.e., three years after his death.  Casal regarded the disease popularly called *"mal de la rosa"* as a peculiar form of leprosy.  He associated it with poverty and with the consumption of spoiled corn (maize).

In 1771, a similar dermatological disorder was described by the Italian physician **Francesco Frapolli**. In his work, _Animadversiones_ in _morbum volgo pelagrum_, he reported the disease to be prevalent in northern Italy. In that region corn, recently introduced from America, had become a popular crop, displacing rye as the major grain. The local name for the disease was _"pelagra"_, meaning rough skin. There is some evidence that it had been seen as early as 1740. At any rate, by 1784, the prevalence of _"pelagra"_ (now spelled pellagra) in that area was so great that a hospital was established in Legano for its treatment. Success in the treatment of pellagra appears to have been attributed to factors other than diet, e.g., rest, fresh air, water, sunshine. Nevertheless, the disease continued to be associated with poverty and the consumption of corn-based diets.

Following the finding of pellagra in Italy, the disease was reported in France by **Hameau** in 1829. It was not until 1845 that the French physician **Roussel** associated pellagra with Casal's _"mal de la rosa"_ and proposed that these diseases, including a similar disease called _"flemma salada"_[2], were related or identical. In order to substantiate his hypothesis, Roussel spent seven months of 1847 in the area where Casal had worked in northern Spain[3] investigating _"mal de la rosa"_ cases; on his return, he presented to the French Academy of Medicine evidence in support of his conclusion. Subsequently, pellagra, as it had come to be called, was reported in Rumania by **Theodari** in 1858, and in Egypt by **Pruner Bey** in 1874. It was a curiosity not to be explained for years that pellagra was never endemic in the Yucatan peninsula where the cultivation of corn originated; the disease was not reported there until 1896.

It is not known how long pellagra had been endemic in the United States; however, in 1912, **J.W. Babcock** examined the records of the state hospital of South Carolina and concluded that the disease had occurred there as early as 1828. It is generally believed that pellagra also appeared during or after the American Civil War (1861-1865) in association with food shortages in the southern states. It is clear from **George Searcy**'s 1907 report to the American Medical Association that the disease was endemic at least in Alabama. By 1909, it had been identified in more than 20 states. Since it first appeared, pellagra was associated with poverty and with the dependence on corn as the major staple food. Ideas arose early on that it was caused by a toxin associated with spoiled corn; yet, by the turn of the century, other hypotheses were also popular. These included the suggestion of an infectious agent with, perhaps, an insect vector.

---

[2] Literally meaning "salty phlegm", _"flemma salada"_ involved gastro-intestinal signs, delirium and a form of dementia. It did not, however, occur in areas where maize was the major staple food; this and disagreement over the similarities of symptoms caused Roussel's proposal of a relationship between these diseases to be challenged by his colleague Arnault Costallat. From Costallat's letters describing _"flemma salada"_ in Spain in 1861, it is apparent that he considered it to be a form of acrodynia, then thought to be due to ergot poisoning.

[3] Casal practiced in the town of Oviedo in the Asturias of northern Spain.

*ideas prevalent
by 1900* Thus, by the beginning of the twentieth century, four different diseases had been linked with certain types of diet. Further, by 1900 it was apparent that at least two, and possibly three, could be cured by changes in diet.

Diet-disease relationships recognized by 1900:

| disease | associated diet | recognized prevention |
|---------|-----------------|------------------------|
| Scurvy | salted foods | fresh fruits, vegetables |
| Beri-Beri | polished rice-based | meats, vegetables |
| Rickets | few *"good"* fats | eggs, cod liver oil |
| Pellagra | corn-based | none |

In addition to this list, other diseases were known since ancient times to respond to what would now be called diet therapy. An example is the disease of *night blindness*, i.e., impaired dark adaptation. The writings of ancient Greek, Roman and Arab physicians show that animal liver was known to be effective in both the prevention and cure of the disease. In fact, the use of liver for the prevention of night blindness became a part of the folk cultures of most seafaring communities. Unfortunately, much of this knowledge was overlooked and its significance was not fully appreciated by a medical community galvanized by the new *"germ theory"* of disease. Alternative theories for the etiologies of these diseases were popular. Thus, as the century began, it was widely held that scurvy, beriberi and rickets were each caused by a bacterium or bacterial toxin rather than by the simple absence of something required for normal health. Some held that rickets might also be due to hypothyroidism, while others thought it to be brought on by lack of exercise or excessive production of lactic acid. These theories died hard and had lingering deaths. In explanation of the lack of interest in the clues presented by the diet-disease associations outlined above, Harris (1955) mused:

> *"Perhaps the reason is that it seems easier for the human mind to believe that ill is caused by some positive evil agency, rather than by any mere absence of any beneficial property".*

*limitations of
empiricism* In actuality, the process of discovery of the vitamins had moved about as far as it could in its empirical phase. Further advances in understanding the etiologies of these diseases would require the rigorous testing of the various hypotheses, i.e., entrance into the deductive phase of nutritional discovery. That movement, however, required *tools* for productive scientific experimentation - tools that had not been available previously.

# THE EXPERIMENTAL PHASE OF VITAMIN DISCOVERY

In a world where one cannot examine all possible cases (i.e., use strictly inductive reasoning), natural truths can be learned only by inference from premises already known to be true (i.e., through deduction).  Both the inductive and deductive approaches may be linked; that is, probable conclusions derived from observation may be used as hypotheses for testing deductively in the process of scientific experimentation.

*requirements of nutrition research*

In order for scientific experimentation to yield informative results, it must be both **repeatable** and **relevant**.  The value of the first point, repeatability, should be self-evident.  In as much as natural truths are held to be constant, non-repeatable results cannot be construed to reveal them.  The value of the second point, relevance, becomes increasingly important when it is infeasible to test an hypothesis in its real-world context.  In such circumstances, it becomes necessary to employ a representation of the context of ultimate interest, a construct known in science as a **model**.  Models are born of practical necessity, but they must be developed carefully in order to serve as analogues of situations that cannot be studied directly.

*defined diets provided repeatability*

Repeatability in nutrition experimentation became possible with the use of **diets of defined composition**.  The most useful type of defined diet that emerged in nutrition research was the **purified diet**.  Diets of this type were formulated using highly refined ingredients (e.g., isolated proteins, refined sugars and starches, refined fats) for which the chemical composition could be reasonably well known.  It was the use of defined diets that facilitated experimental nutrition; such diets could be prepared over and over by the same or other investigators to yield comparable results.  Results obtained through the use of defined diets were repeatable and, therefore, predictable.

*appropriate animal models provided relevance*

Relevance in nutrition research became possible with the identification of **animal models**[4] appropriate to diseases of interest in human medicine or to physiological processes of interest in human medicine or animal production.  The first of these were discovered quite by chance by keen observers studying human disease.  Ultimately, the use of animal models would lead to the discovery of each of the vitamins, as well as to the elucidation of the nutritional roles and metabolic functions of each of the

---

[4]In nutrition and other biomedical research, an animal model consists of the experimental production in a conveniently managed animal species of biochemical and/or clinical changes that are comparable to those occurring in another species of primary interest but that may be infeasible, unethical or uneconomical to study directly.  Animal models are, frequently, species with small body weights (e.g., rodents, chicks, rabbits); however, they may also be larger species (e.g., monkeys, sheep), depending on the target problem and species they are selected to represent.  In any case, background information on the biology and husbandry should be available.  The selection and/or development of an animal model should be based primarily on representation of the biological problem of interest without undue consideration of the practicalities of cost and availability.

approximately 40 nutrients. The careful use of appropriate animal models made possible studies that would otherwise be infeasible or unthinkable in human subjects or in other animal species of interest.

Major forces in the emergence of nutritional science:

| | |
|---|---|
| *i.* | **Recognition** that certain disease were related to diet |
| *ii.* | Development of appropriate **animal models** |
| *iii.* | Use of **defined diets** |

*animal model for beri-beri*
The analytical phase of vitamin discovery, indeed modern nutrition research itself, was entered with the finding of an animal model for beri-beri in the 1890s. In 1886, **Christian Eijkman**, was among a team sent from the Netherlands to a military hospital in what was then Batavia, Dutch East Indies (now Jakarta, Indonesia), for the purpose of finding the cause of beri-beri which was so prevalent in that part of the world. Eijkman, a student of the great bacteriologist **Robert Koch**, expected to find a bacterium and was, therefore, disappointed after many months of searching to uncover no such evidence. Examinations of thousands of blood smears and inoculations of rats with blood, saliva and tissue from patients proved fruitless. But, one day, Eijkman couldn't help but notice an ailment of the chickens kept by his laboratory. Many were too weak to stand and lay twitching on their sides; some walked only with a staggered gait. Some had died. He quickly dismissed the thought that this avian disease might be related to beri-beri.

*serendipity or a keen eye?*
The disease persisted in his flock for some five months before it suddenly disappeared. Then Eijkman considered again the similarities of the signs he had seen among affected chickens and the symptoms of beri-beri patients: neuritis, paralysis, edema. He reviewed his records and found that in June, shortly before the chickens had started to show paralysis, a change in their diet had been occasioned by failure of a shipment of feed-grade brown (unpolished) rice to arrive. His assistant had used, instead, white (polished) rice from the hospital kitchen. It turned out that this extravagance had been discovered a few months earlier by a new hospital superintendent who had ordered it stopped. When Eijkman again fed the chickens brown rice, he found them to recovery completely within days.

With this clue, Eijkman immediately turned to the chicken for his studies. He found the chicken to show signs of polyneuritis within days of being fed polished rice, and that their signs disappeared even more quickly if they were then fed unpolished rice. It was clear that there was something associated with rice husks that protected chickens from the disease. Eijkman then surveyed the use of polished and unpolished rice and the incidence of beri-beri among inmates of the prisons of Java. His results, later to be confirmed in similar epidemiological investigations by other groups, showed an advantage of eating unpolished rice.

Beri-beri statistics from Javanese prisons ca. 1890:

| diet | population | cases/100,000 |
|------|-----------|---------------|
| polished rice | 150,266 | 2795 |
| partially polished rice | 35,082 | 242 |
| unpolished rice | 96,530 | 9 |

When this kind of information was considered in conjunction with his experimental findings with chickens, it was clear that he had a means of investigating by means of bioassay the beri-beri-protective factor apparently associated with rice husks.

Eijkman used this animal model in a series of investigations in 1890-1897 and found that the anti-polyneuritis factor could be extracted from rice hulls with water or alcohol, that it was dialyzable, but that it was rather easily destroyed with moist heat. Eijkman concluded that the water-soluble factor was a *"pharmacological antidote"* to the *"beri-beri microbe"* which, though it was still not identified, he thought to be present in the rice kernel proper. Apparently, his colleague **Grijns** came to interpret their findings somewhat differently, suggesting in 1901 for the first time that beri-beri-producing diets *"lacked a certain substance of importance in the metabolism of the central nervous system."* Subsequently, Eijkman came to share that view. In 1906, the two investigators published a now-classic paper in which they wrote:

*anti-beri-beri factor announced*

> *"There is present in rice polishings a substance different from protein, and salts, which is indispensable to health and the lack of which causes nutritional polyneuritis."*

## THE "VITAMINE" THEORY

*defined diets reveal needs for "accessory factors"*

Eijkman's announcement of the anti-beri-beri factor constituted the first recognition of the concept of the vitamin, although the term itself was yet to be coined. At the time of Eijkman's studies, but a world removed and wholly separate, others were finding that animals would not survive when fed *"synthetic"* or *"artificial"* diets formulated with purified fats, proteins, carbohydrates and salts, i.e., containing all of the nutrients then known to be constituents of natural foods. Such a finding was first reported by the Swiss physiologist, **Lunnin**, in 1888, who found that the addition of milk to a "synthetic" diet supported the survival of mice. Lunnin concluded:

> *"A natural food such as milk must, therefore, contain besides these known principal ingredients small quantities of other and unknown substances essential to life."*

Lunnin's finding was soon confirmed by several other investigators. By 1912, **Rhömann** in Germany, **Socin** in Switzerland, **Pekalharing** in the Netherlands and **Hopkins** in Great Britain had each demonstrated that the addition of milk to purified diets corrected the impairments in growth and survival that were otherwise produced in laboratory rodents. The German physiologist **Stepp** took another experimental approach. He found it possible to extract from bread and milk factors required for animal growth. Though Pekalharing's 1905 comments in Dutch lay unnoticed by most investigators who did not read that language, his conclusions about what Hopkins had called the *"accessory factor"* in milk alluded to the modern concept of a vitamin:

> *"If this substance is absent, the organism loses the power properly to assimilate the well known principal parts of food, the appetite is lost and with apparent abundance the animals die of want. Undoubtedly this substance not only occurs in milk but in all sorts of foodstuffs, both of vegetable and animal origin."*

Perhaps the most important of the early studies with defined diets were those of the Cambridge biochemist Frederick Gowland Hopkins[5]. His studies demonstrated that the growth-promoting activities of *"accessory factors"* were independent of appetite, and that such factors prepared from milk or yeast were biologically active in very small amounts.

*two lines of inquiry*

Therefore, by 1912, two independently developed lines of inquiry had revealed that foods contained beneficial factor(s) in addition to the nutrients known at the time. That these factor(s) were present and active in minute amounts was apparent from the fact that the known nutrients comprised almost all of food mass.

Two lines of inquiry lead to the discovery of the vitamins:

| | |
|---|---|
| i. | the study of substances that prevent *'deficiency diseases'* |
| ii. | the study of *'accessory factors'* required by animals fed purified diets |

Were the *"accessory factors"* related in any way to the *"deficiency diseases"*?

---

[5] Sir Frederick Gowland Hopkins is known for his pioneering work in biochemistry, which involved not only classic work on *"accessory growth factors"* (for which he shared, with Christian Eijkman, the Nobel Prize in Medicine in 1929), but also the discovery of glutathione and tryptophan.

Comments by Hopkins in 1906 indicate that he saw connections; on the subject of the *accessory growth factors* in foods he wrote:

> *"No animal can live on a mixture of pure protein, fat and carbohydrate, and even when the necessary inorganic material is carefully supplied the animal still cannot flourish.  The animal is adjusted to live either on plant tissues or the tissues of other animals, and these contain countless substances other than protein, carbohydrates and fats.  In diseases such as rickets, and particularly scurvy, we have had for years knowledge of a dietetic factor; but though we know how to benefit these conditions empirically, the real errors in the diet are to this day quite obscure . . . They are, however, certainly of the kind which comprises these minimal qualitative factors that I am considering."*

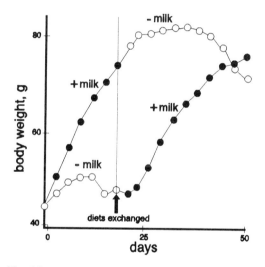

*Hopkins:*  growth of rats fed a purified diet

*the lines converge*

The discovery by Eijkman and Grijns had stimulated efforts by investigators in several countries to isolate the anti-beri-beri factor in rice husks.  Among these was **Casimir Funk**, a Polish biochemist working in the Lister Institute in London, who found that the anti-polyneuritis factor in rice husks was nitrogenous in nature.  When he appeared to have isolated the factor, Funk coined a new word for it, with the specific intent of promoting the new concept in nutrition to which Hopkins had alluded.  Having evidence that the factor was an **amine**, Funk chose the term *"vitamine"*[6] because it was clearly **vital**, i.e., pertaining to life.

---

[6] Harris (1955) reported that the word *"vitamine"* was suggested to Funk by his friend, Dr. Max Nierenstein, Reader in Biochemistry, the University of Bristol.

*Funk's
theory*

In 1912, Funk published his landmark paper in which he pronounced the *"vitamine theory"* in which he proposed four different *"vitamines"*. That not all of these factors later proved to be amines (hence, the change to **"vitamin"**[7]) is far less important than the revolutionary concept that he introduced with the newly coined term. Funk was not unaware of the importance of the term itself; he wrote:

> *"I must admit that when I chose the name 'vitamine' I was well aware that these substances might later prove not all to be of an amine nature. However, it was necessary for me to use a name that would sound well and serve as a 'catch-word'."*

Funk's *"vitamines"*:

| | |
|---|---|
| **anti-beri-beri** "vitamine" | **anti-scurvy** "vitamine" |
| **anti-rickets** "vitamine" | **anti-pellagra** "vitamine" |

*impact of the
new concept*

The *"vitamine theory"* opened new possibilities in nutrition research by providing a new intellectual construct for interpreting observations of the natural world. No longer was the elucidation of the etiologies of diseases to be constrained by the *"germ theory"*. Thus, Funk's greatest contribution involves not the data generated in his laboratory, rather it was the theory produced from his thoughtful review of information already in the medical literature of the time. This fact caused Harris (1955) to write:

> *"The interpreter may be as useful to science as the discoverer. I refer here to any man[8] who is able to take a broad view of what has already been done by others, to collect evidence and discern through it all some common connecting link."*

The real impact of Funk's theory was to provide a new concept for interpreting diet-related phenomena. As **Novak**[9] observed more recently:

> *"As our conceptual and emotional frameworks change, we see different things in the same material."*

Still, it was not clear by 1912 whether the *"accessory factors"* were the same as the *"vitamines"*. In fact, until 1915, there was considerable debate

---

[7]The dropping of the *'e'* from vitamine is said to have been the suggestion of J.C. Drummond.

[8]Harris' word choice reveals him as a product of his times. Because it is clear that the process of intellectual discovery to which Harris refers does not recognize gender, it is more appropriate to read this word as *'person'*.

[9]Novak, J.D. 1977. <u>A Theory of Education</u>, Cornell University Press, Ithaca, NY, 295 pp.

concerning whether the growth factor for the rat was a single or multiple entity (it was already clear that there were more than one "vitamine"). Some investigators were able to demonstrate it in yeast and not butter; others found it in butter and not yeast. Some showed it to be identical with the anti-polyneuritis factor; others showed that it was clearly different.

*more than one*
*"accessory*
*factor"*

The debate was resolved by the landmark studies of the American investigators **E.V. McCollum** and **Marguerite Davis** at the University of Wisconsin in 1913-1915. They demonstrated that there were, indeed, at least two *different* growth factors *both* of which were required to support growth of the rat. One factor could be extracted from certain foods with organic solvents; it appeared to be the factor shown by the German physiologist **Stepp**, earlier and by **Osborne** and **Mendel** at Yale University in the same year, to be required to sustain growth of the rat. The second factor was extractable with water. McCollum's grouped called these factors *"fat-soluble A"* and *"water-soluble B"*.

McCollum's rat growth factors:

| factor | found in | not found in |
|---|---|---|
| *"fat-soluble A"* | milk fat, egg yolk | lard, olive oil |
| *"water-soluble B"* | wheat, milk, egg yolk | polished rice |

*"accessory*
*factors"*
*prevent*
*disease*

Subsequent studies by McCollum's group and others showed that the ocular disorders (i.e., xerophthalmia[10]) which developed in rats, dogs and chicks fed fat-free diets, could be prevented by feeding cod liver oil, butter or preparations of *"fat-soluble A"*, which then became known as the *"anti-xerophthalmic factor"*. Shortly, it was found that the so-called *"water-soluble B"* material was not only required for normal growth of the rat, it also prevented polyneuritis in the chick. Therefore, it was clear that "water-soluble B" was identical to or at least contained Funk's *"anti-beri-beri vitamine"*; hence, it became known as *"vitamine B"*.

*"accessory*
*factors"*
*same as*
*"vitamines"*

With these discoveries, it became apparent that the biological activities of the *"accessory factors"* and the *"vitamines"* were likely to be due to the same compounds. The concept of a "vitamine" was, thus, generalized to include non-nitrogenous compounds, and the *"anti-polyneuritis vitamine"* became *"vitamin B"*.

*elucidation of*
*vitamins*
*begins*

So it was, through the agencies of several factors, a useful new intellectual construct, the use of defined diets and the availability of appropriate animal models, that nutrition emerged as a scientific discipline. By 1915,

---

[10] Xerophthalmia (from the Greek *xeros* = dry and *ophthalmos* = eye) involves dryness of the eyeball due to atrophy of the periocular glands, hyperkeratosis of the conjunctiva and, ultimately, inflammation and edema of the cornea which leads to infection, ulceration and blindness.

thinking about diet and health had been forever changed, and it was clear that the earlier notions about the required nutrients had been incomplete. Therefore, it should not be surprising to find, by the 1920s, mounting interest in the many questions generated by what had become sound nutritional research. That interest and the further research activity it engendered resulted, over the brief span of only five decades, in the development of a fundamental understanding of the identities and functions of about 40 nutrients one-third of which are considered vitamins.

*crooked paths*   The paths leading to the discovery of the vitamins wandered from Java with
*to discovery*    the findings of Eijkman in the 1890s, to England with Funk's theory in 1912, to the United States with the recognition of *"fat-soluble A"* and *"water-soluble B"* in 1915. By that time, the paths had already branched; and, for the next four decades, they would branch again and again as scientists from many laboratories and many nations would pursue many unexplained responses to diet among many types of animal model. Some of these pursuits appeared to fail; but, in aggregate, all laid the groundwork of understanding upon which the discoveries of those factors now recognized to be vitamins were based. When viewed in retrospect, the path to that recognition may seem deceptively straight; but it was most definitely *not* that way. The way was branched and crooked; in many cases, progress was made by several different investigators travelling in apparently different directions. The following recounts the *highlights* of the exciting search for the elucidation of the vitamins.

## THE ELUCIDATION OF THE VITAMINS

*new animal*      Eijkman's report of polyneuritis in the chicken and an animal model for beri-
*model reveals*   beri stimulated researchers **Holst** and **Frolich** in Oslo who were interested
*new vitamin: C*  in *"shipboard beri-beri"*, a common problem among Norwegian seamen. In 1907, they attempted to produce the disease in another experimental animal species, the guinea pig, fed cereal-based diets. Contrary to their expectations, Holst and Frolich failed to produce in that species anything resembling beri-beri; instead, they observed the familiar signs of **scurvy**. Clues from Eijkman's work suggested to them that, like beri-beri, scurvy, too, might be due to a dietary deficiency. Having discovered, quite by chance, one of the few possible animal species in which scurvy could be produced[11], Holst and Frolich had produced something of tremendous value - an animal model of scurvy.

---

[11]Their finding was, indeed, fortuitous, as vitamin C is now known to be an essential dietary nutrient only for the guinea pig, primates, fishes, some fruit-eating bats and some passiform birds. Had they used the rat, the mouse or the chick in their study, vitamin C might have remained unrecognized for, perhaps, quite a while.

This finding led **Chick** and **Hume**, in the 1910s, to develop a bioassay for the determination of the anti-scorbutic activity in foods, and **Zilva** and colleagues at the Lister Institute in London to isolate from lemons the crude factor that had come to be known as *"vitamin C"*. It was soon found that vitamin C could reduce the dye 2,6-dichloroindophenol; but the reducing activity determined with that reagent did not always correlate with the anti-scorbutic activity determined by bioassay. Subsequently, it was found that the vitamin was reversibly oxidized, but that both the reduced and oxidized forms had anti-scorbutic activity. In 1932, two groups, i.e., those of **Szent-Györgi** in Hungary and **King** at the University of Pittsburgh, established that the anti-scorbutic factor was identical with the reductant *"hexuronic acid"*[12] that Szent-Györgi had previously isolated in crystalline form from adrenal cortex and that King had isolated from cabbage and citrus juice[13]. In 1932, **Svirbely** and Szent-Györgi isolated ca. 500 g of crystalline vitamin C from peppers and made samples available to other laboratories. The following year, its chemical structure was elucidated by the groups of **Haworth** in Birmingham and **Karrer** in Zurich, both of which also achieved its synthesis.

*"fat-soluble A"*
*actually*
*two factors*

Pursuing the characterization of *"fat-soluble A"*, by 1919 McCollum's group and others had found that, in addition to supporting growth for the rat, the factor also prevented xerophthalmia and night blindness in that species. In 1920, **Drummond** called this active lipid *"vitamin A"*[14].

*"vitamin A"*
*prevents*
*rickets?*

Undoubtedly influenced by the recent recognition of *"vitamin A"*, Sir Edward **Mellanby** undertook to produce a dietary model of rickets using puppies fed a low-fat diet based on oatmeal. He was successful; when his puppies were not exposed to sunlight, they developed the marked skeletal deformities characteristic of rickets. When Mellanby found that he could effectively prevent rickets in this model by feeding cod liver oil or butterfat, he concluded that rickets, too, was caused by a deficiency of vitamin A discovered by McCollum in those materials.

---

[12] It is said that, when Szent-Györgi first isolated the compound, he was at a loss for a name for it. Knowing it to be a sugar, but otherwise ignorant of its identity, he proposed the name *"ignose"*, which was disqualified by an editor who did not appreciate the humor of the Hungarian chemist. Ultimately, the names *"ascorbic acid"* and *"vitamin C"*, by which several groups had come to refer to the anti-scorbutic factor, were adopted.

[13] The reports of both groups (King and Waugh, 1932; Svirbely and Szent-Györgi, 1932) appeared within two weeks of one another. In fact, Svirbely had recently joined Szent-Györgi's group, having come from King's laboratory. In 1937, King and Szent-Györgi shared the Nobel Prize for their work in the isolation and identification of vitamin C.

[14] In 1920, J.C. Drummond proposed the use of the names *"vitamin A"* and *"vitamin B"* for McCollum's factors, and the use of the letters C, D, etc. for any vitamins subsequently to be discovered.

*new vitamin:*
*"D"*

McCollum, however, suspected the anti-rachitic factor present in cod liver oil of being different from vitamin A. Having moved to the Johns Hopkins University in Baltimore, he conducted an experiment in which he subjected cod liver oil to aeration and heating (100°C for 14 hrs) after which he tested its anti-xerophthalmic and anti-richitic activities with rat and chick bioassays, respectively. He found that heating had destroyed the anti-xerophthalmic (vitamin A) activity, but that cod liver oil had retained anti-richitic activity. McCollum called the heat-stable factor *"vitamin D"*.

*β-carotene*
*a pro-vitamin*

At about the same time (1919) **Steenbock** in Wisconsin, pointed out that the vitamin A activities of plant materials seemed to correlate with their contents of yellow pigments. He suggested that the plant pigment *"carotene"* was responsible for the vitamin A activity of such materials. Yet, the vitamin A-activity in organic extracts of liver was colorless. Therefore, Steenbock suggested that carotene could not be vitamin A, but that it may be converted metabolically to the actual vitamin. This hypothesis was not substantiated until 1929 when **von Euler** and **Karrer** in Stockholm demonstrated growth responses to carotene in rats fed vitamin A-deficient diets. Further, **Moore** in England demonstrated in the rat a dose-response relationship between dietary β-carotene and hepatic vitamin A concentration. This showed that β-carotene is, indeed, a *pro-vitamin*.

*vitamin A link*
*to vision*

In the early 1930s, the first indications of the molecular mechanism of the visual process were produced by **George Wald**, of Harvard University but working in Germany at the time, isolated a chromophore *"retinen"* from bleached retinas[15]. A decade later, **Morton** in Liverpool found that the chromophore was the aldehyde form of vitamin A, i.e., *retinaldehyde*. Just after Wald's discovery, **Karrer**'s group in Zurich elucidated the structures of both β-carotene and vitamin A. In 1937, **Holmes** and **Corbett** succeeded in crystallizing vitamin A from fish liver. In 1942, **Baxter** and **Robeson** crystallized retinol and several of its esters; in 1947, they crystallized the 13-*cis*-isomer. **Isler**'s group in Basel achieved the synthesis of retinol in the same year, and that of β-carotene three years later.

*the nature of*
*vitamin D*

McCollum's discovery of the anti-rachitic factor he called *"vitamin D"* in cod liver oil, which was made possible through the use of animal models, was actually a *"re-discovery"*, as that material had been long recognized as an effective medicine for rickets in children. Still, the nature of the disease was the subject of considerable debate, particularly, after 1919 when **Huldschinsky**, a physician in Vienna, demonstrated the efficacy of ultra-violet light in healing rickets. This confusion was clarified by the findings in 1923 of **Goldblatt** and **Soames**, who demonstrated that when livers from rachitic rats were irradiated with ultra-violet light, they could cure rickets when fed to non-irradiated rats. The next year, Steenbock's group demon-

---

[15]For this and other discoveries of the basic chemical and physiological processes in vision, George Wald was awarded, with Haldan K. Hartline (of the United States) and R. Granit (of Sweden), the Nobel Prize in 1967.

strated the prevention of rickets in rats by UV-irradiation of either the animals, themselves *or* their diet.  Further, the light-produced anti-rachitic factor was associated with the fat-soluble portion of the diet[16].

*vitamers D*    The ability to produce vitamin D, which could be bioassayed using the rat or the chick, by irradiating lipids led to the finding that large quantities of the vitamin could be produced by irradiating the plant sterols.  This, led **Askew**'s and **Windaus**' groups in the early 1930s, to the isolation and identification of the vitamin produced by irradiation of ergosterol. **Steenbock**'s group, however, found that, while the rachitic chick responded appropriately to irradiated products of cod liver oil or the animal sterol cholesterol, that animal did *not* respond to the vitamin D so produced from ergosterol.  On the basis of this apparent lack of equivalence, **Wadell** suggested in 1934 that the irradiated products of ergosterol and cholesterol were different.  Subsequently, Windaus' group synthesized 7-dehydrocholesterol and isolated a vitamin D-active product of its irradiation.  In 1936, they reported its structure, showing it to be a side-chain isomer of the form of the vitamin produced from plant sterols.  Thus, two forms of vitamin D were found: *"ergocalciferol"* (from ergosterol), which was called vitamin $D_2$[17]; and *"cholecalciferol"* (from cholesterol), which was called vitamin $D_3$.  While it was clear that the vitamers D had important metabolic roles in calcification, insights to the molecular mechanisms of the vitamin would not come until the 1960s.  Then, it became apparent that neither vitamer was metabolically active per se; each is converted in vivo to a host of metabolites which participate in a system of calcium homeostasis that continues to be of great interest in the biomedical community.

*multiple*       By the 1920s, it was apparent that the *"anti-polyneuritis factor"* rendered
*identities of*  *"water-soluble B"*, present in such materials as yeasts was not a single
*"water-*        substance.  This was demonstrated by the finding that fresh yeast could
*soluble B"*     prevent both beri-beri and pellagra.   However, the anti-polyneuritis factor in yeast was unstable to heat, while such treatment did not alter the efficacy of yeast to prevent dermititic lesions in rodents.  This caused **Goldberger** to suggest that the so-called *"vitamin B"* was actually at least *two* vitamins: the anti-polyneuritis vitamin and a *new* anti-pellagra vitamin.

In 1926, the heat-labile anti-polyneuritis/beri-beri factor was isolated by **Jansen** and **Donath** working in Eijkman's former laboratory in Java.  They called the factor *"aneurin"*.  Their work was facilitated by the use of the Rice Bird (*Munia maja*) as an animal model in which they developed a

---

[16]This discovery, i.e., that it was possible to induce by UV-irradiation, vitamin D activity in such foods as milk, bread, meats and butter, led to the widespread use of this practice, which has resulted in the virtual eradication of rickets as a public health problem.

[17]Windaus' group had earlier isolated a form of the vitamin he had called vitamin $D_1$, which had turned out to be an irradiation-breakdown product, lumisterol.

rapid bioassay for anti-polyneuritic activity[18]. Six years later, **Windaus'** group isolated the factor from yeast, perhaps the richest source of it. In the same year (1932), the chemical structure was determined by **R.R. Williams** who named it *"thiamin"*. Shortly thereafter, methods of synthesis were achieved by several groups including Williams', **Andersag** and **Westphal**, and **Todd**. In 1937, thiamin diphosphate (thiamin pyrophosphate) was isolated by **Lohmann** and **Schuster**, who showed it to be identical to the *"co-carboxylase"* that had been isolated earlier by **Auhagen**. That many research groups were actively engaged in the research on the anti-polyneuritis/beri-beri factor is evidence of intense international interest due to the widespread prevalence of beri-beri.

The characterization of thiamin clarified the distinction of the anti-beri-beri factor from the anti-pellagra activity, the latter being notably absent in corn which contained appreciable amounts of the former. Goldberger called the two substances the *"A-N (anti-neuritic) factor"* and the *"P-P (pellagra-preventive) factor"*. Others called these factors *vitamins F* (for Funk) and *G* (for Goldberger), respectively; but these terms did not last[19]. By the mid 1920s the terms *vitamins B₁* and *B₂* had been rather widely adapted for these factors, respectively; this practice was codified in 1927 by the Accessory Food Factors Committee, British Medical Research Council.

*vitamin B₂: complex of several factors*   That the thermostable *"second nutritional factor"* in yeast, which by that time was called *"vitamin B₂"*, was not a single substance was not immediately recognized, giving rise to considerable confusion and delay in the elucidation of its chemical identity (identities). It should be noted that efforts to fractionate the *"heat-stable factor"* were guided almost exclusively by bioassays with experimental animal models. Yet, different species yielded discrepant responses to preparations of the *"factor"*. When such variation in responses among species was finally appreciated, it became clear that *"vitamin B₂"* actually included *several* heat-stable factors. *Vitamin B₂*, as then defined, was indeed a *complex*.

The components of the *vitamin B₂ complex* were found to include:

| | |
|---|---|
| i. | the *P-P factor* (prevented pellagra in humans and pellagra-like diseases in dogs, monkeys and pigs) |
| ii. | a *growth factor* for the rat |
| iii. | a *"pellagra"-preventing factor* for the rat |
| iv. | an *anti-dermatitis factor* for the chick |

---

[18]The animals, when fed 2 g polished rice daily, showed a high (98 + %) incidence of polyneuritis within 9-13 days. Anti-polyneuritic activity was based upon the delay in onset of signs of the disease.

[19]In fact, the name *"vitamin F"* was later used, with some debate as to the appropriateness of the term, to describe essential fatty acids. The name *"vitamin G"* has been dropped completely.

*B₂ complex*
*yields*
*riboflavin*

The first substance in the *vitamin B₂ complex* to be elucidated was the heat-stable, water-soluble, rat growth factor, which was isolated by **Kuhn**, **György** and **Wagner-Jauregg** at the Kaiser Wilhelm Institute in 1933. Those investigators found that thiamin-free extracts of yeast, liver or rice bran prevented the growth failure of rats fed a thiamin-supplemented diet. Further, they noted a yellow-green fluorescence in each extract that promoted rat growth, and that the intensity of fluorescence was proportional to the effect on growth. This observation enabled them to develop a rapid chemical assay which, in conjunction with their bioassay, they exploited to isolate in the factor from egg white in 1933. They called it *"ovoflavin"*. The same group then isolated by the same procedure a yellow-green fluorescent growth-promoting compound from whey (which they called *"lactoflavin"*). This procedure involved the adsorption of the active factor on fuller's earth[20] from which it could be eluted with base[21]. At the same time, **Ellinger** and **Koschara** at the University of Düsseldorf isolated similar substances from liver, kidney, muscle and yeast, and **Booher** in the United States isolated the factor from whey. These water-soluble growth factors became designated as *"flavins"*[22]. By 1934, Kuhn's group had determined the structure of the so-called flavins. These substances were thus found to be identical; because each contained a ribose-like (ribotyl) moiety attached to an isoalloxazine nucleus, the term *"riboflavin"* was adopted. Riboflavin was synthesized by Kuhn's group (then at the University of Heidelberg) and by Karrer's group at Zurich in 1935. As the first component of the *vitamin B₂ complex*, it is also referred to as *"vitamin B₂"*; however, that should not be confused with the earlier designation of the pellagra-preventive (P-P) factor.

*B₂ complex*
*yields niacin*

Progress in the identification of the P-P factor was retarded by two factors: pervasive influence of the *"germ theory"* of disease; the lack of an animal model. The former made acceptance of evidence for a nutritional origin to the disease a long and difficult undertaking. The latter precluded the rigorous testing of hypotheses for the etiology of the disease in a timely and highly controlled manner. These challenges were met by **Joseph Goldberger**, a bacteriologist in the U.S. Public Health Service who, in 1914, was assigned the task of identifying the cause of pellagra.

---

[20]Floridin, a nonplastic variety of kaolin containing an aluminum magnesium silicate. The material is useful as a decolorizing medium. Its name comes from an ancient process of cleaning or fulling wool in which a slurry of earth or clay was used to remove oil and particulate dirt.

[21]By this procedure the albumen from 10,000 eggs yielded ca. 30 mg riboflavin.

[22]Initially, the term *"flavin"* was used with a prefix that indicated the source material, e.g., ovoflavin, hepatoflavin and lactoflavin designated the substances isolated from egg white, liver and milk, respectively.

*pellagra:*
*an infection?*

Goldberger's first study[23] is now a classic. He studied a Jackson, Miss., orphanage in which pellagra was endemic. He noted that, while the disease was prevalent among the inmates, it was absent among the staff including the nurses and physicians that cared for patients; this suggested to him that pellagra was not an infectious disease. Noting that the food available to the professional staff was much different from that served to the inmates (the former included meat and milk not available to the inmates), Goldberger secured funds to supply meat and milk to the inmates for a two-year period of study. The results were dramatic: pellagra soon disappeared and no new cases were reported for the duration of the study. However, when funds expired at the end of the study and the institution was forced to return to its former meal program, pellagra reappeared. While the evidence from this uncontrolled experiment galvanized Goldberger's conviction that pellagra was a dietary disease, it was not sufficient to affect a medical community which thought the disease likely to be an infection.

Over the course of two decades, Goldberger undertook to elucidate the dietary basis of pellagra. Among his efforts to demonstrate that the disease was not infectious was the exposure, by ingestion and injection, of himself, his wife and 14 volunteers to urine, feces and biological fluids from pellagrins[24]. The negative results of these radical experiments, plus the finding that therapy with oral supplements of the amino acids cysteine and tryptophan was effective in controlling the disease led, by the early 1920s, to the establishment of a dietary origin of pellagra. Further progress was hindered by the lack of an appropriate animal model. While *"pellagra-like"* diseases had been identified in several species, most proved not to be useful as biological assays (indeed, most of these later proved to be manifestations of deficiencies of other vitamins of the *"$B_2$ complex"* and to be wholly unrelated to pellagra in humans).

The identification of a useful animal model for pellagra came from Goldberger's discovery in 1922 that the feeding to dogs diets essentially the same as those associated with human pellagra resulted in the animals developing a necrotic degeneration of the tongue, *"black tongue disease"*. This animal model for the disease led to the final solution of the problem.

*impact of*
*an animal*
*model*

This finding made possible experimentation that would lead rather quickly to understanding the etiology to the disease. Goldberger's group soon found that yeast, wheat germ and liver would prevent canine black tongue and produce dramatic recoveries in pellagra patients. By the early 1930s, it was established that the human pellagra and canine black tongue curative factor was heat-stable and could be separated from the other *"$B_2$*

---

[23]*See* the list of *"Historically Significant Papers"* at the end of this chapter.

[24]persons suffering from pellagra.

*complex"* components by filtration through fuller's earth which adsorbed only the latter. Thus, the *"P-P factor"* became known as the *"filtrate factor"*. In 1937, **Elvehjem** isolated *nicotinamide* from liver extracts that had high anti-black tongue activity and showed that nicotinamide and *nicotinic acid* each cured canine black tongue. In the same year, several groups went on to show the curative effect of nicotinic acid against human pellagra.

It is ironic that the anti-pellagra factor was already well known to chemists of the time. Some 70 years earlier, the German chemist **Huber** had prepared nicotinic acid by the oxidation of nicotine with nitric acid. **Funk** had isolated the compound from yeast and rice bran in his search for the anti-beri-beri factor; however, because it had no effect on beri-beri, nicotinic acid remained for two decades an entity with unappreciated biological importance. This view changed in the mid-1930s when **Warburg** and **Christian** isolated nicotinamide from the H-transporting co-enzymes I and II[25], giving the first clue to its importance in metabolism. Within a year, Elvehjem had discovered its nutritional significance.

*B₂ complex yields pyridoxine*

During the course of their work leading to the successful isolation of riboflavin, Kuhn and colleagues noticed an anomalous relationship between the growth-promoting and fluorescence activities of their extracts: the correlation of the two activities diminished at high levels of the former. Further, the addition of non-fluorescent extracts were necessary for the growth-promoting activity of riboflavin. They interpreted these findings as evidence for a second component of the heat-stable complex: one that was removed during the purification of riboflavin. These factors were also known to prevent dermatoses in the rat, an activity called *"adermin"*; however, the lack of a critical assay that could differentiate between the various components of the *"B₂ complex"* led to considerable confusion.

In 1934, **György** proffered a definition of what he called *"vitamin B6 activity"*[26] as the factor that prevented what had formerly been called *"acrodynia"* or *"rat pellagra"*, which was a symmetrical florid dermatitis spreading over the limbs and trunk with redness and swelling of the paws and ears. His definition effectively distinguished these signs from those produced by riboflavin deficiency, which involves lesions on the head and chest and inflammation of the eyelids and nostrils. The focus provided by György's definition strengthened the use of the rat in the bioassay of vitamin B₆ activity by clarifying its endpoint. Within two years, partial purification of the vitamin had been achieved by his group; and in 1938 (only 4 years after the recognition of the vitamin), the isolation of vitamin B₆ in crystalline form was achieved by five research groups. The chemical

---

[25]Nicotinamide adenine dinucleotide (NAD) and nicotinamide adenine dinucleotide phosphate (NADP), respectively.

[26]György defined *"vitamin B6 activity"* as *"that part of the vitamin B-complex responsible for the cure of a specific dermatitis developed by rats on a vitamin-free diet supplemented with vitamin B₁, and lactoflavin."*

structure of the substance was quickly elucidated as 3-hydroxy-4,5-bis-(hydroxymethyl)-2-methylpyridine. In 1939, **Folkers** achieved the synthesis of this compound, which György called *"pyridoxine"*.

*B₂ complex yields pantothenic acid*

In the course of studying the growth factor called *"vitamin B₂"*, **Norris** and **Ringrose** at Cornell described, in 1930, a pellagra-like syndrome of the chick. The lesions could be prevented with aqueous extracts of yeast or liver, then recognized to contain the *"B₂ complex"*. In studies of *"B₂ complex"*-related growth factors for chicks and rats, **Jukes** and colleagues at Berkeley found positive responses to a thermostable factor which, unlike pyridoxine, was not adsorbed by fuller's earth from an acid solution. They referred to it as the *"filtrate factor"*.

*microbial growth factor*

At the same time and quite independently, the University of Texas microbiologist **R.J. Williams** was pursuing studies of the essential nutrients for *Saccharomyces cerevisiae* and other yeasts. His group found a potent growth factor which they could isolate from a wide variety of plant and animal tissues[27]. They called it *"pantothenic acid"*, meaning *"found everywhere"* and also referred to the substance as *"vitamin B₃"*. Later in the decade, **Snell**'s group found that several lactic and propionic acid bacteria require a growth factor that had the same properties. Jukes recognized that his *"filtrate factor"*, Norris' chick *"anti-dermatitis factor"*, and the unknown factors required by yeasts and bacteria were identical. He showed that both his *"filtrate factor"* and *"pantothenic acid"* obtained from Williams could prevent dermatitis in the chick. Pantothenic acid was isolated and its chemical structure was determined by Williams' group in 1939. The chemical synthesis of the vitamin was achieved by **Folkers** the following year.

Factors leading to the discovery of pantothenic acid:

| factor | bioassay |
|---|---|
| *"filtrate factor"* | chick growth |
| *"chick anti-dermatitis factor"* | prevention of skin lesions and poor feather development in chicks |
| *"pantothenic acid"* | growth of *S. cerevisiae* and other yeasts |

*a fat-soluble anti-sterility factor: vitamin E*

Interest in the nutritional properties of lipids was stimulated by the resolution of *"fat-soluble A"* into vitamins A and D by the early 1920s. Several groups found that the supplementation with the newly discovered vitamins A, C, D and thiamin markedly improved the performance of animals fed purified diets containing adequate amounts of protein, carbohydrate and known required minerals. But **Evans** and **Bishop**, at the University of

[27]The first isolation of pantothenic acid employed 250 kg sheep liver. The autolysate was treated with fuller's earth; the factor was adsorbed to norite and eluted with ammonia. Brucine salts were formed and were extracted with chloroform:water after which the brucine salt of pantothenic acid was converted to the calcium salt. The yield was 3.0 g of material with ca. 40% purity.

California, observed that rats fed such supplemented diets seldom reproduced normally. They found that fertility was abnormally low in both males, which showed testicular degeneration, and females, which showed impaired placental function and failed to carry their fetuses to term[28]. Dystrophy of skeletal and smooth muscles (i.e., those of the uterus) was also noted. In 1922, those investigators reported that the addition of small amounts of yeast or fresh lettuce to the purified diet would restore fertility to females and prevent infertility in animals of both sexes. They designated the unknown fertility factor *"factor X"*. Using the prevention of *"gestation resorption"* as the bioassay, Evans and Bishop found *"factor X"* activity in such unrelated materials as dried alfalfa, wheat germ, oats, meats and milk fat from which it was extractable with organic solvents. They distinguished the new fat-soluble factor from the known fat-soluble vitamins by showing that single droplets of wheat germ oil administered daily completely prevented this gestation resorption, whereas, cod liver oil, known to be a rich source of vitamins A and D, failed to do so[29]. In 1924, **Sure** at the University of Arkansas, confirmed this work, concluding that the fat-soluble factor was a new vitamin, which he called *"vitamin E"*.

*classical touch in coining "tocopherol"* Soon, Evans was able to prepare a potent concentrate of vitamin E from the unsaponifiable lipids of wheat germ oil; others prepared similar vitamin E-active concentrates from lettuce lipids. By the early 1930s, **Olcott** and **Mattill** at the University of Iowa had found that such preparations, which prevented the gestation resorption syndrome in rats, also had chemical antioxidant properties that could be assayed in vitro[30]. In 1936, Evans isolated from unsaponifiable wheat germ lipids allophanic acid esters of three alcohols, one of which had very high biological vitamin E activity. Two years later, **Fernholz** showed that the latter alcohol had a phytyl side chain and a hydroquinone moiety, and proposed the chemical structure of the new vitamin. Evans coined the term *"tocopherol"* which he derived from the Greek words *tokos* (childbirth) and *pherein* (to bear)[31]; he used the suffix *-ol* to indicate that the factor is an alcohol. He also named the three alcohols *α-*, *β-* and *γ*-tocopherol. In 1938, the synthesis of the most active vitamer, *α*-tocopherol, was achieved by the groups of **Karrer, Smith**

---

[28]The vitamin E-deficient rat carries her fetuses quite well until a fairly late stage of pregnancy at which time they die and are resorbed by her. This syndrome is distinctive and is called *"gestation resorption"*.

[29]In fact, Evans and Bishop found that cod liver oil actually increased the severity of the gestation resorption syndrome, a phenomenon now understood on the basis of the antagonistic actions of high concentrations of the fat-soluble vitamins.

[30]Although the potencies of the vitamin preparations in the in vivo (rat gestation resorption) and in vitro (antioxidant) assays were not always well correlated.

[31]Evans wrote in 1962 that he was assisted in the coining of the name for vitamin E by George M. Calhoun, Professor of Greek and a colleague at the University of California. It was Calhoun who suggested the Greek roots of this now-familiar name.

and **Bergel**.  A decade later another vitamer, $\delta$-tocopherol, was isolated from soybean oil; not until 1959 were the tocotrienols described[32].

*anti-*
*hemorrhagic*
*factor:*
*vitamin K*

In the 1920s, **Henrik Dam**, at the University of Copenhagen, undertook studies to determine whether cholesterol was an essential dietary lipid.  In 1929, Dam reported that chicks fed diets that had been extracted with non-polar solvents to remove sterols developed subdural, subcutaneous or intramuscular hemorrhages, anemia and abnormally long blood clotting times.  A similar syndrome in chicks fed ether-extracted fish meal was reported by **McFarlane**'s group, which was attempting to determine the chick's requirements for vitamins A and D at the time.  They found that non-extracted fish meal completely prevented the clotting defect.  **Holst** and **Holbrook** found that cabbage prevented the syndrome, which they took as evidence of an involvement of vitamin C.  By the mid-1930s Dam had shown that the clotting defect was also prevented by a fat-soluble factor present in green leaves and certain vegetables and distinct from vitamins A, C, D or E.  He named the fat-soluble factor *"vitamin K"* [33].

At that time, **Almquist** and **Stokstad** at the University of California found that the hemorrhagic disease of chicks fed a diet based on ether-extracted fish meal and brewers' yeast, polished rice, cod liver oil and essential minerals was prevented by a factor present in ether extracts of alfalfa that was also produced during microbial spoilage of fish meal and wheat bran. Dam's colleague, **Schønheyder**, discovered the reason for prolonged blood clotting times of vitamin K-deficient animals.  He found that the clotting defect did not involve a deficiency of tissue thrombokinase, plasma fibrinogen or an accumulation of plasma anti-coagulants; that affected chicks showed relatively poor thrombin responses to exogenous thrombo-plastin.  That observation suggested inadequate amounts of the clotting factor prothrombin, which was already known to be important in the prevention of hemorrhages.

In 1936, Dam partially purified chick plasma prothrombin and showed its concentration to be depressed in vitamin K-deficient chicks.  It would be

---

[32]The tocotrienols differ from the tocopherols only by the presence of three conjugated double bonds in their phytyl side chains.

[33]Dam cited the fact that the next letter of the alphabet that had not previously been used to designate a known or proposed vitamin-like activity was also the first letter in the German or Danish phrase *"koagulation facktor"* and was, thus, a most appropriate designator for the anti-hemorrhagic vitamin. The phrase was soon shortened to *"K factor"* and, hence, *"vitamin K"*.

several decades before this finding was fully understood[34].  Nevertheless, the clotting defect in the chick model served as a useful bioassay tool. When chicks were fed foodstuffs containing the new vitamin, their prothrombin values were normalized; hence, clotting time was returned to normal and the hemorrhagic disease was cured.  The productive use of this bioassay led to the elucidation of the vitamin and its functions.

*vitamers K*

Vitamin K was first isolated from alfalfa by Dam in collaboration with **Karrer** at the University of Zurich in 1939.  They showed the active substance, which was a yellow oil, to be a quinone.  The structure of this form of the vitamin (called *"vitamin K₁"*) was elucidated by **Doisy**'s group at the University of St. Louis, and by Karrer's, Almquist's and **Feiser**'s groups in the same year.  Soon Doisy's group isolated a second form of the vitamin from putrified fish meal; this vitamer (called *"vitamin K₂"*) was crystalline. Subsequent studies showed this vitamer to differ from vitamin K₁ by having an unsaturated isoprenoid side chain at the 3-position of the naphthoquinone ring; in addition, putrified fish meal was found to contain several vitamin K₂-substances of differing chain length polyprenyl groups. Syntheses of vitamins K₂ were later achieved by **Isler**'s and **Folker**'s groups.   A strictly synthetic analog of the vitamers K₁ and K₂, the compound consisting of the methylated head group alone (i.e., 2-methyl-1,4-naphthoquinone), was shown by **Ansbacher** and **Fernholz** to have high anti-hemorrhagic activity in the chick bioassay.  It is, therefore, referred to as *"vitamin K₃"*.

*"bios" yields*
*biotin*

During the 1930s, independent studies of a yeast growth factor (called *"bios IIb"*[35]), a growth- and respiration-promoting factor for *Rhizobium trifolii* (called "coenzyme *R"*) and a factor that protected the rat against hair loss

---

[34]It should be remembered that, at the time of this work, the biochemical mechanisms involved in clotting were incompletely understood.  Of the many proteins now known to be involved in the process, only prothrombin, and fibrinogen had been definitely characterized.  It would not be until the early 1950s that the remainder of the now-classical clotting factors would be clearly demonstrated and that, of these, factors VII, IX and X would be shown to be dependent on vitamin K.  While these early studies effectively established that vitamin K deficiency results in impaired prothrombin activity, that finding would be interpreted as indicative of a vitamin K-dependent activation of the protein to its functional form.

[35]*"Bios IIb"* was one of three essential factors for yeasts that had been identified by **Wilders** at the turn of the century in response to the great controversy that raged between **Pasteur** and **Liebig**.  In 1860, Pasteur had declared that yeast could be grown in solutions containing only water, sugar, yeast ash (i.e., minerals) and ammonium tartrate; he noted, however, the growth-promoting activities of *"albuninoid materials"* in such cultures. Liebig challenged the possibility of growing yeast in the absence of such materials.  Though Pasteur's position was dominant through the close of the century, Wilders presented evidence at that time which proved that cultivation of yeast actually did require the presence of a little wort, yeast water, peptone or beef extract. (Wilders showed that an inoculum the size of a bacteriological loopful, which lacked sufficient amounts of these factors, was unsuccessful; whereas, an inoculum the size of a pea grew successfully.)  Wilders used the term *"bios"* to describe the new activity required for yeast growth.  For three decades, investigators undertook to characterize Wilders' *"bios"* factors.  By the mid-1920s, three factors had been identified: *"bios I"*, which was later identified as meso-inositol; *"bios IIa"*, which was replaced by pantothenic acid in some strains and by β-alanine plus leucine in others; and *"bios IIb"*, which was identified with biotin.

and skin lesions induced by raw egg white feeding (called *"vitamin H"[36]*) converged in an unexpected way. **Kögl**'s group isolated the yeast growth factor from egg yolk and named it *"biotin"*. In 1940, **György, du Vigneaud** and colleagues showed that *"vitamin H"* prepared from liver was remarkably similar to Kögl's egg yolk *"biotin"*. Due to some reported differences in physical characteristics between the two factors, the egg yolk and liver substances were called, for a time, *"α-biotin"* and *"β-biotin"[37]*, respectively. These differences were later found incorrect, and the chemical structure of biotin was elucidated in 1942 by du Vigneaud's group at Cornell[38]; its complete synthesis was achieved by Folkers in the following year.

Factors leading to the discovery of biotin:

| factor | bioassay |
|--------|----------|
| *"bios IIb"* | yeast growth |
| *"co-enzyme R"* | *Rhizobium trifolii* growth |
| *"vitamin H"* | prevention of hair loss and skin lesions in rats fed raw egg white |

*anti-anemia factors*

The last discoveries that led to the elucidation of new vitamins involved findings of anemias of dietary origin. The first of these was reported in 1931 by **Wills'** group as a *"tropical macrocytic anemia[39]"* observed in women in Bombay, India, which was often complicated by pregnancy. They found that the anemia could be treated effectively by feeding an extract of autolyzed yeast[40]. Wills and associates found that a macrocytic anemia could be produced in monkeys by feeding a diet similar to that consumed by women in Bombay. Further, the anemia could be cured by feeding the yeast extract or by orally or parenterally administering extracts

---

[36]György used the designation *'H'* after the German word *"haut"* meaning *"skin"*.

[37]The substances derived from each source showed were reported as having different melting points and optical rotations, giving rise to these designations. Subsequent studies, however, have been clear in showing that such differences are not correct, nor do these substances show different biological activities in microbiological systems. Thus, the distinguishing of biotin on the basis of source is no longer valid.

[38]du Vigneaud was to receive a Nobel Prize in Medicine for his work on the metabolism of methionine and methyl groups.

[39]A macrocytic anemia is one in which the number of circulating erythrocytes is below normal, but the mean size of those present is greater than normal (normal range: 82-92 $\mu^3$). Macrocytic anemias occur in such syndromes as pernicious anemia, sprue, celiac disease and macrocytic anemia of pregnancy. Wills' studies of the macrocytic anemia in her monkey model revealed megaloblastic arrest (i.e., failure of the large, nucleated, embryonic erythrocyte-precursor cell type to mature) in the erythropoietic tissues of the bone marrow and a marked reticulocytosis (i.e., the presence of young red blood cells in numbers greater than normal [usually < 1%], occurring during active blood regeneration); both signs were eliminated coincidentally upon the administration of extracts of yeast or liver.

[40]Wills' yeast extract was not particularly potent, as they fed 4 grams of it 2-4 times daily to cure the anemia.

of liver, which also cured human patients. The anti-anemia activity in these materials thus became known as the *"Wills factor"*.

*vitamin M?*  Elucidation of the *"Wills factor"* involved the convergence of several lines of research, some of which appeared to be unrelated. The first of these came in 1935 from the studies of **Day** and colleagues at the University of Arkansas Medical School who undertook to produce riboflavin deficiency in monkeys. They fed their animals a cooked diet consisting of polished rice, wheat, washed casein, cod liver oil, a mixture of salts and an orange; quite unexpectedly, they found them to develop anemia, leukopenia[41], ulceration of the gums, diarrhea and increased susceptibility to bacillary dysentery. They found that the syndrome did not respond to thiamin, riboflavin or nicotinic acid; however, it could be prevented by feeding daily 10 grams of brewer's yeast or 2 grams of a dried hog liver-stomach preparation. Day named the protective factor in brewer's yeast *"vitamin M"*.

*factors U, R*   In the late 1930s, three groups (**Stokstad**'s at the University of California,
*and vitamin B_c*  and **Norris**' at Cornell, and **Hogan**'s at the University of Missouri) reported syndromes characterized by anemia in chicks fed highly purified diets. The anemias were found to respond to dietary supplements of yeast, alfalfa and wheat bran. Stokstad and Manning called this unknown factor *"factor U"*; Baurenfeind and Norris called it *"factor R"*. Shortly thereafter, Hogan and Parrott discovered an anti-anemic substance in liver extracts; they called it *"vitamin B_c"*[42]. At the time (1939) it was not clear the extent to which these factors may have been related.

*yeast growth*    At the same time, the microbiologists **Snell** and **Peterson**, who were study-
*related to*      ing the *"bios"* factors required by yeasts, reported the existence of an
*anemia?*         unidentified water-soluble factor that was necessary for the growth of *Lactobacillus casei*. This factor was present in liver and yeast from which it could be prepared by adsorption to and then elution from norit; for a while, they called it the *"yeast norit factor"*, but it quickly became known as the *"L. casei factor"*. **Hutchings** and colleagues at the University of Wisconsin further purified the factor from liver and found it to stimulate chick growth; this suggested a possible identity of the bacterial and chick factors. The factor from liver was found to stimulate the growth of both *L. helveticus* and *Streptococcus faecalis* R.[43]; whereas the yeast-derived factor was twice as potent for *L. helveticus* as it was for *S. faecalis*. Thus, it became popular to refer to these as the *"liver L. casei factor"* and the *"yeast (or fermentation) L. casei factor"*.

---

[41]Leukopenia refers to any situation in which the total number of leukocytes (i.e., white blood cells) in the circulating blood is less than normal, which is generally ca. 5000 per $mm^3$.

[42]Hogan and Parrott used the subscript *'c'* to designate this factor as one required by the chick.

[43]*S. faecalis* was then called *S. lactis* R.

Factors leading to the discovery of folic acid:

| factor | bioassay |
|---|---|
| "Wills' factor" | cure of anemia in humans |
| "vitamin M" | prevention of anemia in monkeys |
| "vitamin $B_c$" | prevention of anemia in chicks |
| "factor R" | prevention of anemia in chicks |
| "factor U" | prevention of anemia in chicks |
| "yeast Norit factor" | growth of L. casei |
| "L. casei factor" | growth of L. casei |
| "SLR factor" | growth of Rhizobium sp. |
| "rhizopterin" | growth of Rhizobium sp. |
| "folic acid" | growth of S. faecalis and L. casei |

Snell's group found that many green leafy materials were potent sources of something with the microbiological effects of the *"norit eluate factor"*, i.e., extracts promoted the growth of both *S. faecalis* and *L. casei*. They named the factor, by virtue of its sources, ***"folic acid"***. In 1943, a fermentation product was isolated which stimulated the growth of *S. faecalis* but not *L. casei*; this was called the *"SLR factor"* and, later, *"rhizopterin"*.

*Who's on first?* It was far from clear in the early 1940s whether any of these factors were at all related, as *"folic acid"* appeared to be active for both micro-organisms and animals; whereas, concentrates of *"vitamin M"*, factors *"R"* and *"U"*, and *"vitamin $B_c$"* appeared to be effective only for animals. Clues to solving the puzzle came from the studies of **Mims** and associates at the University of Arkansas Medical School who showed that incubation of *"vitamin M"* concentrates in the presence of rat liver enzymes caused a marked increase in the *"folic acid"* activity (i.e., assayed using *S. casei* and *S. lactis* R.) of the preparation. Subsequent work showed such "activation" enzymes to be present in both hog kidney and chick pancreas. **Charkey**, of the Cornell group, found that incubation of their *"factor R"* preparations with rat or chick liver enzymes produced large increases in their *"folic acid"* potencies for micro-organisms. These studies indicated for the first time that at least some of these various substances may be related.

*derivatives of pteroylglutamic acid* The real key to solving what was clearly the most complicated puzzle in the discovery of the vitamins came in 1943 with the isolation of pteroylglutamic acid from liver by Stokstad's group at the Lederle Laboratories of American Cyanamid, and by **Piffner**'s group at Parke-Davis. Stokstad's group achieved the synthesis of the compound in 1946. Soon it was found that pteroylmonoglutamic acid was, indeed, the substance that had been variously identified in liver as *"factor U"*, *"vitamin M"*, *"vitamin $B_c$"*, and the *"liver L. casei factor"*. The *"yeast L. casei factor"* was found to be the diglutamyl derivative (pteroyldiglutamic acid) and that the liver-derived *"vitamin $B_c$"* was the hexaglutamyl derivative (pteroylhexaglutamic acid). Others of these factors (the *"SLR factor"*) were subsequently found to be single-carbon metabolites of pteroylglutamic acid. These various compounds thus became known generically as *"folic acid"*.

*anti-pernicious* The second nutritional anemia that was found to involve a vitamin defi-
*anemia factor* ciency was the fatal condition of human patients that was first described
by **J.S. Combe** in 1822, and became known as *"pernicious anemia"*[44].
The first real breakthrough toward understanding the etiology of pernicious
anemia did not come until 1926 when **Minot** and **Murphy** found that lightly
cooked liver, which the prominent hematologist **G.H. Whipple** had found
to accelerate the regeneration of blood in dogs made anemic by exsan-
guination, was highly effective as therapy for the disease[45,46]. This
indicated that liver contained a factor necessary for hemoglobin synthesis.

*"intrinsic" and* Soon, studies of the anti-pernicious anemia factor in liver revealed that its
*"extrinsic"* enteric absorption depended upon yet another factor in the gastric juice,
*factors* which **W.B. Castle** in 1928 called the *"intrinsic factor"* to distinguish it from
the *"extrinsic factor"* in liver. Biochemists then commenced a long
endeavor to isolate the anti-pernicious anemia factor from liver. The
isolation of the factor was necessarily slow and arduous for the reason that
the only bioassay available was the hematopoietic response of human
pernicious anemia patients, which were frequently not available. No animal
model had been found; and a bioassay could not be replaced by a chemical reaction or physical method because, as is now known, this most
potent vitamin is active at exceedingly low concentrations. Therefore, it
was most important to the elucidation of the anti-pernicious anemia factor
when, in 1947, **Mary Shorb** of the University of Maryland found that it was
also required for the growth of *Lactobacillus lactis* Dorner[47]. Using the
microbiological assay that Shorb developed, isolation of the factor, by that
time called *"vitamin B$_{12}$"*, proceeded rapidly.

*"animal protein* At about the same time, animal growth responses to factors associated with
*factors"* animal proteins or manure were reported as American animal nutritionists
sought to eliminate expensive and scarce animal by-products from the
diets of livestock. **Norris'** group at Cornell attributed responses of this time
to an *"animal protein factor"*; the factor in liver necessary for rat growth
was called *"factor X"* by **Cary** and *"zoopherin"*[48] by **Zucker** and **Zucker**.

---

[44]Pernicious anemia is also called *"Addison's anemia"* after T. Addison who described it in great detail in
1949, and *"Biemer's anemia"* after A. Biemier who reported the disease in Zurich in 1872 and coined the term
"pernicious anemia".

[45]Minot and Murphy treated 45 pernicious anemia patients with 120-240 grams of lightly cooked liver per
day. The patients' mean erythrocyte count increased from $1.47 \times 10^6$ per $\mu l$ before treatment to $3.4 \times 10^6$ per $\mu l$
and $4.6 \times 10^6$ per $\mu l$ after one and two months of treatment, respectively.

[46]Whipple, Minot and Murphy shared the 1934 Nobel Prize in Medicine for the discovery of whole liver
therapy for pernicious anemia.

[47]For a time, this was referred to as the *"LLD factor"*.

[48]The term *"zoopherin"* carries the connotation: *"to carry on an animal species"*.

Soon it became evident that these factors were probably identical. **Stokstad**'s group found the factor in manure and isolated an organism from poultry manure that would synthesize a factor that was effective both in promoting chick growth and in treating pernicious anemia. That the anti-pernicious anemia factor was produced microbiologically was important in that it led to an economical means of industrial production of vitamin $B_{12}$.

Factors leading to the discovery of vitamin $B_{12}$:

| factor | bioassay |
|--------|----------|
| "extrinsic factor" | cure of anemia in humans |
| "LLD factor" | growth of *L. lactis* Dorner |
| "vitamin $B_{12}$" | growth of *L. lactis* Dorner |
| "animal protein factor" | growth of chicks |
| "factor X" | growth of rats |
| "zoopherin" | growth of rats |

*vitamin $B_{12}$ isolated*

By the late 1940s, **Combs**[49] and **Norris**, using chick growth as their bioassay procedure, were fairly close to the isolation of vitamin $B_{12}$. However, in 1948, **Folkers** at Merck, using the *Lactobacillus lactis* Dorner assay, succeeded in first isolating the anti-pernicious anemia factor in crystalline form. This achievement was accomplished in the same year by **Smith**'s group at the Glaxo Laboratories in England; they assayed all of their material on pernicious anemia patients in relapse[50]. The elucidation of the complex chemical structure of vitamin $B_{12}$ was finally achieved in 1955 by **Dorothy Hodgkin**'s group at Oxford with the use of X-ray crystallography. In the early 1960s several groups accomplished the partial synthesis of the vitamin; it was not until 1970 that the *de novo* synthesis of vitamin $B_{12}$ was finally achieved by **Woodward** and **Eschenmoser**.

*vitamins discovered in only five decades*

Beginning with the ***concept*** of a vitamin, which emerged with Eijkman's proposal of an anti-polyneuritis factor in **1906**, the elucidation of the vitamins continued through the isolation of vitamin $B_{12}$ in potent form in **1948**. Thus, the identification of the presently recognized vitamins was achieved within a period of *only 42 years!* For some vitamins (e.g., pyridoxine) for which convenient animal models were available, discoveries came rapidly; for others (e.g., niacin, vitamin $B_{12}$) for which animal models were late to be found, the pace of scientific progress was much slower.

---

[49]The author's father worked on the isolation of the *animal protein factor* as a doctoral student in Norris' laboratory in the late 1940s.

[50]Friedrich (1988) has pointed out that it should be no surprise that the first isolations of vitamin $B_{12}$ were accomplished in industrial laboratories, because the task required industrial-scale facilities to handle the enormous amounts of starting material that were needed. For example, the Merck group used a ton of liver to obtain 20 $\mu$g of crystalline material.

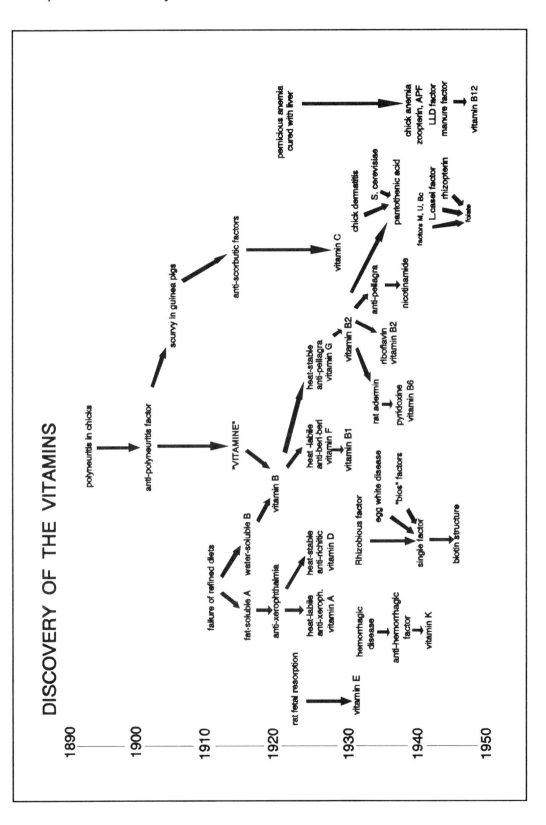

Timelines for the discoveries of the vitamins:

| vitamin | proposed | isolated | structure determined | synthesis achieved |
|---|---|---|---|---|
| thiamin | 1906 | 1926 | 1932 | 1933 |
| vitamin C | 1907 | 1926 | 1932 | 1933 |
| vitamin A | 1915 | 1937 | 1942 | 1947 |
| vitamin D | 1919 | 1932 | 1932 ($D_2$) | 1932 |
|  |  |  | 1936 ($D_3$) | 1936 |
| vitamin E | 1922 | 1936 | 1938 | 1938 |
| niacin | 1926 | 1937 | 1937 | (1867) |
| vitamin $B_{12}$ | 1926 | 1948 | 1955 | 1970 |
| biotin | 1926 | 1939 | 1942 | 1943 |
| vitamin K | 1929 | 1939 | 1939 | 1940 |
| pantothenic acid | 1931 | 1939 | 1939 | 1940 |
| folate | 1931 | 1939 | 1943 | 1946 |
| riboflavin | 1933 | 1933 | 1934 | 1935 |
| vitamin $B_6$ | 1934 | 1936 | 1938 | 1939 |

Nobel Prizes awarded for research on vitamins:

**Prizes in Medicine and Physiology**

| 1929 | Christian Eijkman | *"discovery of the antineuritic vitamin"* |
|---|---|---|
|  | Frederick G. Hopkins | *"discovery of the growth-stimulating vitamins"* |
| 1934 | George H. Whipple | *"discoveries concerning liver therapy against* |
|  | George R. Minot | *pernicious anemia"* |
|  | William P. Murphy |  |
| 1937 | Albert von Szent-Györgi | *"discoveries in connection with the biological combustion, with especial reference to vitamin C and the catalysis of fumaric acid"* |
| 1943 | Henrik Dam | *"discovery of vitamin K"* |
|  | Edward A. Doisy | *"discovery of the chemical nature of vitamin K"* |
| 1953 | Fritz A. Lipmann | *"discovery of coenzyme A and its importance in intermediary metabolism"* |
| 1955 | Hugo Theorell | *"discoveries relating to the nature and mode of action of oxidizing enzymes"* |
| 1964 | Feordor Lynen | *"discoveries concerning the mechanism and regula-* |
|  | Konrad Bloch | *tion of cholesterol and fatty acid metabolism"* |

**Prizes in Chemistry**

| 1928 | Adolf Windaus | *"studies on the constitution of the sterols and their connection with the vitamins"* |
|---|---|---|
| 1937 | Walter N. Haworth | *"researches into the constitution of carbohydrates and vitamin C"* |
|  | Paul Karrer | *"researches into the constitution of carotenoids, flavins and vitamins A and B"* |
| 1938 | Richard Kuhn | *"work on carotenoids and vitamins"* |
| 1967 | George Wald | *"discoveries of the basic chemical and physiological* |
|  | H.K. Hartline | *processes in vision"* |
|  | R. Grant |  |

## THE TERMINOLOGY OF THE VITAMINS

The terminology of the vitamins can be as daunting as that of any other scientific field.  Many vitamins carry alphabetic or alpha-numeric designations, yet the sequence of such designations has an arbitrary appearance by virtue of its many gaps and inconsistent application to all of the vitamins.  This situation not withstanding, the logic underlying the terminology of the vitamins becomes apparent when it is viewed in terms of the history of vitamin discovery.  The familiar designations in use today are, in most cases, the surviving terms coined by earlier researchers on the paths to vitamin discovery.  Thus, because McCollum and Davis used the letters *'A'* and *'B'* to distinguish the lipid-soluble anti-xeropthalmic factor from the water-soluble anti-neuritic and growth activity that was subsequently found to consist of several vitamins, such chemically and physiologically unrelated substances as thiamin, riboflavin, pyridoxine and cobalamins (in fact, all water-soluble vitamins except ascorbic acid, which was designated before the *"vitamin B-complex"* was partitioned) are all called *"B-vitamins"*. In the case of folic acid, certainly the name survived its competitors by virtue of its relatively attractive sound (e.g., *vs. "rhizopterin"*).  Therefore, the accepted designations for the vitamins, in most cases, have relevance only to the history and chronology of their discovery, and *not* to their chemical or metabolic similarities.  The discovery of the vitamins left a path littered with designations of *"vitamins"*, *"factors"* and other terms most of which have been discarded.

Current and obsolete designations of *"vitamins"*[51]:

| name | explanation |
| --- | --- |
| **vitamin A** | accepted designation of retinoids that prevent xerophthalmia and nyctalopia, and are essential for epithelial maintenance |
| vitamin B | original anti-beri-beri factor; now known to be a mixture of factors and designated as the vitamin B complex |
| vit. B complex | term introduced when it became clear that *"water-soluble B"* contained more than one biologically active substance (such preparations were subsequently found to be mixtures of thiamin, niacin, riboflavin, pyridoxine and pantothenic acid); the term has contemporary lay use as a non-specific name for all of the B-designated vitamins |
| **vitamin B$_1$** | synonym for thiamin |
| **vitamin B$_2$** | synonym for riboflavin |
| vit. B$_2$ complex | obsolete term for the thermostable "second nutritional factor" in yeast, which was found to be a mixture of niacin, riboflavin, pyridoxine and pantothenic acid |
| vitamin B$_3$ | infrequently used synonym for pantothenic acid; was also used for nicotinic acid |
| vitamin B$_4$ | unconfirmed activity preventing muscular weakness in rats and chicks; believed to be a mixture of arginine, glycine, riboflavin and pyridoxine |
| vitamin B$_5$ | unconfirmed growth promotant for pigeons; probably niacin |
| **vitamin B$_6$** | synonym for pyridoxine |
| vitamin B$_7$ | unconfirmed digestive promoter for pigeons; may be a mixture; also *"vitamin I"* |
| vitamin B$_8$ | adenylic acid; no longer classified as a vitamin |
| vitamin B$_9$ | unused designation |
| vitamin B$_{10}$ | growth promotant for chicks; likely a mixture of folic acid and vitamin B$_{12}$ |
| vitamin B$_{11}$ | apparently the same as *"vitamin B$_{10}$"* |
| **vitamin B$_{12}$** | accepted designation of the cobalamins (cyano- and aquo-cobalamins) that prevent pernicious anemia and promote growth in animals. |
| vitamin B$_{12a}$ | synonym for aquacobalamin |
| vitamin B$_{12b}$ | synonym for hydroxocobalamin |
| vitamin B$_{12c}$ | synonym for nitritocobalamin |
| vitamin B$_{13}$ | synonym for orotic acid, an intermediate of pyrimidine metabolism; not considered a vitamin |
| vitamin B$_{14}$ | unconfirmed |
| vitamin B$_{15}$ | synonym for "pangamic acid"; no proven biological value |
| vitamin B$_{17}$ | synonym for laetrile, a cyanogenic glycoside with unsubstantiated claims of anti-carcinogenic activity; not considered a vitamin |
| vitamin B$_c$ | obsolete term for pteroylglutamic acid |
| vitamin B$_p$ | activity preventing perosis in chicks; replaceable by choline and Mn |
| vitamin B$_t$ | activity promoting insect growth; identified as carnitine |
| vitamin B$_x$ | activity associated with pantothenic acid and *p*-aminobenzoic acid |
| **vitamin C** | accepted designation of the anti-scorbutic factor, ascorbic acid |
| vitamin C$_2$ | unconfirmed anti-pneumonia activity; also called *"vitamin J"* |
| **vitamin D** | accepted designation of the anti-rachitic factor (the calciferols) |
| **vitamin D$_2$** | accepted designation for ergocalciferol (a vitamin D-active substance derived from plant sterols) |
| **vitamin D$_3$** | accepted designation for cholecalciferol (a vitamin D-active substance derived from animal sterols) |
| **vitamin E** | accepted designation for tocopherols active in preventing myopathies and certain types of infertility in animals |
| vitamin F | obsolete term for essential fatty acids; also an abandoned term for thiamin activity |

---

[51]Currently used names are shown in bold-face print.

Current and obsolete designations of *"vitamins"*[51]:

| name | explanation |
|---|---|
| vitamin G | obsolete term for riboflavin activity; also an abandoned term for the *"pellagra-preventive factor"* (niacin) |
| vitamin H | obsolete term for biotin activity |
| vitamin I | mixture also formerly called *"vitamin $B_7$"* |
| vitamin J | postulated anti-pneumonia factor also formerly called *"vitamin $C_2$"* |
| **vitamin K** | accepted designation for activity preventing hypoprothrombinemic hemorrhage shared by related napthoquinones |
| **vitamin $K_1$** | accepted designation for phylloquinones (vitamin K-active substances produced by plants) |
| **vitamin $K_2$** | accepted designation for prenylmenaquinones (vitamin K-active substances synthesized by micro-organisms and produced from other vitamers K by animals) |
| **vitamin $K_3$** | accepted designation for menadione (synthetic vitamin K-active substance not found in nature) |
| vitamin $L_1$ | unconfirmed liver filtrate activity, probably related to anthranilic acid, proposed as necessary for lactation |
| vitamin $L_2$ | unconfirmed yeast filtrate activity, probably related to adenosine, proposed as necessary for lactation |
| vitamin M | obsolete term for anti-anemic factor in yeast now known to be pteroylglutamic acid |
| vitamin N | obsolete term for a mixture proposed to inhibit cancer |
| vitamin O | unused designation |
| vitamin P | activity reducing capillary fragility related to citrin, which is no longer classified as a vitamin |
| vitamin Q | unused designation (the letter was used to designate coenzyme Q) |
| vitamin R | obsolete term for folic acid; from Norris' chick anti-anemic *"factor R"* |
| vitamin S | chick growth activity related to the peptide *"streptogenin"*; the term was also applied to a bacterial growth activity probably related to biotin |
| vitamin T | unconfirmed group of activities isolated from termites, yeasts or molds and reported to improve protein utilization in rats |
| vitamin U | unconfirmed activity from cabbage proposed to cure ulcers and promote bacterial growth; may have folic acid activity |
| vitamin V | tissue-derived activity promoting bacterial growth; probably related to NAD |

[51] Currently used names are shown in bold-face print.

Older designations of vitamins and vitamin-like *"factors"*:

| factor | explanation |
|---|---|
| aneurin | infrequently used synonym for thiamin |
| A-N factor | obsolete term for the *"anti-neuritic factor"* (thiamin) |
| bios factors | obsolete terms for yeast growth factors now known to include biotin |
| citrovorum factor | infrequently used term for a naturally occurring form of folic acid ($N^5$-formyl-5,6,7,8-tetrahydropteroylmonoglutamic acid) which is required for the growth of *Leuconostoc citrovorum* |
| extrinsic factor | obsolete term for the anti-anemic activity in liver, now called vitamin $B_{12}$ |
| factor U | obsolete term for chick anti-anemic factor now known as a form of folate |
| factor R | obsolete term for chick anti-anemic factor now known as a form of folate |
| factor X | obsolete term used at various times to designate the rat fertility factor now called vitamin E and the rat growth factor now called vitamin $B_{12}$ |
| filtrate factor | obsolete term for the anti-black tongue disease activity, now known to be niacin, that could be isolated from the *"B$_2$ complex"* by filtration through fuller's earth; also used to describe the chick anti-dermatitis factor, now known to be pantothenic acid, isolated from acid solutions of the *"B$_2$ complex"* by filtration through fuller's earth |
| flavin | term originally used to describe the water-soluble fluorescent rat growth factors isolated from yeast and animal tissues; now, a general term for isoalloxazine derivatives including riboflavin and its active forms, FMN and FAD |
| hepatoflavin | obsolete term for the water-soluble rat growth factor, now known to be riboflavin, isolated from liver |
| intrinsic factor | accepted designation for the vitamin $B_{12}$-binding protein produced by gastric parietal cells and necessary for the enteric absorption of the cobalamins |
| lactoflavin | obsolete term for the water-soluble rat growth factor, now known to be riboflavin, isolated from whey |
| LLD factor | obsolete term for the activity in liver that promoted the growth of *Lactobacillus lactis* Dorner, now known to be vitamin $B_{12}$ |
| norit eluate | obsolete term for *Lactobacillus casei* growth-promotant, factor now known as folic acid, that could be isolated from liver and yeasts by adsorption on norit |
| ovoflavin | obsolete term for the water-soluble rat growth factor, now known to be riboflavin, isolated from egg white |
| P-P factor | obsolete term for the thermostable *"pellagra-preventive"* component, now known as niacin, of the *"water-soluble B"* activity of yeast |
| rhizopterin | obsolete synonym for the *"SLR factor"*, i.e., a factor from *Rhizobius* sp. fermentation that stimulated the growth of *Streptococcus lactis* R. (now called *S. faecalis*), which is now known to be a folate activity |
| SLR factor | obsolete term for the *Streptococcus lactis* R. (now called *S. faecalis*) growth promotant later called *"rhizopterin"* and now known to be a folic acid activity |
| streptogenin | a peptide present in liver and in enzymatic hydrolysates of casein and other proteins which promotes growth of mice and certain micro-organisms (hemolytic streptococci and lactobacilli); not considered a vitamin |
| Wills' factor | obsolete term for the anti-anemic factor in yeast now known to be a form of folate |
| zoopherin | obsolete term for a rat growth factor now known as vitamin $B_{12}$ |

# OTHER FACTORS SOMETIMES CALLED VITAMINS

Several other factors have, at various times or are under certain conditions, been called vitamins. Many remain today only as historic markers of once incompletely explained phenomena, now better understood. Today, some would appear to satisfy, for at least some species, the operating definition of a vitamin; although, in practice, that term is restricted to those factors required by higher organisms[52]. Therefore, these are frequently referred to as *quasi-vitamins*.

Quasi-vitamins:

| substance | biological activity |
|---|---|
| choline | Component of the neurotransmitter acetylcholine and the membrane structural component phosphatidylcholine; essential for normal growth and bone development in young poultry; can spare methionine in many animal species and, thus, can be essential in diets that provide limited methyl groups. |
| p-amino-benzoic acid | Essential growth factor for several microbes in which it functions as a pro-vitamin of folic acid; reported to reverse diet- or hydroquinone-induced achromotrichia in rats, and to ameliorate rickettsial infections. |
| myo-inositol | Component of phosphatidylinositol; prevents diet-induced lipo-dystrophies due to impaired lipid transport in gerbils and rats. Essential for some microbes, gerbils and certain fishes. |
| bioflavonoids | Reported to reduce capillary fragility, and inhibit *in vitro* aldolase reductase (has role in diabetic cataracts) and o-methyl-transferase (inactivates epinephrine and norepinephrine). |
| ubiquinones | Group includes a component of the mitochondrial respiratory chain; are antioxidants and can spare vitamin E in preventing anemia in monkeys, and in maintaining sperm motility in birds. |
| lipoic acid | Co-factor in oxidative decarboxylation of $\alpha$-keto acids; essential for growth of several microbes, but inconsistent effects on animal growth. |
| carnitine | Essential for transport of fatty acyl CoA from cytoplasm to mitochondria for $\beta$-oxidation; synthesized by most species except some insects which require a dietary source for growth. |
| pyrroloquinoline quinone | Component of certain bacterial and mammalian metallo-oxido-reductases; deprivation impairs growth, causes skin lesions in mice. |

---

[52]Organic growth-promoting substances required only by micro-organisms are frequently called *"nutrilites"*.

At various times, other factors have been represented as vitamins. For several of these, however, *no solid evidence* supports such claims. These factors have been called *pseudo-vitamins*.

Pseudo-vitamins:

| substance | purported biological activity |
|-----------|-------------------------------|
| laetrile | a cyanogenic glycoside; unsubstantiated claims of anti-tumorigenicity |
| gerovital | unsubstantiated anti-aging elixir |
| orotic acid | normal metabolic intermediate of pyrimidine biosynthesis with hypocholesterolemic activity |
| pangamic acid | ill-defined substance(s), originally derived from apricot kernels, with unsubstantiated claims for a variety of health benefits |

# THE MODERN HISTORY THE VITAMINS

Subsequent to the recognition of the vitamins and the discovery of their identities, it became apparent that a great deal of further information would be needed in order to use fully these substances to improve human and animal health and to optimize the efficiency of producing food animals. Thus, recent research interest in the vitamins has centered on certain foci. This information, much of which is still emerging today, will be the subject of the following chapters.

Foci of modern vitamin research:

| focus | research activities |
|-------|---------------------|
| chemical/physiological characteristics | determining chemical and biological potencies, availabilities, stabilities and requirements of/for the vitamins and their various vitamers and chemical derivatives |
| metabolic functions | elucidating the metabolism of the vitamins and the molecular mechanisms of vitamin action |
| nutritional/metabolic interactions | determining the interactions with other nutrients and/or metabolic factors that affect vitamin functions and needs |
| medical applications | assessing vitamin status; determining roles of vitamins in etiology and/or management of diseases |

## Study Questions and Exercises:

i. How did the *'vitamin theory'* **influence the interpretation** of findings concerning diet and health associations?

ii. For each vitamin, list the **key empirical observations** that led to its initial recognition.

iii. What **general ways** were animal models employed in the discovery of the vitamins?

iv. Which vitamins were discovered as results of efforts to use **chemically defined diets** for raising animals?

v. Which vitamins were discovered primarily through **human experimentation**?

vi. Prepare a **concept map** illustrating the interrelationships of the various prevalent ideas and the many goals, approaches and outcomes that resulted in the discovery of the vitamins.

## Recommended Reading:

**General History of the Vitamins**

Carpenter, K.J. 1986. The History of Scurvy and Vitamin C, Cambridge Univ. Press, Cambridge, 288 pp.

Györgi, P. 1954. Early experiences with riboflavin – a retrospect. Nutr. Rev. 12:97.

Harris, L.J. 1955. Vitamins in Theory and Practice, Cambridge Univ. Press, Cambridge, pp.1-39.

Lepkovsky, S. 1954. Early experiences with pyridoxine – a retrospect. Nutr. Rev. 12:257.

Roe, D.A. 1973. A Plague of Corn: The Social History of Pellagra, Cornell University Press, Ithaca, NY, 217 pp.

Sebrell, Jr., W.H. 1981. History of Pellagra. Federation Proc. 40:1520.

Wald, G. 1968. Molecular Basis of Visual Excitation. Science 162:230-239.

*Recommended Reading (continued):*

**Some Historically Significant Scientific Papers:**

*vitamin concept* Funk,C. 1912. J. State Med. 20:341.

*vitamin A*          McCollum, E.V. and M. Davis. 1913. J. Biol. Chem. 15:167.
                     Osborne, T.B. and L.B. Mendel. 1917. J. Biol. Chem.
                       31:149.
                     Wald, G. 1933. Vitamin A in the retina. Nature (London)
                       132:316.
                     Steenbock, H. 1919. Science 50:352.

*vitamin D*          McCollum, E.V., N. Simmonds and W. Pitz. 1916. J. Biol.
                       Chem. 27:33.

*vitamin E*          Evans, H.M. and K.S. Bishop. 1922. Science 56:650.
                     Olcott, H.S. and H.A. Mattill. 1931. J. Biol. Chem. 93:65-70.

*vitamin K*          Dam. H. 1929. Biochem. Z. 215:475.

*ascorbic acid*      Holst, A. and T. Frolich. 1907. J. Hyg. (Camb.) 7:634.
                     King, C.G. and W.A. Waugh. 1932. Science 75:357.
                     Svirbely, J.L. and A. Szent-Györgi. 1932. Nature (London)
                       129:576.

*thiamin*            Eijkman, C. 1897. Virchow Arch. Pathol. Anat. Physiol.
                       148:523.

*riboflavin*         Kuhn, P., P. Györgi and T. Wagner-Juregg. 1933. Ber.
                       66:317.

*niacin*             Elvehjem, C., R. Madden, F. Strong and D. Wolley. 1937. J.
                       Am. Chem. Soc. 59:1767.
                     Goldberger, J. 1922. J. Am. Med. Assoc. 78:1676.
                     Warburg, O. and W. Christian. 1936. Biochem. Z. 43:287.

*vitamin $B_6$*      Györgi, P. 1934. Nature (London) 133:498.

*biotin*             Kögl, F. and B. Tonnis. 1936. Z. Physiol. Chem. 242:43.

*pantothenic*        Norris, L.C. and A.T. Ringrose. 1930. Science 71:643.
  *acid*             Williams, R.J., C. Lyman, G. Goodyear, J. Truesdail and D.
                       Holaday. 1933. J. Am. Chem. Soc. 55:2912.

*folate*             Jukes, T.H. 1939. J. Am. Chem. Soc. 61:975.
                     Mimms, V., J.R. Totter and P.L. Day. 1944. J. Biol. Chem.
                       155:401.

*vitamin $B_{12}$*   Castle, W.B. 1929. Am. J. Med. Sci. 178:748.
                     Minot, and Murphy 1926 J. Am. Med. Assoc. 87:470.
                     Wills, L., M.A. Contab and B.S. Lond. 1931. Brit. Med. J.
                       1:1059
                     Shorb, M.S. 1948. Science 107:398.

# CHAPTER 3  *CHARACTERISTICS OF THE VITAMINS*

*"La vie est un fonction chemique."*                          A. L. Lavoisier

## *Anchoring Concepts:*

*i.*     The chemical **composition** and **structure** of a substance determines both its physical properties and chemical reactivity.

*ii.*    The **physio-chemical properties** of a substance determine the ways in which it acts and is acted upon in biological systems.

*iii.*   Substances tend to be **partitioned** between hydrophilic regions (plasma, cytosol and mitochondrial matrix space) and hydrophobic regions (membranes, bulk lipid droplets) of biological systems on the basis of their relative solubilities; overcoming such partitioning requires actions of agents (micelles, binding or transport proteins) that serve to alter their effective solubilities.

*iv.*    Isomers and analogues of a given substance may not have equivalent **biological activities**.

## *Learning Objectives:*

*i.*     To understand that the term *vitamin* refers to a family of compounds, i.e., structural analogues, with qualitatively similar biological activities but often with different quantitative potencies.

*ii.*    To become familiar with the **chemical structures** and **physical properties** of the vitamins.

*iii.*   To understand the relationship of the chemical and physical properties of the vitamins and their **stabilities**, and to their means of enteric **absorption**, **transport** and tissue **storage**.

*iv.*    To become familiar with the general nature of vitamin **metabolism**.

*Vocabulary:*

adenosylcobalamin
ascorbic acid
$\beta$-carotene
$\beta$-ionone nucleus
binding proteins
biopotency
biotin
carotenoid
cholecalciferol
chromanol ring
chylomicron
coenzyme A
cobalamin
corrin nucleus
cyanocobalamin
dehydroascorbic acid
ergocalciferol
FAD
FMN
folacin
folic acid
HDL
isoalloxazine nucleus
lipoprotein
menadione
menaquinone
methylcobalamin
micelle
NAD(H)
NADP(H)
naphthoquinone
niacin
nicotinic acid
nicotinamide
pantothenic acid
phylloquinone
portomicron

pteridine
pteroylglutamic acid
pyridine nucleus
pyridoxal
pyridoxal phosphate
pyridoxamine
pyridoxamine phosphate
pyridoxine
pyridoxol
pyrimidine ring
retinal
retinoic acid
retinoid
retinol
riboflavin
steroid
tetrahydrofolic acid
tetrahydrothiophene nucleus
thiamin
thiamin pyrophosphate
tocol
tocopherol
tocotrienol
ureido nucleus
vitamin A
vitamin $B_2$
vitamin $B_6$
vitamin $B_{12}$
vitamin D
vitamin $D_2$
vitamin $D_3$
vitamin E
vitamin K
vitamin $K_1$
vitamin $K_2$
vitamin $K_3$
VLDL

## CHEMICAL AND PHYSICAL PROPERTIES OF THE VITAMINS

*classifying*
*the vitamins*
*by solubility*

The vitamins are organic, low molecular weight substances that have key roles in metabolism. Few of the vitamins are single substances; almost all are families of chemically related substances, i.e., *vitamers*, sharing qualitatively (but not necessarily quantitatively) biological activities. Thus, the vitamers comprising a vitamin family may vary in *biopotency*, and the common vitamin name is actually a generic descriptor for all of the relevant vitamers. Otherwise, vitamin families are chemically heterogeneous; therefore, it is convenient to consider their physical properties, which offer an empirical means of classifying the vitamins broadly[1].

The fat-soluble vitamins (appreciably soluble in non-polar solvents):

| | |
|---|---|
| vitamin A | vitamin D |
| vitamin E | vitamin K |

The water-soluble vitamins  (appreciably soluble in polar solvents):

| | |
|---|---|
| thiamin | riboflavin |
| niacin | vitamin $B_6$ |
| biotin | pantothenic acid |
| folate | vitamin $B_{12}$ |
| vitamin C | |

The fat-soluble vitamins have some traits in common, in that each is comprised either entirely or primarily of five-carbon *isoprenoid* [2] units derived initially from acetyl CoA in those plant and animal species capable of their biosynthesis. In contrast, the water-soluble vitamins have, in general, few similarities of structure. The routes of their biosyntheses in capable species do not share as many common pathways.

*vitamin*
*nomenclature*

The nomenclature of the vitamins is in many cases rather complicated, reflecting both the terminology that evolved non-systematically during the course of their discovery, as well as more recent efforts to standardize the vocabulary of the field. Current standards for vitamin nomenclature policy

---

[1] It is interesting to note that this broad classification of the vitamins recapitulates the history of their discovery, i.e., calling to mind McCollum's *"Fat-Soluble A"* and *"Water-Soluble B"*.

[2] i.e., related to *"isoprene"* (2-methyl-1,3-butadiene)

were established by the International Union of Nutritional Sciences[3]. This policy distinguishes between **generic descriptors** used to describe families of compounds having vitamin activity (e.g., *vitamin D*) and to modify such terms as *activity* and *deficiency*, and **trivial names** used to identify specific compounds (e.g., *ergocalciferol*).

Physical properties of the vitamins:

| vitamin | vitamer | MW | solubility org.[a] $H_2O$[b] | | absorption max, nm | melting pt., °C | color-form |
|---|---|---|---|---|---|---|---|
| vitamin A | retinol | 286.4 | + | - | 325 | 62-64 | yellow crystal |
| | retinal | 284.4 | + | - | 373 | 61-64 | orange crystal |
| | retinoic acid | 300.4 | + | sl | 351 | 180-182 | yellow crystal |
| vitamin D | vitamin $D_2$ | 396.6 | + | - | 265 | 115-118 | white crystal |
| | vitamin $D_3$ | 384.6 | + | - | 265 | 84-85 | white crystal |
| vitamin E | $\alpha$-tocopherol | 430.7 | + | - | 294 | 2.5 | yellow oil |
| | $\gamma$-tocopherol | 416.7 | + | - | 298 | -2.4 | yellow oil |
| vitamin K | vitamin $K_1$ | 450.7 | + | - | 242,248,260, 269,325 | | yellow oil |
| | vitamin $K_{2(35)}$ | 649.2 | + | - | 243,248,261, 270,325-328 | 54 | yellow crystal |
| | vitamin $K_3$ | 172.2 | + | - | | 105-107 | yellow crystal |
| vitamin C | free acid | 176.1 | - | 323 | 245 | 190-192 | white crystal |
| | Na salt | 198.1 | - | 620 | 245 | 218[c] | white crystal |
| thiamin | disulfide form | 562.7 | - | sl | | 177 | yellow crystal |
| | hydrochloride | 337.3 | - | 1000 | | | white crystal |
| | mononitrate | 327.4 | - | 27 | | 196-200[c] | white crystal |
| riboflavin[d] | | 376.4 | - | .33 | 220-225,266, 371,444,475 | 278[c] | orange-yell.crystal |
| niacin | nicotinic acid | 123.1 | - | 16 | 263 | 237 | white crystal |
| | nicotinamide | 122.1 | - | 1000 | 263 | 128-131 | white crystal |
| vitamin $B_6$ | pyridoxal | 167.2 | - | 500 | 293 | 165[c] | white crystal |
| | pyridoxol(HCl) | 205.6 | - | 220 | 255,326 | 160 | white crystal |
| biotin | $d$-biotin | 244.3 | - | .4 | | 167 | white crystal |
| pantothenic | free acid | 219.2 | - | freely | | | clear oil |
| acid | Ca salt | 476.5 | - | 356 | | 195[c] | white crystal |
| folate | monoglutamate | 441.1 | - | .0016 | 256,283,368 | 250[c] | orange-yell. crystal |
| vitamin $B_{12}$ | cyanocobalamin | 1355.4 | - | 12.5 | 278,361,550 | >300 | red crystal |

[a]mg/ml at 25°C   [b]in organic solvents, fats and oils   [c]decomposes at this temperature   [d]fluoresces

---

[3]The 1976 recommendations of the I.U.N.S. Committee on Nomenclature (Nutr. Abstr. Rev. 48A:831-835, 1978) were adopted by the Commission on Nomenclature of the International Union of Pure and Applied Chemists, the International Union of Biochemists, and the Committee on Nomenclature of the American Institute of Nutrition. The latter organization publishes the policy every few years (*see* J. Nutr. 120:12-19, 1990).

## Vitamin A

Essential features of the chemical structure:

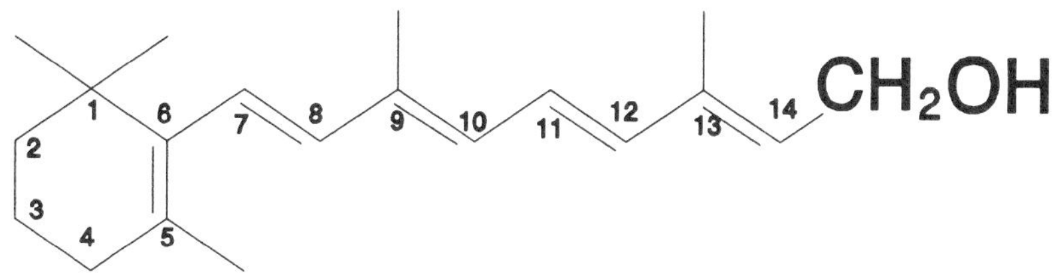

i.    substituted *β-ionone ring* (4-[2,6,6-trimethyl-2-cyclohexen-1-yl]-3-buten-2-one)
ii.   side-chain composed of 3 *isoprenoid units* joined head-to-tail at the 6-position of the *β*-ionone ring
iii.  *conjugated double-bond system* among the side-chain and 5,6-ring carbon atoms

Chemical structures of the vitamin A group:

| | |
|---|---|
| all-*trans*-retinol | 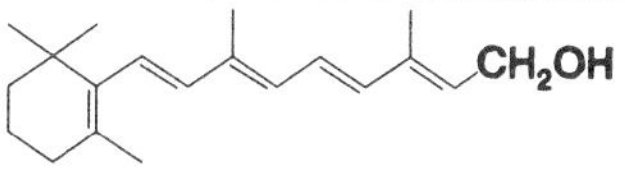 |
| 13-*cis*-retinol | 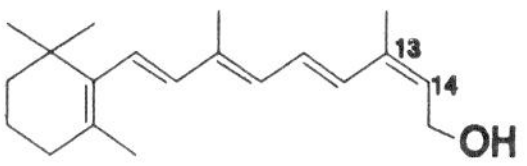 |
| 11-*cis*-retinal | 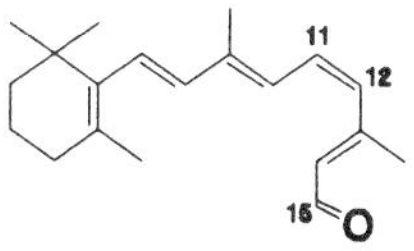 |
| 13-*cis*-retinoic acid | 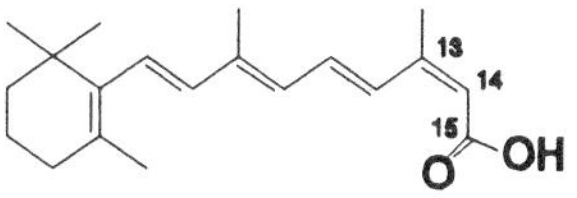 |
| all-*trans*-3-dehydroretinol <br> (sometimes called "vitamin A₂") | |
| all-*trans*-retinoic acid | 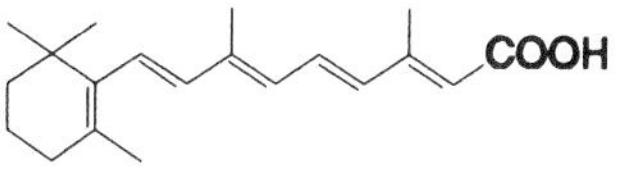 |
| all-*trans*-retinyl phosphate | |

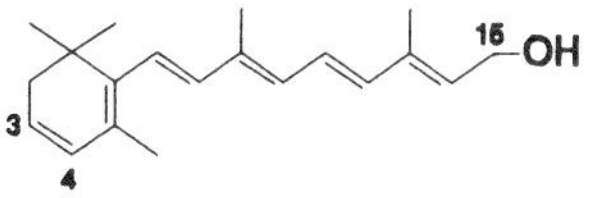

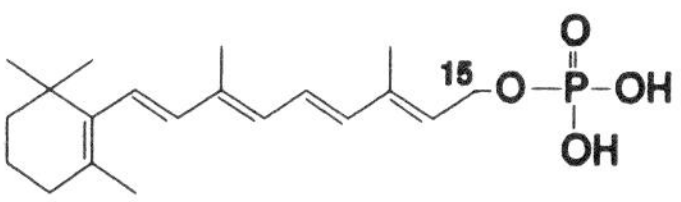

# Vitamin A

Chemical structures of pro-vitamins A:

α-carotene

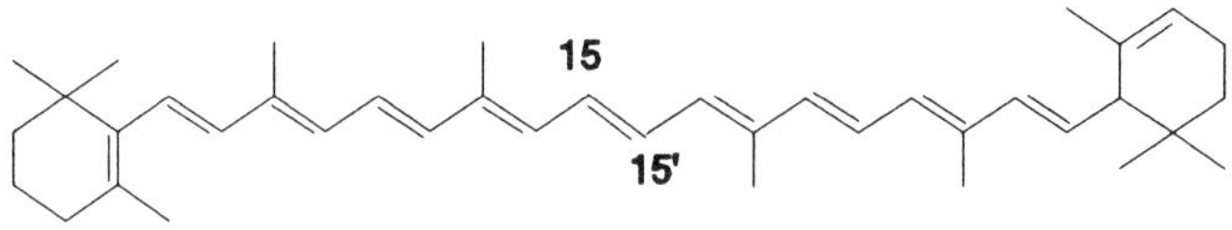

β-carotene

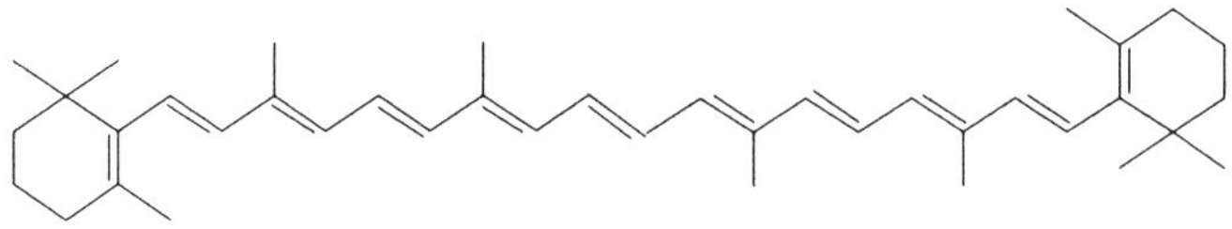

γ-carotene

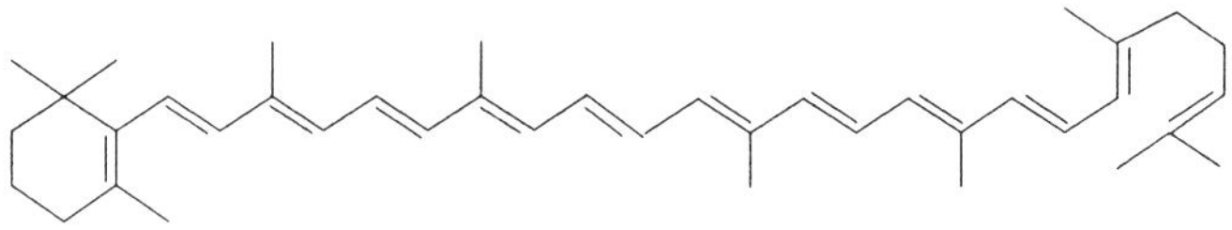

*vitamin A*  
*nomenclature*

Vitamin A is the generic descriptor for compounds with the qualitative biological activity of retinol. These compounds are formally derived from a mono-cyclic parent compound containing five carbon-carbon double bonds and a functional group at the terminus of the acyclic portion. Due to their close structural similarities to retinol, they are called *"retinoids"*.

The vitamin A-active retinoids occur in nature in three forms:

> the alcohol . . . ***retinol***,
> the aldehyde . . . ***retinal*** (also ***retinaldehyde***)
> the acid . . . ***retinoic acid***

All three basic forms are found in two variants: with the ***β-ionone nucleus*** (vitamin A₁) or the ***dehydrogenated β-ionone nucleus*** (vitamin A₂). However, because the former is both quantitatively and qualitatively more important as a source of vitamin A activity, the term *"vitamin A"* is usually taken to mean vitamin A₁. Some compounds of the class of plant pigments called *"carotenoids"* due to their relation to the carotenes yield retinoids upon metabolism and, thus, also have vitamin A activity; these are called *"pro-vitamin A carotenoids"* and include ***β-carotene***, which is actually a tail-conjoined retinoid dimer.

*vitamin A*  
*chemistry*

In solution, retinoids and carotenoids can be converted to geometric isomers by light, heat and iodine through *cis-trans* isomerism of the side-chain double bonds (e.g., in aqueous solution all-*trans*-retinol spontaneously isomerizes to an equilibrium mixture containing one-third *cis*-forms). Of the 16 stereoisomers of vitamin A made possible by the four side-chain double bonds, most of the potential *cis*-isomers are sterically hindered.

## Vitamin A

Thus, only a few isomers are known.  Contrary to what might be expected by their larger number of double bonds, carotenoids in both plants and animals occur almost exclusively in the all-*trans* form.  These conjugated polyene systems absorb light and, in the case of the carotenoids, appear to quench weakly free radicals.  For the retinoids, the functional group at position 15 determines specific chemical reactivity.  Thus, retinol can be oxidized to retinal and retinoic acid or esterified with organic acids; retinal can be oxidized to retinoic acid or reduced to retinol; and retinoic acid can be esterified with organic alcohols.  Retinol and retinal each undergo color reactions with such reagents as antimony trichloride, trifluoroacetic acid, and trichloroacetic acids, which have been used as the basis of their chemical analyses.

Most forms of vitamin A are crystallizable, but have low melting points (e.g., retinol: 62-64°C, retinal: 65°C).  Both retinoids and carotenoids have strong absorption spectra.  Vitamin A and the pro-vitamin A carotenoids are very sensitive to oxygen in air, especially in the presence of light and heat; therefore, isolation of these compounds requires the exclusion of air (e.g., sparging with an inert gas) and the presence of a protective antioxidant (e.g., $\alpha$-tocopherol).  The esterified retinoids are fairly stable.

Relative biopotencies of vitamin A and related compounds:

*vitamin A bioavailability*

| compound | relative biopotency[a] |
|---|:---:|
| all-*trans*-retinol | 100 |
| all-*trans*-retinal | 100 |
| *cis*-retinol isomers | 23-75 |
| retinyl esters | 10-100 |
| 3-dehydrovitamin A | 30 |
| $\beta$-carotene | 50 |
| $\alpha$-carotene | 26 |
| $\gamma$-carotene | 21 |
| cryptoxanthin | 28 |
| zeaxanthin | 0 |

[a]Relative biopotencies were determined by liver storage bioassays with chicks and/or rats with the exception of 3-dehydrovitamin A, which was assessed using liver storage by fish; in each case, the responses were standardized to that of all-*trans*-retinol.

# Vitamin D

Essential features of the chemical structure:

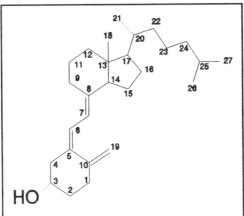

i.      side-chain-substituted, open-ring **steroid** (4-ringed compounds related to the sterols, which serve as hormones and bile acids).
ii.     **cis-triene** structure
iii.    open positions on carbon atoms #1 (ring) and #25 (side-chain)

Chemical structures of the vitamin D group:

vitamin D₂ (ergocalciferol)

vitamin D₃ (cholecalciferol)

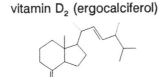

HO

HO

25-OH-vitamin D₃

1,25-(OH)₂ vitamin D₃

OH

OH

HO

HO      OH

# Vitamin D

| | |
|---|---|
| *vitamin D* *nomenclature* | Vitamin D is the generic descriptor for all steroids exhibiting qualitatively the biological activity of cholecalciferol. These compounds contain the intact 'A', 'C' and 'D' steroid rings[4], being ultimately derived *in vivo* by photolysis of the 'B' ring of 7-dehydrocholesterol. These compounds have either of two types of isoprenoid side-chains attached to the steroid nucleus at C-17 of the 'D' ring. One side-chain contains 9 carbons and a single double bond; vitamin D-active compounds with it are called derivatives of *"ergocalciferol"*, which is also called *"vitamin D₂"*. The other type of side-chain consists of 8 carbons and contains no double bonds; vitamin D-active compounds with it are called derivatives of *"cholecalciferol"*, also called *"vitamin D₃"*. The metabolically active forms of vitamin D are ring- (i.e., C-1) and side-chain-hydroxylated derivatives of vitamins $D_2$ and $D_3$. |
| *vitamin D* *chemistry* | Unlike the ring-intact steroids, vitamin D-active compounds tend to exist in extended conformations (shown above) due to the 180° rotation of the 'A' ring about the 6,7 single bond (in solution, the stretched and closed conformations are probably in an equilibrium favoring the former). The hydroxyl group on C-3 is, thus, in the β position (i.e., above the plane of the 'A' ring) in the closed forms and in the α position (i.e., below the plane of the 'A' ring) in the stretched forms. Rotation about the 5,6 double bond can also occur by the action of light or iodine to interconvert the biologically active 5,6-*cis* compounds to 5,6-*trans* compounds which show little of no vitamin D activity. |

Vitamins $D_2$ and $D_3$ are white to yellowish powders which are insoluble in water, moderately soluble in fats, oils and ethanol, and freely soluble in acetone, ether and petroleum ether. Each shows a strong UV absorption, with a maximum at 264 nm. Vitamin D is sensitive to oxygen, light and iodine. Heating or mild acidity can convert it to the 5,6-*trans* and other inactive forms. Whereas the vitamin is stable in dry form, in organic solvents and most plant oils (due to the presence of α-tocopherol, which serves as a protective antioxidant), its thermal- and photo-lability can result in losses during such procedures as saponification with refluxing. Therefore, it is often necessary to use inert gas environments, light-tight sealed containers and protective antioxidants in isolating the vitamin.

---

[4] Steroids contain a polycyclic hydrocarbon cyclopentanaperhydrophenanthrene nucleus consisting of three 6-carbon rings (referred to as the *"A"*, *"B"* and *"C"* rings) and a 5-carbon ring (the *"D"* ring).

## Vitamin D

*vitamin D bioavailability*

Relative biopotencies of vitamin D-active compounds:

| compound | relative biopotency[a] |
|---|---|
| vitamin $D_2$ (ergocalciferol) | $100^b$, $10^c$ |
| vitamin $D_3$ (cholecalciferol) | 100 |
| dihydrotachysterol[d] | 5-10 |
| 25-OH-cholecalciferol[e] | 200-500 |
| 1,25-$(OH)_2$-cholecalciferol[e] | 500-1000 |
| 1$\alpha$-OH-cholecalciferol[f] | 500-1000 |

[a]Results of bioassays of rickets prevention in chicks and/or rats.
[b]For mammalian species, the biopotencies of vitamins $D_2$ and $D_3$ are equivalent.
[c]The biopotency of vitamin $D_2$ is very low for chicks, which cannot use this vitamer effectively.
[d]i.e., a sterol generated by the irradiation of ergosterol
[e]Normal metabolite of vitamin $D_3$; the analogous metabolite of vitamin $D_2$ is also formed and is comparably active in non-avian species.
[f]a synthetic analog

# Vitamin E

Essential features of the chemical structure:

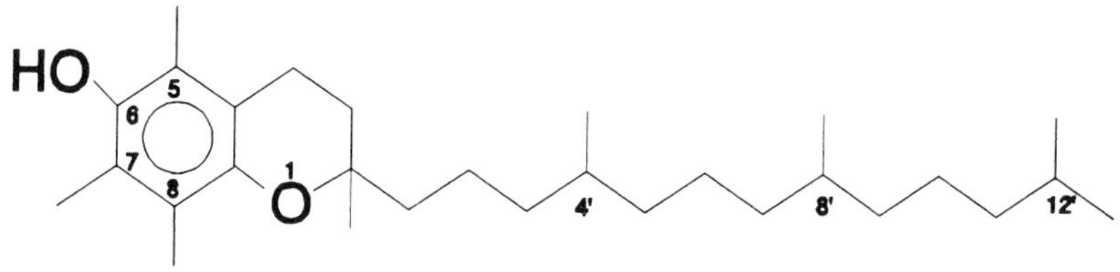

i. side-chain-derivative of a **ring-methylated 6-chromanol** (3,4-di-hydro-2H-1-benzopyran-6-ol)
ii. side-chain consists of three **isoprenoid units** joined head-to-tail
iii. **free hydroxyl or ester linkage** on carbon #6 of chromanol ring

Chemical structures of the vitamin E group:

the tocopherols

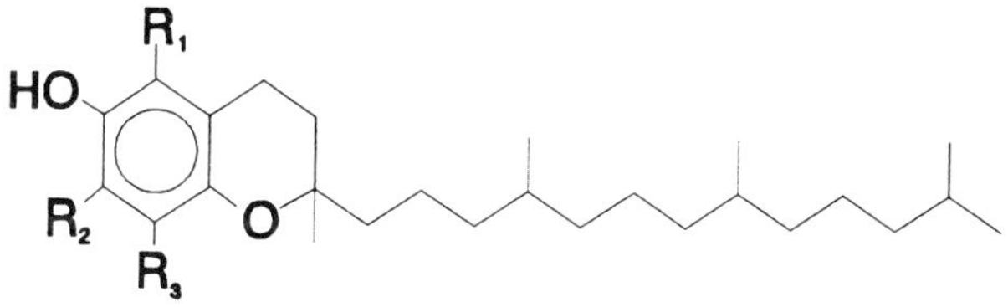

| vitamer | $R_1$ | $R_2$ | $R_3$ |
|---|---|---|---|
| α-tocopherol | $CH_3$ | $CH_3$ | $CH_3$ |
| β-tocopherol | $CH_3$ | H | $CH_3$ |
| γ-tocopherol | H | $CH_3$ | $CH_3$ |
| δ-tocopherol | H | H | $CH_3$ |
| tocol | H | H | H |

the tocotrienols

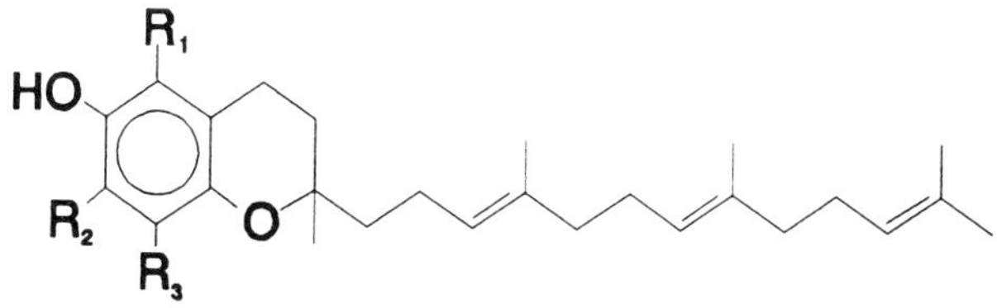

| vitamer | $R_1$ | $R_2$ | $R_3$ |
|---|---|---|---|
| α-tocotrienol | $CH_3$ | $CH_3$ | $CH_3$ |
| β-tocotrienol | $CH_3$ | H | $CH_3$ |
| γ-tocotrienol | H | $CH_3$ | $CH_3$ |
| δ-tocotrienol | H | H | $CH_3$ |
| tocotrienol | H | H | H |

# *Vitamin E*

*vitamin E
nomenclature*

Vitamin E is the generic descriptor for all tocol and tocotrienol derivatives that exhibit qualitatively the biological activity of *a*-tocopherol. These compounds are isoprenoid side-chain derivatives of 6-chromanol. The term *"tocol"* is the trivial designation for the derivative with a side chain consisting of three fully saturated isopentyl units; *"tocopherol"* denotes generically the mono-, di- and tri-methyl tocols irrespective of biological activity. *"Tocotrienol"* is the trivial designation of the 6-chromanol derivative with a similar side chain containing three double bonds. Individual tocopherols and tocotrienols are named according to the position and number of methyl groups on their chromanol rings.

Because the tocopherol side chain contains two anomeric carbons (C-4', C-8') in addition to the one at the point of its attachment to the ring (C-2), eight stereoisomers are possible. However, only one stereoisomer occurs naturally: the R,R,R- form. The chemical synthesis of vitamin E produces mixtures of other stereoisomers, depending on the starting materials. For example, through the early 1970s the commercial synthesis of vitamin E used as the source of the side-chain iso-phytol isolated from natural sources (which has the R-configuration at both the 4- and 8-carbons); tocopherols so produced were racemic at only the C-2 position. Such a mixture of 2RS-*a*-tocopherol was then called *"dl-a-tocopherol"*; its acetate ester was the form of commerce and was adopted as the international standard upon which the biological activities of other forms of the vitamin are still based. In recent years, however, the commercial synthesis of vitamin E has turned away from using iso-phytol in favor of a fully synthetic side-chain. Therefore, synthetic preparations of vitamin E presently available are mixtures of all eight possible stereoisomers, i.e., 2RS,4'RS,8'RS-compounds, which are designated more precisely with the prefix *"all-rac-"*. The acetate esters of vitamin E are used in medicine and animal feeding; whereas, the unesterified (i.e., free alcohol forms) are used as antioxidants in foods and pharmaceuticals. Other forms (e.g., *a*-tocopheryl hydrogensuccinate, *a*-tocopheryl polyethylene glycol-succinate) are used in multi-vitamin preparations.

*vitamin E
chemistry*

The tocopherols are light yellow oils at room temperature. They are insoluble in water, but readily soluble in non-polar solvents. Being monoethers of a hydroquinone with a phenolic hydrogen on the C-6 ring-hydroxyl group and the ability to accommodate an unpaired electron within the resonance structure of the ring (undergoing transition to a semi-stable chromanoxyl radical before being converted to tocopheryl quinone), they are good quenchers of free radicals and, thus, serve as antioxidants. They are, however, easily oxidized and can be destroyed by peroxides, ozone and permanganate in a process catalyzed by light and accelerated by poly-unsaturated fatty acids and metal salts. They are very resistant to acids

## Vitamin E

and, only under anaerobic conditions, to bases. Tocopheryl esters, by virtue of the blocking of the C-6 hydroxyl group, are very stable in air and are, therefore, the forms of choice as food/feed supplements. Because tocopherol is liberated by the saponification of its esters, all extraction and isolation of vitamin E calls for the use of protective antioxidants (e.g., propyl gallate, ascorbic acid), metal chelators, inert gas environments and subdued light. The UV absorption spectra of tocopherols and their acetates in ethanol have maxima of 280-300 nm ($a$-tocopherol: 292 nm); however, their extinction coefficients are not great. Because their fluorescence is significant (294 nm excitation, 330 nm emission), this property has analytical utility.

*vitamin E bioavailability*

Relative biopotencies of vitamin E-active compounds:

| trivial designation | systematic name | biopotency |
|---|---|---|
| R,R,R-$a$-tocopherol[a] | 2R-(4'R,8'R)-5,7,8-trimethyltocol | 1.49[b] |
| R,R,R-$a$-tocopheryl acetate | 2R-(4'R,8'R)-5,7,8-trimethyltocol acetate | 1.36 |
| all-*rac*-$a$-tocopherol[c] | 2RS-(4'RS,8'RS)-5,7,8-trimethyl-tocol | 1.1 |
| all-*rac*-$a$-tocopheryl acetate | 2RS-(4'RS,8'RS)-5,7,8-trimethyl-tocol acetate | 1.0 |
| R,R,R-$\beta$-tocopherol | 2R-(4'R,8'R)-5,8-dimethyltocol | .12 |
| R,R,R-$\gamma$-tocopherol | 2R-(4'R,8'R)-5,7-dimethyltocol | .05 |
| R-$a$-tocotrienol | *trans*-2R-5,7,8-trimethyltocotrienol | .32 |
| R-$\beta$-tocotrienol | *trans*-2R-5,8-dimethyltocotrienol | .05 |
| R-$\gamma$-tocotrienol | *trans*-2R-5,7-dimethyltocotrienol | - |

[a]Formerly called *d*-$a$-tocopherol
[b]International Units per mg material, based chiefly on rat gestation-resorption bioassay data
[c]Formerly called *dl*-$a$-tocopherol; this form remains the international standard despite the fact that it has not been produced commercially for several years.

# *Vitamin K*

Essential features of the chemical structure:

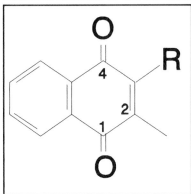

i.      derivative of **2-methyl-1,4-naphthoquinone**
ii.     ring structure can be **alkylated with an isoprenoid side-chain**

Chemical structures of the vitamin K group:

the phylloquinones

the menaquinones

menadione

## Vitamin K

*vitamin K*
*nomenclature*

Vitamin K is the generic descriptor for 2-methyl-1,4-naphthoquinone and all of its derivatives exhibiting qualitatively the biological (anti-hemorrhagic) activity of phylloquinone. Naturally occurring forms of the vitamin have an unsaturated isoprenoid side chain at C-3 of the naphthoquinone nucleus; the type and number of isoprene units (*not* carbon atoms) is the basis of the characterization of the side chain and, hence, the designation of the vitamer. The ***phylloquinone*** group includes forms with phytyl side-chains and side chains that are further alkylated, thus, consisting of several iso-prenoid units. The vitamers of this group have only one double bond in their side-chains, i.e., on the proximal isoprene unit. These vitamers are synthesized by green plants. They are properly referred to as *"phylloquin-ones"* [5] and are abbreviated as *"K"*. The ***menaquinone*** group also includes vitamers with side chains consisting of variable numbers of iso-prenoid units; however, *each* isoprene unit has a double bond. These vitamers are synthesized by bacteria. They are abbreviated as *"MK"* [6]. For each of these groups of vitamers, a numeric system is used to indicate side-chain length, e.g., the abbreviations **K-*n*** and **MK-*n*** are used for the phylloquinones and menaquinones, respectively, to indicate specific vita-mers with side chains consisting of *n* isoprenoid units. The compound 2-methyl-1,4-naphthoquinone, i.e., without a side chain, is called *"menadione"*[7]. It does not exist naturally, but has biological activity by virtue of the fact that animals can alkylate it to produce such metabolites as MK-4. Menadione is the compound of commerce; it is made in several forms (e.g., menadione sodium bisulfite complex, menadione dimethyl-pyrimidinol bisulfite).

Systems of vitamin K nomenclature:

| chemical name | IUPAC[a] system[b] | IUNS[c] system | old tradition |
|---|---|---|---|
| 2-methyl-3-phytyl-1,4-naphthoquinone | phylloquinone (K) | phytylmenaquinone (PMQ) | $K_1$ |
| 2-methyl-3-multiprenyl-1,4-naphthoquinone (class) | menaquinone-n (MK-n) | prenylmenaquinone-n (MQ-n) | $K_{2(n)}$ |
| 2-methyl-1,4-naphthoquinone | menadione | menaquinone | $K_3$ |
| [a]Internat. Union of Pure and Applied Chemists [b]preferred system [c]Internat. Union of Nutritional Sciences | | | |

[5] These vitamers were formerly called the *"phytylmenaquinones"*, or *"vitamin $K_1$"*; the latter term is still encountered.

[6] Formerly referred to as the *"prenylmenaquinones"*.

[7] Formerly referred to as *"vitamin $K_3$"*.

## Vitamin K

*vitamin K*
*chemistry*

Phylloquinone ($K_1$) is a yellow oil at room temperature, but the other vitamers K are yellow crystals. The vitamers K, MK and most forms of menadione are insoluble in water, slightly soluble in ethanol and readily soluble in ether, chloroform, fats and oils. The vitamers K are sensitive to light and alkali, but are relatively stable to heat and oxidizing environments. Their oxidation proceeds to produce the 2,3-epoxide form. Being naphthoquinones, they can be reduced to the corresponding naphthohydroquinones (e.g., with sodium hydrogen sulfite) which can be re-oxidized with mild oxidizing agents. The vitamers K show the characteristic UV spectra of the naphthoquinones, i.e., their oxidized forms having four strong absorption bands in the 240-270 nm range. The reduced (hydroquinone) forms show losses of the band near 270 nm and increases of the band around 245 nm. Extinction decreases with increasing side-chain length.

Relative biopotencies of vitamin K-active compounds:

*vitamin K*
*bioavailability*

| compound | biopotency[a] |
|---|---|
| *phylloquinones (formerly $K_1$)* | |
| K-1[b] | 5 |
| K-2 | 10 |
| K-3 | 30 |
| K-4 | 100 |
| K-5 | 80 |
| K-6 | 50 |
| *menaquinones (formerly $K_2$)* | |
| MK-2[b] | 15 |
| MK-3 | 40 |
| MK-4 | 100 |
| MK-5 | 120 |
| MK-6 | 100 |
| MK-7 | 70 |
| *forms of menadione (formerly $K_3$)* | |
| menadione | 40-150[c] |
| " sodium bisulfite complex | 50-150[c] |
| " dimethylpyrimidinol bisulfite | 100-160[c] |

[a]Relative biopotency is based on chick prothrombin/clotting time bioassays using phylloquinone (K-1) as the standard.
[b]For both the phylloquinones (K) and menaquinones (MK), the number of side-chain isoprenoid units (each containing five carbons) is indicated in parentheses.
[c]Activities of the menadiones tend to be variable, as they depend in part on the stabilities of the preparations and whether the vitamin K-antagonist sulfaquinoxaline was used in the assay diet.

## Vitamin C

Essential features of the chemical structure:

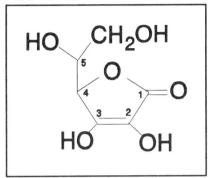

i.      6-carbon *lactone*
ii.     *2,3-endiol* structure

Chemical structure of vitamin C:

| | |
|---|---|
| ascorbic acid | |
| semidehydroascorbic acid | |
| dehydroascorbic acid | |

*vitamin C*      *"Vitamin C"* is the generic descriptor for all compounds exhibiting
*nomenclature*  qualitatively the biological activity of ascorbic acid.  The terms *"L-ascorbic acid"* and *"ascorbic acid"* are both trivial designators for the compound 2,3-didehydro-L-threo-hexano-1,4-lactone, which was formerly known as *"hexuronic acid"*.   The oxidized form of this compound is called *"L-dehydroascorbic acid"* or *"dehydroascorbic acid"*.

## Vitamin C

*vitamin C*
*chemistry*

Ascorbic acid is a dibasic acid (with $pK_a$s of 4.1 and 11.8), because both enolic hydroxyl groups can dissociate. It forms salts, the most important being with sodium and calcium; aqueous solutions of these are strongly basic. A strong reducing agent, ascorbic acid is oxidized under mild conditions to dehydroascorbic acid via the radical intermediate semi-dehydroascorbic acid (*"monodehydroascorbic acid"*). The semiquinoid ascorbic acid radical is a strong acid (pK = -.45); after the loss of a proton, it becomes a radical anion which, due to resonance stabilization, is relatively inert but disproportionates to ascorbic acid and dehydro-ascorbic acid. Thus, the three forms (ascorbic acid, semidehydroascorbic acid and dehydroascorbic acid) comprise a reversible redox system making the vitamin an effective quencher of free radicals such as singlet oxygen ($^1O_2$). It reduces ferric ($Fe^{+++}$) to ferrous ($Fe^{++}$) iron (and other metals analogously), and the superoxide radical ($O_2^{\cdot}$) to $H_2O_2$, being oxidized to monodehydroascorbic acid in the process. Ascorbic acid complexes with disulfides (e.g., oxidized glutathione, cystine), but does not reduce those disulfide bonds. Dehydroascorbic acid is not ionized near physiological pH; thus, it is relatively hydrophobic and is better able to penetrate membranes than ascorbic acid. In aqueous solution, dehydro-ascorbic acid is unstable and is degraded by hydrolytic ring opening to yield 2,3-dioxo-L-gulonic acid. Dehydroascorbic acid reacts with several amino acids to form brown-colored products, a reaction contributing to the spoilage of food. Some synthetic analogues of ascorbic acid have biological activity (e.g., 6-deoxy-L-ascorbic acid), while others (e.g., D-isoascorbic acid and L-glucoascorbic acid) have little or none. Several esters of ascorbic acid are converted to the vitamin *in vivo* and, thus, have good biological activity (e.g., ascorbyl-5,6-diacetate, ascorbyl-6-palmitate, 6-deoxy-6-chloro-L-ascorbic acid); esters of the C-2 position show variable vitamin C activity among different species.

Relative biopotency of vitamin C-active substances:

| compound | relative biopotency |
|---|---|
| ascorbic acid | 100 |
| ascorbyl-5,6-diacetate | 100 |
| ascorbyl-6-palmitate | 100 |
| 6-deoxy-6-chloroascorbic acid | 70-98 |
| dehydroascorbic acid | 80 |
| 6-deoxyascorbic acid | 33 |
| ascorbic acid 2-sulfate | -,+[a] |
| isoascorbic acid | 5 |
| L-glucoascorbic acid | 3 |

[a]This form is active in fishes, whose intestinal sulfohydrase releases ascorbic acid; it is inactive in guinea pigs, rhesus monkeys and humans, which lack that enzyme.

## Thiamin

Essential features of the chemical structure:

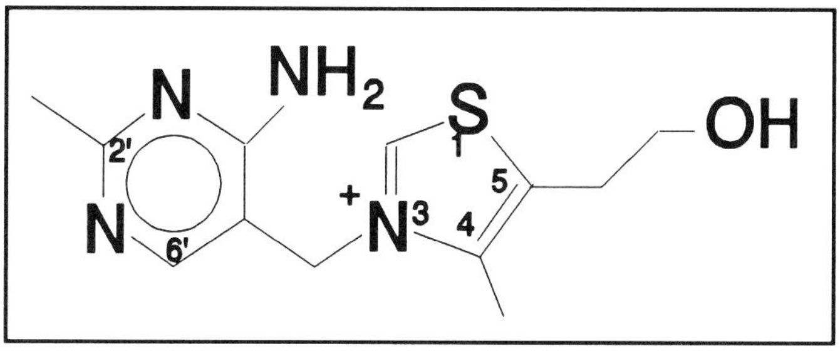

i.      conjoined *pyrimidine* and *thiazole* rings
ii.     thiazole ring contains a *quartenary nitrogen*, an *open carbon #2*, and a *phosphorylatable alkyl group* on carbon #5
iii.    *amino group* on carbon #4 of the pyrimidine ring

Chemical structure of thiamin and derivatives:

thiamin (free base)

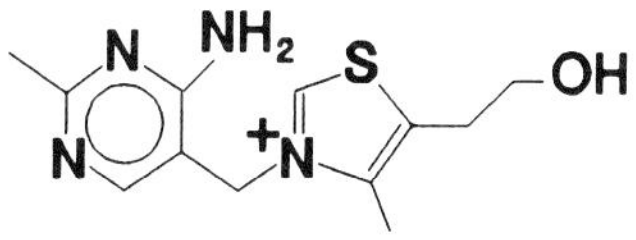

thiamin pyrophosphate

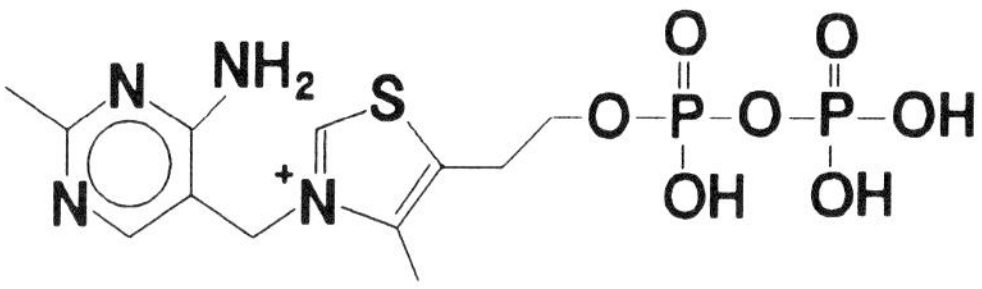

thiochrome

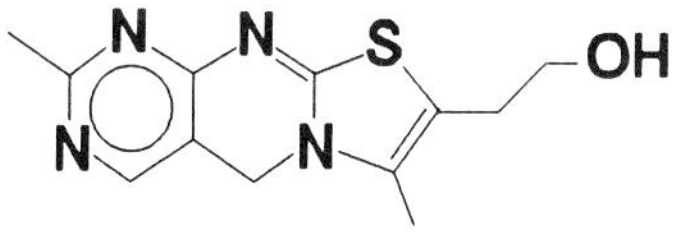

# Thiamin

thiamin
nomenclature

The term *thiamin* is the trivial designation of the compound 3-(4-amino-2-methylpyrimidin-5-ylmethyl)-4-methyl-5-(2-hydroxyethyl)-thiazolium, which was known formerly as *"vitamin B₁"*, *"aneurin"* and *"thiamine"*.

thiamin
chemistry

Free thiamin is unstable because of its quartenary N; in water it is cleaved to the thiol form. For this reason the hydrochloride and mononitrate forms are used in commerce. Thiamin hydrochloride (actually, thiamin chloride hydrochloride) is a colorless crystal which is very soluble in water[7] (thus, making it a very suitable form for parenteral administration), soluble in methanol and glycerol, but practically insoluble in acetone, ether, chloroform or benzene. The protonated salt has two positive charges: one associated with the pyrimidine ring and one associated with the thiazole ring. The mononitrate form is more stable than the hydrochloride, but it is less soluble in water[8]. It is used in food/feed supplementation and in dry pharmaceutical preparations.

Free thiamin is easily oxidized to thiamin disulfide and other derivatives including thiochrome, a yellow biologically inactive product with strong blue fluorescence that can be used for the quantitative determination of thiamin. The thiazole hydroxyethyl group can be phosphorylated *in vivo* to form thiamin mono-, di- and tri-phosphates. Thiamin diphosphate, also called *"**thiamin pyrophosphate**"*, is the metabolically active form sometimes referred to as *"co-carboxylase"*. Thiamin antagonists of experimental significance include pyrithiamin (the analog consisting of a pyridine moiety replacing the thiazole ring) and oxythiamin (the analog consisting of an hydroxyl group replacing the C-4 amino group on the pyrimidine ring).

---

[7]ca. 1 g per ml

[8]27 mg per ml

## Riboflavin

Essential features of the chemical structure:

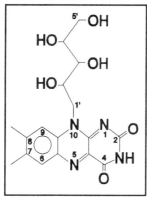

i.      substituted *isoalloxazine ring*
ii.     *D-ribityl side-chain*
iii.    *reducable ring nitrogen atoms*

Chemical structure of riboflavin:

riboflavin (interconversion of oxidized, radical anion and reduced forms)

flavin mononucleotide (FMN)

flavin adenine dinucleotide (FAD)

# Riboflavin

*riboflavin nomenclature*

Riboflavin is the trivial designation of the compound 7,8-dimethyl-10-(1'-D-ribityl)isoalloxazine, formerly known as vitamin $B_2$, vitamin G, lactoflavin or riboflavine. The metabolically active forms are commonly called flavin mononucleotide (FMN) and flavin adenine dinucleotide (FAD). Despite their acceptance, each is a misnomer as FMN is not a nucleotide and FAD is not a dinucleotide. More properly, these compounds should be called riboflavin monophosphate and riboflavin adenine diphosphate, respectively.

*riboflavin chemistry*

Riboflavin is a yellow tricyclic molecule that is usually phosphorylated (to FMN) and subsequently adenylated (to FAD) in biological systems. In FAD, the isoalloxazine and adenine ring systems are arranged one above the other and are nearly co-planar. The flavins are light-sensitive, undergoing photochemical degradation of the ribityl side-chain resulting in the formation of such breakdown products as lumiflavin and lumichrome. Therefore, the handling of riboflavin must be done in the dark or under subdued red light.

Riboflavin is moderately soluble in water (10-13 mg/dl) and ethanol, but insoluble in ether, chloroform or acetone. It is soluble but unstable under alkaline conditions. Because riboflavin cannot be extracted with the usual organic solvents, it is extracted with chloroform as lumiflavin after photochemical cleavage of the ribityl side-chain. Flavins show two absorption bands at ca. 370 nm and ca. 450 nm. This chromophore produces fluorescence with an emission maximum at ca. 520 nm.

The catalytic functions of riboflavin are carried out primarily at positions N-1, N-5 and C-4 of the isoalloxazine ring. In addition, the methyl group at C-8 participates in covalent bonding with enzyme proteins. The flavin coenzymes are highly versatile redox cofactors because they can participate in either one- or two-electron redox reactions, thus, serving as switching sites between obligate two-electron donors (e.g., NADH, succinate) and obligate one-electron acceptors (e.g., iron-sulfur proteins, heme proteins). They serve this function by undergoing reduction through a two-step sequence involving a radical anion intermediate. Because the latter can also react with molecular oxygen, flavins can also serve as cofactors in the two-electron reduction of $O_2$ to $H_2O$, and in the reductive four-electron activation and cleavage of $O_2$ in the monooxygenase reactions. In these redox reactions, riboflavin undergoes changes in its molecular shape, i.e., from a planar oxidized form to a folded reduced form. Differences in the affinities of the associated apoprotein for each shape affect the redox potential of the bound flavin. Riboflavin antagonists include analogues of the isoalloxazine ring (e.g., diethylriboflavin, dichloro-riboflavin) and the ribityl side-chain (e.g., D-araboflavin, D-galactoflavin).

## Niacin

Essential features of the chemical structure:

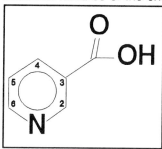

i.      **pyridine ring** substituted with a β-carboxylic acid or a corresponding amide
ii.     pyridine-N undergoes **reversible oxidation/reduction** (i.e., quartenary pyridinium ion to/from tertiary amine)
iii.    open sites at pyridine carbons #2-6

Chemical structure of niacin:

nicotinic acid

nicotinamide

nicotinamide adenine dinucleotide (NAD$^+$) *and*
nicotinamide adenine dinucleotide phosphate (NADP$^+$)

*NADH:* R=H   *NADPH:* R=PO$_3$H$_2$

## Niacin

*niacin*
*nomenclature*

Niacin is the generic descriptor for pyridine 3-carboxylic acid and derivatives exhibiting qualitatively the biological activity of nicotinamide[9].

*niacin*
*chemistry*

Nicotinic acid and nicotinamide are colorless crystalline substances. Each
is insoluble or only sparingly soluble in organic solvents. Nicotinic acid is
slightly soluble in water and ethanol; nicotinamide is very soluble in water
and moderately soluble in ethanol. The two compounds have similar
absorption spectra in water, with an absorption maximum at ca. 262 nm.

Nicotinic acid is amphoteric and forms salts with acids as well as bases.
Its carboxyl group can form esters and anhydrides and can be reduced.
Both nicotinic acid and nicotinamide are very stable in dry form, but in
solution nicotinamide is hydrolyzed by acids and bases to yield nicotinic
acid.

The coenzyme forms of niacin are the pyridine nucleotides, NAD and
NADP. In each of these compounds, the electron-withdrawing effect of the
N-1 and the amide group of the oxidized pyridine ring enables the pyridine
C-4 to react with many nucleophilic agents (e.g., sulfite, cyanide and
hydride ions). It is the reaction with hydride ions (H⁻) that is the basis of
the enzymatic hydrogen transfer by the pyridine nucleotides; the reaction
involves the transfer of two electrons in a single step[10]. The hydride
transfer of non-enzymatic reactions of the pyridine nucleotides are not
usually very stereospecific, though a secondary effect may be caused by
weak and reversible association between the adenine and pyridine rings.
In contrast, enzyme-catalyzed reactions are stereospecific for both
substrate and coenzyme, involving the binding of the latter in relatively
open (extended) conformation.

Several substituted pyridines are antagonist of niacin in biological systems:
pyridine-3-sulfonic acid, 3-acetylpyridine, isonicotinic acid hydrazide[11] and
6-aminonicotinamide.

---

[9]This compound is sometimes referred to as *"niacinamide"* which, because its use would suggest that
nicotinic acid should be called *"niacin"*, invites confusion and is not recommended.

[10]It has been argued that the enzyme-catalyzed oxidation of NADH occurs in two steps with the intermediate
formation of the NAD⁻ radical. Such a radical has been demonstrated, but is spontaneously dimerizes to an
enzymatically inactive form $(NAD)_2$, thus making it unlikely that such a mechanism plays a significant role in the
redox functions of the pyridine nucleotides.

[11]Also called *"isoniazid"*, this compound (4-pyridinecarboxylic acid hydrazide) is used as an antituberculous
and anti-actinomycotic agent.

## Vitamin $B_6$

Essential features of the chemical structure:

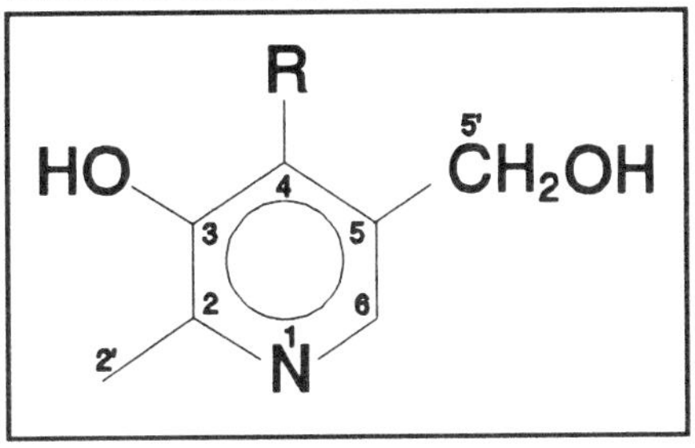

i.      a *pyridine* derivative[12]
ii.     phosphorylatable *5-hydroxymethyl group*
iii.    substituent at carbon #4 must be convertible metabolically to an *aldehyde*

Chemical structures of vitamin $B_6$ and metabolites:

general structure
R = $CH_2OH$    pyridoxine
  = CHO           pyridoxal
  = COOH          pyridoxic acid
  = $CH_2NH_2$    pyridoxamine

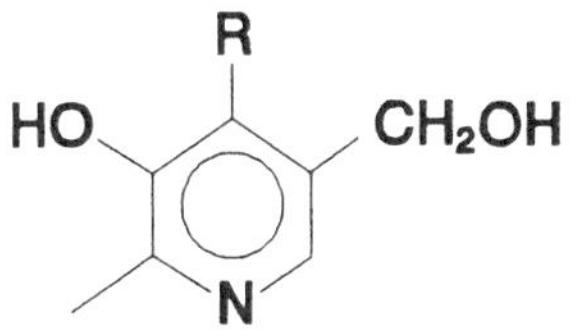

pyridoxal 5'-phosphate

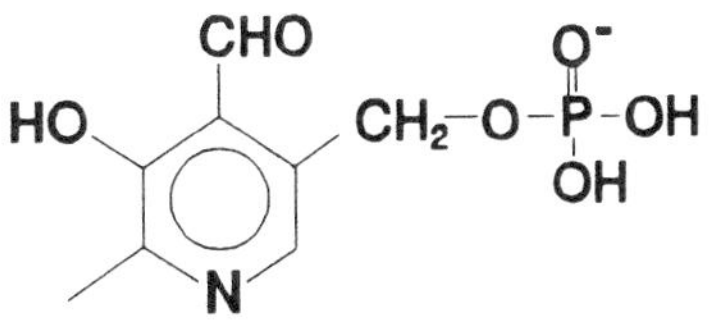

pyridoxamine 5'-phosphate

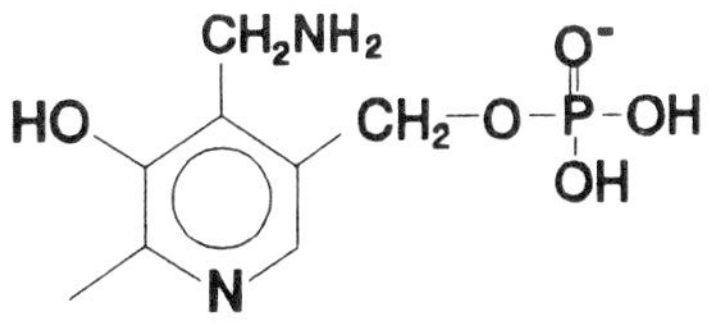

[12]More appropriately, derivatives of 2-methyl-3-hydroxy-pyridine.

## Vitamin $B_6$

| | |
|---|---|
| *vitamin $B_6$* *nomenclature* | Vitamin $B_6$ is the generic descriptor for all 2-methyl-3,5-dihydroxy-methylpyridine derivatives exhibiting the biological activity of pyridoxine in rats. The term *"pyridoxine"* is the trivial designation of one vitamin $B_6$-active compound, 2-methyl-3-hydroxy-4,5-*bis*(hydroxymethyl)-pyridine, which was formerly called *"adermin"* or *"pyridoxol"*. The biologically active analogues of pyridoxine are the aldehyde *"pyridoxal"* and the amine *"pyridoxamine"*. |
| *vitamin $B_6$* *chemistry* | The vitamers $B_6$ are colorless crystals at room temperature. Each is very soluble in water, weakly soluble in ethanol, and either insoluble or sparingly soluble in chloroform. Each is fairly stable in dry form and in solution. |
| | Pyridoxine is converted *in vitro* under mild oxidizing conditions to the aldehyde form, pyridoxal. *In vivo*, such a direct oxidation is not significant; instead, pyridoxine is first phosphorylated (by a kinase) to the 5'-phosphate, which is then oxidized enzymically to yield **pyridoxal 5'-phosphate**[13]. The prominent feature of the chemical reactivity of pyridoxal phosphate is the ability of its aldehyde group to react with primary amino groups (e.g., of amino acids) to form Schiff bases[14]. The electron-withdrawing effect of the resulting Schiff base labilizes the other bonds on the bound carbon, thus, serving as the basis of the catalytic roles of enzyme-bound pyridoxal phosphate. |

---

[13]Pyridoxamine is similarly phosphorylated *in vivo* to the 5'-phosphate, which functions interchangeably with pyrixodal phosphate in aminotransferases. Additionally, it is oxidized to pyridoxal phosphate.

[14]This reaction can occur with tris(hydroxymethyl)amino methane (i.e., Tris) and may, thus, affect results of biochemical studies of vitamin $B_6$ in which this common buffering agent is employed.

## Biotin

Essential features of the chemical structure:

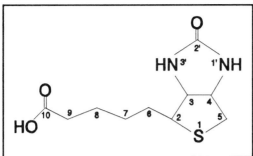

i.     conjoined *ureido* and *tetrahydrothiophene (thiophane) rings*
ii.    ureido 3'-N is *sterically hindered*, preventing substitution
iii.   ureido 1'-N is poorly nucleophilic

Chemical structure of biotin:

enzyme-bound biotin (i.e., *"biocytin"*)

| biotin nomenclature | Biotin is the trivial designation of the compound *cis*-hexahydro-2-oxo-1*H*-thieno[3,4-d]imidazole-4-pentanoic acid, formerly known as *"vitamin H"* or *"coenzyme R"*. |

| biotin chemistry | Biotin is a white crystalline substance that, in dry form, is fairly stable to air, heat and light. In solution, however, it is sensitive to degradation under strongly acidic or basic conditions. Its structure consists of a planar ureido ring and a folded thiophane ring which results in a boat configuration with a plane of symmetry passing through S-1, C-2' and O in such a way as to elevate the sulfur atom above the plane of the four carbons. The molecule has three asymmetric centers; however, of the eight possible stereoisomers, only the (+)-isomer (called *"d-biotin"*) has biological activity. Biotin is covalently bound to its enzymes by an amide bond to the ε-amino group of a lysine residue and C-2 of the thiophane nucleus. This bond is flexible, allowing the coenzyme to move between the active centers of some enzymes. The biotin molecule is activated by polarization of the O and N-1' of the ureido ring. This leads to increased nucleophilicity at N-1', which promotes the formation of a covalent bond between the electrophilic carbonyl phosphate formed from bicarbonate and ATP, and allows biotin to serve as a transport agent for $CO_2$. |

## Pantothenic Acid

Essential features of the chemical structure:

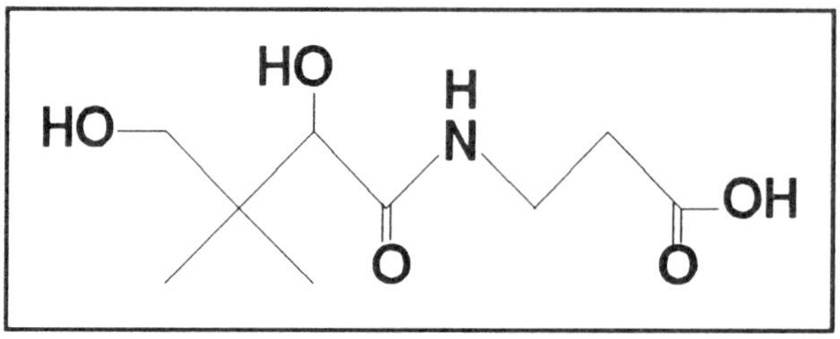

i.      formal derivative of **pantoic acid** and **alanine**
ii.     **optically active**


Chemical structure of pantothenic acid:

pantothenic acid

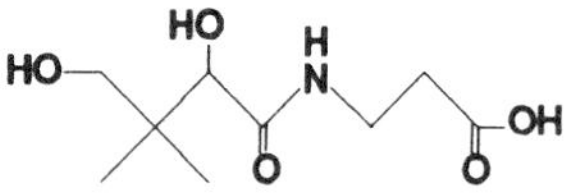

coenzyme A (showing its constituent parts)

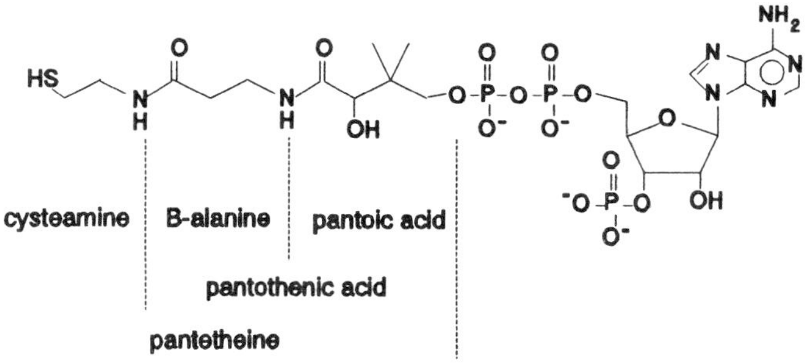

acyl-carrier protein

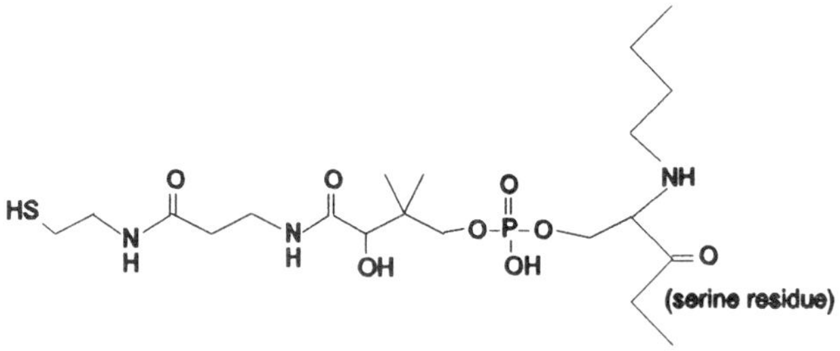

## Pantothenic Acid

*pantothenic*
*acid*
*nomenclature*

Pantothenic acid is the trivial designation for the compound dihydroxy-$\beta,\beta$-dimethylbutyryl-$\beta$-alanine, which was formerly known as "*pantoyl-$\beta$-alanine*". It has two metabolically active forms: **coenzyme A** in which the vitamin is linked *via* a phosphodiester group with adenosine-3',5'-diphosphate, and **acyl-carrier protein** in which it is linked *via* a phosphodiester to a serinyl residue of the protein.

*pantothenic*
*acid*
*chemistry*

Pantothenic acid is composed of $\beta$-alanine joined to 2,4-dihydroxy-3,3-di-methylbutyric acid *via* an amide linkage. The molecule has an asymmetric center, and only the R-enantiomer, usually called "*D(+)-pantothenic acid*" is biologically active and occurs naturally. Pantothenic acid is a yellow, viscous oil. Its calcium and other salts, however, are colorless crystalline substances; calcium pantothenate is the main product of commerce. Neither form is soluble in organic solvents, but each is soluble in water and ethanol. Aqueous solutions of pantothenic acid are unstable to heating under acidic or alkaline conditions, resulting in the hydrolytic cleavage of the molecule (to yield $\beta$-alanine and 2,4-dihydroxy-3,3-dimethylbutyrate)[13]. The analogue *panthenol* (in which the carboxyl group is replaced by an hydroxymethyl group) is fairly stable in solution. In dry form, the salts are stable to air and light; but they, particularly sodium pantothenate, are hygroscopic.

---

[13]This reaction is often used in the chemical determination of pantothenic acid by quantifying colorimetrically the $\beta$-alanine released upon alkaline hydrolysis using reagents such as 1,2-naphthoquinone 4-sulfonic acid or ninhydrin.

## Folate

Essential features of the chemical structure:

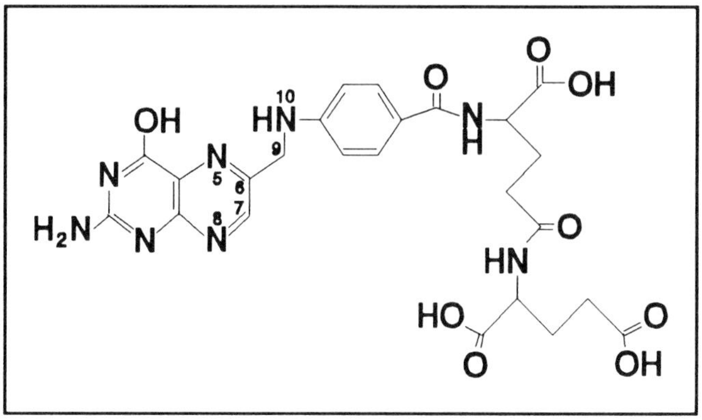

i.      **pteridine** derivative
ii.     **variable degree of hydrogenation** of pteridine ring
iii.    **single carbon units can bind** at #5 and/or #10 nitrogens
iv.     one or more **glutamyl residues** linked via peptide bonds

Chemical structures of the folate group:

pteroylglutamic acid

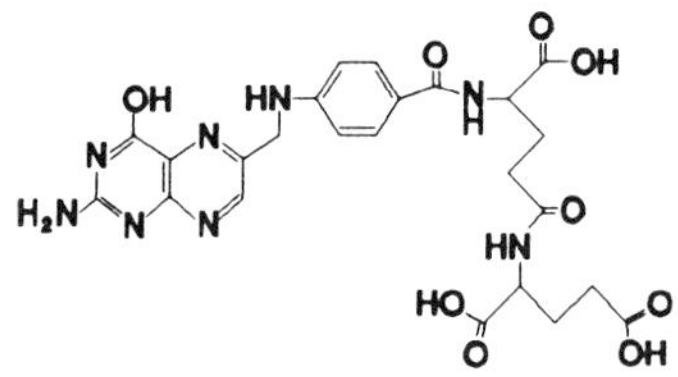

tetrahydrofolic acid and its derivatives

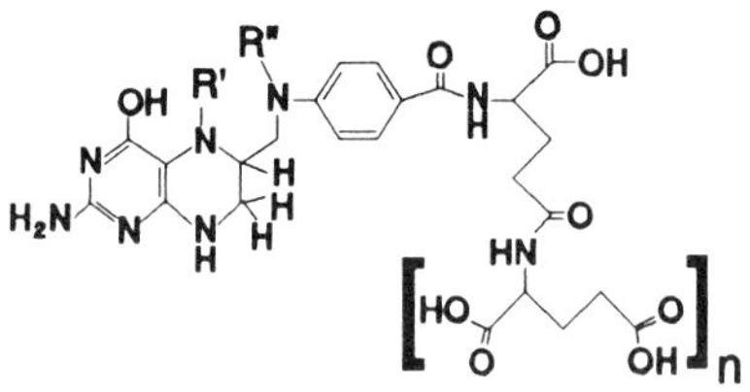

| vitamer | abbreviation | R'(#5-N) | R" (#10-N) |
|---|---|---|---|
| tetrahydrofolic acid | FH$_4$ | -H | -H |
| 5-methyl- " | 5-CH$_3$-FH$_4$ | -CH$_3$ | -H |
| 5,10-methenyl- " | 5,10-CH$^+$-FH$_4$ | -CH$^+$- | |
| 5,10-methylene- " | 5,10-CH$_2$=FH$_4$ | -CH$_2$= | |
| 5-formyl- " | 5-HCO-FH$_4$ | -HCO | -H |
| 10-formyl- " | 10-HCO-FH$_4$ | -H | -HCO |
| 5-forminin- " | 5-HCNH-FH$_4$ | -HCNH | -H |

# Folate

|  |  |
|---|---|
| *folate*<br>*nomenclature* | Folate is the generic descriptor for folic acid (pteroylmonoglutamic acid) and related compounds exhibiting the biological activity of folic acid. The plural terms *"folic acids"* and *"folates"* are used only as general terms for this group of heterocyclic compounds based on the N-[(6-pteridinyl)-methyl]-*p*-aminobenzoic acid skeleton conjugated with one or more L-glutamic acid residues. Folates can consist of a mono- or poly-glutamyl conjugate; these are named for the number of glutamyl residues (*n*) using such notations as PteGlu$_n$.[14] The reduced compound tetrahydropteroyl-glutamic acid is called *"tetrahydrofolic acid"*; its single-carbon derivatives are named according to the specific carbon moiety bound. |
| *folate*<br>*chemistry* | The folates include a large number of chemically related species each differing with respect to the variable substituents possible at three sites on the pteroylglutamic acid basic structure. Each is a formal derivative of pteridine[15]. With three known reduction states of the pyrazine ring, six different single carbon substituents on N-5 and/or N-10, and as many as eight glutamyl residues on the benzene ring, more than 170 different folates are theoretically possible[16]. Not all of these occur in nature; but it has been estimated that as many as 100 different forms are found in animals. The compound called *"folic acid"*, i.e., pteroylglutamic acid, is probably not present in living cells, being rather an artifact of isolation of the vitamin. The folates from most natural sources usually have a single carbon unit at N-5 and/or N-10; these forms participate in the metabolism of the *"single carbon pool"*. The single carbon units that may be transported and stored by folates can vary in oxidation state from the methyl (e.g., 5-CH$_3$-FH$_4$), to the formyl (e.g., 5-HCO-FH$_4$, 10-HCO-FH$_4$). Intracellular folates contain poly-$\gamma$-glutamyl chains usually of 2-8 glutamyl residues, which sometimes extend to 12 in bacteria. Tissues contain enzymes called *"conjugases"* that hydrolytically remove glutamyl residues to release the monoglutamyl form, i.e., folic acid. While the actual biochemical role of the polyglutamyl side-chain is not presently clear, it appears that the folylpolyglutamates are the actual coenzyme forms active intracellularly, and that the monoglutamates, which can pass through membranes, are transport forms. |

---

[14]Although they are still frequently used, the abbreviations using *PteGlu* to indicate pteroylglutamic acid are not suggested by current IUPAC-IUNS recommendations for vitamin nomenclature.

[15]More specifically, the folates are *pterins*, namely 2-amino-4-hydroxypteridies. The pteridines are yellow compounds first isolated from butterfly wings from which they were named (i.e., *"pteron"* is the Greek word meaning *"wing"*); many are folate antagonists.

[16]This estimate is low, as bacteria are known to have as many as 12 residues in their polyglutamyl chains.

## Folate

The folates have an asymmetric center at the #6-carbon. This introduces stereospecificity in the orientation of hydrogen atoms upon reduction of the pteridine system; that is, they add to carbons #6 and #7 in positions below the plane of the pyrazine ring. The UV absorption spectra of the folates is characterized by the independent contributions of the pterin and 4-aminobenzoyl moieties; most have absorption maxima in the region of 280-300 nm.

Folic acid (pteroylglutamic acid) is an orange-yellow crystalline substance that is soluble in water but insoluble in ethanol or less polar organic solvents. It is unstable to light, to acidic or alkaline conditions, to reducing agents and, except in dry form, to heat. It is reduced *in vivo* enzymatically (or *in vitro* with a reductant such as dithionite) first to 7,8-dihydrofolic acid ($FH_2$) and then to $FH_4$, which are each unstable in aerobic environments and must be protected by using an antioxidant (e.g., ascorbic acid, 2-mercaptoethanol).

Two derivatives of folic acid, each having an amino group in the place of the hydroxyl at C-4, are folate antagonists of biomedical use: **aminopterin** (4-aminofolic acid) and **methotrexate** (4-amino-$N^{10}$-methylfolic acid). Aminopterin is used as a rodenticide; methotrexate is an anti-neoplastic agent.

Essential features of the chemical structure:

| | |
|---|---|
| *i.* | Cobalt (Co)-centered **corrin ring** |
| *ii.* | Co $\alpha$-position (below the plane of the corrin ring as shown) may be open or occupied by a side-chain heterocyclic N, or solvent |
| *iii.* | Co $\beta$-position (above the plane of the corrin ring as shown) may be occupied by an hydroxo, aqua, methyl, 5-deoxyadenosyl, CN⁻, Cl⁻, Br⁻, nitro, sulfito or sulfato group.[17] |

Chemical structures of vitamin $B_{12}$:

5'-deoxyadenosylcobalamin                    cyanocobalamin

| | |
|---|---|
| *vitamin B₁₂* | Vitamin $B_{12}$ is the generic descriptor for all corrinoids (i.e., compounds |
| *nomenclature* | containing the corrin nucleus) exhibiting the qualitative biological activity of cyanocobalamin. **"Cyanocobalamin"** is the trivial designation of the vitamin $B_{12}$-active corrinoid with a cyano- ligand (CN⁻) at the $\beta$-position of the Co atom. The analogues containing methyl-, 5'-deoxyadenosyl-, |

[17] Only the first four liganded forms of vitamin $B_{12}$ are found in biological systems.

# Vitamin $B_{12}$

hydroxo- (OH⁻), nitrito- or aqua- ($H_2O$) groups at that position are called *"methylcobalamin"*, *"adenosylcobalamin"*, *"hydroxocobalamin"* (formerly "vitamin $B_{12b}$"), *"nitritocobalamin"* (formerly "vitamin $B_{12c}$") or *"aquacobalamin"* (formerly "vitamin $B_{12a}$"), respectively.

*vitamin $B_{12}$*
*chemistry*

Vitamin $B_{12}$ is an octahedral cobalt complex consisting of a porphyrin-like, Co-centered macro-ring (called a *"corrin ring"*), a nucleotide and a second Co-bound group (e.g., $CH_3$, $H_2O$, CN⁻). The corrin ring consists of four reduced pyrrole rings linked by three methylene bridges and one direct bond. The Co atom, which is triply ionized (i.e., $Co^{+++}$), can form up to 6 coordinate bonds, is tightly bound to the four pyrrole N atoms and can also bond a nucleotide and a small ligand below and above, respectively, the plane of the ring system. The Co atom is removed *in vitro* only with difficulty, resulting in loss of biological activity.

The corrinoids are red, red-orange or yellow crystalline substances that show intense absorption spectra above 300 nm due to the $\pi$-$\pi$ transitions of the corrin ring. They are soluble in water and are fairly stable to heat but decompose at temperatures above ca. 210°C without melting.

Vitamin $B_{12}$ reacts with ascorbic acid, which results in the reduction and subsequent degradation of the former which releases its Co atom as the free ion. Cobalamins with relatively strongly bound ligands (e.g., cyano-, methyl- and adenosylcobalamin) are less reactive and are, therefore, more stable in the presence of ascorbic acid. The cobalamins are unstable to light. Cyanocobalamin undergoes a photo-replacement of the CN⁻ ligand with water; the organocobalamins (methyl- and adenosylcobalamin) undergo photoreduction of the Co-C bond resulting in the loss of the ligand and the reduction of the corrin-Co.

## GENERAL PROPERTIES OF THE VITAMINS

*multiple forms* Few of the vitamins are active in biological systems without conversion to
*of the vitamins* another species and/or binding to a protein.  Thus, any consideration of
the vitamins in nutrition involves, for each vitamin group, a number of
vitamers and metabolites some of which are important in the practical
sense for food and diet supplementation, while others are important in the
physiological sense as they participate in metabolism.

The most important forms of the vitamins:

| vitamin | representative | metabolically active forms | important dietary forms |
|---|---|---|---|
| vitamin A | retinol | retinol<br>retinal<br>retinoic acid | retinyl palmitate and acetate, pro-vitamins<br>($\beta$-carotene, other carotenoids) |
| vitamin D | cholecalciferol | 25-OH-cholecalciferol<br>1,25-(OH)$_2$-cholecalciferol | cholecalciferol, ergocalciferol |
| vitamin E | $\alpha$-tocopherol | $\alpha$-, $\beta$-, $\gamma$- and $\delta$-<br>tocopherols | R,R,R-$\alpha$-tocopherol; all-*rac*-$\alpha$-tocopheryl<br>acetate |
| vitamin K | phylloquinone | phylloquinones (K)<br>menaquinones (MK) | K, MK, menadione, menadione Na-bisulfite<br>complex |
| vitamin C | ascorbic acid | ascorbic acid<br>dehydroascorbic acid | L-ascorbic acid, Na-ascorbate |
| thiamin | thiamin | thiamin pyrophosphate | thiamin;thiamin-pyrophosphate,-disulfide,<br>-HCl, -mononitrate |
| riboflavin | riboflavin | FMN, FAD | FMN, FAD, flavoproteins, riboflavin |
| niacin | nicotinamide | NAD, NADP | NAD, NADP, nicotinamide, nicotinic acid |
| vitamin B$_6$ | pyridoxine | pyridoxal 5'-phosphate<br>pyridoxamine 5'-phosphate | pyridoxal HCL, pyridoxal- and pyridoxamine-<br>5'-phosphates |
| biotin | d-biotin | *d*-biotin | biocytin, *d*-biotin |
| pantothenic<br>acid | pantothenic acid | coenzyme A | Ca-pantothenate, coenzyme A, acyl CoAs |
| folate | pteroylglutamic<br>acid | pteroylpolyglutamates | pteroyl poly- and mono-glutamates |
| vitamin B$_{12}$ | cyanocobalamin | methylcobalamin<br>5'-deoxyadenosylcobalamin | cyano-, aquo-, hydroxo-, methyl-, and<br>5'-deoxyadenosyl-cobalamins |

*vitamin*        For the use of vitamins as feed additives, in diet supplements, and as
*stability*      pharmaceuticals, stability is a prime concern.  In general, the fat-soluble
vitamins are poorly stable to oxidation.  They must be protected from heat,
oxygen, metal ions and UV light; antioxidants are frequently used in their
formulations.  For vitamins A and E, the more stable esterified forms are
used for these purposes.  Because of the instabilities of their naturally
occurring vitamers, the amounts of the fat-soluble vitamins in natural foods
and feedstuffs are highly variable, being greatly affected by the conditions
of food production and processing.  The water-soluble vitamins tend to be
more stable under most practical conditions, exceptions being riboflavin,
and vitamins B$_6$ and B$_{12}$ which are degraded by light, and thiamin which is
sensitive of mildly alkaline conditions.

Stabilities of the vitamins:

| vitamin | vitamer | UV light | heat[a] | O$_2$ | acid | base | metals[b] | most stable |
|---|---|---|---|---|---|---|---|---|
| vitamin A | retinol | + | | + | + | | + | dark, seal |
| | retinal | | | + | + | | + | seal |
| | retinoic acid | | | | | | | good stability |
| | dehydroret. | | | + | | | | seal |
| | ret. esters | | | | | | | good stability |
| | β-carotene | | | + | | | | seal |
| vitamin D | D$_2$ | + | + | + | + | | + | dark, cool, seal |
| | D$_3$ | + | + | + | + | | + | dark, cool, seal |
| vitamin E | tocopherols | | + | + | + | + | + | cool, neutral pH |
| | tocoph.esters | | | | + | + | | good stability |
| vitamin K | K | + | | + | | + | + | avoid reductants[c] |
| | MK | + | | + | | + | + | avoid reductants[c] |
| | menadione | + | | | | + | + | avoid reductants[c] |
| vitamin C | ascorbic acid | | | +[b] | | + | + | seal, neutral pH |
| thiamine | disulfide form | | + | + | + | + | + | neutral pH[c] |
| | hydrochloride[d] | | + | + | + | + | + | seal, neutral pH[c] |
| riboflavin | riboflav. | +[e] | + | | | + | + | dark, pH 1.5-4[c] |
| niacin | nicotinic acid | | | | | | | good stability |
| | nicotinamide | | | | | | | good stability |
| vit. B$_6$ | pyrid.-al | + | + | | | | | cool |
| | pyrid.-ol (HCl) | | | | | | | good stability |
| biotin | biotin | | | + | | + | | seal, neutral pH |
| pantoth. | free acid[f] | + | | + | | + | | cool, neutral pH |
| acid | Ca salt[d] | | | + | | | | seal, pH 6-7 |
| folate | FH$_4$ | + | + | + | +[g] | | + | good stability[c] |
| vit. B$_{12}$ | CN-B$_{12}$ | + | | | +[h] | | +[i] | good stability[c] |

[a]i.e., 100°C   [b]in solution with Fe$^{+++}$ and Cu$^{++}$   [c]unstable to reducing agents
[d]slightly hygroscopic   [e]especially in alkaline solution   [f]very hygroscopic   [g]pH<5
[h]pH<3   [i]pH>9

*vitamin analysis*

Several methods are available for the determination of the vitamins. In recent years, chromatographic separations of vitamins have proven useful for the analysis of vitamin supplements or other preparations in which the concentrations of the vitamins are of interest. Of these, high-performance liquid-liquid partition chromatographic (HPLC) techniques are most useful; they depend on the separation technique itself for specificity and a suitable means of detection (e.g., UV-Vis absorption, fluorescence, electrochemical) for sensitivity. Because such methods are not routinely available for all of the vitamins, other established techniques continue to be useful.

Methods of vitamin analysis:

| method | vitamins determined |
|---|---|
| HPLC[a] | fat-soluble vitamins (A, D, E, K), riboflavin, thiamin, pantothenic acid, niacin, folic acid, vitamin $B_6$, biotin |
| TLC[b] | fat-soluble vitamins, thiamin, riboflavin, vitamin $B_6$, biotin, vitamin C |
| mass spectroscopy | several vitamins |
| radioimmunoassay | folate, vitamin $B_{12}$ and vitamin D metabolites |
| chemical colorimetry | the fat-soluble vitamins |
| microbiological assay | thiamin, riboflavin, vitamin $B_6$, vitamin $B_{12}$, folate, pantothenic acid, biotin, niacin |

[a]high-performance liquid chromatography    [b]thin-layer chromatography

*physico-chemical properties determine vitamin utilization*

The ways in which the vitamins are utilized by and function in biological systems are determined by their chemical and associated physical properties.  In the cases of the isoprenoid-based fat-soluble vitamins, enteric absorption depends on micellar dispersion[18] in the aqueous environment of the intestinal lumen.  By this phenomenon, these and other hydrophobic substances can be delivered to the absorptive surfaces of the mucosal brush border for uptake by diffusion across the phospholipid membranes of enterocytes.

---

[18]Hydrophobic substances including the fat-soluble vitamins, cholesterol, carotenoids, etc., which are not soluble in the aqueous environment of the alimentary canal, are associated with and dissolved in other lipid materials.  In the upper portion of the gastro-intestinal tract, they are dissolved in the bulk lipid phases of the emulsions that are formed by the mechanical actions of mastication and gastric churning. Emulsion oil droplets, however, are generally too large (e.g., $10^3$ Å) to gain the intimate proximity to the absorptive surfaces of the small intestine that is necessary to facilitate the diffusion of these substances into the hydrophobic environment of the brush border membranes of intestinal mucosal cells.  However, lipase which is present in the intestinal lumen, having been synthesized in and exported from the pancreas via the pancreatic duct, binds to the surface of the emulsion oil droplet where it catalyzes the hydrolytic removal of the $a$- and $a'$-fatty acids from triglycerides which make up the bulk of the lipid material in these large particles. The products of this process (i.e., free fatty acids and $\beta$-monoglycerides) have strong polar regions or charged groups and, thus, will dissolve to some extent monomerically in this aqueous environment. However, they also have long-chain hydrocarbon non-polar regions; therefore, when certain concentrations (*'critical micellar concentrations'*) are achieved, these species and bile salts, which have similar properties, combine spontaneously to form small particles called *'mixed micelles'*. Mixed micelles thus contain free fatty acids, $\beta$-monoglycerides and bile salts in which the non-polar regions of each are associated interiorly and the polar or charged regions of each are oriented externally and are associated with the aqueous phase.  The core of the mixed micelle is hydrophobic and, thus, serves to solubilize the fat-soluble vitamins and other non-polar lipid substances.  Because they are small (10-50 Å in diameter), mixed micelles can gain close proximity to microvillar surfaces of intestinal mucosa, thus, facilitating the diffusion of their contents into and across those membranes. Because the enteric absorption of the fat-soluble vitamins depends on micellar dispersion, it is impaired under conditions of lipid malabsorption.

Enteric absorption of the vitamins:

| vitamer | digestion | site[a] | enterocytic metabolism | efficiency % | conditions of potential malabsorption |
|---|---|---|---|---|---|
| **Micelle-Dependent Diffusion** | | | | | |
| retinol | - | D,J | esterification | 80-90 | pancreatic insufficiency (pancreatitis, |
| retinyl esters | de-esterified | D,J | re-esterification | | Se-deficiency, cystic fibrosis, cancer) |
| β-carotene | cleavage | D,J | esterification | 50-60 | biliary atresia, obstructive jaundice, |
| celiac disease, very low fat diet | | | | | |
| vitamins D | - | D,J | - | ~50 | pancreatic or biliary insufficiency |
| tocopherols | - | D,J | - | 20-80 | "          "          " |
| tocoph. esters | de-esterified[b] | D,J | - | 20-80 | "          "          " |
| MK's | - | D,J | - | 10-70 | "          "          " |
| menadione | - | D,J | - | 10-70 | "          "          " |
| **Active Transport** | | | | | |
| phylloquinone | - | D,J | - | ~80 | pancreatic or biliary insufficiency |
| ascorbic acid | - | I | - | 70-80 | D-isoascorbic acid |
| thiamin | - | D | phosphorylation | | pyrithiamin, excess ethanol |
| thiamin di-P | de-phosphor.[b] | D | " | | "          " |
| riboflavin | - | J | " | | |
| FMN, FAD | hydrolysis[b] | J | " | | |
| flavoproteins | hydrolysis[b] | J | " | | |
| folylmono-glu | - | J | glutamation | | celiac sprue |
| folylpoly-glu | hydrolysis[b] | J | " | | celiac sprue |
| vitamin $B_{12}$ | hydrolysis[b] | I | adenosinylation, methylation | >90 | intrinsic factor deficiency (pernicious anemia) |
| **Facilitated Diffusion[c]** | | | | | |
| nicotinic acid | - | J | | >90[d] | |
| nicotinamide | - | J | | ~100[d] | |
| niacytin | hydrolysis[b] | J | | | |
| NAD(P) | hydrolysis[b] | J | | | |
| biotin | - | J | | | biotinidase deficiency, avidin |
| biocytin | hydrolysis[b] | J | | | "          " |
| pantothenate | - | | | | |
| coenzyme A | hydrolysis[b] | | | | |
| **Simple Diffusion** | | | | | |
| ascorbic acid[e] | - | D,J,I | - | <50 | |
| thiamin[e,f] | - | J | phosphorylation | | |
| nicotinic acid | - | J | - | | |
| nicotinamide | - | J | - | | |
| pyridoxol | - | J | phosphorylation | | |
| pyridoxal | - | J | " | | |
| pyridoxamine | - | J | " | | |
| biotin | - | D,J | - | >95 | raw egg white (avidin) |
| pantothenate | - | | - | | |
| folylmono-glu[e] | - | J | glutamation | | |
| vitamin $B_{12}$[e] | - | D,J | adenosination, methylation | ~1 | |

[a]Duodenum, **J**ejunum or **I**leum   [b]yields vitamin in absorbable form   [c]Na$^+$-dependent saturable processes
[d]estimate may include contribution of simple diffusion   [e]simple diffusion important only at high doses
[f]symport with Na$^+$

Other vitamins that are soluble in the intestinal lumen can be taken up by the absorptive surface of the gut more directly. Some, therefore, are absorbed as the result of diffusion; whereas others are absorbed *via* specific carriers as means of overcoming concentration gradients not favorable to simple diffusion. Some water-soluble vitamins (e.g., vitamin C, vitamin $B_{12}$, thiamin, folate) are absorbed *via* carrier-dependent mechanisms at low doses, and by simple diffusion (albeit at lower efficiency) at high doses.

*vitamin transport*

Similarly, the mechanisms of post-absorptive transport of the vitamins vary according to their particular physical and chemical properties. Again, therefore, the problem of solubility in the aqueous environments of the blood plasma and lymph is a major determinant of ways in which the vitamins are transported from the site of absorption (the small intestine) to the liver and peripheral organs. The fat-soluble vitamins, because they are insoluble in these transport environments, depend on carriers that are soluble there. These vitamins, therefore, are associated with the lipid-rich **chylomicrons**[19] that are elaborated in intestinal mucosal cells largely of re-esterified triglycerides from free fatty acids and $\beta$-monoglycerides that have just been absorbed. As the lipids in these particles are transferred to other **lipoproteins**[20] in the liver, some of the fat-soluble vitamins (vitamins E and K) are also transferred to those carriers. Others (vitamins A and D) are transported from the liver to peripheral tissues by specific carriers of hepatic origin. Some of the water-soluble vitamins are transported by protein carriers in the plasma and, therefore, are not found free in solution. Some (riboflavin, vitamin $B_6$) are carried *via* weak, non-specific binding to albumin and may, thus, be displaced by other substances (e.g., ethanol) that also bind to that protein. Others are tightly associated with certain immunoglobulins (riboflavin) or bind to specific proteins involved in their transport (riboflavin, vitamins A, D, E and $B_{12}$). Several vitamins (e.g., vitamin C, thiamin, niacin, riboflavin, pantothenic acid, biotin, folate) are transported in free solution in the plasma.

---

[19]Chylomicrons are the largest (ca. 1 $\mu$ in diameter) and the lightest of the blood lipids. They consist mainly of triglyceride with smaller amounts of cholesterol, phospholipid, protein and the fat-soluble vitamins. They are normally synthesized in the intestinal mucosal cell and serve to transport lipids to tissues. In mammals, these particles are secreted into the lymphatic drainage of the small intestine (hence, their name). However, in birds, fishes and reptiles, they are secreted directly into the renal portal circulation; therefore, in these species they are referred to as *"portomicrons"*. In either case, they are cleared from the plasma by the liver and their lipid contents are either deposited in hepatic stores (e.g., vitamin A) or are released back into the plasma bound to more dense particles called *"lipoproteins"*.

[20]As the name would imply, a lipoprotein is a lipid-protein combination with the solubility characteristics of a protein (i.e., soluble in the aqueous environment of the blood plasma) and, hence, involved in lipid transport. Four classes of lipoproteins, each defined empirically on the basis of density, are found in the plasma: chylomicrons/portomicrons, *high density lipoproteins* (**HDL**), *low density lipoproteins* (**LDL**) and *very low density lipoproteins* (**VLDL**). The latter three classes are also known by names derived from the method of electrophoretic separation, i.e., $\alpha$-, $\beta$- and pre-$\beta$-lipoproteins, respectively.

Post-absorptive transport of the vitamins in the body:

| vehicle | vitamin | form transported | distribution |
|---|---|---|---|
| **Lipoprotein-Bound** | | | |
| chylomicrons[e] | vitamin A | retinyl esters | lymph[e] |
| " | | β-carotene | " |
| | vitamin D | vitamin D[b] | " |
| | vitamin E | tocopherols | " |
| | vitamin K | K, MK, menadione | " |
| VLDL[c]/HDL[d] | vitamin E | tocopherols | plasma |
| | vitamin K | mainly MK-4 | " |
| **Associated Non-Specifically with Proteins** | | | |
| albumin | riboflavin | free riboflavin | plasma |
| | | flavin mononucleotide | " |
| | vitamin B$_6$ | pyridoxal | " |
| | | pyridoxal phosphate | " |
| immunoglobulins[e] | riboflavin | free riboflvin | " |
| **Bound to Specific Binding Proteins** | | | |
| retinol BP (RBP) | vitamin A | retinol | plasma |
| cellular RBP (CRBP) | " | " | intracellular |
| cellular RBP, type II (CRBPII) | " | " | enterocytic |
| interstitial RBP (IRBP) | " | " | interstitial spaces |
| cellular retinal BP (CRALBP) | " | retinal | intracellular |
| cellular retinoic acid (CRABP) | " | retinoic acid | " |
| transcalciferin | vitamin D | D$_2$; D$_3$; 25-OH-D; 1,25-(OH)$_2$-D; 24,25-(OH)$_2$-D | plasma |
| vitamin D receptor | vitamin D | 1,25-(OH)$_2$-D | enterocyte |
| vitamin E BP | vitamin E | tocopherols | intracellular |
| riboflavin BP | riboflavin | riboflavin | plasma |
| flavoproteins | " | flavin mononucleotide | intracellular |
| | " | flavin adenine dinucleotide | " |
| transcobalamin I | vitamin B$_{12}$ | vitamin B$_{12}$ | " |
| transcobalamin II | " | methylcobalamin | plasma |
| transcobalamin III | " | vitamin B$_{12}$ | " |
| **Erythrocyte-Carried** | | | |
| erythrocyte membranes | vitamin E | tocopherols | blood |
| erythrocytes | vitamin B$_6$ | pyridoxal phosphate | " |
| erythrocytes | pantothenic acid | coenzyme A | " |
| **Free in Plasma** | | | |
| - | vitamin C | ascorbic acid | plasma |
| - | thiamin | free thiamin | " |
| " | " | thiamin pyrophosphate | " |
| - | riboflavin | flavin mononucleotide | " |
| - | pantothenic acid | pantothenic acid | " |
| - | biotin | free biotin | " |
| - | niacin | nicotinic acid | " |
| " | " | nicotinamide | " |
| - | folate | pteroylmonoglutamates[f] | " |

[e]In mammals, lipids are absorbed into the lymphatic circulation where they are transported to the liver and other tissues as large lipoprotein particles called *"chylomicra"* (*"chylomicron"*, s.); in birds, reptiles and fishes lipids are absorbed directly into the hepatic portal circulation and the analogous lipoprotein particle is called a *"portomicron"*.  [b]Representation of vitamin D without a subscript is meant to refer to both major forms of the vitamin: ergocalciferol (D$_2$) and cholecalciferol (D$_3$).  [c]i.e., **Very Low Density Lipoproteins**  [d]i.e., **High Density Lipoproteins**  [e]e.g., IgG, IgM and IgA  [f]especially 5-CH$_3$-tetrahydrofolic acid

*tissue distribution of the vitamins*

The retention and distribution of the vitamins among the various tissues varies also according to their general physical and chemical properties. In general, the fat-soluble vitamins are well retained; they tend to be stored in association with tissue lipids. For that reason, such lipid-rich tissues as adipose and liver, frequently have appreciable stores of the fat-soluble vitamins. Storage of these vitamins means that animals may be able to accommodate widely variable intakes without consequence by mobilizing their tissue stores in times of low dietary intakes.

In contrast, the water-soluble vitamins tend to be excreted rapidly and not retained well. Few of this group of vitamins are stored to any appreciable extent. The notable exception is vitamin $B_{12}$ which, under normal circumstances, can accumulate in the liver in amounts adequate to satisfy the nutritional needs of the host for periods of years.

Tissue distribution of the vitamins:

| vitamin | predominant storage form(s) | depot(s) |
|---|---|---|
| vitamin A | retinyl esters (e.g., palmitate) | liver |
| vitamin D | $D_3$; 25-OH-D | plasma, adipose, muscle |
| vitamin E | $\alpha$-tocopherol | adipose, adrenal, testes, platelets, other tissues |
| vitamin K[a] | K: K-4,K-4 | liver |
| | MK: MK-4 | all tissues |
| | menadione: MK-4 | all tissues |
| vitamin C | ascorbic acid | adrenals, leucocytes |
| thiamin | thiamin pyrophosphate[b] | heart, kidney, brain, muscle |
| riboflavin | flavin adenine dinucleotide[b] | liver, kidney, heart |
| vitamin $B_6$ | pyridoxal phosphate[b] | liver[c], kidney[c], heart[c] |
| vitamin $B_{12}$ | methylcobalamin | liver[d], kidney[c], heart[c], spleen[c], brain[c] |
| niacin | no appreciable storage | - |
| biotin | no appreciable storage[b] | - |
| pantothenic acid | no appreciable storage | - |
| folate | no appreciable storage | - |

[a]The predominant form of the vitamin is shown for each major form of dietary vitamin K consumed. [b]The amounts in the body are comprised of the enzyme-bound coenzyme. [c]Small amounts of the vitamin are found in these tissues. [d]Predominant depot.

## *METABOLISM OF THE VITAMINS*

*some vitamins have limited biosynthesis*

By definition, the vitamins as a group of nutrients are obligate factors in the diet (i.e., the chemical environment) of an organism. Nevertheless, some vitamins do not quite fit that general definition by being synthesized by certain species regularly or in many species in certain circumstances (see discussion in Chapter 1). The biosynthesis of those vitamins for which this occurs, thus depends on the availability, either from dietary or metabolic sources of appropriate precursors (e.g., adequate free tryptophan for niacin production; presence of 7-dehydrocholesterol in the surface layers of the skin for its conversion to vitamin $D_3$), as well as the presence of the appropriate metabolic and/or chemical catalytic activities (e.g., the several enzymes involved in the tryptophan-niacin conversion; exposure to UV light for the photolysis of 7-dehydrocholesterol to produce vitamin $D_3$; the several enzymes of the gulonic acid pathway including L-gulonolactone oxidase for the formation of ascorbic acid).

Vitamins that can be biosynthesized:

| vitamin | precursor | route | limitation | bases of dietary needs |
|---|---|---|---|---|
| niacin | tryptophan | conversion to NMN *via* picco-linic acid | 3-OH-anthranilic acid oxidase | high piccolinic acid carboxylase activity low dietary TRY high dietary LEU[a] |
| vitamin $D_3$ | 7-dehydro-cholesterol | UV-photolysis | photolysis | insufficient UV |
| vitamin C | glucose | gulonic acid pathway | L-gulonolactone oxidase | L-gulonolactone oxidase deficiency |

[a]The role of leucine as an effector of the conversion of tryptophan to niacin is controversial (*see* Chapter 12). [b]*via* S-adenosylmethionine.

Vitamins that are direct-acting:

vitamin E
vitamin C
vitamin K[a]

[a]Some forms of vitamin K (e.g., MK-4) are metabolically active *per se*; although most other forms undergo some dealkylation/realkylation in order to be converted to metabolically active vitamers.

*most vitamins must be metabolized*

Whereas a few of the vitamins function in biological systems without some sort of metabolic activation or linkage to a co-functional species (e.g., an enzyme), most require such metabolic conversions.

*vitamin*
*activation*

The metabolic transformation of dietary forms of the vitamins into the forms that are active in metabolism may involve substantive modification of a vitamin's chemical structure and/or its combination with another metabolically important species. Thus, some vitamins are *"activated"* to their functional species; factors that may affect their metabolic (i.e., enzymatic) activation can have profound influences on their nutritional efficacy.

Vitamins that must be activated metabolically:

| vitamin | active form(s) | activation step | conditions increasing need |
|---|---|---|---|
| vitamin A | retinol | retinal reductase | protein insufficiency |
| | | retinol hydrolase | |
| | 11-cis-retinol | retinyl isomerase | |
| | 11-cis-retinal | alcohol dehydrogenase | Zn insufficiency |
| vitamin D | $1,25\text{-}(OH)_2\text{-}D$ | vit. D 25-hydroxylase | hepatic failure |
| | | 25-OH-D 1-hydroxylase | renal failure |
| | | | Pb exposure |
| | | | estrogen deficiency |
| | | | anti-convulsant drugs |
| vitamin K | all forms | dealkylation of K's, MK's | hepatic failure |
| | | alkylation of K's, MK's, | |
| | | menadione | |
| thiamin | thiamin-diP[a] | phosphorylation | high carbohydrate intake |
| riboflavin | FMN, FAD | phosphorylation | |
| | | adenosylation | |
| vitamin $B_6$ | pyridoxal-P | phosphorylation | high protein intake |
| | | oxidation | |
| niacin | NAD(H) | amidation (nicotinic ac.) | low tryptophan intake |
| | NADP(H) | | |
| pantothenic acid | coenzyme A | phosphorylations, decarboxyl- | |
| | | lation, ATP-condensation, | |
| | | peptide bond formation | |
| | ATP | phosphorylation, peptide | |
| | | bond formation | |
| folate | $C_1\text{-}FH_4$[b] | reduction; addition of $C_1$ | |
| vitamin $B_{12}$ | methyl-$B_{12}$ | cobalamin methylation | folate deficiency |
| | | | $CH_3$-group insufficiency |
| | 5'-deoxy- | adenosylation | |
| | adenosyl-$B_{12}$ | | |

[a]i.e., thiamin pyrophosphate.     [b]i.e., tetrahydrofolic acid.

*vitamin binding*
*to proteins*

Some vitamins, even some requiring metabolic activation, are biologically active only when bound to a protein. In most cases, this happens when the vitamin serves as the prosthetic group of an enzyme, remaining bound to the enzyme protein during catalysis[21].

---

[21]Vitamins of this type are properly called *"co-enzymes"*; those that participate in enzymatic catalysis but are not firmly bound to enzyme protein during the reaction are, more properly, *"co-substrates"*. This distinction, however, does not address mechanism, but only tightness of binding. For example, the associations of NAD and NADP with certain oxidoreductases are weaker than those of FMN and FAD with the flavoprotein oxidoreductases. Therefore, the term *"co-enzyme"* has come to be used to describe enzyme cofactors of both types.

Vitamins that must be linked to enzymes and other proteins:

| vitamin | form(s) linked |
|---|---|
| biotin | biotin |
| vitamin $B_{12}$ | methylcobalamin, adenosylcobalamin |
| vitamin A | 11-*cis*-retinal |
| thiamin | thiamin pyrophosphate |
| riboflavin | FMN, FAD |
| niacin | NAD, NADP |
| vitamin $B_6$ | pyridoxal phosphate |
| pantothenic acid | acyl carrier protein |
| folate | tetrahydrofolic acid ($FH_4$) |

*vitamin*
*excretion*

In general, the fat-soluble vitamins, which tend to be retained in hydrophobic environments, are excreted with the feces via enterohepatic circulation[22]. Exceptions include vitamins A and E which, to some extent, have water-soluble metabolites (e.g., short-chain derivatives of retinoic acid; the so-called *"Simon's metabolites"* of vitamin E) and menadione (which can be metabolized to a polar salt), which are excreted in the urine. In contrast, the water-soluble vitamins are generally excreted in the urine, intact (riboflavin, pantothenic acid) and as water-soluble metabolites (vitamin C, thiamin, niacin, riboflavin, pyridoxine, biotin, folate, vitamin $B_{12}$).

## METABOLIC FUNCTIONS OF THE VITAMINS

*vitamins serve*
*4 basic*
*functions*

The thirteen families of nutritionally important substances called vitamins comprise two to three times that number of practically important vitamers and function in metabolism in four general (and not mutually exclusive) ways. The type of metabolic function of any particular vitamer or vitamin family, of course, is dependent on its tissue/cellular distribution and its chemical reactivity, both of which are direct or indirect functions of its chemical structure.

General functions of the vitamins:

| | |
|---|---|
| membrane stabilizer | $H^+/e^-$ donors/acceptors |
| hormone | co-enzymes |

---

[22]i.e., these substances are discharged from the liver with the bile; the amounts that are not subsequently reabsorbed are eliminated with the feces.

Excretory forms of the vitamins:

| vitamin | urinary form(s) | fecal form(s) |
|---------|-----------------|---------------|
| vitamin A | retinoic acid<br>acidic short-chain forms | retinoyl glucuronides<br>intact-chain products |
| vitamin D | | 25,26-$(OH)_2$-D<br>25-$(OH)_2$-D-23,26-lactone |
| vitamin E | | tocopheryl quinone<br>tocopheronic acid and its lactone |
| vitamin K<br>  K, MK, and<br>    menadione | | vitamin K-2,3-epoxide<br>2-$CH_3$-3,(5'-carboxy-3'-$CH_3$-2'-pentenyl)-<br>  1,4-naphthoquinone<br>2-$CH_3$-3(3'-carboxy-3'-methylpropyl)-1,4-<br>  napthoquinone<br>other unidentified metabolites |
|   menadione | menadiol-phosphate, -sulfate | menadiol glucuronide |
| vitamin C[a] | ascorbate-2-sulfate; oxalic acid<br>2,3-diketogulonic acid | |
| thiamin | thiamin, thiamin disulfide<br>thiamin pyrophosphate, thiochrome<br>2-methyl-4-amino-5-pyrimidine carboxylic acid<br>4-methyl-thiazole-5-acetic acid<br>2-methyl-4-amino-5-hydroxymethyl pyrimidine<br>5-(2-hydroxyethyl)-4-methylthiazole<br>3-(2'-methyl-4-amino-5'-pyrimidinyl-<br>  methyl)-4-methylthiazole-5-acetic acid<br>2-methyl-4-amino-5-formylaminomethylpyrimidine<br>(several other minor metabolites) | |
| riboflavin | riboflavin, 7- and 8-hydroxmethylriboflavins,<br>8$\beta$-sulfonylriboflavin, riboflavinyl peptide ester,<br>10-hydroxyethylflavin, lumiflavin, 10-formylmethylflavin<br>10-carboxymethylflavin, lumichrome | |
| niacin | $N^1$-methylnicotinamide<br>nicotinuric acid<br>nicotinamide-$N^1$-oxide<br>$N^1$-methylnicotinamide-$N^1$-oxide<br>$N^1$-methyl-4-pyridone-3-carboxamide<br>$N^1$-methyl-2-pyridone-5-carboxamide | |
| vitamin $B_6$ | pyridoxol, pyridoxal, pyridoxamine and phosphates<br>4-pyridoxic acid and its lactone<br>5-pyridoxic acid | |
| biotin | biotin; bis-nor-biotin; a ketone<br>biotin d- and l-sulfoxide | |
| pantothenic acid | pantothenic acid | |
| folate | pteroylglutamic acid<br>5-methyl-pteroylglutamic acid<br>10-formyl-THFA[b], pteridine<br>acetamidobenzoylglutamic acid | intact folates |
| vitamin $B_{12}$ | cobalamin | cobalamin |

[a]Substantial amounts also oxidized to $CO_2$ and is excreted across the lungs.   [b]i.e., tetrahydrofolic acid.

Metabolic functions of the vitamins:

| vitamin | activities |
|---|---|
| **Membrane stabilizer** | |
| vitamin E | antioxidant protection of polyunsaturated phospholipids |
| **Hormone** | |
| vitamin D | several metabolites important in Ca homeostasis |
| **$H^+/e^-$ donors/acceptors** | |
| vitamin E | quenching of free radicals *via* conversion of tocopherol to the tocopheroxyl radical and, then, to the quinone |
| vitamin K | conversion to the epoxide form in the carboxylation of peptide glutamyl residues |
| vitamin C | oxidation to dehydroascorbic acid in hydroxylations |
| niacin | interconversion of the $NAD^+/NADH$ and $NADP^+/NADPH$ couples in several dehydrogenases |
| riboflavin | interconversion of the $FMN/FMNH/FMNH_2$ and $FAD/FADH/FADH_2$ systems in several oxidases |
| pantothenic acid | oxidation of CoA in the synthesis/oxidation of fatty acids |
| **Co-enzymes** | |
| vitamin A | rhodopsin conformational change following light-induced bleaching |
| vitamin K | vitamin K-dependent peptide-glutamyl carboxylase |
| vitamin C | cytochrome $P_{450}$-dependent oxidations (drug and cholesterol metabolism, steroid hydroxylations) |
| thiamin | co-factor of $\alpha$-keto acid decarboxylases and transketolase |
| niacin | NAD(H)/NADP(H) used by 30+ dehydrogenases in the metabolism of carbohydrates (e.g., glucose-6-P dehydrogenase), lipids (e.g., $\alpha$-glycerol-P dehydrogenase), protein (e.g., glutamate dehydrogenase); Krebs cycle, rhodopsin synthesis (alcohol dehydrogenase) |
| riboflavin | FMN: L-amino acid oxidase, lactate dehydrogenase, pyridoxine (pyridoxamine) 5'-phosphate oxidase |
| | FAD: D-amino acid and glucose oxidases, succinic and acetyl CoA dehydrogenases; glutathione, vitamin K and cytochrome reductases |
| vitamin $B_6$ | metabolism of amino acids (aminotransferases, deaminases, decarboxylases, desufhydratases), porphyrins ($\delta$-aminolevulinic acid synthase), glycogen (glycogen phosphorylase) and epinephrine (tyrosine decarboxylase) |
| biotin | carboxylations (pyruvate, acetyl CoA, propionyl CoA, 3-methylcrotonyl CoA carboxylases) and transcarboxylations (methylmalonyl CoA carboxymethyl transferase) |
| pantothenic acid | fatty acid synthesis/oxidation |
| folate | single-carbon metabolism (serine-glycine conversion, histidine degradation, purine synthesis, methyl-group synthesis) |
| vitamin $B_{12}$ | methylmalonyl CoA mutase, $N^5$-$CH_3$-$FH_4$:homocysteine methyl transferase |

## Study Questions and Exercises:

i.      Prepare a *concept map* of the **relationships** between the chemical structures, the physical properties and the modes of absorption, transport and tissue distributions of the vitamins.

ii.     For each vitamin, identify the **key feature(s)** of its chemical structure. How is/are this/these feature(s) related to the stability and/or biologic activity of the vitamin?

iii.    Prepare **general classifications** of the vitamins by prominent physical properties, by key chemical properties and by stability.

iv.     Which vitamins would you *suspect* might be in shortest supply in the diets of livestock? in your own diet? *Explain your answer* in terms of the physico-chemical properties of the vitamins.

## Recommended Reading:

*Vitamin Nomenclature:*
    Anonymous. 1987. Nomenclature Policy: Generic Descriptors and Trivial Names for Vitamins and Related Compounds. J. Nutr. 120:12-19.

*Vitamin Chemistry:*
    Friedrich, W. 1988. Vitamins. Walter de Gruyter, New York. 1058 pp.

# CHAPTER 4 *AVITAMINOSES*

*"These diseases . . . were considered for years either as intoxication by food or as infectious diseases, and twenty years of experimental work were necessary to show that diseases occur which are caused by a deficiency of some essential substance in the food."*     C. Funk

## Anchoring Concepts:

| | |
|---|---|
| *i.* | A **disease** is an interruption or perversion of function of any of the organs with characteristic signs and/or symptoms caused by specific biochemical and morphological changes. |
| *ii.* | **Deficient intakes** of essential nutrients can cause disease. |

## Learning Objectives:

| | |
|---|---|
| *i.* | To understand the concept of *"vitamin deficiency"*. |
| *ii.* | To understand that deficient intakes of vitamins lead to **sequences of lesions** involving changes starting at the biochemical level, progressing to affect cellular and tissue function and, ultimately, resulting in morphological changes. |
| *iii.* | To understand the range of possible morphological changes in **organ systems** that can be caused by vitamin deficiencies. |
| *iv.* | To understand the **specific morphological signs** and/or symptoms of deficiencies of each vitamin in animals including humans. |

## Vocabulary:

achlorhydria
achromatrichia
acrodynia
age pigments
alopecia
anemia
anorexia
arteriosclerosis
ataxia
avitaminosis
beri-beri
bradycardia
brown bowel disease
brown fat disease
caged layer fatigue
capillary fragility
cardiomyopathy
caries
cataract
cervical paralysis
cheilosis
chondrodystrophy
cirrhosis
clinical sign
clubbed down
convulsion
cornification
curled toe paralysis
dementia
dermatitis
desquamation
diarrhea
dystrophy
edema
encephalomalacia
encephalopathy
exudative diathesis
fatty liver and kidney syndrome
geographical tongue
gizzard myopathy

glossitis
hemorrhage
hyperkeratosis
hypoprothrombinemia
hypovitaminosis
inanition
inflammation
keratomalacia
leucopenia
lipofuscin(osis)
malabsorption
mulberry heart disease
myopathy
necrosis
nephritis
neuropathy
night blindness
nyctalopia
nystagmus
opisthotonos
osteomalacia
osteoporosis
paralysis
pellagra
perosis
photophobia
polyneuritis
retrolental fibroplasia
rickets
scurvy
steatitis
stiff lamb disease
stomatitis
symptom
ulcer
vitamin deficiency
Wernicke-Korsakoff syndrome
white muscle disease
xerophthalmia
xerosis

# DEFICIENCIES OF THE VITAMINS

*what is meant by the term "vitamin deficiency"?*

Because the gross functional and morphological changes caused by deprivation of the vitamins were the source of their discovery as important nutrients, these signs have become the focus of attention by many with interests in human and/or veterinary health.  Indeed, freedom from clinical diseases caused by insufficient vitamin nutriture has generally been used as the main criterion by which vitamin requirements have been defined.

*vitamin deficiencies involve cascades of progressive changes*

Yet, the diseases associated with low intakes of particular vitamins typically represent clinical manifestations of a progressive sequence series of lesions that result from biochemical perturbations (e.g., diminished enzyme activity due to lack of a co-enzyme or co-substrate; membrane dysfunction due to lack of a stabilizing factor) that lead first to cellular and then to tissue and organ dysfunction.  Thus, the clinical signs of a vitamin deficiency are actually the end result of a chain of events that starts with the diminution in cells and tissues of the metabolically active form of the vitamin.

Stages of vitamin deficiency:

| | |
|---|---|
| i. | ***depletion*** of vitamin stores, which leads to . . . |
| ii. | cellular ***metabolic changes***, which lead to . . . |
| iii. | ***clinical defects***, which ultimately produce . . . |
| iv. | ***morphological changes*** |

Marks[1] illustrated this point with the results of a study of thiamin depletion of human volunteers.  When the subjects were fed a thiamin-free diet, no changes of any type were detected for 5-10 days, after which the first signs of decreased saturation of erythrocyte transketolase with its essential cofactor, thiamin pyrophosphate (TPP), were noted.  Not for nearly 200 days of depletion, i.e., long after tissue thiamin levels and transketolase-TPP saturation had declined, were classical clinical signs of thiamin deficiency (anorexia, weight loss, malaise, insomnia, hyperirritability) detected.

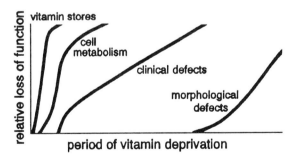

[1]Marks, J. 1968. The Vitamins in Health and Disease: a Modern Reappraisal.  J. & A. Churchill, Ltd., London. 183 pp.

*intervention most effective in early stages of deficiency*

That vitamin deficiencies[2] are not simply specific morphological events but, rather, *cascades of biochemical, physiological and anatomical changes* is the key point in both the assessment of vitamin status and the effective treatment of hypovitaminoses. Because the early biochemical and metabolic effects of specific vitamin deficiencies are almost always readily reversed by therapy with the appropriate vitamin, in contrast to the later functional and anatomical changes which may be permanent, intervention to correct hypovitaminoses is most effective when the condition is detected in its early and less severe stages. In this respect, the management of the vitamin deficiencies is not different from that of other diseases for which treatment is generally most effective when given at the stage of cellular biochemical abnormality, rather than waiting for the appearance of the ultimate clinical signs[3]. For this reason, the early detection of insufficient vitamin status using biochemical indicators has been and will continue to be a very important activity in the clinical assessment of vitamin status.

*"vitamin deficiency" defined*

The expression *"vitamin deficiency"*, therefore, simply refers to the basic condition distinct from but underlying the various biochemical changes, functional impairment or other overt disease signs by which the need for a vitamin is defined.

A **vitamin deficiency** is . . .

> the shortage of supply of a vitamin relative to its needs by a particular organism.

*primary and secondary vitamin deficiencies*

**Vitamin status** is, therefore, the balance of vitamin supply and need for a particular individual at a given point in time. Shifts in this balance by either reduced effective vitamin supply or increased effective vitamin need produce vitamin deficiencies. When these come about as the result of the failure to ingest a vitamin in sufficient amounts to meets physiological needs, the condition is called a *"primary deficiency"*. When these come about as a result of the failure to absorb or otherwise utilize a vitamin due to an environmental condition or physiological state and *not* to insufficient consumption of the vitamin, the condition is called a *"secondary deficiency"*. Therefore, vitamin deficiencies can be caused in several ways.

*causes of vitamin deficiency in humans*

Many of the ways in which vitamin deficiencies can come about are interrelated. For example, poverty is often accompanied by gross ignorance of what constitutes a nutritionally adequate diet. People living alone, and especially the elderly and others with chronic disease, tend to consume

---

[2]This discussion, of course, is pertinent to *any* class of nutrients.

[3]Marks makes this point clearly with the example of diabetes, which should be treated once hypoglycemia is detected, thus reducing the danger of diabetic arteriosclerosis and retinopathy.

foods that require little preparation but which may not provide good nutrition. Despite these potential causes of vitamin deficiency, in most of the technologically developed parts of the world, the general level of nutrition is high. In those areas relative few persons can be expected to show signs of vitamin deficiency; those that do present such signs will most frequently be found to have a potentiating condition that affects either their consumption of food or their utilization of nutrients. In the developing parts of the world, however, famine is still the largest single cause of general malnutrition today. People affected by famine show signs of multiple nutrient deficiencies including those of total energy, protein and several vitamins.

*causes of vitamin deficiency in animals*

Many of the same primary and secondary factors can lead to vitamin deficiencies in animals. In livestock, however, most of these factors are related to human errors involving improper or careless animal husbandry.

Potential causes of vitamin deficiency in humans:

| primary deficiency | secondary deficiency |
|---|---|
| poor food habits | poor digestion (e.g., achlorhydria) |
| poverty (i.e., low food-purchasing power) | malabsorption (e.g., pancreatic dysfunction, diarrhea, intestinal infection, parasitism) |
| ignorance (i.e., lack on sound nutrition information) | impaired utilization (e.g., drug therapy) |
| lack of total food (e.g., crop failure) | increased requirement (e.g., infection, increased work, pregnancy, lactation, rapid growth, nutrient imbalance) |
| lack of vitamin-rich foods (e.g., consumption of highly refined foods) | vitamin destruction (i.e., storage, cooking) |
| anorexia (e.g., homebound elderly, infirm, dental problems) | increased vitamin excretion (e.g., excessive sweating, diuresis, lactation) |
| food taboos and fads (e.g., fasting, avoidance of certain foods) | |
| apathy (lack of incentive to prepare adequate meals) | |

Potential causes of vitamin deficiency in animals[4]

| primary deficiency | secondary deficiency |
|---|---|
| improperly formulated diet | poor digestion |
| feed mixing error (e.g., omission of vitamin premix) | malabsorption (e.g., diarrhea, parasitism, intestinal infection) |
| poor access to feed (e.g., competition for limited feeder space, improper feeder placement, breakdown of feed delivery system) | impaired post-absorptive utilization (e.g., drug therapy) |
| anorexia | increased requirement (e.g., infection, change in environmental temperature, egg/milk production, rapid growth, pregnancy, lactation) |
| | vitamin destruction in feed (e.g., feed storage, pelleting, extrusion) |

---

[4] livestock and other managed animal species

## CLINICAL MANIFESTATIONS OF VITAMIN DEFICIENCIES

*organ systems* Every organ system of the body can be the target of a vitamin deficiency.
*affected by* While the individual vitamins each tend to affect only certain organs, it is
*vitamin* useful to consider the morphologic lesions caused by vitamin deficiencies
*deficiencies* from the standpoint of the organ systems themselves, for the reason that
it is anatomical and/or functional changes in particular organs that are the
initial presentations of deficiencies of each of the vitamins.

Dermatologic disorders of vitamin deficiencies:

| signs/symptoms | vitamins involved | species affected | specific diseases |
|---|---|---|---|
| skin | | | |
|   subcut. hemorrhage | vitamin K | poultry | |
|   dermatitis | | | |
|     scaly | vitamin A | cattle | |
| | pantothenic acid | rat | |
| | biotin | rat, mouse, hamster, mink, fox, cat | |
| | riboflavin | pig | |
| | pyridoxine | rat | acrodynia |
|     cracking | niacin | human, chick | pellagra |
| | pantothenic | chick (feet) | |
| | biotin | monkey (feet, hands), pig, poultry (feet) | |
|     desquamation | niacin | human, chick | |
| | biotin | rat | |
| | riboflavin | rat, poultry, dog, monkey, human | |
| | pyridoxine | human | |
|     hyperkeratosis | niacin | human, chick | pellagra |
| | biotin | rat, mouse, hamster, mouse | |
| | riboflavin | rat | |
|     hyperpigmentation | niacin | human | pellagra |
|     photosensitization | niacin | human | pellagra |
|     stomatitis | niacin | human | pellagra |
| | pantothenic acid | chick | |
| | biotin | chick | |
| | riboflavin | calf, human | |
|     edema | thiamin | human | beri-beri |
| hair | | | |
|   rough | vitamin A | cattle | |
|   achromatrichia | pantothenic acid | rat | |
| | biotin | rat, rabbit, mink, fox, cat, monkey | |
|   alopecia | pantothenic acid | rat | |
| | niacin | pig, rat | |
| | biotin | rat, mouse, hamster, pig, rabbit, cat, mink, fox | "spectacle" eye |
| | riboflavin | rat, pig, calf | |
|   "blood"-caked whiskers | pantothenic acid | rat | |
| feathers | | | |
|   rough | vitamin A | poultry | |
| | biotin | poultry | |
|   impaired growth | folic acid | poultry | |
| | biotin | poultry | |

Muscular disorders of vitamin deficiencies:

| signs/symptoms | vitamin involved | species affected | specific disease |
|---|---|---|---|
| general weakness | vitamin A | cat | |
| | vitamin D | human | osteomalacia |
| | pantothenic acid | human | |
| | ascorbic acid | human | scurvy |
| | thiamin | rat | |
| | | human | beri-beri |
| | riboflavin | dog, fox, pig | |
| | pyridoxine | rat, chick | |
| skeletal myopathy | vitamin E | monkey, pig, rat, rabbit, guinea pig, horse, goat, mink, duckling, salmon, catfish | |
| | | calf, chick | "white muscle" disease |
| | | lamb | "stiff lamb" disease |
| | ascorbic acid | guinea pig, human | scurvy |
| | thiamin | rat, human | beri-beri |
| hemorrhage of skeletal muscles | vitamin K | poultry | |
| | pantothenic | pig | |
| cardiomyopathy | vitamin E | pig | "mulberry heart" disease |
| | | rat, dog, rabbit, guinea pig, calf, lamb, goat | |
| | thiamin | human, rat | beri-beri |
| gizzard myopathy | vitamin E | turkey poults, ducklings | |

Reproductive disorders of vitamin deficiencies:

| signs/symptoms | vitamin involved | species affected | specific disease |
|---|---|---|---|
| female | | | |
| vaginal cornification | vitamin A | human, rat | |
| ovarian degeneration | vitamin A | poultry | |
| thin egg shell | vitamin D | poultry | |
| low rate of egg production | vitamin A | poultry | |
| | riboflavin | poultry | |
| | pyridoxine | poultry | |
| uterine lipofucsinosis | vitamin E | rat | |
| anestrus | riboflavin | rat | |
| male | | | |
| degen. of germinal epithelium | vitamin A | rat, bull, cat | |
| | vitamin E | rat, rooster, dog, pig, monkey, rabbit, guinea pig, hamster | |
| fetus | | | |
| death | vitamin A | poultry | |
| | vitamin E | rat | |
| | riboflavin | chick | |
| | folate | chick | |
| | vitamin $B_{12}$ | poultry | |
| abnormalities | riboflavin | rat | |
| | | chick | "clubbed down" |
| | folate | chick | "parrot beak" |

Vascular disorders of vitamin deficiencies:

| signs/symptoms | vitamin involved | species affected | specific disease |
|---|---|---|---|
| blood vessels | | | |
| increased capillary permeability | vitamin E | chick | exudative diathesis |
| | | pig | visceral edema |
| capillary fragility | vitamin C | human | scurvy |
| hemorrhage | | guinea pig, monkey | scurvy |
| arteriosclerosis | pyridoxine | monkey | |
| blood cells | | | |
| anemia | vitamin E | human, monkey, pig | |
| | vitamin K | chick, rat | |
| | niacin | pig | |
| | folate | chick, rat, human | |
| | riboflavin | monkey, baboon | |
| | pyridoxine | human | |
| erythrocyte fragility | vitamin E | human, rat, monkey, pig | |
| leucopenia | folate | guinea pig, rat | |
| excess platelets | vitamin E | rat | |
| increased platelet aggregation | vitamin E | rat | |
| impaired blood clotting | vitamin K | chick, rat, pig, calf, human | |

Gastro-intestinal disorders of vitamin deficiencies:

| signs/symptoms | vitamin involved | species affected | specific disease |
|---|---|---|---|
| intestine | | | |
| lipofuscinosis | vitamin E | dog | "brown bowel" disease |
| hemorrhage | vitamin K | poultry | |
| | niacin | dog | |
| | thiamin | rat | |
| ulcer | thiamin | rat | |
| diarrhea | niacin | dog, pig, poultry | |
| | | human | pellagra |
| | riboflavin | calf, dog, pig, chick | |
| | vitamin B$_{12}$ | young pigs | |
| constipation | niacin | human | pellagra |
| inflammation | niacin | chick | |
| | thiamin | rat | |
| | riboflavin | dog, pig, chick | |
| stomach | | | |
| achlorhydria | niacin | human | pellagra |
| gastric distress | thiamin | human | beri-beri |
| mouth | | | |
| inflammation | niacin | poultry | |
| glossitis | niacin | human | pellagra |
| abnormal tongue | riboflavin | rat, human | "geographical tongue" |
| papillae | niacin | human | |
| stomatitis | niacin | human | pellagra |
| | riboflavin | human | |
| cheilosis | riboflavin | human | |

Vital organ disorders of vitamin deficiencies:

| signs/symptoms | vitamin involved | species affected | specific disease |
|---|---|---|---|
| liver | | | |
| necrosis | vitamin E | rat, mouse | dietary liver necrosis |
| | | pig | "hepatosis dietetica" |
| steatosis | pantothenic acid | chick, dog | |
| | biotin | chick | fatty liver and kidney syndrome* |
| | thiamin | rat | |
| cirrhosis | choline | rat, dog, monkey | |
| kidney | | | |
| nephritis | vitamin A | human | |
| steatosis | biotin | chick | fatty liver and kidney syndrome |
| | riboflavin | pig | |
| hemorrhagic necrosis | choline | rat, mouse, pig, rabbit, calf | |
| calculi | pyridoxine | rat | |
| thymus | | | |
| lymphoid necrosis | pantothenic acid | chick, dog | |
| adrenal glands | | | |
| hypertrophy | pantothenic acid | pig | |
| hemorrhage | riboflavin | pig | |
| necrosis | pantothenic acid | rat | |
| | riboflavin | baboon | |
| adipose | | | |
| lipofuscinosis | vitamin E | rat, mouse, cat, hamster, mink, pig | "brown fat" disease |
| pancreas | | | |
| insulin insufficiency | pyridoxine | rat | |

*This condition is generally referred to as "FLKS" by poultry pathologists and nutritionists.

Ocular disorders of vitamin deficiencies:

| signs/symptoms | vitamin involved | species affected | specific disease |
|---|---|---|---|
| retina | | | |
| night blindness | vitamin A | rat, pig, sheep, cat, human | nyctalopia |
| retinal degeneration | vitamin E | rat, dog, cat, monkey | |
| | | human | retrolental fibroplasia* |
| cornea | | | |
| xerophthalmia[b] | vitamin A | human, calf, rat | |
| keratomalacia[c] | vitamin A | human, calf, rat | |
| lens | | | |
| cataract | vitamin E | turkey embryo, rabbit | |
| photophobia | riboflavin | human | |

*There is considerable debate as to the role of vitamin E status in the etiology of this condition involving the abnormal growth of fibrous tissue behind the crystalline lens. The condition, occurring in premature infants maintained in high-$O_2$ environments, has been reported to be reduced in severity or prevented by treatment with vitamin E, which is known to be at low levels in such infants.
[b]Xerophthalmia is characterized by extreme dryness (i.e., xerosis) of the conjunctiva.
[c]xerotic keratitis, i.e., dryness with ulceration and perforation of the cornea resulting in blindness.

Nervous disorders of vitamin deficiencies:

| signs/symptoms | vitamin involved | species affected | specific disease |
|---|---|---|---|
| excessive CSF[a] pressure | vitamin A | calf, pig, chick | |
| ataxia[b] | vitamin A | calf, pig, chick, sheep | |
| | thiamin | calf, pig, rat, chick, rabbit, mouse, monkey | |
| | | human | Wernicke-Korsakoff synd.[c] |
| | riboflavin | pig, rat | |
| tremors | niacin | human | pellagra |
| tetany | vitamin D | pig, chick, children | rickets |
| encephalopathy | vitamin E | chick | encephalomalacia |
| | thiamin | human | Wernicke-Korsakoff synd.[c] |
| nerve degeneration | riboflavin | rat, pig | |
| | | chick | "curled-toe" paralysis |
| | vitamin E | monkey, rat, dog, duck | |
| | niacin | pig, rat | |
| | pyridoxine | rat | |
| | vitamin B$_{12}$ | human | |
| peripheral neuropathy | thiamin | human | beri-beri |
| | | chick | polyneuritis |
| | riboflavin | human | |
| | pantothenic acid | human | "burning feet"[d] |
| | vitamin B$_{12}$ | human | |
| abnormal gait | pantothenic acid | pig, dog | "goose-stepping" |
| seizures | pyridoxine | rat, human infant | |
| opisthotonos[e] | thiamin | chicken, pigeon | "star-gazing" |
| paralysis | pantothenic acid | chick | |
| | | poult | cervical paralysis |
| | riboflavin | rat | |
| | | chick | "curled-toe" paralysis |
| | pyridoxine | chick | |
| nystagmus[f] | thiamin | human | Wernicke-Korsakoff synd.[c] |
| depression | niacin | human | pellagra |
| | thiamin | human | beri-beri |
| anxiety | thiamin | human | beri-beri |
| dizziness | niacin | human | pellagra |
| irritability | niacin | human | pellagra |
| | thiamin | human | beri-beri |
| | pyridoxine | rat, human | |
| | vitamin B$_{12}$ | pig | |
| dementia | niacin | human | pellagra |
| psychosis | thiamin | human | Wernicke-Korsakoff synd.[c] |

[a]cerebrospinal fluid
[b]poor coordination
[c]condition, most frequent among alcoholics, characterized by Wernicke's syndrome (presbyophrenia, i.e., loss of memory, disorientation and confabulation but integrity of judgment) and Korsakoff's psychosis (polyneuritic psychosis, i.e., imaginary reminiscences and agitated hallucinations)
[d]parathesia of the feet
[e]tetanic spasm with spine and extremities bent with convexity forward, i.e., severe head retraction.
[f]rhythmical oscillation of the eyeballs, either horizontal, rotary or vertical.

Skeletal disorders of vitamin deficiencies:

| signs/symptoms | vitamin involved | species affected | specific disease |
|---|---|---|---|
| excess periosteal growth | vitamin A | calf, pig, dog, horse, sheep | blindness |
| undermineralization (epiphyseal abnormality) | vitamin D | children, chick puppy, rat, calf | rickets[a] rickets |
| demineralization (bone deformation) | vitamin D | human adult | osteomalacia[b] |
| increased fractures | vitamin D | human adult laying hen | osteoporosis[c] "cage layer fatigue" |
| dental caries | vitamin D pyridoxine | human child human | rickets |
| chondrodystrophy | niacin biotin | chick, poult chick, poult | perosis[d] perosis |
| congenital deformities | riboflavin pyridoxine | rat rat | |

[a]*Rickets* is the disease of infants and young characterized by softening of bones, epiphyseal abnormalities, enlargement of liver and spleen, profuse sweating, and general tenderness.
[b]*Osteomalacia* is the disease characterized by gradual softening and bending of bones with more or less severe pain; bones are soft because they contain osteoid tissue that has failed to calcify.
[c]*Osteoporosis* involves the reduction in the quantity of bone, i.e., skeletal atrophy; usually, the remaining bone normally mineralized.
[d]*Perosis* is the condition of slippage of the Achilles tendon such that extension of the foot and, therefore, walking is impossible; it occurs as the result of twisting of the tibial and/or metatarsal bones due to their improper development.

*deficiency diseases grouped by vitamin*

It is also useful to consider the clinical signs of vitamin deficiencies according to the various vitamins.  While this means of categorizing vitamin deficiency disorders has little relevance to the practical diagnosis of vitamin deficiencies, it is a most convenient way to systematize this information for the purpose of learning about the vitamins.

Summary of organ systems affected by vitamin deficiencies *(part 1)*:

| organ system | vitamin A | vitamin D | vitamin E | vitamin K |
|---|---|---|---|---|
| general | | | | |
| appetite | decrease | decrease | decrease | |
| growth | decrease | decrease | decrease | decrease |
| immunity | decrease | | decrease[a] | |
| dermatologic | scaly rough hair | | | hemorrhage[b] |
| muscular | weakness | weakness | myopathy | hemorrhage[c] |
| gastro-intestinal | | | lipofuscinosis[d] | hemorrhage |
| adipose | | | lipofuscinosis[d] | |
| skeletal | periosteal overgrowth | rickets[e] osteomalacia[f] | | |
| vital organs | nephritis | | liver necrosis | |
| vascular | | | | |
| vessels | | exudative diathesis[g] | | |
| erythrocytes | | | anemia | anemia |
| platelets | | | incr. no. & aggreg. | decr. clotting |
| nervous | incr. CSF pressure ataxia | tetany ataxia | encephalopathy[h] axonal dystrophy | |
| reproductive | | | | |
| male | decr. sperm motility | decr. sperm motility | | |
| female | vaginal cornification[i] | decr. eggs, shell | uterine lipofuscinosis[d] | |
| fetal | death | | death, resorption | |
| ocular | | | | |
| retinal | nyctalopia[j] | | | |
| corneal | xerophthalmia[k] keratomalacia[l] | | | |
| lens | | | cataract[m] retrolental fibroplasia[n] | |

[a]Some aspects of immune function can be impaired, especially if Se is also deficient.
[b]subcutaneous
[c]intramuscular
[d]accumulation of ceroid (*"age"* pigments), which are adducts of lipid breakdown products and proteins
[e]impaired production of growing bone
[f]loss of mineralization of mature bone
[g]edema resulting from loss of plasma through abnormally permeable capillaries
[h]disease of the brain
[i]replacement of normal vaginal mucosa with a horny layer of cells
[j]night blindness (impaired dark adaptation)
[k]severe dryness of the conjunctiva
[l]xerotic keratitis, i.e., dryness with ulceration and perforation of the cornea resulting in blindness
[m]lens opacity
[n]abnormal growth of fibrous tissue behind the lens

Summary of organ systems affected by vitamin deficiencies *(part 2)*:

| organ system | vitamin C | thiamin | riboflavin | vitamin B₆ |
|---|---|---|---|---|
| <u>general</u> | | | | |
| appetite | decrease | sev. decrease | decrease | decrease |
| growth | decrease | decrease | decrease | decrease |
| immunity | decrease[a] | | | |
| heat resistance | decrease | | | |
| dermatologic | | edema | cheilosis[b] stomatitis[c] | acrodynia |
| muscular | skeletal muscle atropy | cardiomyopathy bradycardia[d] heart failure weakness | weakness | weakness |
| gastro-intestinal | | inflammation ulcer | inflammation | |
| adipose | | | | |
| skeletal | | | deformities | dental caries |
| vital organs | | fatty liver[e] | fatty liver[e] | |
| <u>vascular</u> | | | | |
| vessels | capillary fragility hemorrhage | | | arteriosclerosis |
| erythrocytes platelets | | | anemia | anemia |
| nervous | tenderness | periph. neuropathy opisthotonos[f] | paralysis ataxia[g] | paralysis convulsions |
| <u>reproductive</u> | | | | |
| male | | | sterility | |
| female | | | decr. eggs | decr. eggs |
| fetal | | | death, malformations | |
| <u>ocular</u> | | | | |
| retinal | | | photophobia | |
| corneal | | | decr. vascularization | |
| lens | | | retrolental fibroplasia | |

[a]Some aspects of immunity may be affected by vitamin C status.
[b]cracks and fissures at the corners of the mouth
[c]inflammation of the oral mucosa (soft tissues of the mouth)
[d]abnormally slow heartbeat
[e]hepatic steatosis
[f]severe head retraction
[g]poor coordination

Summary of organ systems affected by vitamin deficiencies *(part 3)*:

| organ system | niacin | folate | pantothenic acid | biotin | vitamin B$_{12}$ |
|---|---|---|---|---|---|
| general | | | | | |
|   appetite | decrease | | | decrease | |
|   growth | decrease | decrease | decrease | decrease | decrease |
|   immunity | | | | | |
| dermatologic | dermatitis photosensitization | alopecia[a] | scaly dermatitis achromatrichia[b] alopecia[a] | dermatitis alopecia[a] | |
| muscular | | | hemorrhage weakness | | |
| gastro-intestinal | diarrhea glossitis[c] | | | | diarrhea |
| adipose | | | | | |
| skeletal | perosis[d] | | | perosis[d] | |
| vital organs | | | fatty liver thymus degen. | FLKS[e] | |
| vascular | | | | | |
|   vessels | | | | | |
|   erythrocytes | anemia | anemia | | | anemia |
|   platelets | | | | | |
| nervous | ataxia[f] dementia[g] | | abnormal gait paralysis | | peripheral neuropathy |
| reproductive | | | | | |
|   male | | | | | |
|   female | | | | | |
|   fetal | | | | | death |
| ocular | | | | | |
|   retinal | | | | | |
|   corneal | | | | | |
|   lens | | | | | |

[a]baldness, or loss of hair or feathers
[b]loss of normal pigment from hair or feathers
[c]inflammation of the tongue
[d]slipped Achilles tendon, *"hock disease"* in birds, resulting in crippling
[e]fatty liver and kidney syndrome involving both hepatic and renal steatosis
[f]poor coordination
[g]mental deterioration

# VITAMIN DEFICIENCY DISEASES:
# MANIFESTATIONS OF BIOCHEMICAL LESIONS

*relationship between biochemical lesions and clinical disease*

That impairments in biochemical function (i.e., biochemical lesions) resulting from insufficient vitamin supply are causally related to the morphological and/or functional changes (i.e., the clinical signs) associated with the latter stages of the vitamin deficiency is a fundamental concept in understanding the nutrition of the vitamins.  While the validity of this concept is readily apparent in the abstract, documentary evidence for it in the case of *each* of the vitamin deficiency diseases is not available and, thus, offers opportunities for achieving through continued discovery better understanding of the biochemical bases for vitamin activity.

*need for more information on modes of vitamin action*

Vitamin A offers a case in point of this fact.  While the role of vitamin A in preventing nyctalopia (night blindness) is clear from presently available knowledge of the essentiality of retinal as the prosthetic group of rhodopsin and several other photosensitive visual receptors in the retina, the amount of vitamin A in the retina and thus available for visual function is only ca. 1% of the total amount of vitamin A in the body.  Further, it is clear from the clinical signs of vitamin A deficiency that the vitamin has other essential functions unrelated to vision, especially some relating to the integrity and differentiation of epithelial cells.  However, though evidence indicates that vitamin A is involved in the metabolism of mucopolysaccharides and other essential intermediates, present knowledge cannot adequately explain the mechanism(s) of action of vitamin A in supporting growth, in maintaining epithelia, etc.  It has been said that 99% of our information about the mode of action of vitamin A concerns only 1% of the vitamin A in the body.

The ongoing search for understanding of the mechanisms of vitamin action is, therefore, largely based on the study of biochemical correlates of changes in physiological function or morphology effected by changes in vitamin status.  The following table summarizes in general terms current information concerning these correlates.  In this regard, naturally occurring hereditary anomalies involving vitamin-dependent enzymes, transport proteins, etc., can be most useful.  Those inborn metabolic *"errors"* relevant to the vitamins are listed on page 115.

Important biological functions of the vitamins:

| vitamin | metabolically active form(s) | deficiency disorders | important biological function(s) or reaction(s) catalyzed |
|---|---|---|---|
| vitamin A | retinol, retinal, retinoic acid | night blindness, xerophthalmia, keratomalacia | photosensitive retinal pigment, regulation of epithelial cell differentiation |
| vitamin D | $1,25\text{-}(OH)_2\text{-}D$ | rickets, osteomalacia | promotion of intestinal Ca absorption, mobilization of Ca from bone, stimulation of renal Ca resorption, regulation of PTH secretion, possible function in muscle |
| vitamin E | $\alpha$-tocopherol | nerve, muscle degen. | antioxidant protector for membranes |
| vitamin K | K, MK | impaired blood coagulation hemorrhage | co-substrate for $\gamma$-carboxylation of glutamyl residues of several clotting factors and other Ca-binding proteins |
| vitamin C | ascorbic acid dehydroascorbic acid | scurvy | co-substrate for hydroxylations in collagen synthesis, drug and steroid metabolism |
| thiamin | thiamin pyro-phosphate | beri-beri, polyneuritis, Wernicke-Korsakoff syndrome | co-enzyme for oxidative decarboxylation of 2-ketoacids (e.g., pyruvate and 2-keto-glutarate); co-enzyme for pyruvate decarboxylase and transketolase |
| riboflavin | FMN, FAD | dermatitis | co-enzymes for numerous flavoproteins that catalyze redox reactions in fatty acid degradation/synthesis, TCA cycle |
| niacin | NAD(H), NADP(H) | pellagra | co-substrates for H-transfer catalyzed by many dehydrogenases, e.g., TCA cycle respiratory chain |
| pyridoxine | pyridoxal-5'-phosphate | signs vary with species | co-enzyme for metabolism of amino acids, e.g., side-chain, decarboxylation, transamination, racemization |
| folate | polyglutamyl tetrahydrofolates | megaloblastic anemia | co-enzyme for transfer of single-C units, e.g., formyl and hydroxymethyl groups in purine synthesis |
| biotin | 1'-N-carboxybiotin | dermatitis | co-enzyme for carboxylations, e.g., acetyl-CoA/malonyl-CoA conversion |
| pantothenic acid | Coenzyme A | signs vary with species | co-substrate for activation/transfer of acyl groups to form esters, amides, citrate, triglycerides, etc. |
| | acyl carrier protein | | co-enzyme for fatty acid biosynthesis |
| vitamin $B_{12}$ | 5'-deoxyadenosyl-$B_{12}$ | pernicious, megaloblastic anemias | co-enzyme for conversion of methyl-malonyl-CoA to succinyl-CoA |
| | methyl-$B_{12}$ | | methyl group transfer from $CH_3\text{-}FH_4$ to homocysteine in methionine synthesis |

Vitamin-responsive inborn metabolic lesions:

| curative vitamin | missing protein or metabolic step affected | clinical condition |
|---|---|---|
| vitamin A | apolipoprotein B | abetalipoproteinemia; low tissue levels of retinoids |
| vitamin D | receptor | unresponsive to $1,25(OH)_2$-D; osteomalacia |
| vitamin E | apolipoprotein B | abetalipoproteinemia; low tissue levels of tocopherols |
| thiamin | branched-chain 2-oxo-acid dehydrogenase | "maple syrup urine" disease |
| | pyruvate metabolism | lactic acidemia; neurological anomalies |
| riboflavin | methemoglobin reductase | methemoglobinemia |
| | electron transfer flavoprotein | multiple lack of acyl-CoA dehydrogenations, excretion of acyl-CoA metabolites, i.e., metabolic acidosis |
| niacin | abnormal neurotransmission | psychiatric disorders, tryptophan malabsorption, abnormal tryptophan metabolism |
| pyridoxine | cystathionine $\beta$-synthase | homocysteinuria |
| | cystathionine $\gamma$-lyase | cystathioninuria; neurological disorders. |
| | kynureninase | xanthurenic aciduria |
| folate | enteric absorption | megaloblastic anemia, mental disorder |
| | methylene-$FH_4$-reductase | homocysteinuria, neurological disorders |
| | glutamic-formimino-trans. | urinary excretion of formininoglutamic acid (FIGLU) |
| | homocysteine/methionine conversion | schizophrenia |
| | tetrahydrobiopterin-phenylalanine hydrolase | mental retardation, phenylketonuria (PKU) |
| | dihydrobiopteridine reductase | PKU, severe neurological disorders |
| | tetrahydrobiopterin formation | PKU, severe neurological disorders |
| biotin | biotinidase | alopecia, skin rash, cramps, acidemia, developmental disorders, excess urinary biotin and biocytin |
| | propionyl-CoA carboxylase | propionic acidemia |
| | 3-methylcrotonyl CoA carbox. | 3-methylcrontonylglycinuria |
| | pyruvate carboxylase | Leigh syndrome, accumulation of lactate and pyruvate |
| | acetyl-CoA carboxylase | severe brain damage |
| | holocarboxylase synthase | lack of multiple carboxylase activities, urinary excretion of metabolites |
| vitamin $B_{12}$ | intrinsic factor | juvenile pernicious anemia |
| | enteric absorption | Imerslund-Gräsbeck syndrome |
| | transcobalamin | megaloblastic anemia, growth impairment |
| | methylmalonyl-CoA mutase | methylmalonic acidemia |

## Study Questions and Exercises:

i.      For each *major organ system*, list the vitamin deficiencies that may affect its
        function.

ii.     List the ***clinical signs*** that have special diagnostic value (i.e., are specifically
        associated with insufficient status with respect to certain vitamins) for *specific*
        vitamin deficiencies.

iii.    List the ***clinical signs*** that are produced by, but are not diagnostic for,
        specific vitamin deficiencies.

iv.     List the ***animal species*** and ***deficiency diseases*** that, because they show
        specificity for certain vitamins, might be particularly useful in vitamin research.

## Recommended Reading:

Friedovich, W. 1988. Vitamins. Walter de Gruyter, New York. 1058 pp.

Marks, J. 1968. The Vitamins in Health and Disease. J. & A. Churchill, London, 183
pp.

McDowell, L.M. 1989. Vitamins in Animal Nutrition, Comparative Aspects to Human
Nutrition, Academic Press, New York, 486 pp.

# SECTION II

## CONSIDERING THE INDIVIDUAL VITAMINS

# CHAPTER 5 *VITAMIN A*

*"In . . . four [southeast Asian] countries alone at least 500,000 preschool age children every year develop active xerophthalmia involving the cornea. About half of this number will be blind and a very high proportion, probably in excess of 60% will die. The annual prevalence for these same countries of noncorneal xerophthalmia is many times higher, probably on the order of 5 million. . . . There can be no doubt about the claim that vitamin A deficiency is the most common cause of blindness in children and one of the most prevalent and serious of all nutritional deficiency diseases."* — D. S. McLaren

## Anchoring Concepts:

i. **Vitamin A** is the generic descriptor for compounds with the qualitative biological activity of retinol, i.e., retinoids and some (pro-vitamin A) carotenoids.

ii. Vitamin A-active substances are **hydrophobic** and, thus, are insoluble in aqueous environments (intestinal lumen, plasma, interstitial fluid, cytosol).

iii. Vitamin A was discovered by its ability to prevent **night blindness** (nyctalopia) and xerophthalmia.

## Learning Objectives:

i. To understand the nature of the various **sources** of vitamin A in foods.

ii. To understand the means of vitamin A **absorption** from the small intestine.

iii. To become familiar with the various **carriers** involved in the extra- and intra-cellular transport of vitamin A.

iv. To understand the **metabolic conversions** involved in the activation and degradation of vitamin A in its absorption, transport and storage, cellular function and excretion.

v. To become familiar with current knowledge of the **biochemical mechanisms of action** of vitamin A and their relationships to vitamin A-deficiency diseases.

vi. To understand the physiologic implications of **high doses** of vitamin A.

## Vocabulary:

abetalipoproteinemia
acyl CoA:cholesterol acyltransferase
alcohol dehydrogenase
all-*trans*-retinal
*apo*-RBP
*β*-carotene
*β*-carotene-15,15'-dioxygenase
*"bleaching"*
carotenoid
chylomicron remnant
11-*cis*-retinal
CRABP
CRBP
CRBP (II)
glycoproteins
*holo*-RBP
hyperkeratosis
iodopsins
IRBP
I.U.
keratomalacia
metarhodopsin II
night blindness
nyctalopia
pancreatic nonspecific lipase

protein-calorie malnutrition
opsin
RBP
retinal
retinal isomerase
retinal oxidase
retinal reductase
retinoic acid
retinoic acid receptors
retinoid
retinol
retinol dehydrogenase
retinol equivalent (R.E.)
retinol phosphorylase
retinyl ester hydrolase
retinyl ester synthase
retinyl-*β*-glucuronide
retinyl palmitate
retinyl phosphate
retinyl stearate
rhodopsin
transducin
transthyretin
xerophthalmia
xerosis

# SOURCES OF VITAMIN A

*distribution*
*in foods*
The ***retinoids*** are isoprenoid compounds found in animal products and the ***carotenoids*** are isoprenoid pigments produced by plants. Vitamin A exists in several forms in animal products, but mainly as long-chain fatty acid esters the predominant one being ***retinyl palmitate***. The carotenoids are present in both plant and animal food products; in animal products their occurrence results from dietary exposure. Carotenoid pigments are widespread among diverse animal species, with over 500 different compounds estimated. About 60 of these have pro-vitamin A activity, i.e., those that can be cleaved by animals to yield at least one molecule of retinol. In practice, however, only 5 to 6 of these pro-vitamins A are commonly encountered in foods. Therefore, the reporting of vitamin A activity from its various forms in foods requires some means of standardization. Two systems are used for this purpose: ***international units*** (IU) and ***retinol equivalents*** (RE).

Reporting food vitamin A activity:

| 1 *International Unit (IU)* | = | 0.3 | $\mu$g retinol |
|---|---|---|---|
| | = | 0.344 | $\mu$g retinyl acetate |
| | = | 0.6 | $\mu$g $\beta$-carotene |
| | = | 1.2 | $\mu$g other pro-vitamin A carotenoids |
| 1 *Retinol Equivalent (RE)* | = | 1 | $\mu$g retinol |
| | = | 6 | $\mu$g $\beta$-carotene |
| | = | 12 | $\mu$g other pro-vitamin A carotenoids |

In the calculation of RE values, it is assumed that retinol is completely absorbed (i.e., absorption efficiency is 100%). Although one mole of $\beta$-carotene can theoretically be converted (by cleavage of the C15=C15' bond) to yield two moles of retinal, the physiological efficiency of this process appears to be only 50%. Therefore, the conversion of $\beta$-carotene to RE values employs this discount for inefficiency of cleavage, as well as a discount of two-thirds to account for the observed average efficiency of intestinal absorption. Thus, factors of one-sixth and one-twelfth are used to calculate RE values from the $\beta$-carotene and other pro-vitamin A carotenoids, respectively, in foods. In addition, the term ***$\beta$-carotene equivalent*** ($\beta$-CE) is often used; it is defined as the sum of the amount of $\beta$-carotene and one-half of the amounts of other provitamin A carotenoids present in a food. These three systems are employed in the most widely used tables of nutrient composition of foods[1].

---

[1] USDA Handbook 8-9 lists both IU and RE; The FAO Tables list $\mu$g retinol and $\beta$-CE. The INCAP tables (Instituto de Nutricion de Centro America y Panama) list vitamin A as $\mu$g retinol; however, those values are not the same as RE values for the reason that a factor of one-half has been used to convert $\beta$-carotene to retinol, instead of the more common factor of one-sixth used to calculate RE values.

*dietary sources of vitamin A*

Actual intakes of vitamin A, therefore, depend on the patterns of consumption of vitamin A-bearing animal food products and pro-vitamin A-bearing plant food products. In American diets, it appears that each group contributes roughly comparably to vitamin A nutriture; however, this is greatly influenced by personal food habits and food availability. In many countries meat and meat products comprise such a low percentage of the diet that the only sources of vitamin A come from plant foods. In such cases, the use of RE values, the calculation of which downgrades the contributions of carotenoids to total dietary vitamin A, may underestimate true dietary status of vitamin A.

Sources of vitamin A in foods:

| food | percentage distribution of vitamin A activity | | |
|---|---|---|---|
| | retinol | β-carotene | non-β-carotenoids |
| animal foods | | | |
| red meats | 90 | 10 | |
| poultry meat | 90 | 10 | |
| fish and shellfish | 90 | 10 | |
| eggs | 90 | 10 | |
| milk, milk products | 70 | 30 | |
| fats and oils | 90 | 10 | |
| | | | |
| plant foods | | | |
| maize, yellow | | 40 | 60 |
| legumes and seeds | | 50 | 50 |
| green vegetables | | 75 | 25 |
| yellow vegetables[a] | | 85 | 15 |
| pale sweet potatoes | | 50 | 50 |
| yellow fruits[b] | | 85 | 15 |
| other fruits | | 75 | 25 |
| red palm oil | | 65 | 35 |
| other vegetable oils | | 50 | 50 |

source:   Leung, W.T.W, and M. Flores. 1980. *"Table de composicion de Alimentos para uso en America  Latina"*, INCAP.

[a]e.g., carrots, deep-orange sweet potatoes      [b]e.g., apricots

*foods rich in vitamin A*

Several foods contain vitamin A activity; however relatively few are rich dietary sources, those being green and yellow vegetables[2], liver, oily fishes and vitamin A-fortified products such as margarine. It should be noted that, for vitamin A and other vitamins that are susceptible to breakdown during storage and cooking, values given in food composition tables are probably high estimates of amounts actually encountered in practical circumstances.

[2]It is estimated that carotene from vegetables contribute two-thirds of dietary vitamin A world-wide, and over 80% in developing countries.

Vitamin A activities of foods:

| food | IU/100 g | RE(μg)/100 g |
|---|---|---|
| animal products | | |
| red meats | - | - |
| beef liver | 10,503 | 35,346 |
| poultry meat | 41 | 140 |
| mackerel | 130 | 434 |
| herring | 28 | 94 |
| egg | 552 | 1,839 |
| swiss cheese | 253 | 856 |
| butter | 754 | 3058 |
| | | |
| plant products | | |
| corn | - | - |
| peas | 15 | 149 |
| beans | 171 | 171 |
| chick peas | 7 | 67 |
| lentils | 4 | 39 |
| soybeans | 2 | 24 |
| green peppers | - | 420 |
| red peppers | - | 21,600 |
| carrots | - | 11,000 |
| peach | - | 1,330 |
| pumpkin | - | 1,600 |
| yellow squash | - | - |
| orange sweet potatoes | - | - |
| margarine[a] | 993 | 3,307 |

source:    USDA Handbook 8 series
[a]fortified with vitamin A

# ABSORPTION OF VITAMIN A

*absorption of retinoids and carotenoids*
Most of the pre-formed vitamin A in the diet is in the form of retinyl esters; however, the major sources of vitamin A activity for most populations are the pro-vitamin A carotenoids.  Retinyl esters are hydrolyzed to yield retinol by hydrolases produced from the pancreas[3] or situated on the mucosal brush border.   The retinyl esters as well as the carotenoids, are hydrophobic and thus depend on micellar solubilization for their dispersion in the aqueous environment of the small intestinal lumen.  This process facilitates access of soluble hydrolytic enzymes to their substrates (i.e., the retinyl esters), and provides a means for the subsequent presentation of retinol to the mucosal surface across which free retinol and intact β-carotene diffuse passively into the mucosal epithelial cell.  The overall

---

[3]This appears to be the same enzyme that catalyzes the intraluminal hydrolysis of cholesteryl esters; it is a relatively non-specific carboxylic ester hydrolase. It has been given various names in the literature, the most common being *pancreatic non-specific lipase* and *cholesteryl esterase*.

absorption of vitamin A esters appears to be high (e.g., 80-90%), but this process is necessarily affected by the level and type of dietary fat and protein (which exerts surfactant effects), and by the amount of the vitamin itself (i.e., less efficient absorption occurs at very high vitamin A doses).

*metabolism linked to absorption*

That some carotenoids[4] can be pro-vitamins A is due to their being metabolized to yield retinal. This step involves the cleavage of the polyene moiety by a soluble enzyme, **β-carotene 15,15′-dioxygenase**, found in the intestinal mucosa, liver and corpus luteum. In the case of β-carotene, the products of this enzymatic cleavage are two molecules of retinal; other carotenoids have pro-vitamin A activities only to the extent that they yield retinal by the action of the dioxygenase (this is determined by both the chemical structure of the carotenoid and the efficiency of its enzymatic cleavage). The reaction requires molecular oxygen, which reacts with the two central carbons (C15 and C15′), followed by cleavage of the C-C bond. It is inhibited by sulfhydryl group inhibitors and by chelators of ferrous iron ($Fe^{++}$). The enzyme, sometimes also called the "**carotene cleavage enzyme**", has been found in a wide variety of animal species[5]; enzyme activities were found to be greatest in herbivores (e.g., guinea pig, rabbit), intermediate in omnivores (e.g., chicken, tortoise, fish), and *absent* in the only carnivore studied (cat). The latter finding corresponds to the fact that β-carotene cannot support the vitamin A needs of cats fed diets devoid of the pre-formed vitamin.

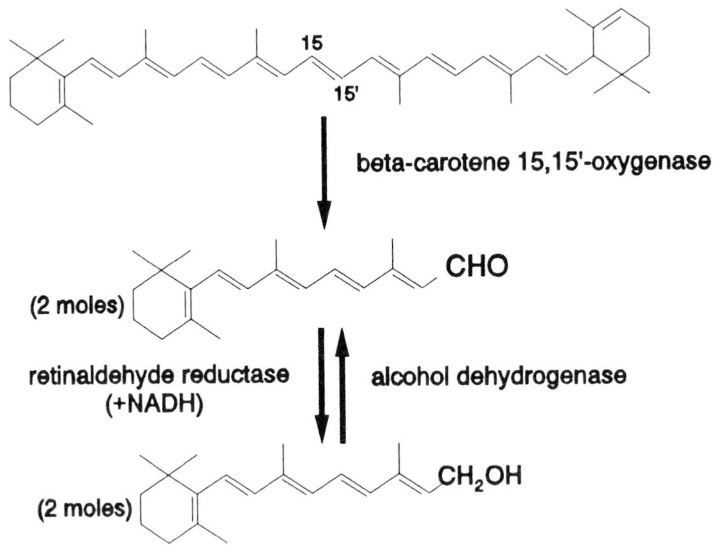

15

15′

beta-carotene 15,15′-oxygenase

CHO

(2 moles)

retinaldehyde reductase (+NADH)          alcohol dehydrogenase

$CH_2OH$

(2 moles)

---

[4] Fewer than 10% of naturally occurring carotenoids are pro-vitamins A.

[5] The β-carotene 15,15′-dioxygenase has also been identified in *Halobacterium halobium* and related halobacteria, which use retinal, coupled with an opsin-like protein, to form bacteriorhodopsin, an energy-generating light-dependent proton pump.

The carotene cleavage activity is highly variable between individuals. In the bovine corpus luteum, which also contains a high amount of $\beta$-carotene, it has been shown to vary with the estrus cycle, showing a maximum on the day of ovulation. Studies with the rat indicate that the activity is stimulated by vitamin A deprivation and reduced by dietary protein restriction. Retinal produced by this cleavage step in the intestinal mucosa is reduced there to retinol by another enzyme, ***retinaldehyde reductase***, which is also found in the liver and eye. The reduction requires a reduced pyridine nucleotide (NADH/NADPH) as a cofactor, and has an apparent $K_m = 20~\mu M$; this step can be catalyzed by ***alcohol dehydrogenase*** and there is some debate concerning whether the two activities reside on the same enzyme.

Retinol, formed either from the hydrolysis of dietary retinyl esters or from the reduction of retinal cleaved from $\beta$-carotene, is quickly re-esterified with long-chain fatty acids in the intestinal mucosa. Thus, vitamin A is transported to the liver mainly (i.e., 80-90% of a retinol dose[6]) in the form of retinyl esters. The composition of lymph retinyl esters is remarkably independent of the fatty acid composition of the most recent meal. ***Retinyl palmitate*** typically comprises about one-half of the total esters, with ***retinyl stearate*** comprising about one-quarter and ***retinyl oleate*** and ***retinyl linoleate*** being present in small amounts.

*re-esterification by two routes* Two pathways for the enzymatic re-esterification of retinol have been identified in the microsomal fraction of the intestinal muscosa. The first, a high-affinity route, involves retinol complexed with a specific binding protein, ***cellular retinol-binding protein (type II)***[7]; it is catalyzed by ***lecithin:retinol acyl-transferase (LRAT)***. The second, a low-affinity route, involves retinol apparently bound non-specifically to cellular proteins; it is catalyzed by ***acyl co-enzyme A:retinol acyl-transferase (ARAT)***.

Intestinal Metabolism of Vitamin A:

$$\beta\text{-carotene} \xrightarrow{\text{dioxygenase}} \text{retinal} \xrightarrow{\text{reductase}} \text{retinol} \xrightarrow{\text{ARAT}} \text{retinyl esters}$$

$$\beta\text{-carotene} \xrightarrow{\text{dioxygenase}} \text{CRBPII-retinal} \xrightarrow{\text{reductase}} \text{CRBPII-retinol} \xrightarrow{\text{LRAT}} \text{retinyl esters}$$

---

[6] Humans fed radiolabeled $\beta$-carotene showed the ability to absorb some of the unchanged compound directly in the lymph, with only 60-70% of the label appearing in the retinyl ester fraction.

[7] CRBP-II is a low molecular weight (15.6 kD) protein with a distribution apparently limited to the enterocyte (mainly of the jejunum), and to fetal and neonatal liver. In enterocytes of the rat, CRBP-II constitutes ca. 1% of the total soluble protein. Like the other retinoid binding proteins, it is thought to have the same general tertiary structure as a class of low-molecular weight proteins that bind hydrophobic ligands (e.g., fatty acids, cholesterol, biliverdin). While crystallographic structures of the retinoid-binding proteins have not been determined to date, the inference by analogy to the other proteins in this class is that they have a multi-stranded $\beta$-sheet that is folded to yield a deep hydrophobic pocket suitable for binding appropriate hydrophobic ligands.

## TRANSPORT OF VITAMIN A

*retinyl esters conveyed by chylomicra in lymph*

Retinyl esters are secreted from the intestinal mucosal cells in the hydrophobic cores of chylomicron particles by way of which absorbed vitamin A is transported to the liver through the lymphatic circulation, ultimately entering the plasma[8] compartment through the thoracic duct. Retinyl esters are almost quantitatively retained in the extrahepatic processing of chylomicra to their remnants; therefore, remnants are richer in vitamin A than chylomicra. Retinyl and cholesteryl esters can undergo exchange reactions between lipoproteins including chylomicra in rabbit and human plasma by virtue of a *cholesteryl ester transfer protein* peculiar to those species[9]. While this kind of lipid transfer between lipoproteins is probably physiologically important in those species, the demonstrable transfer involving chylomicra is unlikely to be a normal physiological process.

The absorption of vitamin A (as well as the other fat-soluble vitamins) is a particular problem in patients with *abetalipoproteinemia*, a rare genetic disease characterized by general lipid malabsorption. These patients lack apo-B and, consequently cannot synthesize any of the apo-B-containing lipoproteins (i.e., LDL, VLDL and chylomicra). Having no chylomicra, they show hypolipidemia and low plasma vitamin A levels; however, when given oral vitamin A supplementation, their plasma levels are normal. While the basis of this response is not clear, it has been suggested that these patients can transport retinol from the absorptive cell via their remaining lipoprotein (HDL), possibly by the portal circulation.

Studies have shown that vitamin A can also be absorbed via a nonlymphatic pathway. Rats with ligated thoracic ducts retain the ability to deposit retinyl esters in their livers. That such animals fed retinyl esters show greater concentrations of retinol in their portal blood than in their aortic blood suggests that, in mammals, the portal system may be an important alternative route of vitamin A absorption when the normal lymphatic pathway is blocked. This phenomenon corresponds to the route of vitamin A absorption in birds, fishes and reptiles which, lacking lymphatic drainage of the intestine, rely strictly upon portal absorption.

---

[8]Upon entering the plasma, chylomicra acquire apolipoproteins C and E from the plasma high-density lipoproteins (HDL). Acquisition of one of these (*apo*-CII) activates lipoprotein lipase at the surface of extrahepatic capillary endothelia, which hydrolyses the core triglycerides, thus, causing them to shrink and transfer surface components (e.g., *apo*-AI, *apo*-AII, some phospholipid) to HDL and fatty acids to serum albumin, and lose *apo*-AIV and fatty acids to the plasma or other tissues. These processes leave a smaller particle called a *chylomicron remnant* which is depleted of triglyceride but relatively enriched in cholesteryl esters, phospholipids and proteins (including *apo*-B and *apo*-E). Chylomicron remnants are almost entirely removed from the circulation by the liver, which takes them up by a rapid, high-affinity receptor-mediated process stimulated by *apo*-E.

[9]This protein has not been found in several other mammalian species examined.

*vitamin A*
*stored in the*
*liver*

Newly absorbed retinyl esters are taken up by the liver in association with chylomicron remnants by receptor-mediated[10] endocytosis on the part of liver ***parenchymal cells***[11]. Within those cells, remnants are degraded by lysosomal enzymes. It appears that intact retinyl esters are taken up and are subsequently hydrolyzed to yield retinol. Retinol can be transferred from the parenchymal cells to ***stellate cells***[12] where it is re-esterified. It is likely that the re-esterification proceeds by a reaction similar to that of the intestinal microsomal acyl CoA:retinol acyltransferase (ARAT). The liver thus serves as the primary storage depot for vitamin A, normally containing more than 90% of the total amount of the vitamin in the body. Most of this (ca. 80%) is stored in stellate cells (which account for only ca. 2% of total liver volume), with the balance stored in parenchymal cells (these two cell types are the only hepatocytes that contain retinyl ester hydrolase activities). Almost all (ca. 95%) of hepatic vitamin A occurs as long-chain retinyl esters, the predominant one being retinyl palmitate. Kinetic studies of vitamin A turnover indicate the presence, in both liver and extrahepatic tissues, of two effective pools (i.e., fast- and slow-turning over pools) of the vitamin. Of rat liver retinoids, 98% were in the slow pool (retinyl esters of stellate cells), with the balance corresponding to the retinyl esters of parenchymal cells.

*retinol*
*conveyed*
*protein-bound*
*in plasma:*

Vitamin A is mobilized as retinol from the liver by hydrolysis of hepatic retinyl esters. This mobilization accounts for ca. 55% of the retinol discharged to the plasma (the balance comes from recycling from extrahepatic tissues). The ***retinyl ester hydrolase*** involved in this process shows extreme variation between individuals[13]. The activity of this enzyme is known to be low in protein-deficient animals, and has been found to be inhibited, at least *in vitro*, by vitamins E and K[14]. Once mobilized from liver stores, retinol is transported to peripheral tissues by means of a specific carrier protein, plasma ***retinol binding protein*** (***RBP***). Human RBP consists of a single polypeptide chain of 182 amino acid residues, with a molecular weight of 21 kD; it has a single binding site for retinol. It is

---

[10]Chylomicron remnants are recognized by high-affinity receptors for their apo-E moiety.

[11]The parenchymal cell is the predominant cell type of the liver, comprising in the rat over 90% of the volume of the organ.

[12]These are also known as *pericytes*, *fat-storing cells*, *interstitial cells*, *lipocytes*, *Ito cells*, or *vitamin A-storing cells*.

[13]In the rat, hepatic retinyl ester hydrolase activities can vary by 50-fold among individual rats and 60-fold among different sections of the same liver.

[14]Each vitamin has been shown to act as a competitive inhibitor of the hydrolase. This effect may explain the observation of impaired hepatic vitamin A mobilization (i.e., increased total hepatic vitamin A and hepatic retinyl esters with decreased hepatic retinol) of animals fed very high levels of vitamin E.

synthesized as a 24 kD **pre-RBP** by parenchymal cells which also convert it to RBP by the co-translational removal of a 3.5 kD polypeptide[15]. The product (*apo*-RBP) is secreted from the liver cell in a 1:1 complex with all-*trans*-retinol (*holo*-RBP). The secretion of RBP from the liver is regulated in part by estrogen levels[16], and by vitamin A status (i.e., liver vitamin A stores) protein, and Zn status; deficiencies of each markedly reduce RBP secretion[17] and, thus, reduce circulating levels of retinol. In healthy human adults, plasma RBP is 40-50 $\mu$g/ml; newborn infants typically have about half that. In the plasma, RBP forms a 1:1 complex with **trans-thyretin**[18] (a tetrameric, 55 kD protein which strongly binds four thyroxine molecules). The formation of the RBP-transthyretin complex appears to reduce the glomerular filtration of RBP and, thus, its renal catabolism[19]. The kidney appears to be the only site of the catabolism of RBP, which turns over rapidly[20,21]. Contrary to previous thinking, recent computer modeling studies indicate that more than half of hepatically released *holo*-RBP comes from *apo*-RBP recycled from RBP-transthyretin complexes.

---

[15]RBPs isolated from several species, including rat, chick, dog, rabbit, cow, monkey and human, have been found to have similar sizes and binding properties.

[16]Seasonally breeding animals show three-fold higher plasma RBP levels in during estrus than in the anestrus phase. Women using oral contraceptive steroid frequently show plasma RBP levels that are greater than normal.

[17]*Apo*-RBP is not secreted from the liver. Vitamin A-deficient animals continue to synthesize *apo*-RBP, but the absence of retinol inhibits its secretion (a small amount of denatured *apo*-RBP is always found in the plasma). Due to this hepatic accumulation of apo-RBP, vitamin A-deficient individuals may show a transient overshooting of normal plasma RBP levels upon vitamin A re-alimentation. Other factors including protein (e.g., protein-calorie malnutrition) and Zn deficiencies can inhibit the synthesis of *apo*-RBP and, thus, reduce the amount of the carrier available for binding retinol and secretion into the plasma. Thus, dietary deficiencies of protein or Zn can reduce plasma retinol (i.e, RBP) concentrations, rendering those parameters not strictly indicative of dietary vitamin A deficiency. Also, because vitamin A deprivation leads to reductions of plasma RBP only after the depletion of hepatic retinyl ester stores (i.e., reduce retinol availability), the use of plasma RBP/retinol as a parameter of nutritional vitamin A status can yield false negative results in cases of vitamin A deprivation of short duration.

[18]previously called *prealbumin*

[19]Studies have shown *holo*-RBP bound to transthyretin to have a half-life in human adult males of 11-16 hours; that of free RBP was only 3.5 hours. These half-lives increase (i.e., turnover decreases) under conditions of severe protein-calorie malnutrition.

[20]For this reason, patients with chronic renal disease show greatly elevated plasma levels of both RBP (which shows a half-life 10-15 fold that of normal) and retinol, while concentrations of transthyretin remain normal.

[21]Turnover studies of RBP and retinol in the liver and plasma suggest that some retinol does indeed recirculate to the liver; however the mechanism of such recycling, perhaps involving transfer to lipoproteins, is unknown.

Percentage distribution of vitamin A in serum of fasted humans:

| fraction | retinol | retinyl palmitate |
|----------|---------|-------------------|
| VLDL | 6 | 71 |
| LDL | 8 | 29 |
| HDL | 9 | - |
| RBP | 77 | - |
| total: | 100 | 100[a] |

[a]This represents only ca. 5% of the total circulating vitamin A.

The retinol ligand of *holo*-RBP is taken into cells *via* specific receptor-mediated binding of RBP.  Apparently, RBP binding facilitates the release of retinol to the target cell;  this is accompanied by an increase in the negative charge of *apo*-RBP which reduces its affinity for transthyretin, which is subsequently lost.  The residual *apo*-RBP is filtered by the kidney where it is degraded.  Thus, plasma *apo*-RBP levels are elevated (by ca. 50%) under conditions of acute renal failure.  Studies have shown that *apo*-RBP can be recycled to the *holo*- form; indeed, injections of *apo*-RBP into rats produced marked (70-164%) elevations in serum retinol levels.  It is thought, therefore, that circulating *apo*-RBP may be a positive feedback signal from peripheral tissues for the hepatic release of retinol, the extent of which response is dependent upon the size of hepatic vitamin A stores.

Retinoic acid is not transported by RBP, but it is normally present in the plasma, albeit at very low concentrations (1-3 ng/ml), tightly bound to albumin.  Because this form of vitamin A appears to be important in cell growth and differentiation, it is presumed that its cellular uptake from serum albumin is very efficient.

*other binding proteins*

Upon entry into the target cell, retinol combines to another carrier, ***cellular retinol-binding protein*** (**CRBP**).  Like RBP in the plasma, this intracellular binding protein is a single polypeptide chain that binds one molecule of all-*trans*-retinol.  Intestinal enterocytes have a CRBP (called "**CRBP type II**") of similar size but distinct from the CRBP of other tissues.  Cells of many tissues also contain ***cellular retinoic acid-binding proteins*** (**CRABP**, **CRABP-II**), a ***cellular retinal-binding protein*** (**CRALBP**), and ***nuclear retinoic acid receptor proteins*** (**RARα and RARβ**).  Other vitamin A-binding proteins, with narrow tissue distributions, have been identified: an ***interphotoreceptor retinol-binding protein*** (**IRBP**) in the retina, retinoic acid-binding proteins of the lumen of the epididymus, and retinol-binding proteins in the uterus of the pregnant sow.  These binding proteins are thought to be involved in the transport of the hydrophobic retinoids within and between cells, and to effect presentation of their retinoid ligands to enzymes.

Vitamin A-binding proteins of animals[22]:

| binding protein | abbrev. | MW (kD) | endogenous ligand | location |
|---|---|---|---|---|
| retinol-BP | RBP | 21 | all-*trans*-retinol | plasma |
| cellular retinol-BP | CRBP | 15.7 | all-*trans*-retinol | cytosol: most tissues except heart, adrenal, and ileum |
| cellular retinol-BP, type II | CRBP(II) | 15.6 | all-*trans*-retinol all-*trans*-retinal | cytosol: enterocytes, fetal and neonatal liver |
| cellular retinal-BP | CRALBP | 36 | 11-*cis*-retinal | cytosol: retina |
| cellular retinoic acid-BP | CRABP | 15.5 | all-*trans*-retinoic acid | cytosol: most tissues except liver, jejunum, and ileum |
| cellular retinoic acid-BP, type II | CRABP(II) | 15 | all-*trans*-retinoic acid | cytosol: embryo limb bud |
| epididymal retinoic acid-BP 1,2 | EBP 1,2 | 18.5 | all-*trans*-retinoic acid | lumen of epididymus |
| uterine retinol-BP | - | 22 | all-*trans*-retinol | cytosol: uterus (sow) |
| interphotoreceptor retinol-BP | IRBP | 135 | all-*trans*-retinol 11-*cis*-retinol | retinal interphotoreceptor space |
| nuclear retinoic acid receptors | RARα,β | 50 | all-*trans*-retinoic acid | nucleus: most tissues except adult liver |
| opsin | - | 41 | 11-*cis*-retinal | cytosol: retina |

*transport roles of binding proteins*    The intracellular vitamin A-binding proteins appear to be important in the intracellular and transcellular transport of various vitamin A metabolites. Both **CRBP** and **CRABP** have been shown to serve as carriers of their ligands (retinol and retinoic acid, respectively) from the cytoplasm into the nucleus where the latter are transferred to the chromatin such that the binding proteins are released, possibly to return to the cytoplasm.

In addition, the CRBP appears to have more specialized transport functions in certain tissues. In the liver, CRBP concentrations increase with the retinyl ester contents, suggesting that the binding protein may function in the transport of retinol from parenchymal cells into the stellate cells which store retinyl esters. Specific and rich localization of CRBP has been identified in endothelial cells of the brain microvasculature, in cuboidal cells of the choroid plexus, in the Sertoli cells of the testis, and in the pigment epithelium of the retina. Because these tight-junctioned cells also have surface receptors for the plasma *holo*-RBP-transthyretin complex, it is thought that their abundant CRBP concentrations are involved in the transport of retinal across the blood-brain, blood-testis and retinal blood-pigment epithelium barriers.

---

[22] Retinal-binding proteins (*bacterioopsin, haloopsin, P575, P370 and "slow-cycling rhodopsin"*) have been identified in bacteria. Each has structural similarities, but no significant sequence homology, to the vitamin A-dependent visual pigment opsin.

The *CRBP(II)* appears to be restricted largely to the enterocytes of the small intestine (particularly, jejunum)[23]. Its abundance in mature enterocytes, where it comprises 1% of the total soluble protein, as well as the absence of CRBP in those cells, suggest that CRBP(II) is involved in enteric absorption of vitamin A, presumably by transporting it across the cell.

Some retinoid-binding proteins found extracellularly are believed to serve similar transport functions. These include two low molecular weight retinoic acid-binding proteins generally related to RBP and are secreted into the lumen of the epididymus; they (the *EBPs*) are thought to participate in the delivery of all-*trans*-retinoic acid to sperm in that organ, which also contain a particularly abundant supply of CRBP[24]. Other retinol-binding proteins are synthesized in the uterine endometrium and secreted into the uterus; these show some sequence homology with RBP, but are slightly larger. They are thought to be involved in the transport of retinol to the fetus. The IRBP of the retinal interphotoreceptor space is thought to function in the transport of retinol between the pigment epithelium and photoreceptor cells. It is synthesized by the latter, in which its mRNA has been detected. Unlike the other retinoid-binding proteins, the IRBP is a large (135 kD) glycoprotein; it binds 6 moles of fatty acid in addition to 2 moles of retinol. It has been suggested that its relatively low affinity for retinol, in comparison to the other retinol-binding proteins, facilitates rapid high-volume transport of that ligand along a series of IRBPs. That IRBP is involved in the visual process, perhaps by delivering the chromophore, is indicated by the finding that its binding specificity shifts from mainly 11-*cis*-retinol to mostly all-*trans*-retinol as eyes are more completely light-adapted[25].

---

[23]Ong and colleagues have identified in hepatic parenchymal cells of fetal and newborn rats both CRBP (II), as well as a high-capacity esterase that esterifies retinol bound to CRBP (II). After birth, CRBP(II) appears to be replace by CRBP, such that mature animals show none of the former binding protein in that organ. The presence of CRBP (II) in fetal liver corresponds to the increased concentration of retinyl palmitate in that organ at birth. They have found that CRBP (II) and CRBP have ca. 50% sequence homology.

[24]The initial segment of the epididymus contains the greatest concentration of CRBP found in any tissue.

[25]IRBP is also found in another photosensitive organ, the pineal gland.

## METABOLISM OF VITAMIN A

*fates of*     The metabolism of vitamin A centers around the transport form, retinol, and
*retinol*      the various routes of conversion available to it: ***esterification***, ***conjugation***,
               ***oxidation*** and ***isomerization***.

*esterification*   As discussed above (see p. 125), retinol is esterified in the cells of the
                   intestine and most other tissues *via* enzymes of the endoplasmic reticulum
                   which use acyl groups from either phosphatidylcholine (***lecithin-retinol***
                   ***acyl-transferase, LRAT***) or acylated coenzyme A (***acyl CoA:retinol acyl-***
                   ***transferase, ARAT***).   These systems show marked specificities for
                   saturated fatty acids, in particular, palmitic acid; thus, the most abundant
                   product is ***retinyl palmitate***.

*conjugation*   Retinol may also be conjugated in either of two ways.  The first entails the
                reaction catalyzed by ***retinol-UDP-glucuronidase***, present in the liver and
                probably other tissues, which yields ***retinyl β-glucuronide***, a metabolite
                that is excreted in the bile[26].  The second path of conjugation involves the
                ATP-dependent phosphorylation to yield ***retinyl phosphate*** catalyzed by
                ***retinol phosphorylase***.  That product, in the presence of guanosine-
                diphosphomannose (GDP-man) can be converted to the glycoside ***retinyl***

---

[26]About 30% of the retinyl β-glucuronide excreted in the bile is reabsorbed from the intestine and is
recycled in an enterohepatic circulation back to the liver.  For this reason, it was originally thought to be an
excretory form of the vitamin.  That view has changed with the findings that retinyl β-glucuronide is biologically
active in supporting growth and tissue differentiation, and that it is formed in many extrahepatic tissues.

*phosphomannose*, which can transfer its sugar moiety to glycoprotein receptors.  However, because only a small amount of retinol appears to undergo phosphorylation *in vivo*, the physiological significance of this pathway is not clear.

*oxidation*

Retinol can also be reversibly oxidized to *retinal* by NADH- or NADPH-dependent *retinol dehydrogenase*[27].  This activity is found in many tissues, the greatest being in the testis[28].  Retinal can be *irreversibly* oxidized by *retinal oxidase* to *retinoic acid*.  The rate of that reaction is several fold greater than that of retinol dehydrogenase; that, plus the fact that the rate of reduction of retinal back to retinol is also relatively great, results in retinal being present at very low concentrations in tissues.

*fates of retinoic acid*

Once retinoic acid is formed from retinol, it is converted to forms that are readily excreted.

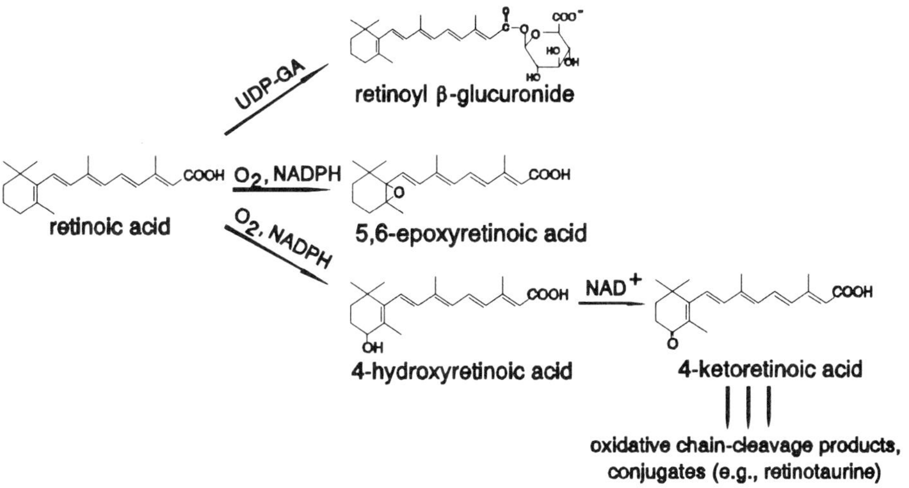

retinoyl β-glucuronide

retinoic acid

5,6-epoxyretinoic acid

4-hydroxyretinoic acid

4-ketoretinoic acid

oxidative chain-cleavage products, conjugates (e.g., retinotaurine)

Retinoic acid can be *conjugated* by glucuronidation in the intestine, liver and possibly other tissues to *retinoyl β-glucuronide*.  Alternatively, it can be catabolized by further *oxidization* to several excretory end products including several oxidative chain-cleavage metabolites that are conjugated

---

[27]There is some debate as to whether this is actually an activity of *alcohol dehydrogenase*, which can catalyze the reaction.  The latter enzyme is known to be Zn-dependent, and nutritional deprivation of Zn appears to impair the utilization of vitamin A.  However, the crude activity from rat testis shows only weak inhibition by a large excess of ethanol, suggesting the presence of *specific* retinol dehydrogenases.

[28]Curiously, male rats fed retinoic acid instead of retinol become aspermatogenic and experience testicular atrophy.  It has been proposed that retinoic acid is, indeed, required for spermatogenesis, but that in cannot cross the blood-testis barrier; this hypothesis is further supported by the fact that the rat testis is also rich in CRABP.

with glucuronic acid, taurine[29], or other polar molecules. It should be noted that both the production and catabolism of retinoic acid involve uni-directional processes; therefore, while the reduced forms of vitamin A (retinol, retinyl esters, retinal) can be converted *in vivo* to retinoic acid, the latter cannot be converted to any of the reduced forms.

*isomerizations*  Interconversion of the most common all-*trans*- forms of vitamin A and various *cis*- forms occurs in the eye and is a key aspect of the visual function of the vitamin, as the conformational change caused by the isomerization alters the binding affinity of retinal for the visual pigment protein opsin. In the eye, light induces the conversion of 11-*cis*-retinal to all-*trans*-retinal; the conversion back to the 11-*cis*- form is catalyzed by the enzyme **retinal isomerase**, which also catalyzes the analogous isomeriza-tion (in both directions) of 11-*cis*- and all-*trans*-retinol. Some isomers (e.g., 13-*cis*-) tend to be isomerized to the all-*trans*- form more rapidly than others.

all-trans-retinal                    11-cis-retinal

*role of binding proteins in vitamin A metabolism*  The finding that the esterification of retinol (by LRAT) occurs while the substrate is bound to CRBP or CRBP (II), stimulated Ong and Chytil to suggest that at least some of the retinoid binding proteins may have impor-tant functions in the enzymatic reactions of the intermediary metabolism of vitamin A. They proposed that substrate accessibility for at least some of the retinoid-metabolizing enzymes is determined by characteristics of their binding protein complexes. This appears to be the case for CRBP: its abundance in the liver and its high affinity for retinol suggest that its presence directs the esterification of the retinoid ligand to the reaction catalyzed by LRAT, rather than that catalyzed by ARAT, which can only use free retinol. It also appears to be the case for CRBP (II), which, unlike CRBP, can bind both retinol *and* retinal. In fact, only when retinal is bound to CRBP (II) can the reducing enzyme retinal reductase use it as substrate; in addition, the binding of retinol or retinal to CRBP (II) greatly reduces the reverse reaction (oxidation to retinal). Thus, by facilitating retinal formation and inhibiting its loss, CRBP (II) seems to direct the retinoid to the appropriate enzymes which sequentially convert retinal to the esterified form in which it is exported from the enterocyte. The preferential binding of 11-*cis*-retinal by CRALBP and not CRBP, appears to be another example of compartmentalization directing the ligand to its appropriate enzyme, i.e., a microsomal NAD-dependent retinal reductase in the pigment epithelium of the retina which uses only the carrier-bound substrate.

---

[29]Significant amount of retinotaurine are excreted in the bile.

*excretion of*
*vitamin A*

Vitamin A is excreted in various forms in both the urine and feces. Under normal physiological conditions, the efficiency of enteric absorption of vitamin A in high (i.e., 80-95%), with 30-60% of the absorbed amount being deposited in esterified form in the liver. The balance of absorbed vitamin A is catabolized (mainly at C4 of the ring and C15 at the end of the side chain[30]) and is released in the bile or plasma, where they are removed by the kidney and excreted in the urine (i.e., short-chain, oxidized, conjugated products). About 30% of the biliary metabolites (i.e., retinoyl $\beta$-glucuronides) are reabsorbed from the intestine in an enterohepatic circulation back to the liver, but most are excreted in the feces with unabsorbed dietary vitamin A. In general, vitamin A metabolites with intact carbon chains are excreted in the feces, whereas, the chain-shortened, acidic metabolites are excreted in the urine. The relative amounts of vitamin A metabolites in the urine and feces, thus, vary with vitamin A intake (i.e., at high intakes fecal excretion may be twice that of the urine) and the hepatic vitamin A reserve (i.e., when reserves are above the low-normal level of 20 $\mu g/g$, both urinary and fecal excretion varies with the amount of vitamin A in the liver).

## *METABOLIC FUNCTIONS OF VITAMIN A*

*vitamin A in*
*vision*

The best elucidated function of vitamin A is in the visual process where, as 11-*cis*-retinal, it serves as the photosensitive chromophoric group of the visual pigments of rod and cone cells of the retina. Rod cells contain the pigment ***rhodopsin***; cone cells contain one of three possible ***iodopsins***. In each case, 11-*cis*-retinal is bound (*via* formation of a Schiff's base) to a specific lysyl residue of the respective protein (collectively referred to as *"opsins"*).

etc.

(opsin)

The visual functions of rhodopsin and the iodopsins differ only with respect to their properties of light absorbency[31], which are conferred by the different opsins involved. In each, photo-reception is effected by the rapid,

---

[30]The chain terminal carbon atoms (C14 and C15) can be oxidized to $CO_2$; retinoic acid is oxidized to $CO_2$ to a somewhat greater extent than retinol.

[31]The absorbance maxima of the pigments from the human retina are: rhodopsin (rods), 498 nm; iodopsin (blue cones), 420 nm; iodopsin (green cones), 534 nm; iodopsin (red cones), 563 nm.

light-induced isomerization of 11-*cis*-retinal to the all-*trans*-form. That product, present as a protonated Schiff base of a specific lysyl residue of the protein, produces a highly strained conformation. This results in the dissociation of the retinoid from the opsin complex. This process (*"bleaching"*) is a complex series of reactions, involving progression of the pigment through a series of unstable intermediates of differing conformations[32] and, ultimately, to *N-retinylidene opsin* which dissociates to all-*trans*-retinal and opsin.

The dissociation of all-*trans*-retinal and opsin is coupled nervous stimulation of the vision centers of the brain. The bleaching of rhodopsin causes the closing of $Na^+$ channels in the rod outer segment, thus, leading to hyperpolarization of the membrane. This change in membrane potential is transmitted as a nervous impulse along the optic neurons. This response appears to be stimulated by the reaction of an unstable *"activated"* form on rhodopsin, *metarhodopsin II*, which reacts with *transducin*, a membrane-bound G-protein of the rod outer segment discs. This results in the binding of the transducin *a*-subunit with *cGMP phosphodiesterase*, which activates the latter to catalyze the hydrolysis of cGMP to GMP. Because cGMP maintains $Na^+$ channel of the rod plasma membrane in the open state, the resulting decrease in its concentration causes a marked reduction in $Na^+$ influx. This results in hyperpolarization of the membrane and the generation of a nerve impulse through the synaptic terminal of the rod cell.

---

[32]The conformation of *rhodopsin* is changed to yield a transient photopigment, *bathorhodopsin*, which, in turn, is converted sequentially to *lumirhodopsin*, *metarhodopsin I*, and (by deprotonation) *metarhodopsin II*.

The visual process is a cyclic one, in that its constituents are regenerated. All-*trans*-retinal can be converted enzymatically in the dark back to the 11-*cis* form. After bleaching, all-*trans*-retinal is rapidly reduced to all-*trans*-retinol, which is isomerized to the 11-*cis* form in the *rod outer segment*. Retinol is then transferred (presumably *via* **IRBP**) into the retinal pigment epithelial cells where it is esterified (again, predominantly with palmitic acid) and stored in the bulk lipid of those cells. The regeneration of rhodopsin, which occurs in the dark-adapted eye, involves the hydrolysis of retinyl esters to yield retinol which is transferred (probably *via* IRBP) into the rod outer segment where it is oxidized to 11-*cis*-retinal, which can then react with an opsin-lysyl residue. Nervous recovery is effected by the GTPase activity of the transducin *α*-subunit which, by hydrolyzing GTP to GDP, causes the re-association of transducin subunits and, hence, the loss of its activating effect on cGMP phosphodiesterase. Metarhodopsin II is also removed by phosphorylation to a form incapable of activating transducin, and by dissociation to yield opsin and all-*trans*-retinal.

*"systemic" functions incompletely understood*

Though they are much less well understood, the extra-retinal functions of vitamin A are clearly of *greater* physiological impact than the visual function. Collectively, these are called the *"systemic"* functions of the vitamin; more specifically, they include roles in the differentiation and growth of epithelial cells and on growth in general. While deprivation of vitamin A disrupts the visual cycle resulting in impaired dark adaptation (*night blindness*, or *nyctalopia*), the disruption of the *"systemic"* functions of the vitamin are far more severe and often life-threatening (e.g., corneal destruction, infection, stunted growth).

> *Vitamin A-deficient animals die, but not from lack of visual pigments.*

That the biochemical bases of the systemic functions of vitamin A are quite different from that of the visual function is evidenced by the fact that the visual function employs retinal exclusively, whereas the systemic functions are effectively supported by **retinoic acid**. Because retinol can be oxidized metabolically to retinal and, then, to retinoic acid, either of the reduced forms of the vitamin can support *both* the visual and systemic functions. However, because the oxidation of retinal to retinoic acid is *irreversible*, retinoic acid can support *only* the systemic functions. Animals fed diets containing retinoic acid as the sole source of vitamin A grow normally and appear healthy in every way except that they go blind.

*role in cell differentiation*

Vitamin A has a clearly vital role in the **differentiation of epithelial cells**. It is well documented that vitamin A-deficient individuals (humans or animals) experience replacement of normal mucus-secreting cells by cells that produce keratin, particularly in the conjunctiva and cornea of the eye, the trachea, the skin and other ectodermal tissues. Less severe effects are also produced in tissues of mesodermal or endodermal origin. It appears that retinoids affecting cell differentiation through actions analogous to those of the steroid hormones, i.e., that they bind to the nuclear chromatin to signal transcriptional processes. In fact, studies have revealed that the differentiation of cultured cells can be stimulated by exposure to retinoids, and that abnormal mRNA species are produced by cells cultured in vitamin A-deficient media[33]. Further, retinoic acid has been found to stimulate, synergistically with thyroid hormone, the production of growth hormone in cultured pituitary cells.

That vitamin A plays such a role in cell differentiation has been supported by the recent discovery of a family of nuclear receptors for steroid hormones, $1,25-(OH)_2$-vitamin $D_3$, thyroid hormone $(T_3)$ and retinoic acid, which appear to have similar ligand-binding and DNA-binding regions and substantial sequence homology. The receptor-ligand complexes of two of these which bind retinoic acid ("RARα", "RARβ") have been shown to bind to the promoter region of specific genes, thus, activating their transcription. Both receptors and their respective mRNAs have been found in most tissues[34]. The RARs have been found to bind both the gene element responsive to RAR, as well as the one responsive to thyroxine, suggesting that retinoic acid and thyroid hormone control overlapping networks of genes. Many proteins are known to appear during retinoic acid-induced cell differentiation. Of these, it is established that three are, indeed, induced by the activation by RAR-binding: *growth hormone* (in cultured pituitary cells), the protein *laminin* (in mouse embryo cells), and the *RARs*. The latter finding indicates autoregulation, i.e., retinoic acid induces its own receptor (RAR). In fact, the induction of RARs appears to be differentially selective among various tissues; retinoic acid has been found to induce mainly RARα in hemopoietic cells, but RARβ in other tissues.

The morphogenic role of retinoic acid in embryonic tissues appears to be effected by the establishment of concentration gradients of RARβ due to the differential induction of the receptor by the retinoid[35]. Studies have found that CRABP-mRNA is not transcribed in tissues expressing the RAR-mRNAs, suggesting that CRABP is involved in regulating differentiation by

---

[33] Epidermal keratinocytes cultured in a vitamin A-deficient medium made keratins of higher molecular weight than those made by vitamin A-treated controls; this shift toward larger keratins was corrected by treatment with vitamin A. Different mRNA species were identified, which coded for the different proteins produced under each condition.

[34] Greatest concentrations have been found in adrenals, hippocampus, cerebellum, hypothalamus and testis.

[35] Indeed, the mRNAs of three RARs (α, β and γ) have been found to appear at different times in limb development in mouse embryos. The expression of one of these, RARβ, has been proposed to be associated with the programming of cell death, as in the developing mouse embryonic limb its mRNA has been found only in interdigital mesenchymal cells at the time of digit separation.

controlling available free retinoic acid. Recent evidence indicates that, in addition to retinoic acid, the morphogenic role of vitamin A may also be discharged by one of its metabolites, **all-*trans*-3,4-didehydroretinoic acid**. That compound has been shown to be produced by differentiating epithelial cells of the chick embryonic central nervous system[36], which also respond to treatment with the compound. It appears, therefore, that vitamin A effects cell differentiation thought the actions of two morphogens, all-*trans*-retinoic acid and its oxidation product all-*trans*-didehydroretinoic acid as well as at least three nuclear receptors.

It has also been proposed that vitamin A has a co-enzyme-like role as a sugar carrier in the synthesis of glycoproteins, which function on the surfaces of cells to effect intercellular adhesion, aggregation, recognition and other interactions. This hypothesis is supported by the findings that retinol can be phosphorylated to give **retinyl phosphate** that will accept **mannose** from its carrier **GDP-mannose** (to form **retinyl phospho-mannose**) and donate it to a membrane-resident acceptor for the production of glycoproteins. Further, vitamin A-deficient animals show general diminution of glycoprotein synthesis (particularly in plasma, intestinal goblet cells, and corneal and trachea epithelial cells) with the production of abnormal glycoproteins.

While changes in the glycan moieties of glycoproteins can certainly have great effects on cell functions, the actual physiologic significance of this sugar carrier role of vitamin A is not as clear for the reason that the form that supports the *"systemic"* functions of vitamin A, retinoic acid, cannot serve as a sugar carrier because it cannot be reduced to form retinol. Further, retinoyl phosphate does not accept mannose. This problem has not been resolved; however, it has been proposed that retinoic acid may actually be hydroxylated *in vivo* to a derivative capable of being phosphorylated and, thus, serving as a sugar carrier.

*role in reproduction*    Vitamin A is necessary for reproduction, but the biochemical basis of this function is not known. It is apparent, however, that this role is different from the *"systemic"* one, as maintenance of reproduction is discharged by retinol and *not* retinoic acid, at least in mammals[37]. For example, rats maintained with retinoic acid grow well and appear healthy, but lose reproductive ability, i.e., males show impaired spermatogenesis and females abort and resorb their fetuses. Injection of retinol into the testis restores spermatogenesis, indicating that vitamin A has a direct role in that organ. It has been proposed that these effects are secondary to lesions in cellular differentiation and/or hormonal sensitivity.

---

[36]*"Floor plate"* cells, i.e., epithelial cells at the ventral midline, derived from cells of *"Hensen's node"*.

[37]In the chicken, retinoic acid supports normal spermatogenesis, but in all mammalian species examined this function is supported only by retinol or retinal.

*role in*
*immunity*

Vitamin A is clearly important in supporting immunocompetence, although the nature of its role in this process is also not clear. Vitamin A-deficient animals and humans are typically more susceptible to infection than are individuals of adequate vitamin A nutriture. Epidemiologic studies have found that low vitamin A status is frequently associated with increased disease incidence and mortality rates. A large longitudinal study of preschool children in Indonesia revealed that the overall mortality rate in children with xerophthalmia was four times that of children with no ocular lesions. Further, mortality increased with increasing severity of the eye disease, with xerophthalmic children having a rate nine times that of normal children. Further, active infection appears to alter the utilization or, at least, the distribution of vitamin A among tissues; plasma retinol concentrations have been found to drop during malarial attacks in children, and the manifestation of ocular signs of xerophthalmia has been documented in children following outbreaks of measles. That such insults on vitamin A status are of clinical significance is indicated by the results of intervention studies that have shown treatment with vitamin A to greatly reduce the case fatality rate in measles and respiratory diseases[38].

Vitamin A deficiency appears to affect immunity in several ways[39]. It is thought, at present, that retinoids and carotenoids affect the immune system differently. Retinoids seem to act on the differentiation of immune cells, increasing mitogenesis of lymphocytes and phagocytosis of monocytes and macrophages. Carotenoids seem to affect immunosurveillance of activated NK cells and T-helper cells by modifying the release of at least some cytokine-like products by activated lymphocytes and monocytes.

*role in*
*bone*

Vitamin A has an essential role in the normal metabolism of bone; however, this role is not at all understood at a mechanistic level. What is clear is that vitamin A affects osteoclasts, which are reduced in vitamin A deficiency, resulting in excessive deposition of periosteal bone by the apparently unchecked function of osteoblasts. This effect is associated with a reduction in the degradation of glycosaminoglycans.

*role in*
*cancer*

Because vitamin A deficiency characteristically results in a failure of differentiation of epithelial cells without impairment of proliferation (i.e., the keratinizing of epithelia), it has been reasonable to question the possible role of the vitamin in the etiology of epithelial cell tumors, i.e., carcinomas. The squamous metaplastic changes seen in vitamin A deficiency are morphologically similar to pre-cancerous lesions induced experimentally. From this theoretical basis, studies with animal tumor models have found vitamin

---

[38]Of course, the first line of defense against such diseases as measles should be immunologic.

[39]In practice, it is difficult to ascribe such effects simply to the lack of vitamin A for the reason that individuals showing nutritional vitamin A deficiency generally also have protein-calorie malnutrition which, itself, leads to impaired immune function.

A deficiency to enhance susceptibility to chemical carcinogenesis and large doses of vitamin A (i.e., supranutritional levels) to inhibit carcinogenesis in some models.  On the basis of these findings, it was proposed that retinol can be anti-carcinogenic by competing at high levels in the cell, with carcinogens to prevent expression of malignant phenotypes and, thus, reinforce expression of the normal one.  However, the fact that high doses of vitamin A serve best to increase only the hepatic stores of retinyl esters rather than retinol concentrations in target extrahepatic tissues, retinoic acid and, later, other retinoids were examined in animal tumor models.

Studies with retinoic acid indicated that it, too, could reduce to some extent some kinds of tumors in animals and humans.  While the use of retinoic acid, which is rapidly degraded and eliminated from the body, avoids the problem of chronic hyper-vitaminosis, its substantial toxicity makes it unsuitable for regular clinical use.  Therefore, more than 1500 retinoids have been synthesized and tested for potential anti-carcino-genicity[40].  A number of these[41] have been found to effectively inhibit experimentally induced tumors in several organs of animals, and have yielded hopeful results in clinical trials.  Several have also been shown to inhibit the induction of *ornithine decarboxylase*, an enzyme the induction of which appears to be essential in the development of neoplasia.  The consensus, however, is that while retinoids currently available can delay tumorigenesis, they cannot do so at doses that are not, themselves, toxic.

Epidemiological investigations of vitamin A intake and human cancer have produced results that support the plausibility of the hypothesis that low vitamin A status may increase cancer risk[42].  Among the problems that usually attend epidemiologic studies have been the variable and often imprecise ways of reporting the dietary intakes of vitamin A in free-living people.  The results of these surveys have fostered many hypotheses, including the proposal that *β-carotene* may have some beneficial effect *unrelated* to its role as a pre-vitamin A.  While this hypothesis has been seized by some as though it were a fact, it has also been the subject of much debate.  Supporting evidence comes from still-limited findings of tumor inhibition by β-carotene in animal models, and from the demonstration that β-carotene can function as an antioxidant perhaps analogously to vitamin E.  Nevertheless, the correlations on which the hypothesis was based make it possible (perhaps even probable) that β-carotene as

---

[40] These compounds are formal derivatives of retinal differing by changes in the isoprenoid side-chain (including modification of the polar end and cyclization of the polyene structure), or modifications of the cyclic head group (including replacement with other ring systems).

[41] e.g., 13-*cis*-retinoic acid, N-ethylretinamide, N-(2-hydroxyethl)-retinamide, N-(4-hydroxyphenyl)-retinamide, etretinate, N-(pivaloyloxyphenyl)-retinamide, N-(2,3-dihydroxypropyl)-retinamide.

[42] See review by Peto, R., R. Doll, J.D. Buckley and M.B. Sporn. 1981. Nature 290:201.

*role in*
*dermatology*

assessed in those epidemiological studies was actually a proxy variable for some other factor(s) related to causality[43]. In addition, two facts weaken that argument: the antioxidant activity of $\beta$-carotene is much weaker than that of vitamin E (which is more abundant in tissues); its antioxidant activity appears to be greatest at low oxygen tension.

Due to their similarities to changes observed in vitamin A-deficient animals, certain dermatologic disorders of keratinization (e.g., ichthyosis, Darier's disease, pityriasis, rubra pilaris) have been treated with large doses of vitamin A. Clinical success rates of such treatments generally appear to be variable, and the high doses of the vitamin needed for efficacy commonly produce unacceptable side effects. Therefore, the synthetic retinoids have commanded attention in the hope of finding therapeutically effective compounds of low toxicity. Of these, the most effective ones have been 13-*cis*-retinoic acid[44] and etretinate[45]. The most successful of these has been 13-*cis*-retinoic acid for the treatment of acne in which it dramatically reduces sebum production. However, it is also teratogenic and, as acne patients will include women of child-bearing age, the compound must be used with strict medical supervision. Vitamin A appears to have a role in the normal health of the skin. Vitamin A (and carotenoids) are typically found in greater concentrations in the subcutis than in the plasma (significant amounts are also found in the dermis and epidermis), indicating the uptake of retinol from plasma RBP. Vitamin A deficiency not only affects the terminal differentiation of human keratinocytes (as mentioned above) and causes the skin to be thick, dry and scaly, but it also results in obstruction and enlargement of the hair follicles[46].

Functional forms of vitamin A:

| function | active form(s) |
| --- | --- |
| transport | retinol |
| storage | retinyl esters |
| vision | retinal |
| "systemic" | retinoic acid, didehydroretinoic acid? |
| reproduction | retinol (mammals); retinoic acid (birds) |
| other (immunity, bone, etc.) | retinol? |

---

[43]For example, $\beta$-carotene may be a proxy for any of several other constituents of foods including but not limited to the non-$\beta$-carotenoids; accordingly, many studies show the apparent inverse effect on cancer incidence to be greater for total fruits and vegetables than for $\beta$-carotene.

[44]13-*cis*-retinoic acid is effective in the treatment of ichthyosis, pityriasis rubra pilaris, Darier's disease and keratosis palmaris et plantaris, and acne vulgaris.

[45]An aromatic analog of retinoic acid effective in the treatment of Darier's disease and psoriasis.

[46]i.e., follicular hyperkeratosis; this condition can also be caused by deficiencies of niacin and vitamin A.

## EXTREMES IN VITAMIN A INTAKE

*vitamin A*
*deficiency*

The appreciable storage of vitamin A in the body tends to mitigate against the effects of low dietary intakes of the vitamin, as tissue stores are mobilized when conditions of low vitamin A demand. However, because there are two effective pools of vitamin A in the body, the rate of mobilization varies between tissues according to their respective proportions of fast- and slow-turning over pools. For this reason, rats showed faster losses of vitamin A from intestine than liver (71% vs. 53%) after being fed a vitamin A-deficient diet. It should be noted that, while hepatic stores are great enough to provide retinol, plasma retinol level is only minimally affected by vitamin A deprivation (e.g., in the same experiment, it decreased by only 8%). Cellular functions of vitamin A can be expected to change only *after* transport of the vitamin is reduced, i.e., after vitamin A stores have dropped to such levels as to reduce plasma retinol-RBP concentrations.

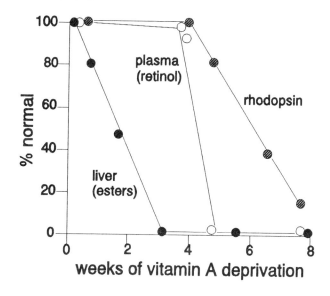

Vitamin A appears to function in a variety of ways in many organs of the body. Therefore, the consequences of vitamin A deficiency include many non-specific signs. In fact, the only unequivocal signs of vitamin A deficiency are the ocular lesions, **nyctalopia** and **xerophthalmia**. The former retinal disorder responds rapidly to vitamin A treatment, whereas the latter disorder of the anterior segment of the eye involves permanent morphological changes that are not correctable without scarring. Early intervention is, however, very important in cases of xerophthalmia in order to interrupt the progressive lesions in early stages before permanent blindness occurs.

Signs of vitamin A deficiency:

| organ system | sign |
|---|---|
| general | loss of appetite, retarded growth, drying and keratinization of membranes, infection, death |
| dermatologic | rough scaly skin, rough hair/feathers |
| muscular | weakness |
| skeletal | periosteal overgrowth, restriction of cranial cavity and spinal cord, narrowing of foramina |
| vital organs | nephritis |
| nervous system | increased cerebrospinal fluid pressure, ataxia, constricted optic nerve at foramina |
| reproduction | aspermatogenesis, vaginal cornification, fetal death and resorption |
| ocular | nyctalopia, xerophthalmia, keratomalacia, constriction of optic nerve |

Stages of xerophthalmia in vitamin A deficiency:

| stage | signs |
|---|---|
| 1. xerosis | dryness of conjunctiva<br>Bitot's spots°<br>ultimate extension to cornea |
| 2. keratomalacia | softening of cornea<br>ultimate involvement of iris/lens<br>secondary infection |

°lusterless, gray-white, foamy, greasy, *"cheesy"* deposits on the conjunctiva near the cornea; the secretion contains fatty degenerated epithelial cells and leukocytes. There is some question about the relation of this sign, which can also occur in vitamin A-adequate individuals, to the deficiency.

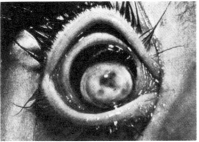
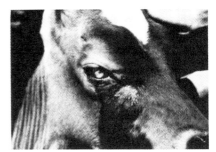

Keratomalacia in a vitamin A-deficient child (courtesy D.S. McLaren, American University of Beirut)

Vitamin A-deficient calf: blind with copious lacrimation (courtesy J.K. Loosli, University of Florida)

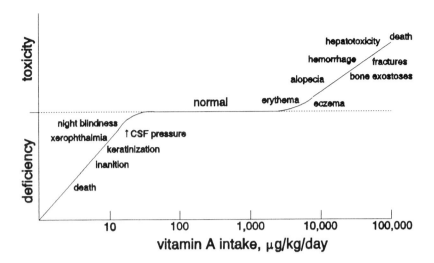

*hyper-*
*vitaminosis*

The hepatic storage of vitamin A tends to mitigate against the development of intoxication due to intakes in excess of physiological needs.  However, persistent large overdoses (more than 1000-times nutritionally required amounts) can exceed the capacities of liver to store and catabolize and will, thus, produce intoxication.  This is marked by the appearance in the plasma of high levels of retinyl esters which, because they are associated with lipoproteins rather than RBP, are outside of the normal strict control of vitamin A transport to extrahepatic tissues.  Two other aspects of vitamin A metabolism tend to protect against hypervitaminosis: relatively inefficient conversion of the pro-vitamins A in the gut, and the unidirectional oxidation of the vitamin to a form (retinoic acid) that is rapidly catabolized and excreted.  Signs of hypervitaminosis A are usually reversed upon cessation of exposure.  In humans, these effects are manifest mainly in the skin and mucous membranes.  Animals frequently show bone abnormalities that apparently result from changes in osteoclastic and osteoblastic activities.  Congenital malformations in animals and humans have been associated with maternal overexposure to the vitamin.  Because retinol has potent membranolytic activity, it has been proposed that disruption of cellular and subcellular membranes, with the consequent release of lysosomal enzymes, may be involved in these lesions.

Signs of hypervitaminosis A:

| organ affected | signs |
| --- | --- |
| general | muscle and joint pains, headache |
| skin | erythema, desquamation, alopecia |
| mucous membranes | cheilitis, stomatitis, conjunctivitis |
| liver | dysfunction |
| skeletal | thinning and fracture of long bones |

## CASE STUDY

*Instructions:*  *Review each of the following case reports paying special attention to the diagnostic indicators upon which the respective treatments were based. Then answer the questions that follow.*

case 1  The physical examination of a 5-month-old boy with severe **marasmus**[47] showed extreme wasting, apathy and ocular changes: in the left eye, **Bitot's spots**, and conjunctival and corneal **xerosis**; in the right eye, corneal liquefaction and **keratomalacia** with subsequent prolapse of the iris, extrusion of lens and loss of vitreous humor. The child was 65 cm tall and weighed 4.5 kg. His malnutrition had begun at cessation of breast-feeding at 4 months, after which he experienced weight loss and diarrhea.

Laboratory results:

| parameter | patient | normal range |
|---|---|---|
| Hb (hemoglobin) | 10.7 g/dl | 12-16 g/dl |
| HCT (hematocrit) | 36 ml/dl | 35-47 mg/dl |
| WBC (white blood cells) | 15,000/$\mu$l | 5,000-9,000/$\mu$l |
| serum protein | 5.6 g/dl | 6-8 g/dl |
| serum albumin | 2.49 g/dl | 3.5-5.5 g/dl |
| plasma Na | 139 mEq/l | 136-145 mEq/l |
| plasma K | 3.5 mEq/l | 3.5-5.0 mEq/l |
| blood glucose | 70 mg/dl | 60-100 mg/dl |
| total bilirubin | 1.1 mg/dl | <1 mg/dl |
| serum retinol | 5.5 $\mu$g/dl | 30-60 $\mu$g/dl |
| serum $\beta$-carotene | 10.7 $\mu$g/dl | 50-250 $\mu$g/dl |
| serum vitamin E | 220 $\mu$g/dl | 500-1,500 $\mu$g/dl |

The child had an infection, showing otitis media[48] and *salmonella* septicemia[49], which responded to antibiotic treatment in the first week. The patient was given by nasogastric tube an aqueous dispersion of **retinyl palmitate** (with a non-ionic detergent) at the rate of 3,000 $\mu$g/kg per day for 4 days. This increased his plasma retinol concentration from 5 $\mu$g/dl to 35 $\mu$g/dl by the second day at which level it was maintained for the next 12 days. The child responded to general nutritional rehabilitation with a high-protein, high-energy formula which was followed by whole milk supplemented with solid foods. He recovered, but was permanently blind in the right eye and was left with a mild corneal opacity in the left eye. He returned to his family after 10 weeks of hospitalization.

---

[47] extreme emaciation or general atrophy, occurring especially in young children, due to extreme undernutrition, primarily, lack of energy and protein.

[48] inflammation of the middle ear

[49] presence in the blood of pathogenic, gram-negative, rod-shaped bacteria of the genus *Salmonella*

*case 2*

An obese 15-year-old girl, 152 cm tall and weighing 100 kg, was admitted to the hospital for partial jejuno-ileal bypass surgery for morbid obesity. She had past history of obsessive eating that had not been correctable by diet. Except for massive obesity, her physical examination was negative.

Initial laboratory results:

| parameter | patient | normal range |
|---|---|---|
| Hb | 14 g/dl | 12-15 g/dl |
| RBC | $4.5 \times 10^6/\mu l$ | $4-5 \times 10^6/\mu l$ |
| WBC | $8,000/\mu l$ | $5,000-9,000/\mu l$ |
| serum retinol | 38 $\mu g$/dl | 30-60 $\mu g$/dl |
| serum β-carotene | 12 $\mu g$/dl | 50-300 $\mu g$/dl |
| serum vitamin E | 580 $\mu g$/dl | 500-1,500 $\mu g$/dl |
| serum 25-OH-$D_3$ | 11 ng/dl | 8-40 ng/dl |

Serum electrolytes, Ca, P, triglycerides, cholesterol, total protein, albumin, total bilirubin, Fe, TBIC (total serum Fe-binding capacity), Cu, Zn, folic acid, thiamin and vitamin $B_{12}$ were within the normal ranges.

The patient encountered few post-operative complications except for mild bouts of diarrhea and some fatigue. Over the next year, she lost 45 kg of body weight while ingesting a liberal diet. She reported having 3-4 stools daily, but denied having any objectionable diarrhea or changes in stool appearance. Two years after surgery, she noted the onset of inflammatory horny lesions above her knees and elbows, and she experienced some difficulty in seeing at dusk. The skin lesions failed to respond to topical corticosteroids and oral antihistamine therapy. Because of intensification of these signs, she sought the medical help; however, the cause was not determined.

She was readmitted to the hospital complaining of her skin disorder and night blindness. At that time, she showed evidence of mild liver dysfunction and her serum concentrations of retinol and β-carotene were 16 $\mu g$/dl and 14 $\mu g$/dl, respectively. Her fecal fat was 70 g per day (normal: <7g per day). Biopsies of the skin of her left thigh and right upper arm each showed hyperkeratosis and horny plugging of dilated follicles. She was treated with 15,000 $\mu g$ of retinyl palmitate given orally three times daily for six months. By one month, the follicular hyperkeratosis had cleared and healed with residual pigmentation. By two months, the night blindness had subsided. At that time her serum retinol concentration was 54 $\mu g$/dl, β-carotene was 7 $\mu g$/dl, α-tocopherol was 1.6 $\mu g$/ml, and urinary $^{57}$Co-$B_{12}$ was 6.7% (normal: 7-8%). She has been well on a daily oral supplement of 1,500 $\mu g$ of retinyl palmitate.

*case 3*

A 41-year-old man was housed on a metabolic ward for two years during a clinical investigation of vitamin A deficiency. He weighed 77.3 kg and was healthy by standard criteria (history, physical examination and laboratory studies). For 505 days, he was fed a casein-based formula diet that contained <10 μg of vitamin A per day. His initial plasma retinol concentration was 58 μg/dl, and his body vitamin A pool, determined by isotope dilution, was 766 mg (10 mg/kg). At the end of one year, his plasma retinol had declined to 25 μg/dl and he began to show follicular hyperkeratosis. On the 300th day his plasma retinol was 20 μg/dl, and he showed a mild anemia (Hb = 12.6 mg/dl). Two months later, by which time his plasma retinol had dropped to 10 μg/dl, he developed night blindness evidenced by changes in dark adaption and electroretinogram. When his plasma retinol reached 3 μg/dl, his body vitamin A pool was 377 mg and repletion with vitamin A was begun with increasing doses starting with 150 μg and increasing to 1,200 μg retinol per day over a 145-day period. After receiving 150 μg retinol per day for 82 days, his night blindness was partially repaired, but his skin keratinization remained and his plasma retinol level was only 8 μg/dl. Then, after receiving 300 μg retinol per day for 42 days, his follicular hyperkeratosis resolved and his plasma retinol level was 20 μg/dl. At the 600 μg retinol per day level, his plasma retinol was in the normal range and all signs of vitamin A deficiency disappeared.

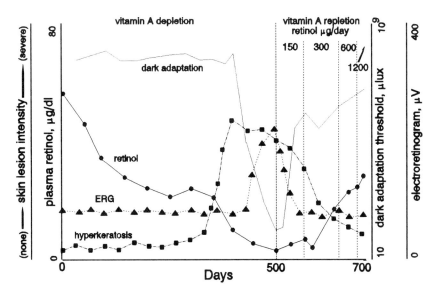

*Questions:*    *i.*    For each case, what signs/symptoms indicated vitamin A deficiency?

               *ii.*    Propose hypotheses to explain why the patients of cases 1 and 2, each responded to oral vitamin A treatment even though they had very different medical conditions. Outline tests of those hypothesis.

               *iii.*   Comment on the value of serum retinol concentration for the diagnosis of nutritional vitamin A status.

## Study Questions and Exercises:

i.     Discuss how the *absorption, transport, tissue distribution* and *intracellular activities* of vitamin A *relate* to the **concept** of solubility.

ii.     Construct a **flow diagram** showing vitamin A, in its various forms, as it passes from ingested food, through the body where it functions in its various physiologic roles, and ultimately to its routes of elimination.

iii.     Construct a **"decision tree"** for the diagnosis of vitamin A deficiency in a human or animal.

iv.     *Night blindness* is particularly prevalent among alcoholics.  Propose an **hypothesis** for the metabolic basis of this phenomenon and outline an experimental approach to **test** it.

## Recommended Reading:

Baurenfeind, J.C. (ed.). 1986. Vitamin A Deficiency and Its Control. Academic Press, New York. 530 pp.

Bendich, A., and L. Langseth. 1989. Safety of Vitamin A. Am. J. Clin. Nutr. 49:358-371.

Chytil, F., and D.E. Ong. 1984. Cellular Retinoid-Binding Proteins, Chapter 9 in The Retinoids (J.C. Baurenfeind, ed.), Academic Press, New York, pp. 89-123.

Friedrich, W. 1988. Vitamin A and Its Provitamins. Chapter 2 in Vitamins. Walter de Gruyter, New York. pp. 65-140.

Frolick, C.A. 1984. Metabolism of Retinoids, Chapter 11 in The Retinoids (J.C. Baurenfeind, ed.), Academic Press, New York, pp. 177-208.

Goodman, D.S. 1984. Plasma Retinol-Binding Proteins, Chapter 8 in The Retinoids (J.C. Baurenfeind, ed.), Academic Press, New York, pp. 41-87.

Hathcock, J.N., D.G. Hattin, M.Y. Jenkins, J.T. McDonald, P.R. Sundarsan and V.L. Wilkening. 1990. Evaluation of vitamin A toxicity. Am. J. Clin. Nutr. 52:183-202.

Lippman, S.M. and F.L. Meyskens, Jr. 1989. Retinoids for the Prevention of Cancer. Chapter 9 in Nutrition and Cancer Prevention (T.E. Moon and M.S. Miccozzi, eds.). Marcel Dekker, New York, pp. 243-272.

Olson, J.A. 1991. Vitamin A, Chapter 1 in Handbook of Vitamins, 2nd edition (L.J. Machlin, ed.), Marcel Dekker, New York, pp.1-57.

## Recommended Reading (continued):

Pitt, G.A.J. 1985. Vitamin A, Chapter 1 in Fat-Soluble Vitamins (A.T. Diplock, ed.). Technomic Publ. Co., Basel, pp. 1-75.

Prabhala, R.H., H.S. Garewal, F.L. Meyskens, Jr., and R.R. Watson. 1990. Immunomodulation in humans caused by beta-carotene and vitamin A. Nutr. Res. 10:1473-1486.

Roberts, A.B., and M.B. Sporn. 1984. Cellular Biology and Biochemistry of the Retinoids, Chapter 12 in The Retinoids (J.C. Baurenfeind, ed.), Academic Press, New York, pp. 209-280.

Temple, N.J. and T.K. Basu. 1988. Does beta-carotene prevent cancer? A critical appraisal. Nutr. Rev. 8:685-701.

Tompkins, A., and G. Hussey. 1989. Vitamin A, Immunity and Infection. Nutr. Res. Rev. 2:17-28. Underwood, B.A. 1990. Vitamin A prophylaxis programs in developing countries: past experiences and future prospects. Nutr. Rev. 48:265-274.

West, Jr., K.P., G.R. Howard and A. Sommer. 1989. Vitamin A and Infection: Public Health Implications. Ann. Rev. Nutr. 9:63-86.

Willett, W.C., 1990. Vitamin A and Lung Cancer. Nutr. Rev. 48:201-211.

Wolf, G. 1991. The intracellular vitamin A-binding proteins: an overview of their functions. Nutr. Rev. 49:1-12.

Zeigler, R.G. 1989. A review of the epidemiological evidence that carotenoids reduce the risk of cancer. J. Nutr. 119:116-122.

# CHAPTER 6  *VITAMIN D*

*"By following the reasoning that vitamin D is not required in the diet under conditions of adequate ultraviolet irradiation of skin and that it is the precursor of a hormone, it is likely that the vitamin is not truly a vitamin but must be regarded as a pro-hormone. These arguments, however, are only semantic; the fact remains the vitamin D is taken in the diet and is an extremely potent substance which prevents a deficiency disease."*

H.F. DeLuca

## Anchoring Concepts:

| | |
|---|---|
| *i.* | Vitamin D is the generic descriptor for **steroids** exhibiting qualitatively the biological activity of cholecalciferol (i.e., vitamin $D_3$). |
| *ii.* | Most vitamers D are **hydrophobic** and, thus, are insoluble in aqueous environments (e.g., plasma, interstitial fluids, cytosol). |
| *iii.* | Vitamin D is *not* required in the diets of animals or humans adequately exposed to sources of **ultraviolet light** (e.g., sunlight). |
| *iv.* | Deficiencies of vitamin D lead to structural lesions of **bone**. |

## Learning Objectives:

| | |
|---|---|
| *i.* | To understand the nature of the various **sources** of vitamin D. |
| *ii.* | To understand the means of **endogenous production** of vitamin D. |
| *iii.* | To understand the means of **enteric absorption** of vitamin D. |
| *iv.* | To understand the **metabolism** involved in the **activation** of vitamin D to its functional forms. |
| *v.* | To understand the role of vitamin D and other endocrine factors in **calcium homeostasis**. |
| *vi.* | To understand the physiologic implications of **high doses** of vitamin D. |

## Vocabulary:

CaBP
cage layer fatigue
calbindin
calcinosis
calcitonin
carcinomedin
cholecalciferol
DBP
7-dehydrocholesterol
diuresis
ergocalciferol
ergosterol
genu varum
hypercalcemia
hyperphosphatemia
hypocalcemia
hypoparathyroidism
hypophosphatemia
1,25-$(OH)_2$-vitamin D
24,25-$(OH)_2$-vitamin D
25,25,26-$(OH)_3$-vitamin D
25-OH-vitamin D
25-OH-vitamin D 1-hydroxylase

osteoblast
osteocalcin
osteoclast
osteomalacia
osteoporosis
parathyroid gland
parathyroid hormone (PTH)
previtamin D
privational rickets
privational osteomalacia
prolactin
pro-vitamin $D_2$
pro-vitamin $D_3$
pseudofracture
pseudohypoparathyroidism
rickets
tibial dyschondroplasia
transcalciferin
varus deformity
vitamin D 25-hydroxylase
vitamin D-dependent rickets
vitamin D-dependent osteomalacia

## *SOURCES OF VITAMIN D*

*distribution*
*in foods*

Vitamin D, as either ***ergocalciferol*** (vitamin $D_2$) or ***cholecalciferol*** (vitamin $D_3$), is rather sparsely represented in nature; however, its pro-vitamins are common is both plants and animals.  Ergocalciferol and its pro-vitamin D form ***ergosterol*** are found in plants, fungi[1], molds, lichens and some invertebrates (e.g., snails and worms).  In fact, some microorganisms are quite rich in ergosterol, in which it may comprise as much as 10% of the total dry matter[2].  Ergosterol does not occur naturally in higher vertebrates, but it can be present adventitiously in low amounts in tissues of those species.  The actual distribution of ergocalciferol in nature is much more limited and variable than that of ergosterol (e.g., grass hays and alfalfa contain vitamin D only after they have been cut and left to dry in the sun).  While vitamin $D_2$ is, thus, probably only present in small amounts from natural sources, it has been the major synthetic form used in animal and human nutrition for four decades.

Cholecalciferol is widely distributed in animals, in which its pro-vitamin D form ***7-dehydrocholesterol*** is a normal metabolite, but has an extremely limited distribution in plants.  In animals, tissue cholecalciferol concentrations are dependent upon the vitamin D content of the diet and/or the exposure to sunlight.  Fish liver and oils[3] are particularly rich sources of vitamin $D_3$, which occurs in those materials in free form as well as esters of long-chain fatty acid esters.  With a few notable exceptions, vitamin $D_3$ is not found in plants.  Those exceptions include the species[4] *Solanum glaucophyllum*, *Solanum malacoxylon*, *Cestrum diurnum* and *Trisetum flavescens* in which vitamin D occurs as water-soluble $\beta$-glycosides of vitamin $D_3$, 25-OH-vitamin $D_3$ and $1,25(OH)_2$-vitamin $D_3$[5].

Because most foods contain only very low amounts of vitamin D, it has become the practice in many countries to fortify certain common and frequently consumed foods (e.g., baked goods, grain products, milk and

---

[1] Ergosterol was named for the parasitic fungus, ergot, from which the sterol was first isolated.

[2] Pro-vitamin $D_2$ accounts for virtually all of the sterols in *Aspergillus niger* and 80% of those in *Saccharomyces cerevisiae* (i.e., brewer's yeast).

[3] Fish oils typically have vitamin $D_3$ concentrations of ca. 50 $\mu$g/g, but tuna or mackerel oils can contain 20-fold that level.

[4] Consumption of these plants has been associated with calcinosis in grazing ruminants; this observation was the basis of the discovery that they contained vitamin D.

[5] Both vitamin $D_3$-25-hydroxylase and 25-OH-vitamin $D_3$-1-hydroxylase activities have been found in *S. malacoxylon*, indicating that its ability to metabolize vitamin D is similar to that of higher animals.

milk products, infant foods) to prevent rickets. Both vitamin $D_2$ and vitamin $D_3$ are used in the fortification of foods. Other foods are enriched indirectly as the result of the supplementation of animal feeds with the vitamin.

*biosynthesis of vitamin $D_3$ by animals*

Vitamin D is formed in animals by the action of ultraviolet light (285-315 nm) on **7-dehydrocholesterol** in the skin. The activation reaction depends upon the absorption of UV light by the $\Delta^{5\text{-}7}$-double bond system in the B ring of the sterol nucleus, and involves the opening of that ring in the formation of **pre-vitamin $D_3$**, which is in thermal equilibrium with vitamin $D_3$. This physio-chemical reaction appears to convert only 5-15% of the available 7-dehydrocholesterol to vitamin $D_3$[6]. That efficiency is affected by the physical properties of the skin and of the environment; it, thus, differs between individuals and species, and shows great variation according to time of day, season and latitude.

The pro-vitamin D sterol, 7-dehydrocholesterol, is both a precursor to and product of cholesterol (*via* different pathways); it is synthesized in the sebaceous glands of the skin and it is secreted rather uniformly on to the surface where it is re-absorbed into the various layers of the epidermis. Thus, the skin contains very high concentrations of the sterol (e.g., 200-fold that of liver). The distribution of 7-dehydrocholesterol in the epidermis varies according to its penetration from the surface. In humans, greatest concentrations are found in the deeper *Malpighian layer*; whereas, in the rat it is distributed more superficially in the *stratum corneum*. In consequence of such a difference in pro-vitamin $D_3$ distribution, the rat can undergo the photo-production in the stratrum corneum itself, while this reaction in humans occurs deeper and is, therefore, subject to the loss of

---

[6]Excess irradiation does little to increase the efficiency of this activation step. Instead, it increases the photo-production of biologically inactive forms, e.g., lumisterol₃, tachysterol₃ and 5,6-*trans*-vitamin $D_3$.

UV due to absorption by the stratum corneum layer. In fact, the thickness of that layer is a primary determinant of its transmission of UV light; the stratum corneum of black human skin is thicker than that of white human skin and transmits only ca. 40% of the UV light of the latter.

Physical factors that reduce the exposure of the skin to UV light also reduce the biosynthesis of vitamin D. These include factors associated with lifestyle of humans (e.g., clothing, indoor living, use of sun screens) and practical management of livestock (e.g., confined indoor housing). In addition, variations in environmental exposure to UV light result in corresponding variations in vitamin D biosynthesis. Vitamin D-producing UV irradiation is greatest at noon (60% occurs between 10 am and 2 pm), reaches an annual peak at mid-summer, and declines with the distance from the earth's equator (e.g., in winter there is almost no UV light at latitudes above 50°[7]). These factors interact to result in substantial variation in vitamin D biosynthesis among people and animals. For many individuals the aggregate effect of these factors is to render a need for exogenous (dietary) vitamin D.

## ABSORPTION OF VITAMIN D

micelle-
dependent
passive
diffusion

Vitamin D is absorbed from the small intestine by non-saturable passive diffusion that is dependent upon micellar solubilization and, hence, the presence of bile salts. The fastest absorption appears to be in the upper portions of the small intestine (i.e., the duodenum and ileum) but, due to the longer transit time of food in the distal portion of the small intestine, the greatest amount of vitamin D absorption probably occurs there. Like other hydrophobic substances absorbed by micelle-dependent passive diffusion in mammals, vitamin D enters the lymphatic circulation[8] predominantly (ca. 90% of the total amount absorbed) in association with chylomicra with most of the balance being associated with the $\alpha$-globulin fraction[9]. The efficiency of this absorption process for vitamin D appears to be ca. 50%.

---

[7] i.e., that of Winnipeg, Frankfurt, Prague and Kiev

[8] In birds, reptiles and fishes vitamin D, like other lipids, is absorbed into the portal circulation via portomicra.

[9] This is probably identical to the carrier, vitamin D-binding protein (DBP), in the plasma.

Vitamin D activities in foods:

| food | | vitamin D, I.U.*/100 g |
|---|---|---|
| animal products | | |
| dairy products: | butter | 35 |
| | cheese | 12 |
| | cream | 50 |
| eggs | | 28 |
| fish products: | cod | 85 |
| | cod liver oil | 10,000 |
| | herring | 330 |
| | herring liver oil | 140,000 |
| | mackerel | 120 |
| | salmon | 220-440 |
| | sardines | 1,500 |
| | shrimp | 150 |
| liver: | beef | 8-40 |
| | chicken | 50-65 |
| | pork | 40 |
| milk (100 ml): | cow | .3-4 |
| | human | 0-10 |
| meats: | beef | 13 |
| | pork | 84 |
| | poultry | 80 |
| | poultry skin | 900 |
| plant products | | |
| cabbage | | 0.2 |
| corn oil | | 9 |
| spinach | | 0.2 |

*1 I.U. = .025 $\mu$g vitamin $D_2$ or vitamin $D_3$

## TRANSPORT OF VITAMIN D

*transfer from chylomicra to binding protein*  Almost all absorbed vitamin D is retained in non-esterified form which is thought to be associated with the chylomicron surface for the reason that a portion of it can be transferred from that lipoprotein particle to a binding protein in the plasma either directly or during the process of chylomicron degradation. Vitamin D which is not transferred in the plasma is taken up with chylomicra remnants by the liver where it is transferred to the same binding protein and released to the plasma.

Like other steroids, vitamin D is transported in the plasma strictly in association with protein. In most of the species surveyed[10], (i.e., the bony fishes, all amphibians and reptiles, most birds and mammals), the carrier is a protein in the $\alpha$- or, occasionally, $\beta$-globulin families; this has been called *"transcalciferin"* and, more commonly, *"DBP"* (vitamin D-

---

[10] At least 140 different species in five classes have been examined.

binding protein).  Some birds and mammals transport vitamin D in association with serum albumin, and fishes with cartilaginous skeletons (e.g., sharks and rays) transport it in association with plasma lipoproteins.  The DBP of mammals is a single 55 kD protein which binds stoichiometrically vitamins $D_2$ and $D_3$, and their metabolites; but the chicken has *two* distinct DBPs (54 kD and 60 kD) each of which binds vitamin $D_3$ and its metabolites preferentially to vitamin $D_2$ and its metabolites.  Human DBP shows genetic polymorphism[11] due to differences in both the primary structure of the protein and the carbohydrate moiety that is added after translation.  That no person, in a large survey[12], was found to lack plasma DBP suggests that it must, indeed, have a critical metabolic function.

Studies of DBP from humans and rats reveal it to be a monomeric glycoprotein that depends on the *cis*-triene structure and C3-hydroxyl group of the vitamin for binding.  It binds both vitamin D[13] and its hydroxylated metabolites, but shows a markedly greater affinity to 25-OH-D than any of the other forms.  The concentration of DBP in the plasma is greatly in excess of that of 25-OH-D (e.g., 9 $\mu$M *vs.* 50 nM) and is remarkably constant, being unaffected by sex, age or vitamin D status.  Being synthesized by the liver, however, it is depressed in patients with hepatic disease; in addition, it is increased during estrogen therapy or pregnancy.  It does not appear to cross the placenta; fetal DBP is immunologically distinct from the maternal protein.  The effect of having in the plasma an excess of DBP is that, in individuals of normal vitamin D status, less than 5% of the available binding sites are occupied by vitamin D compounds.  Because its binding affinity for 25-OH-D is very high, that metabolite accumulates in the plasma rather than other tissues[14]; however, the protein-binding in the plasma results in a regulation of the free metabolite at very low levels.  In contrast, DBP levels are correlated with the plasma concentrations of 1,25-$(OH)_2$-D. The effect is similar, in that increasing plasma levels of that metabolite are accommodated by increased protein binding, maintaining very low circulating concentrations of the free form of this metabolite also[15].

---

[11]In humans, DBP is identical with group-specific component ($G_c$ protein), a genetic marker of use in population studies and forensic medicine.

[12]More than 80,000 individuals were examined.

[13]The use of the letter D without a subscript is meant to indicate *either* vitamin $D_2$ or vitamin $D_3$.

[14]DBP also has a high affinity for actin, the reasons for which are unclear.  (The formation of this complex can interfere with the assay of 25-OH-D-1-hydroxylase in kidney homogenates.) It is likely, however, that the interaction of DBP with this widely distributed cellular protein may be the basis of reports of an intracellular 25-OH-D-binding protein.

[15]This may be a very important aspect of the function of DBP, i.e., in regulating the availability to cells of 1,25-$(OH)_2$-D, which appears to be the most metabolically active as well as toxic metabolite.

In addition to facilitating the peripheral distribution of vitamin D from dietary origin, DBP functions to mobilize the vitamin produced endogenously in the skin. Indeed, vitamin $D_3$ is found in the skin bound to DBP[16]. It has been suggested that the efficiency of endogenously produced vitamin $D_3$ is greater than that given orally for the reason that the former enters the circulation strictly via DBP, whereas the latter enters as complexes of DBP as well as chylomicra. This would indicate that oral vitamin D remains longer in the liver and is, thus, more quickly catabolized to excretory forms. In support of this hypothesis, it has been noted that high oral doses of vitamin D can lead to very high levels of 25-OH-D ($>400$ ng/ml) associated with intoxication; whereas, intensive UV-irradiation can rarely produce plasma 25-OH-$D_3$ concentrations greater than one-fifth that level, and that hypervitaminosis D has never been reported from excessive irradiation.

Distribution of vitamin D metabolites in human plasma:

| metabolite | percentage distribution | | | normal |
|---|---|---|---|---|
| | DBP | lipoprotein | albumin | concentration |
| vitamin $D_3$ | 60 | 40 | 0 | 2-4 ng/ml |
| 25-OH-$D_3$ | 98 | 2 | 0 | 15-38 ng/ml |
| 24,25-$(OH)_2$-$D_3$ | 98 | 2 | 0 | - |
| 1,25-$(OH)_2$-$D_3$ | 62 | 15 | 23 | 20-40 pg/ml |

*tissue distribution*

Unlike the other fat-soluble vitamins, vitamin D is *not* stored by the liver[17], but is distributed relatively evenly among the various tissues where it resides in the lipid phases. Therefore, fatty tissues such as adipose show slightly greater concentrations. However, in that tissue the vitamin is found in the bulk lipid phase from which it is only slowly mobilized. About half of the total vitamin D in the tissues occurs as the parent vitamin $D_3$ species, with the next most abundant form, 25-OH-$D_3$ accounting for ca. 20% of the total. In the plasma, however, the latter metabolite predominates by several fold[18,19]. Tissues including those of the kidneys, liver, lungs, aorta and heart also tend to accumulate 25-OH-$D_3$[20]. It is thought that the uneven tissue distribution of vitamin D, in its various forms, relates to differences in both tissue lipid contents as well as tissue-associated

---

[16] DBP has practically no affinity for lumisterol$_3$ or tachysterol$_3$; therefore, these forms produced under conditions of excessive irradiation are not well mobilized from the skin.

[17] The high concentrations of vitamin D found in the livers of some fishes are important exceptions.

[18] The next most abundant form is 24,25-$(OH)_2$-vitamin D.

[19] The plasma concentrations of 25-OH-$D_3$ and 24,25-$(OH)$-$D_3$ of free-living persons vary seasonally, showing maxima in the summer months and minima in the winter. In contrast, plasma levels of 1,25-$(OH)$-$D_3$ are rather constant, indicating an effective regulatory mechanism for that metabolite.

[20] These organs are also prone to calcification in hypervitaminosis D.

vitamin D-binding proteins, the latter fraction being the smaller of the two intracellular pools of the vitamin.

*intracellular*
*receptor*

In contrast to 25-OH-D, the further hydroxylated metabolite 1,25-$(OH)_2$-D is distributed largely intracellularly where, like other steroid hormones, it is present exclusively in the nucleus and cytoplasm bound to a specific protein. Using the terminology of endocrinology, this binding protein is usually referred to as the **1,25-(OH)_2-D-receptor**. Intracellular 1,25-$(OH)_2$-D-receptors have been identified in a wide variety of organs in mammals and birds[21], and in fishes and amphibians[22], as well as in tumors, suggesting that 1,25-$(OH)_2$-vitamin D functions in those tissues. Its function in the intestinal cell is associated with the induction of the synthesis of **calcium-binding proteins** (**CaBP**); in that tissue the concentration of the receptor is surprisingly low, i.e., fewer than 2000 binding sites per cell. In neonates, the intestinal receptor is absent until weaning, being induced upon the feeding of solid foods, by a process that apparently involves cortisol. In at least some organs the receptor appears to be inducible by estrogen treatment and affected by vitamin C status[23].

The 1,25-$(OH)_2$-D-receptor is a 60 kD sulfhydryl protein that binds 1,25-$(OH)_2$-vitamin D with high affinity, utilizing the three hydroxyl groups of the ligand. That the receptor-ligand complex is less readily extractable from the nucleus than the free receptor suggests that binding to 1,25-$(OH)_2$-vitamin D causes a conformational change in the protein which increases its affinity for DNA. It is thought that, after the manner of the other steroid hormone receptors, the intracellular vitamin D-receptor mediates the effect of 1,25-$(OH)_2$-vitamin D in initiating the translational processes involved in the biosynthesis of CaBP and, perhaps, other proteins. Indeed, there is a high correlation between the receptor and CaBP levels in tissues.

*nuclear*
*localization*

Studies have revealed that 1,25-$(OH)_2$-vitamin D is localized in the nucleus not only in the target tissues of classical action of vitamin D (bone, kidney, intestine) but also in other tissues (placenta, parathyroid, pancreatic islets, gastric endocrine cells, certain cells of the brain). In all of these cases, the presence of the vitamin corresponds to that of its receptor. The finding of both 1,25-$(OH)_2$-vitamin D and its receptor in a wide variety of tissues, including several not involved in calcium homeostasis, strongly indicates that the active vitamer must have additional functions.

---

[21] e.g., bones, colon, kidney, mammary gland, ovary, pancreas, parathyroid gland, pituitary, placenta, skin, shell gland, small intestine, testes, thymus, uterus.

[22] e.g., brain, intestine, liver

[23] Guinea pig intestinal 1,25$(OH)_2$-$D_3$-receptors (occupied and unoccupied) were reduced by vitamin C deprivation. Whether this finding relates to the rickets-like bone changes observed in vitamin C-deficient guinea pigs and humans is not clear.

## METABOLISM OF VITAMIN D

*metabolic*
*activation*

The metabolism of vitamin D (i.e., cholecalciferol/ergocalciferol) involves its conversions to a variety of hydroxylated products each of which is more polar than the hydrophobic parent[24]. The discovery of these metabolites, some of which are the actual metabolically active forms of the vitamin, explain the lag time that is commonly observed between the administration of vitamin $D_3$ and the earliest biological response. The metabolism of vitamin D, therefore, includes reactions that effect the metabolic activation of the ingested or endogenously produced vitamin.

*conversion to*
*25-OH-D*

Most of the vitamin D taken up by the liver from either DBP or lipoproteins is converted by hydroxylation of side-chain carbon C25 to yield 25-OH-D[25], which is the major circulating form of the vitamin. This reaction is catalyzed by an enzyme activity limited to the liver in mammals but occurring in both liver and kidney in birds. That activity, **vitamin D-25-hydroxylase**, involves cytochrome $P_{450}$-dependent mixed-function oxygenases[26] of two types: a low affinity, high capacity enzyme associated with the endoplasmic reticulum; a high affinity, low capacity enzyme located in the mitochondria[27]. The 25-hydroxylase activity appears to be only poorly regulated, that by the hepatic concentration of vitamin D, with little or no inhibition by 25-OH-vitamin D. It is increased by inducers of cytochrome $P_{450}$ (phenobarbital, diphenylhydantoin)[28], and is inhibited by isoniazid[29]. The product, 25-OH-D, is not retained in the cell, but is released to the plasma where it accumulates by the binding with DBP. At normal plasma concentrations of this metabolite, only small amounts of 25-OH-D are released from this pool to enter tissues. Therefore, the circulating level of 25-OH-D is a good indicator of vitamin D status.

---

[24]In fact, it was the finding in the late 1960s of radioactive peaks migrating ahead (more polar) of vitamin D in gel filtration of plasma from animals given radiolabeled cholecalciferol that first evidenced the conversion of vitamin D to other species, some of which have subsequently been found to be the metabolically active forms of the vitamin.

[25]Also called "calcidiol".

[26]i.e., an oxygenase that uses molecular oxygen ($O_2$) but incorporates only one oxygen atom into the substrate; a mono-oxygenase

[27]The utility of having two different enzymes to catalyze this hydroxylation would appear to be in having highly efficient reactions under both deficient and excessive conditions of vitamin D status.

[28]Anti-epileptic agents such as these reduce the half-life if vitamin D apparently *via* enhancing its conversion to 25-OH-D and other hydroxylated products.

[29]This appears to be the basis for the development of bone disease among patients on long-term isoniazid therapy.

*conversion to* | The initial hydroxylation product of vitamin D (25-OH-vitamin D) is further
*1,25-(OH)₂-D* | hydroxylated at the C1 position of the A-ring to yield $1,25\text{-}(OH)_2$-vitamin

$D^{30}$. This reaction is catalyzed by **25-OH-vitamin D 1-hydroxylase**, which is located primarily in renal cortical mitochondria[31]. The 1-hydroxylase uses $NADPH_2$ as the electron donor and has three constituent proteins: ferridoxin reductase, ferridoxin, and cytrochrome $P_{450}$. The activity is widely distributed among animal species, being found in all but two of 28 species surveyed, with highest activities in rachitic chicks.

Regulation of the vitamin D endocrine system is effected by tight control of the activity of the 1-hydroxylase by several factors: $1,25\text{-}(OH)_2$-D, **parathyroid hormone** (PTH), **calcitonin** (CT), several other hormones[32], as well as circulating levels of $Ca^{++}$ and phosphate. The hormones PTH and CT appear to stimulate different 1-hydroxylase enzymes, the effect of the former being rapid and mediated by cAMP, while the effect of the latter being relatively slow, apparently acting at the level of transcription[33]. The 1-hydroxylase is inhibited by strontium and is feedback-inhibited by $1,25\text{-}(OH)_2$-vitamin $D^{34}$. It is stimulated by prolactin, hypocalcemia (which elicits PTH secretion by the parathyroid gland), and hypophosphatemia (which acts independently of PTH). Thus, when circulating levels of $1,25\text{-}(OH)_2$-D are low, the renal production of $1,25\text{-}(OH)_2$-D are high; when circulating levels of that metabolite are high, its synthesis in the kidney is low. These factors combine, in some cases (PTH and CT) additively, to effect tight regulation of the hydroxylase activity resulting in the maintenance of nearly constant plasma concentrations of $1,25\text{-}(OH)_2$-vitamin D. Reports of the formation of $1,25\text{-}(OH)_2$-vitamin D in anephric rats and humans, and in human patients with chronic renal insufficiency, suggest that the 25-OH-vitamin D 1-hydroxylase might also occur in extrarenal tissues. Hydroxylase activities have been confirmed in placenta and in cultured cell lines (skin, bone, embryonic intestine, calvarial cells).

---

[30] Also called *"calcitriol"*.

[31] Although 25-OH-vitamin D 1-hydroxylase activity has been detected in several extrarenal tissues (e.g., bone cells), it does not appear that such sources are physiologically important. Evidence for this conclusion includes the findings that anephric rats cannot form $1,25\text{-}(OH)_2$-vitamin $D_3$ from either 25-OH-vitamin $D_3$ or vitamin $D_3$, and that only $1,25\text{-}(OH)_2$-vitamin $D_3$ (and not 25-OH-vitamin $D_3$ or vitamin $D_3$) is effective in stimulating Ca absorption in anephric rats. An exception may be placental tissue which has been shown to contribute to the $1,25\text{-}(OH)_2$-vitamin D pool of the fetal rat.

[32] e.g., prolactin, estradiol, testosterone, growth hormone.

[33] It has been suggested that the function of the CT-sensitive 1-hydroxylase, which is elevated in the fetus, may be to accommodate situations of increased need for $1,25\text{-}(OH)_2$-vitamin D.

[34] The hydroxylase is also inhibited by the 25-OH-vitamin D-binding protein-actin complex. The effect of this inhibitor *in vitro* can be overcome by using large amounts of 25-OH-vitamin D to saturate the binding protein; otherwise, it masks the 1-hydroxylase activity in kidney homogenates.

*conversion to* A second hydroxylation of 25-OH-vitamin D can occur at C24 of the side-
*24,25-(OH)₂-D* chain to produce the dihydroxy metabolite **24,25-(OH)₂-vitamin D**. This
reaction is catalyzed by **25-OH-vitamin D 24-hydroxylase**, an activity
thought to be an alternate one of the 25-OH-vitamin D 1-hydroxylase, that
has been found in all tissues that have receptors for 1,25-(OH)₂-D. Like the
1-hydroxylase, the 24-hydroxylase is a cytochrome $P_{450}$-dependent enzyme
requiring NADPH; but, unlike the former activity which is inhibited by
hypercalcemia and hyperphosphatemia, the 24-hydroxylase activity is
increased under these conditions and it is very strongly induced by 1,25-
(OH)₂-vitamin D. Thus, 24,25-(OH)₂-vitamin D appears to be the alternative
metabolite of vitamin D, produced under conditions of vitamin D-adequacy
and normal Ca homeostasis.

*other* More than sixteen other metabolites of vitamin D have been identified; most,
*metabolites* if not all, of which appear to be physiologically inactive excretory forms[35].
One of these, **1-OH-24,25,26,27-tetranor-23-carboxycholecalciferol**, is
produced in the kidney and intestine by the oxidation of the side chain of
1,25-(OH)₂-vitamin D; it accounts for nearly one-fifth of the biliary excretion
of the vitamin. Another of these, 1,24,25-(OH)₃-vitamin D, is produced in
the kidney and, perhaps, intestine, probably by the action of the 1/24-
hydroxylase on 25-OH-vitamin D. Other reactions involving chain-shorten-
ing of 1,25-(OH)₂-vitamin D have been demonstrated in intestine and are
thought to account for the rapid turnover of that metabolite. These metabolites appear in the bile mainly as glucuronide conjugates. Small amounts
of vitamin D esters (with both saturated and unsaturated fatty acids) occur
in all tissues; these are produced by the **cholesterol-esterifying enzyme**.

*distinguishing* The metabolic basis of the discrimination of vitamin D₂ in favor of vitamin
*D₂ and D₃* D₃, which occurs in birds and some mammals involves the enhanced rates
of clearance of the mono- and di-hydroxylated metabolites of the former

---

[35]It should be noted that ca. 95% of vitamin D excretion occurs via the bile; of that amount, only 2-3% of
an oral or parenteral dose of vitamin D appears as vitamin D or the mono- or di-hydroxy metabolites.

vitamer, i.e., in the chick, the plasma turnover rates of vitamin $D_2$, 25-OH-vitamin $D_2$ and 1,25-$(OH)_2$-vitamin $D_2$ were 1.5-, 11- and 33-fold faster than those of the respective vitamin $D_3$ analogues.  Because these differences in turnover rates are greater than those for the binding affinities to DBP (5-, 3.6- and 3-fold, respectively), it is thought that the relatively poor utilization of vitamin $D_2$ by these species is due to their abilities to clear it and its metabolites very rapidly.

*degradation*  Vitamin D is catabolized in several different ways: oxidative cleavage of the side-chain; hydroxylation of 1,25-$(OH)_2$-D to produce the tri-hydroxylated products 1,24,25-$(OH)_3$-D and 1,25,26-$(OH)_3$-D; formation of the 1,25-$(OH)_2$-D-23,26-lactone.  Many other products, including glucuronides and sulfates, have also been identified.  Most are excreted in the feces *via* the bile.

## METABOLIC FUNCTIONS OF VITAMIN D

*1,25-$(OH)_2$-D*  The clearest physiological role of vitamin D is in the maintenance of Ca and
*as the active*  phosphate homeostasis, impairment of which produces the lesions in bone
*form*  called rickets or osteomalacia.  In addition, other roles (e.g., induction of cell differentiation) have been proposed.  In these roles, it is clear that vitamin D itself is not the functionally active form, but that it must be converted metabolically to a form(s) that exert its biological activity.  That form appears to be 1,25-$(OH)_2$-vitamin D.

*vitamin D as*  At least some, if not all, of the mechanisms of action of 1,25-$(OH)_2$-vitamin
*a steroid*  D appears to fit the classical model of a **steroid hormone**.  That is, it has
*hormone*  specific cells in target organs with specific receptor proteins; the receptor-ligand complex moves to the nucleus where it binds to the chromatin and stimulates the transcription of particular genes to produce specific mRNAs which code for the synthesis of specific proteins.  Autoradiographic studies have demonstrated that 1,25-$(OH)_2$-vitamin D is localized in intestinal mucosal epithelial cells (which contain the 1,25-$(OH)_2$-vitamin D-receptor) exclusively in the nucleus.  The receptor has been characterized and the cDNA for it has been cloned; it has been found to have substantial sequence homology with receptors for other steroids, thyroid hormone and retinoic acid.  The binding of this active form of the vitamin in the rat or chick duodenum has been shown to induce the synthesis of mRNA that codes for several proteins including the Ca-binding proteins called **"calbindins"**.

The vitamin D-dependent calbindins are widespread in animal tissues, with greatest concentrations found in avian and mammalian duodenal mucosa where it can comprise 1-3% of the total soluble protein of the cell.  The next greatest concentrations are found in kidney (distal convoluted tubules) and pancreas ($\beta$-cells), in that order.  They are also found in shell gland (i.e., uterus), brain, retina, ovary, pituitary, bone, cartilage, splenic macrophages and thymus. These vitamin D-dependent calbindins are different from the vitamin K-dependent, γ-glutamate-containing Ca-binding proteins found in these and other tissues, although the finding that vitamin D-deficient rats have reduced amounts of these calbindins in bone and renal cortex suggests that some of these may also be induced by vitamin D. It is generally believed that the intestinal calbindin has some role in the enteric absorption of Ca[36].

Proteins known to be regulated by vitamin D:

| protein | tissue demonstrated |
|---|---|
| *induced* | |
| calbindin-$D_{28kD}$[a,b,c] | chick: intestine, kidney, brain, shell gland (uterus) |
| | rat: kidney, brain |
| calbindin-$D_{9kD}$[a,b,d] | chick: kidney, skin, bone |
| | rat: intestine, skin, bone |
| fibronectin[e] | human: fibroblasts |
| osteocalcin[e] | rat: osteosarcoma cells |
| c-fos[e] | human: HL-60 myeloid leukemic cells |
| c-fms[e] | human: HL-60 myeloid leukemic cells |
| 1,25-$(OH)_2$-$D_3$-receptor[e] | mouse: fibroblasts |
| prolactin[e] | rat: pituitary cells |
| | |
| *suppressed* | |
| pre-pro-PTH[e] | rat: parathyroid glands |
| calcitonin[e] | rat: thyroid gland |
| type I collagen[e] | rat: fetal calvaria |
| interleukin-2[e] | human: activated lymphocytes |
| γ-interferon[e] | human: activated lymphocytes |
| GM-CSF[b] | human: activated lymphocytes |
| c-myc[e] | human: HL-60 myeloid leukemic cells |

[a]1,25-$(OH)_2$-$D_3$ regulates expression *via* affecting transcription.
[b]1,25-$(OH)_2$-$D_3$ regulates expression *via* post-translational effects on mRNA expression.
[c]*"avian type"* calbindin; a 28kD protein that binds 4 moles of $Ca^{++}$
[d]*"mammalian type"* calbindin; a 8-11kD protein that binds 2 moles of $Ca^{++}$
[e]It is known that vitamin D affects the level of mRNA for this protein; however, it is not known whether that effect occurs *via* the modulation of gene transcription or post-transcriptional effects on mRNA accumulation.

---

[36]The absorption of Ca across the intestine is a complex phenomenon involving an active transport process (important at low luminal concentrations of Ca) as well as a passive diffusional one (important at luminal Ca concentrations above 2-5 mM). Both processes appear to contribute to enteric Ca absorption in a differential manner related to Ca intake; thus, the efficiency of net Ca uptake across the gut can vary from ca. 25% at high Ca intakes to ca. 60% at low Ca intakes. In any case, the initial movement of $Ca^{++}$ across the brush border of the mucosal epithelial cell occurs by diffusion, as the cytosolic concentration of $Ca^{++}$ is low (i.e., in the $\mu$molar range) and the cell interior has a negative potential difference relative to the cell exterior. However, the same electrochemical gradient makes the movement of $Ca^{++}$ across the baso-lateral membrane an energy-dependent step, i.e., active transport. This is accomplished by a saturable (i.e., carrier-mediated) process which is not sensitive to such metabolic inhibitors as $CN^-$ and $N_2$. Vitamin D stimulates Ca absorption by increasing the flux of $Ca^{++}$ across the mucosal cell, thus, increasing the flux of $Ca^{++}$ from the intestinal lumen to the plasma (and also the flux in the reverse direction) by way of both a Ca-Mg-ATPase and a $Ca^{++}$-$Na^+$ exchange (in which three $Na^+$ are transported across the baso-lateral membrane for one $Ca^{++}$). Both transport systems are stimulated by 1,25-$(OH)_2$-vitamin D, but it is not known in either case whether the effect of the steroid is direct or indirect.

*intestinal*
*absorption*
*of Ca$^{++}$*

Vitamin D stimulates the enteric absorption of Ca. The active form in this function appears to be 1,25-(OH)$_2$-vitamin D, as the lag-time after exposure is shortest, and the stimulation of Ca-absorption is greatest for this metabolite. Because 1,25-(OH)$_2$-vitamin D induces calbindin in the intestinal mucosa, it has been proposed that the latter factor mediates the effect of vitamin D on the absorption of Ca across the gut. However, although intestinal levels of 1,25-(OH)$_2$-vitamin D, calbindin-mRNA and Ca uptake are highly correlated, the temporal changes in intestinal calbindin concentrations in response to a dose of 1,25-(OH)$_2$-vitamin D are *not* correlated with these other changes. Thus, exposure to the active metabolite increases Ca absorption *before* calbindin is induced, and the stimulatory effect of a single dose on Ca absorption decays long *before* intestinal calbindin levels start to fall[37]. Therefore, it is not clear whether the effect on vitamin D on the enteric absorption of Ca is mediated by calbindin. It has been suggested that calbindin may have a second role in mucosal cells in addition to binding Ca, i.e., that of directly activating the ATPase and/or exchange reactions involved in moving Ca$^{++}$ across the baso-lateral membrane during absorption.

*intestinal*
*phosphate*
*absorption*

Vitamin D also increases the mucosal uptake of phosphorus and enhances its absorption from the lumen of the gut. The active metabolite in this process is 1,25-(OH)$_2$-vitamin D, which appears to modulate the number of carrier sites available at the mucosal membrane for Na-dependent phosphate entry[38]. At least in the duodenum, this process is independent of any role of Ca absorption. The mechanism of vitamin D function in this process has not been elucidated.

*renal*
*resorption of*
*phosphate*
*and Ca$^{++}$*

Vitamin D, as 1,25-(OH)$_2$-vitamin D, stimulates the resorption of both phosphate and Ca$^{++}$ in the distal renal tubule. The quantitative significance of this effect is greater for phosphate than it is for Ca$^{++}$, as nearly all (99%) of the latter is resorbed independently of vitamin D. It appears that vitamin D functions in the kidney again as a steroid hormone, as nuclear localization, receptors and a protein product (calbindin) have all been found there. Calbindin appears to be required for the transcellular movement of both phosphate and Ca$^{++}$ in that organ.

*bone mineral*
*turnover*

Bone is the largest target organ for vitamin D, accumulating more than one-quarter of a single dose of the vitamin within a few hours of its administration. That lesions in bone mineralization (rickets, osteomalacia) occur in vitamin D deficiency, has long indicated its vital function in the metabo-

---

[37]This effect has been called *"transcaltachia"*; it is thought to involve the interaction of Ca$^{++}$ in the endocytic vesicles at the brush border where they fuse with lysosomes to travel along the microtubules to the basal lateral border where excytosis occurs.

[38]Phosphate uptake by the brush border membrane takes place against an electrochemical gradient via a saturable Na$^+$-phosphate synport (common transport). The rate-limiting and regulated step for phosphate absorption appears to be as the brush-border membrane entry.

lism of this organ[39]. The pattern of vitamin D metabolites in bone differs from that in intestine; whereas the latter is comprised mainly of 1,25-(OH)$_2$-vitamin D, bone contains mainly 25-OH-vitamin D (accounting for >50% of the vitamin D metabolites present, with 1,25-(OH)$_2$-vitamin D comprising less than 35%). As in plasma, the level of 24,25-(OH)$_2$-vitamin D in bone is fairly constant in proportion to that of 25-(OH)-vitamin D.

Vitamin D plays roles both in the formation (mineralization) of bone as well as in the mobilization of bone mineral (de-mineralization). Some evidence suggests that bone mineralization may be mediated through 1,25-(OH)$_2$-vitamin D, which is localized in the nuclei of the cells (*osteoblasts* and osteoprogenitor cells) that lay down bone mineral. These cells have been found to have 1,25-(OH)$_2$-vitamin D receptors that are stimulated by gluco-corticoids. However, it is generally thought that 24,25-(OH)$_2$-vitamin D is also involved in this process; though the mechanism remains unclear, it appears to involve PTH. Interestingly, 1,25-(OH)$_2$-vitamin D has been found both to stimulate bone growth *in vivo* but to inhibit bone accretion in tissue culture. The synthesis of the vitamin K-dependent Ca$^{++}$-binding protein *osteocalcin* is increased by 1,25-(OH)$_2$-vitamin D both *in vivo* and in cultured cells, but the relevance of this finding to bone mineralization is unclear as osteocalcin is known to inhibit hydroxyapatite formation. It is possible that 1,25-(OH)$_2$-vitamin D may both stimulate *and* repress bone mineralization, according to such factors as its concentration, the presence of 24,25-(OH)$_2$-vitamin D, etc.

Vitamin D stimulates *osteoclast*-mediated bone resorption. This process appears to be mediated by 1,25-(OH)$_2$-vitamin D, as it is the only form of vitamin D that is effective in anephric rats. It appears that, in this process, vitamin D has a role in the differentiation of macrophages to osteoclasts, as the number of these giant multinucleated bone-degrading cells is very low in bone from vitamin D-deficient animals. The demineralization of bone serves to mobilize Ca$^{++}$ and phosphate from that reserve, thus, maintaining the homeostasis of those minerals in the plasma[40]. The process of bone resorption involves *parathyroid hormone (PTH)*, which appears to act *via* cAMP (i.e., PTH stimulates adenylcyclase activity) in a mechanism involving a 1,25-(OH)$_2$-vitamin D-dependent factor. Because PTH is secreted in response to hypophosphatemia, nutritional deprivation of phosphate, too, can lead to bone demineralization[41]. The stimulation in bone cells of alkaline phosphatase activity, by a process inhibited by cycloheximide and

---

[39]Thus, the involvement of vitamin D in the metabolism of Ca and P was clear, as structural bone contains 95% of total body Ca and 90% of total body P which, in a 70 kg man are ca. 1200 g and 770 g, respectively.

[40]The normal ranges of these parameters in human adults are Ca: 8.5-10.6 mg/dl and P: 2.5-4.5 mg/dl.

[41]Hypophosphatemia also increases the activity of 25-OH-vitamin D 1-hydroxylase and the accumulation of 1,25-(OH)$_2$-vitamin D in target tissues. These effects are associated with bone demineralization. In addition, hypophosphatemia can lead to bone resorption directly by a process that is independent of vitamin D.

actinomycin D and, therefore, involving *de novo* protein synthesis, has been demonstrated for 1,25-(OH)$_2$-vitamin D.

*Ca$^{++}$ and*
*phosphate*
*homeostasis*

The most clearly elucidated (and probably the most physiologically important) function of vitamin D is in the homeostasis of Ca$^{++}$ and phosphate in the system involving regulation at the points of intestinal absorption, bone accretion and mobilization and renal excretion.  As described above, regulation at these points is effected by the controlled metabolism of vitamin D to its active form 1,25-(OH)$_2$-vitamin D.  That control involves Ca$^{++}$, parathyroid hormone (PTH) and calcitonin (CT).

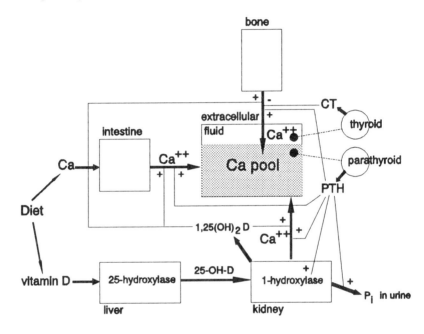

The normal concentration of Ca$^{++}$ in the serum of most species is ca. 10 mg/dl; the vitamin D-dependent homeostatic system responds to perturbations of that level.  For example, when serum Ca$^{++}$ concentration falls below this target level (i.e., the development of **hypocalcemia**), PTH is secreted by the parathyroid glands which function to detect hypocalcemia. The kidney responds to PTH in two ways:  phosphate diuresis and stimulation of 25-OH-vitamin D 1-hydroxylase.  The latter effect increases the production of 1,25-(OH)$_2$-vitamin D which acts (probably by inducing calbindin) in the intestine to increase the enteric absorption of both Ca$^{++}$ and phosphate.  In addition, 1,25-(OH)$_2$-vitamin D acts jointly with PTH in bone to promote the mobilization of Ca$^{++}$ and phosphate.  The aggregate result of these responses is to increase the concentrations of Ca$^{++}$ and phosphate in the plasma.

Under conditions of increased circulating concentrations of Ca$^{++}$ (**hypercalcemia**), calcitonin (CT) is secreted by the thyroid gland (i.e., "C" cells).

That hormone suppresses bone mobilization and is also thought to increase the renal excretion of both $Ca^{++}$ and phosphate. In that situation, the 25-OH-vitamin D 1-hydroxylase may be feedback-inhibited by 1,25-$(OH)_2$-vitamin D, and may actually be converted to the catalysis of the 24-hydroxylation of 25-OH-vitamin D. In the case of egg-laying birds, which show relatively high circulating concentrations of 1,25-$(OH)_2$-vitamin D, the 1-hydroxylase activity remains stimulated by the hormone **prolactin**.

Experimental evidence for *"non-classical"* functions of vitamin D:

| putative role | observations |
|---|---|
| cell differentiation | promotion by 1,25-$(OH)_2$-$D_3$ of myeloid leukemic precursor cells to differentiate to cells resembling macrophages |
| membrane structure | alteration of the fatty acid composition of enterocytes, reducing their membrane fluidity |
| mitochondrial metabolism | rachitic chicks show decreases in isocitrate lyase and malate synthase |
| muscular function | stimulation of $Ca^{++}$ transport into the sarcoplasmic reticulum of cultured myloblasts by 1,25-$(OH)_2$-$D_3$ |
| | electrophysiological abnormalities in muscle contraction and relaxation in vitamin D-deficient humans; these respond to vitamin D |
| | positive responses to vitamin D treatment for muscular weakness in humans |
| pancreatic function | stimulation of insulin production by pancreatic $\beta$-cells in rats by 1,25-$(OH)_2$-$D_3$ |
| | vitamin D-deficient humans show impaired insulin secretion unrelated to the level of circulating Ca |
| immunity | stimulation of immune cells functions by 1,25-$(OH)_2$-$D_3$ |
| neural function | region-specific enhancement of choline acetyltransferase in rat brain by 1,25-$(OH)_2$-$D_3$ |
| skin | inhibition of DNA synthesis in mouse epidermal cells by 1,25-$(OH)_2$-$D_3$ |
| parathyroid function | inhibition of transcription of PTH gene *via* interaction of 1,25-$(OH)_2$-$D_3$ and DNA in parathyroid cells. |

*functions in other tissues*

The finding of 1,25-$(OH)_2$-vitamin D in tissues not involved in Ca homeostasis (e.g., $\beta$-cells of the pancreas[42], malpighian layer of the skin, specific cells of the brain, the pituitary, the mammary gland, endocrine cells of the stomach, the chorioallantoic membrane surrounding chick embryos)[43] suggests that this form of the vitamin may have a more general function in many cells. The nature of such a function is still speculative; however, it seems reasonable to propose that 1,25-$(OH)_2$-vitamin D may be involved in regulating the temporal/spatial distribution of intracellular Ca. Whatever

---

[42]It is of interest to note that circulating insulin levels are reduced in vitamin D-deficiency and respond quickly to treatment with 1,25-$(OH)_2$-vitamin D.

[43]Cytologic localization of 1,25-$(OH)_2$-vitamin D has been achieved by the technique of frozen section autoradiography made possible by the availability of radiolabeled 1,25-$(OH)_2$-vitamin D of high specific activity.

its function in such tissues, it would appear that the role of vitamin D may not be obligatory, as the physiologic functions of these organs are not affected in vitamin D deficiency and that other tissues appear not to have any 1,25-$(OH)_2$-vitamin D (e.g., smooth muscle, heart, liver, spleen).

*anti-tumor effects*

The recent identification of an abnormal vitamin D metabolite in serum of cancer patients has focused attention on the possibility of a role of the vitamin in carcinogenesis. That metabolite, 1-*keto*-24-$CH_3$-25-OH-vitamin $D_3$, appears very infrequently (ca. 3%) in sera from healthy individuals, but in as much as 96% of sera from cancer patients and, thus, has been suggested as a cancer marker[44]. This finding, along with others showing vitamin D treatment to inhibit growth of tumor cells[45] in culture, and carcinogenesis in a couple of animal tumor models, have prompted a consideration of a role of vitamin D in cancer. Tests of this hypothesis have not been conducted in human subjects, but at least one clinical study has found Ca supplements to have anti-cancer effects.

## EXTREMES IN VITAMIN D INTAKE

*deficiency*

Vitamin D deficiency can result from inadequate irradiation of the skin, from insufficient intake from the diet, or from impairments in the metabolic activation (hydroxylation) of the vitamin. While sunlight can provide the means of biosynthesis of vitamin $D_3$, it is a well documented fact that many persons, particularly those in extreme latitudes during the winter months, do not receive adequate solar irradiation to support adequate vitamin D status. Even people in sunnier climates may not produce adequate vitamin D if their lifestyles keep them indoors, or if such factors as air pollution reduce their exposure to UV light. Most persons, therefore, show strong seasonal fluctuations in plasma 25-OH-vitamin $D_3$ concentrations; for some, this can be associated with considerable periods of suboptimal vitamin D status if not corrected by an adequate dietary source of the vitamin. Until the practice of vitamin D-fortification of foods became widespread, at least in technologically developed countries, it was difficult to obtain adequate vitamin D from the diet, as most foods contain only minuscule amounts[46].

Regardless of its cause, vitamin D deficiency leads to skeletal diseases: *rickets* in children and *osteomalacia* in adults. When these diseases are due to inadequate vitamin D supplies, they are described as *privational*.

---

[44]The name *'carcinomedin'* has been proposed.

[45]murine myeloid leukemic cells

[46]Eggs are the notable exception. Even cows' milk and human milk contain only very small amounts of vitamin D.

***Rickets*** first appears in children 6-24 months of age with the impaired mineralization of the growing bones and accompanying bone pain, muscular tenderness and hypocalcemic tetany. Tooth eruption may be delayed. Other signs include late closure of the fontanelle, and enlargement of the joints particularly of the long bones. Older children show skeletal deformations under the weight of the body, i.e., *"bow-leg"*[47] or *"knock-knee"*[48]. Radiography reveals enlarged epiphyseal growth plates.

***Osteomalacia*** occurs in adults with formed bones. Its signs and symptoms are more generalized than those of rickets, e.g., muscular weakness and bone tenderness, particularly in the spine, shoulder, ribs or pelvis. Radiographic examination reveals abnormally low bone density and the presence of pseudo-fractures, especially in the spine, femur and humerus. Patients with osteomalacia are at increased risk to fractures of all types, but particularly to those of the wrist and pelvis.

*non-privational causes of deficiency*   Rickets and osteomalacia can attend several other diseases that affect the absorption or metabolic activation of vitamin D. These include several diseases of the gastrointestinal tract (e.g., small bowel disease, gastrectomy, pancreatitis), which involve malabsorption of the vitamin from the diet, diseases of the liver (biliary cirrhosis, hepatitis) which involve reduced activities of the 25-hydroxylase, and diseases of the kidney (e.g., nephritis, renal failure) which involve reduced activities of the 1-hydroxylase. Especially important to the function of vitamin D are conditions that affect renal function, as this organ is the major site of production of $1,25\text{-}(OH)_2\text{-}$vitamin D[49].

Functional vitamin D deficiency can be caused by exposure to certain ***drugs*** and is seen among epileptic patients maintained with anti-convulsives (e.g., phenobarbital, diphenylhydantoin). These drugs induce the catabolism of 25-OH-vitamin D and $1,25\text{-}(OH)_2\text{-}$vitamin D and, thus, result in reduced circulating levels of the former. Affected children often show signs of rickets and have elevated PTH levels[50].

Individuals with ***hypoparathyroidism*** (reduced production of PTH resulting from the surgical removal or disease of the parathyroid glands), lack the

---

[47] *genu varus*

[48] *genu valgum*

[49] Chronic kidney disease leading to bone disease is called ***renal osteodystrophy***. It is a frequent complication in renal dialysis patients in which its severity varies directly with the reduction in glomerular filtration rate. It is more common among children than adults, presumably due to the greater sensitivity of growing bone to the deprivation of vitamin D, phosphate and PTH which occurs in renal disease.

[50] Vitamin D supplements (up to 4000 IU/day) are recommended to prevent rickets in children on long-term anti-convulsant therapy.

signal (PTH) to respond to hypocalcemia by increasing the conversion of 25-OH-vitamin D to 1,25-$(OH)_2$-vitamin D. Thus, they show continued hypocalcemia which leads to hyperphosphatemia responding to treatment with 1,25-$(OH)_2$-vitamin $D_3$ or high levels of vitamin $D_3$. Individuals with *nephrotic syndrome*[51] commonly are hypocalcemic and vitamin D-deficient. Their nephrosis results in losses of 25-(OH)-D along with its globulin binding protein into the urine; this results in depressed plasma levels of 25-(OH)-D which can, in turn, lead to depressed Ca absorption, hypocalcemia, secondary hyperparathyroidism and osteomalacia.

*osteoporosis*    Although the etiology of *osteoporosis* (loss of trabecular bone with retention of bone structure) is not fully understood, it appears to involve impairment in vitamin D metabolism and/or function associated with decreasing estrogen levels. The disease occurs mainly in older people[52] (e.g., non-ambulatory geriatrics, post-menopausal women) and in persons on chronic steroid therapy, both of which groups show high incidence of fractures, especially of the vertebrae[53], hip, distal radius and proximal femur[54,55]. Affected individuals show abnormally low circulating levels of 1,25-$(OH)_2$-vitamin D, suggesting that estrogen loss may impair the renal 1-hydroxylation step, i.e., that the disease may involve a bi-hormonal deficiency. Patients treated with either 25-OH-vitamin $D_3$, 1,25-$(OH)_2$-vitamin $D_3$ or 1$\alpha$-OH-vitamin $D_3$ have shown increased bone mass; those with highest serum concentrations of 24,25-$(OH)_2$-vitamin $D_3$ at outset showed the best responses to treatment. Osteoporosis is seen in the high-

---

[51]A clinical condition, involving renal tubular degeneration, characterized by edema, albuminuria, hypoalbuminemia and usually hypercholesterolemia.

[52]In women, bone loss generally begins in the third and fourth decades and accelerates after menopause; in men, bone loss begins about a decade later.

[53]Fractures of the vertebrae are probably the most common, although in many cases they may be asymptomatic. In 1984, vertebral fractures in the U.S. accounted for an estimated 160,000 physician office visits and 5 million patient-days of restricted activity.

[54]It is estimated that 13,000,000 fractures, including 200,000 hip fractures, occur annually in the U.S. The associated mortality rate (due to peri- and post-operative complications) within 3 months of the fracture has been estimated to be ca. 10%, i.e., 12-20% higher than that of other fracture patients. Survivors often have permanent disabilities. As the U.S. population ages, these rates can be expected to increase; for example, the incidence of hip fractures is expected to triple by the year 2050.

[55]Osteoporotic fractures appear to involve different syndromes. Type I osteoporosis is characterized by distal radial and vertebral fractures and occurs primarily in women aged 50-65; it is probably due to post-menopausal decreases in the amount of calcified bone at the fracture site. Type II osteoporosis occurs primarily in patients over 70 years and is characterized by fractures of the hip, proximal humerus and pelvis, where there has been loss of both cortical and trabecular bone. Where there is considerable overlapping of these types of osteoporosis, it is thought that different mechanisms may play roles in the pathophysiology of each.

producing laying hen[56] in which it is called *"cage layer fatigue"*.

There appear to be other situations of impaired renal 1-hydroxylation of 25-OH-vitamin D, thus, limiting the physiological function of the vitamin. One is the failure of bone mineralization seen in rapidly growing heavy-bodied chickens called *"tibial dyschondroplasia"*; this disease responds, at least in part, to treatment with 1,25-$(OH)_2$-vitamin $D_3$ or 1$a$-OH-vitamin $D_3$ but not vitamin $D_3$. Another situation involves exposure to lead (Pb) the absorption of which is increased by treatment with 1,25-$(OH)_2$-vitamin $D_3$. In children, blood levels of 1,25-$(OH)_2$-vitamin $D_3$ and Pb are inversely related[57], suggesting that Pb may inhibit the renal 1-hydroxylation of the vitamin perhaps constituting an adaptation to protect against lead toxicity.

Several *inherited conditions* are known to affect directly or indirectly vitamin D metabolism. The first is *vitamin D-resistant rickets* (in children) or osteomalacia (in adults)[58]. It involves impaired phosphate transport in the intestine and reabsorption in the proximal renal tubules and is not responsive to vitamin D; it also involves hypersensitivity to PTH and impaired 1-hydroxylation of 25-OH-vitamin D in spite of hypophosphatemia. The condition responds to treatment with phosphate (e.g. 1-4 g/day) plus either high doses of vitamin $D_3$ (e.g., 25,000-50,000 IU/d) or low doses of 1,25-$(OH)_2$-vitamin $D_3$ or 1$a$-OH-vitamin $D_3$ (e.g., .25-3 µg/day). Another hereditary abnormality of vitamin D metabolism is *vitamin D-dependent rickets*, i.e., a hypocalcemic rickets that responds to vitamin D *only* at very high doses. Two types of the disease have been described: type I involves defective 1-hydroxylation of 25-OH-vitamin D; type II involves defective receptors for 1,25-$(OH)_2$-vitamin D. Type I patients can be managed using low levels of 1,25-$(OH)_2$-vitamin $D_3$ or 1$a$-OH-vitamin $D_3$; whereas, much higher doses are required to manage type II patients. A third related hereditary abnormality is *pseudohypoparathyroidism*, which involves a resistance of target cells to PTH. In these patients, drops in serum $Ca^{++}$ are not responded to by either the kidneys or bone, despite the fact that secretion of PTH is normal (unlike patients with hypoparathyroidism). The hypocalcemia responds to 1,25-$(OH)_2$-vitamin $D_3$ or 1$a$-OH-vitamin $D_3$.

---

[56]In well managed flocks, it is not uncommon for a hen to lay more than 300 eggs in a year, with 40 of these laid during the first 40 days after commencing egg-laying. As each eggshell contains ca. 2 g Ca and the hen is only able to absorb 1.8-1.9 g Ca from the diet each day, she experiences a Ca-debt of .1-.2 g per day in that period. She accommodates this by mobilizing medullary bone; but, as her total skeleton contains only 35 g Ca, chronic demineralization at that rate without either decreasing the rate of egg production or increasing the efficiency of Ca absorption, leads to osteoporosis characterized by fractures of the ribs and long bones.

[57]The prevalence of Pb toxicity among children is seasonal, i.e., greatest in the summer months.

[58]This is also called *hypophosphatemic rickets/osteomalacia* and *phosphate diabetes*.

Signs of vitamin D deficiency:

| organ system | sign in rickets | sign in osteomalacia |
| --- | --- | --- |
| general | loss of appetite, retarded growth | none |
| dermatologic | none | none |
| muscular | weakness | weakness |
| skeletal | failure of bone to mineralize: deformation, swollen joints, delayed tooth eruption, bone pain and tenderness | demineralization of formed bone: fractures, pseudo-fractures, bone pain and tenderness |
| vital organs | none | none |
| nervous | tetany, ataxia | none |
| reproduction | - | low sperm motility and number birds: thin egg shells |
| ocular | none | none |

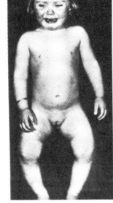

Rickets in a child, showing *varus* deformities of the legs

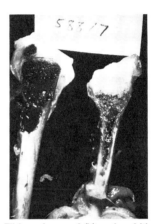

Tibiae of normal (l.) and rachitic (r.) chicks

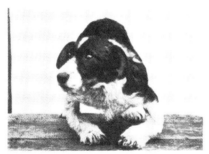

Rachitic puppy

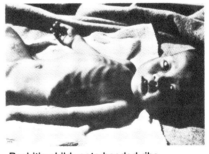

Rachitic child; note beaded ribs

*vitamin D in the treatment of skin diseases*

The findings that 1,25-$(OH)_2$-vitamin $D_3$ can inhibit proliferation and induce terminal differentiation of cultured keratinocytes has stimulated study of its potential value in the treatment of proliferative skin disorders. Clinical studies have shown that both oral and topical applications of that form of the vitamin can be safe and effective in the treatment of psoriasis[59]. Because the use of 1,25-$(OH)_2$-vitamin $D_3$ carries associated risks of hypercalcemia and hypercalciuria, there is interest in developing treatment regimens for such diseases involving the application of high doses of the vitamin in safe and effective manners.

*hyper-*
*vitaminosis*
Excessive intakes of vitamin D are associated with increases in circulating levels of 25-OH-vitamin D; this is especially true for vitamin $D_3$, exposure to high levels of which produce higher serum levels of the 25-OH-metabolite than do comparable intakes of vitamin $D_2$[60]. The 25-OH-metabolite is believed to be the critical metabolite in vitamin D intoxication. At high levels[61], it appears to compete successfully for intracellular receptors for 1,25-$(OH)_2$-vitamin D, thus, inducing the responses normally produced by the latter metabolite. Thus, hypervitaminosis D involves increased enteric absorption and bone resorption of Ca producing hypercalcemia, with attendant decreases in serum PTH and glomerular filtration rate and, ultimately loss of Ca homeostasis. The result is *calcinosis*, i.e., the deposition of Ca and phosphate in soft tissues, especially heart and kidney but also the vascular and respiratory systems and practically all other tissues. It is not known whether calcinosis involves specific tissue lesions induced by high levels of vitamin D metabolites or whether it is simply a consequence of the induced hypercalcemia.

Calcinosis in grazing livestock has been traced to the consumption of water-soluble glycosides of 1,25-$(OH)_2$-vitamin $D_3$ present in some plants. There are no documented cases of hypervitaminosis D due to excessive sunlight exposure. The availability of synthetic 1$\alpha$-OH-vitamin $D_3$ in recent years has meant that it can be used at very low doses to treat vitamin D-dependent or -resistant osteopathies, thus reducing the risks of hypervitaminosis attending the use of massive doses of vitamin $D_3$ needed for therapy in such cases.

Signs of hypervitaminosis D:

| |
|---|
| anorexia |
| gastro-intestinal distress |
| headache |
| lameness |
| polyuria |
| hypercalcemia |
| calcinosis |

---

[59]Results of one clinical series showed that topical application of 1,25-$(OH)_2$-vitamin $D_3$ caused complete clearing of lesions in 60% of patients, with an additional 30% of patients showing significant decreases in scale, plaque thickness and erythema.

[60]Vitamin $D_3$ is 10-20 times more toxic than vitamin $D_2$.

[61]i.e., 100 times normal physiological requirements.

## CASE STUDY

*Instructions*    *Review each of the following case reports paying special attention to the diagnostic indicators upon which the respective treatments were based. Then answer the questions that follow.*

*case 1*    When the patient was first evaluated at the National Institutes of Health, he was a thin, short, bow-legged, 20-year-old male.  His height at that time was 159 cm (below the 1st percentile) and he weighed 52 kg.  In addition to his **dwarfism**, he showed a **varus deformity**[62] of both knees, and he walked with a waddling gait.  Radiographs showed diffusely **decreased bone density, subperiosteal resorption** and a **pseudofracture**[63] of the left ischiopubic ramus[64].

Laboratory results:

| parameter | patient | normal range |
|---|---|---|
| serum Ca | 8.0 mg/dl | 8.5-10.5 mg/dl |
| serum P | 2.2 mg/dl | 3.5- 4.5 mg/dl |
| serum alkaline phosphatase | 152 U/ml | <77 U/ml |

Urine chromatography showed a generalized aminoaciduria.

The patient's history revealed that he had been a normal, full-term infant weighing 3.2 kg.  He had been breast-fed and had been given supplementary vitamin D.  At 20 months, however, he failed to walk unsupported and was diagnosed as having active **rickets**, as revealed by **genu varum**[62], irregular **cupped metaphyses** and **widened growth plates**[65] , with reductions of both Ca and P in his blood.  The rickets did not respond to oral doses of ergocalciferol (normally effective in treating nutritional rickets), but healing was observed radiographically after intramuscular administration of 1,500,000 IU (37.5 mg) of vitamin $D_2$ weekly for five months. The patient continued to receive vitamin D in the form of cod liver oil, approximately 5,000-20,000 units per day.  At 4 years of age, corrective surgery was performed for deformities of the tibias and femurs.  At age 14, the patient's height was in the 15th percentile.  Additional surgery was performed, after which vitamin D therapy was stopped and, over the next 2 years, weakness and severe bone pain became evident.  At age 19, bilateral femoral

---

[62]i.e., bow leg.

[63]i.e., new bone detected radiographically as thickening of the periosteum at the site of an injury to the bone.

[64]i.e., a narrow process of the pelvis.

[65]i.e., failure of mineralization of the growing ends of long bones.

osteotomies[66] were performed again. As an outpatient at the NIH Clinical Center, the patient received oral ergocalciferol, 50,000 IU daily, for the next 6 yrs. and experienced remission of pain and weakness and normalization of serum Ca and P levels. His height reached 161 cm (63.3 in), i.e., still below the 1st percentile. At 27 years of age, his radiographs showed improved density of the skeletal cortices and healing of the pseudofractures, but the patient still showed the clinical stigmata[67] of rickets.

Laboratory results:

| parameter | patient | normal range |
|---|---|---|
| serum PTH | .31 ng/ml | <.22 ng/ml |
| urine cAMP | 6 nmol/dl | 2.3 ± 1.2 nmol/dl |
| $^{47}$Ca absorption | 19% | 33-43% |
| plasma 25-OH-$D_3$ | 25 ng/ml | 10-40 ng/ml |
| plasma 1,25-$(OH)_2$-$D_3$ | 213 pg/ml | 20-60 pg/ml |
| plasma 24,25-$(OH)_2$-$D_3$ | 1.0 ng/ml | 0.8-3 ng/ml |

Two hundred $\mu$g of 25-OH-$D_3$ were then given orally daily for 2 weeks. Ca retention improved, urinary cAMP fell and plasma P and Ca rose, each to the normal level. Vitamin $D_3$ maintenance doses (ca. 40,000 IU, i.e., 1 mg per day) were given periodically to prevent recurrent osteomalacia.

case 2
This patient was a sister of the patient described above. She was first evaluated at NIH when she was 18 years old. She was a thin female dwarf 147 cm tall (below the 1st percentile), and weighing 44.8 kg. She walked with a waddling gait and had mild bilateral varus deformities of the knees. **Chvostek sign**[68] was present bilaterally. Analyses of her serum showed 7.0 mg Ca and 3.0 mg P per dl and alkaline phosphatase at 110 U/ml. Skeletal radiographs showed delayed ossification of several epiphyses and a pseudofracture in the left tibia. Her plasma 25-OH-D was 44 ng/ml, 1,25-$(OH)_2$-$D_3$ was 280 pg/ml and 24,25-$(OH)_2$-$D_3$ was 2.5 ng/ml.

Her history showed that she had been a normal, full-term infant who weighed 3.8 kg at birth. At 5 months of age, she showed radiographic features of *rickets*. During infancy and childhood, she received vitamin D as cod liver oil, in doses of 2,000-10,000 IU/day. She began to walk at 9 months and developed slight *varus deformity* of both legs. Her rate of growth was at the 5th percentile until the vitamin D was discontinued when she was 11 years old. Within 3 years, her height fell below the 1st percentile. From ages 15 to 16, the bowing of her legs progressed moderately.

---

[66]i.e., surgical correction of bone shape.

[67]i.e., abnormalities.

[68]i.e., facial irritability in tetany induced by a slight tap over the facial nerve.

When she was 18 years old, at the time of her first admission to the NIH Clinical Center, she was treated with 200 $\mu$g 25-OH-$D_3$ per day for 2 weeks. During this time, her Ca retention improved, and her serum Ca and P increased.   Studies showed that 500 $\mu$g of vitamin $D_3$ per day were required to maintain her plasma Ca in the normal range.  At this dose, her 25-OH-$D_3$ was 141 ng/ml, 1,25-$(OH)_2$-$D_3$ was 640 pg/ml and 24,25-$(OH)_2$-$D_3$ was 3.6 ng/ml (above normal).  When she was 24 years old, i.e., 6 years after her first admission to the Center, she was readmitted for studies of the effectiveness of oral 1,25-$(OH)_2$-$D_3$ with a supplement of 800 mg Ca per day.  Serum Ca remained below normal on doses of 2-10 $\mu$g 1,25-$(OH)_2$-$D_3$ per day.  Only when the dose was increased to 14-17 $\mu$g 1,25-$(OH)_2$-$D_3$ per day did her plasma Ca reach the normal range.   PTH remained elevated at 0.40 ng/ml.  At these high doses of 1,25-$(OH)_2$-$D_3$, her plasma 25-OH-$D_3$ was 26 ng/ml, and her 1,25-$(OH)_2$-$D_3$ was 400 pg/ml. While on 1,25-$(OH)_2$-$D_3$, her osteomalacia improved, and serum Ca and P entered normal ranges.

Questions     i.     What are the common clinical features (physical and biochemical observations, response to treatment, etc.) of these two cases?

               ii.     What can you infer about the nature of vitamin D metabolism in these siblings?

               iii.     Propose an hypothesis to explain these cases of vitamin D-resistant rickets.  How might you test this hypothesis?

## Study Questions and Exercises:

i.     Construct a **flow diagram** showing the **metabolism** of vitamin D to its physiologically active and excretory forms.

ii.    Construct a *"decision tree"* for the **diagnosis** of vitamin D deficiency in a human or animal. How can deficiencies of vitamin D and Ca be distinguished?

iii.   How does the concept of **solubility** related to vitamin D utilization? What *features* of the **chemical structure** of vitamin D relate to its *utilization*?

iv.    Relate the concept of **organ function** to the concept of vitamin D utilization/status?

v.     Discuss the concept of **homeostasis**, using vitamin D as an example.

## Recommended Reading:

Collins, E.D. and A.W. Norman. 1991. Vitamin D, Chapter 2 in <u>Handbook of Vitamins</u>, 2nd edition (L.J. Machlin, ed.), Marcel Dekker, New York, pp. 59-98.

DeLuca, H.F. 1986. Vitamin D, in <u>Nutrition and the Adult: Micronutrients</u>. (R.B. Alfin-Slater and D. Kritchevsky, eds.), Plenum Press, New York. pp. 205-244.

Friedrich, W. 1988. <u>Vitamins</u>, Walter de Gruyter, New York, pp. 141-216.

Henry, H.L., and A.W. Norman. 1984. Vitamin D: Metabolism and Biological Actions. Ann. Rev. Nutr. 4:493-520.

Lawson, E. 1985. Vitamin D, Chapter 2 in <u>Fat-Soluble Vitamins</u> (A.T. Diplock, ed.), Technomic Publ. Co., Basal, pp. 76-153.

Marx, S.J., U.A. Liberman and C. Eil. 1983. Calciferols: Actions and Deficiencies in Action. Vit. Horm. 40:235-308.

Norman, A.W. 1990. Vitamin D, Chapter 12 in <u>Present Knowledge in Nutrition</u>, 6th edition (M. Brown, ed.), International Life Sciences Inst.-Nutrition Found., Washington, D.C., pp. 108-116.

Suda, T., T. Shinki and N. Takahashi. 1990. The role of vitamin D in bone and intestinal cell differentiation. Ann. Rev. Nutr. 10:195-212.

# CHAPTER 7  *VITAMIN E*

*"Vitamin E is a focal point for two broad topics, namely, biological antioxidants and lipid peroxidation damage. Vitamin E is related by its reactions to other biological antioxidants and reducing compounds (which) stabilize polyunsaturated lipids and minimize lipid peroxidation damage. In vivo lipid peroxidation has been identified as a basic deteriorative reaction in cellular mechanisms of aging processes, in some phases of atherosclerosis, in chlorinated hydrocarbon hepatotoxicity, in ethanol-induced liver injury and in oxygen toxicity. These processes may be a universal disease of which the chemical deteriorative effects might be slowed by use of increased amounts of antioxidants."*      A.L. Tappel

## Anchoring Concepts:

| | |
|---|---|
| *i.* | Vitamin E is the generic descriptor for all tocol and trienol derivatives exhibiting qualitatively the biological activity of *α*-tocopherol. |
| *ii.* | The vitamers E are hydrophobic and, thus, are insoluble in aqueous environments (e.g., plasma, interstitial fluids, cytosol). |
| *iii.* | By virtue of the phenolic hydrogen on the C-6 ring-hydroxyl group, the vitamers E have antioxidant activities *in vitro*. |
| *iv.* | Deficiencies of vitamin E have a wide variety of clinical manifestations in different species. |

## Learning Objectives:

| | |
|---|---|
| *i.* | To understand the various *sources* of vitamin E. |
| *ii.* | To understand the means of *enteric absorption* and *transport* of vitamin E. |
| *iii.* | To understand the *metabolic interrelationships* of vitamin E and other nutrients. |
| *iv.* | To understand the physiologic implications of *high doses* of vitamin E. |

*Vocabulary:*

| | |
|---|---|
| abetalipoproteinemia | membrane |
| anemia | mulberry heart disease |
| antioxidant | myopathy |
| areflexia | pentane |
| ataxia | peroxide |
| catalase | peroxy radical |
| chylomicron | prooxidant |
| conjugated diene | PUFA |
| cysteine | resorption-gestation syndrome |
| encephalomalacia | selenium |
| ethane | Simon's metabolites |
| exudative diathesis | steatorrhea |
| free radical | superoxide dismutase |
| glutathione | superoxide radical |
| glutathione peroxidase | TBP |
| glutathione reductase | $\alpha$-tocopherol |
| HDL | $\beta$-tocopherol |
| hemolysis | $\gamma$-tocopherol |
| hydroperoxide | $\delta$-tocopherol |
| hydroxyl radical | tocopheronic acid |
| $H_2O_2$ | tocopherylhydroquinone |
| intraventricular hemorrhage | tocopherylquinone |
| LDL | tocotrienol |
| lipid peroxidation | VLDL |
| liver necrosis | white muscle disease |
| malonyldialdehyde | |

# SOURCES OF VITAMIN E

*distribution*
*in foods*

Vitamin E is synthesized only by plants and, therefore, is found primarily in plant products, the richest sources being plant oils. All higher plants appear to contain $a$-tocopherol in their leaves and other green parts; while $\gamma$-tocopherol is generally present in lower concentrations; like the $a$-vitamer it is generally considered always to be present in plant tissues. Because $a$-tocopherol is contained mainly in the chloroplasts of plant cells (while the $\beta$-, $\gamma$- and $\delta$-vitamers are usually found outside of these particles), green plants tend to contain more vitamin E than yellow ones. In contrast, the tocotrienols are not found in green leaves but, rather, in the bran and germ fractions of certain plants. Unlike the tocopherols which exist only as free alcohols, the tocotrienols can occur naturally in esterified form. Animal tissues tend to have low amounts of vitamin E. The highest levels occur in fatty tissues and vary according to the dietary intake of the vitamin.

*expressing*
*vitamin E*
*activity*

Vitamin E activity is shown by several side-chain isomers and methylated analogues of tocopherol and tocotrienol. These various compounds differ in their vitamin E activities, the epimeric configuration at the 2-position being important in determining biological activity. Therefore, the use of an international standard facilitated the referencing of these various sources of vitamin E activity which, presumably, relates to differences in their absorption, transport, retention and/or metabolism. Although the original preparation[1] that was the international standard has not been extant for over 30 years, the US Pharmacopoeia has recommended standardized unitage[2,3] which is generally used as an international standardization.

Biopotencies of tocopherols and tocotrienols by different bioassays:

| compound | fetal resorption (rat) | hemolysis (rat) | myopathy prevention (chick) | myopathy cure (rat) |
|---|---|---|---|---|
| $a$-tocopherol | 100 | 100 | 100 | 100 |
| $\beta$-tocopherol | 25-40 | 15-27 | 12 | - |
| $\gamma$-tocopherol | 1-11 | 3-20 | 5 | 11 |
| $\delta$-tocopherol | 1 | .3-2 | - | - |
| $a$-tocotrienol | 28 | 17-25 | - | 28 |
| $\beta$-tocotrienol | 5 | 1-5 | - | - |

---

[1] At the time, the standard was called *d,l-a*-tocopheryl acetate; now it would be called *2RS-a*-tocopheryl acetate. Because of uncertainty about the proportions of the two diastereoisomers in that mixture, once the supply was exhausted it was impossible to replace it.

[2] *see* Chapter 3, p.65

[3] It should be noted that this system distinguishes only the methylated analogues and not the particular diastereoisomers possible for each.

It is important to note that some of the vitamers E common in foods (β- and γ-tocopherols, tocotrienols) have little biological activity. The vitamer of greatest interest in nutrition is the most biopotent one, α-tocopherol, which occurs naturally as the *RRR*-stereoisomer (*RRR*-α-tocopherol).

*dietary sources of vitamin E*

The important sources of vitamin E in human diets and animal feeds are vegetable oils and, to lesser extents, seeds and cereal grains. Wheat germ oil is the richest natural source, containing 0.85-1.28 mg/g α-tocopherol, i.e., ca. 60% of its total tocopherols. The seeds and grains from which these oils are derived also contain appreciable amounts of vitamin E; accordingly, cereals in general and wheat germ in particular are good sources of the vitamin. Foods that are formulated (e.g., margarine, baked products) with vegetable oils tend to vary greatly in vitamin E content due to differences in the types of oils used and to the thermal stabilities of the vitamers E present[4]. Processing of foods and feedstuffs can reduce vitamin E contents, especially with exposure to peroxidizing lipids, formed during the development of oxidative rancidity of fats. Other treatments that can lead to destruction of vitamin E include drying in the presence of sunlight and air, addition of organic acids[5], milling and refining[6], irradiation, and canning. Some foods (e.g., milk and milk products) also show marked seasonal fluctuations in vitamin E content related to variations in vitamin E intake of the host (e.g., vitamin E intake is greatest when fresh forage is consumed). The many potential sources of vitamin E loss, mean that the vitamin E contents of foods and feedstuffs vary considerably[7].

Vitamin E in grains:

| Item | tocopherols, μg/g | | | | tocotrienols, μg/g | |
|---|---|---|---|---|---|---|
| | α- | β- | γ- | δ- | α- | γ- |
| maize | 6-15 | | 29-55 | | 5-10 | 34-77 |
| soybean | 1- 3 | | 3-33 | 2-6 | | tr. |
| cotton | 1-18 | | 5-18 | | | 1-2 |
| oats | 4- 8 | <1 | | | 10-22 | |
| milo | 4- 7 | | 14-17 | | <1 | |
| barley | 8-10 | 1-2 | 3-4 | | 23-28 | 3 |
| wheat | 8-12 | 4-6 | | | 2-3 | |
| source: Cort, et al. 1983. J. Agric. Food Chem. 31:1330. | | | | | | |

[4]Tocotrienols tend to be less stable to high temperatures than tocopherols; therefore, baking tends to destroy them selectively.

[5]The addition of 1% propionic acid (as an anti-fungal agent) to fresh grain can destroy up to 90% of its vitamin E.

[6]Vitamin E losses occur both due to removal of tocopherol-rich bran and germ, but also due to the use of oxidants (e.g., $ClO_2$) to improve the baking characteristics of the flour.

[7]e.g., refining losses in edible plant oils are typically 10-40%, but can sometimes be much greater.

Vitamin E in fats and oils:

| Item | total vitamin E mg/100 g | tocopherols, % α- | γ- | δ- | tocotrienols, % α- | β- | γ- | δ- |
|------|--------------------------|-------------------|----|----|--------------------|----|----|----|
| **animal fats:** | | | | | | | | |
| lard | 0.6-1.3 | >90 | <5 | | <5 | | | |
| butter | 1-5 | >90 | <10 | | | | | |
| tallow | 1.2-2.4 | >90 | <10 | | | | | |
| **plant oils:** | | | | | | | | |
| soybean | 56-160 | | 4-18 | 58-69 | | | | |
| cotton | 30-81 | 51-67 | 33-49 | | | | | |
| maize | 53-162 | | 11-24 | 76-89 | | | | |
| coconut | 1-4 | 14-67 | | <17 | <14 | <3 | <53 | <17 |
| peanut | 20-32 | 48-61 | 39-52 | | | | | |
| palm | 33-73 | 28-50 | | <9 | 16-19 | 4 | 34-39 | <9 |
| safflower | 25-49 | 80-94 | 6-20 | | | | | |
| olive | 5-15 | 65-85 | | | | 15-35 | | |

source: Chow, C.K. 1985. World Rev. Nutr. Diet. 45:133.

# ABSORPTION OF VITAMIN E

*micelle-dependent passive diffusion*

Vitamin E is absorbed from the small intestine by non-saturable passive diffusion dependent upon micellar solubilization and, hence, the presence of bile salts and pancreatic juice. The primary site of absorption appears to be the medial small intestine. Esterified forms of the vitamin E are hydrolyzed, probably by a duodenal mucosal *esterase*; the predominant forms absorbed are free alcohols. At nutritionally important intakes, the efficiency of vitamin E absorption appears to be low and variable (35-50%[8]) with a large proportion of the intake of vitamin E appearing in the feces. Vitamin E absorption shows biphasic kinetics apparently reflecting initial uptake of the vitamin by existing chylomicra followed by a lag due to the assembly of new chylomicra. Tocopherols are better absorbed from an aqueous environment than an oily one. They interact with *polyunsaturated fatty acids (PUFAs)* in the lumen of the gut such that absorption can be stimulated by intragastric *medium-chain triglycerides* and inhibited by linoleic acid. Absorbed vitamin E, like other hydrophobic substances, enters the lymphatic circulation[9] in association with chylomicra. Because the enteric absorption of vitamin E is dependent on the adequate absorption of lipids, individuals with lipid malabsorption syndromes (e.g., cystic fibrosis, biliary atresia, premature infants) typically have low vitamin E status if not treated with higher levels of the vitamin.

---

[8] The enteric absorption of γ-tocopherol appears to be only 85% of that of α-tocopherol.

[9] i.e., the portal circulation in birds, fishes and reptiles.

## TRANSPORT OF VITAMIN E

*absorbed*
*vitamin E*
*transferred to*
*lipoproteins,*
*erythrocytes*

Unlike vitamins A and D, vitamin E does not appear to have a specific carrier protein in the plasma. Instead, it is rapidly transferred from chylomicra to plasma lipoproteins to which it binds non-specifically. The vitamin is taken up by the liver and is released in LDL (with selectivity in favor of α-tocopherol over the γ-vitamer); therefore, plasma tocopherol levels tend to correlate with those of total lipids and cholesterol[10]. Tocopherol exchanges rapidly between the lipoproteins[11] and erythrocytes (about one-fourth of total erythrocyte vitamin E turns over per hour); thus, the concentrations of vitamin E in plasma and erythrocytes are highly correlated[12] (the latter having 15-25% of the plasma concentration). As vitamin E is membrane-protective, plasma tocopherol levels are inversely related to susceptibility to oxidative hemolysis. This relationship makes plasma α-tocopherol level useful as a parameter of vitamin E status; in healthy people, values $\geq 0.5$ mg/dl are associated with protection against hemolysis and are taken to indicate nutritional adequacy. Maternal tocopherol levels increase during pregnancy, but fetal levels remain low[13], suggesting a barrier to transplacental movement of the vitamin.

Serum α-tocopherol concentrations in humans:

| group | α-tocopherol mg/dl | group | α-tocopherol mg/dl |
|---|---|---|---|
| healthy adults | .85 ± .03 | infants | |
| postpartum mothers | 1.33 ± .40 | full term | .22 ± .10 |
| children, 2-12 yrs. | .72 ± .02 | premature | .23 ± .10 |
| cystic fibrotics | | premature at 1 mo. | .13 ± .05 |
| 1-19 yrs. | .15 ± .15 | 2 mos., bottle-fed | .33 ± .15 |
| biliary atresiacs | | 2 mos., breast-fed | .71 ± .25 |
| 3-15 mos. | .10 ± .10 | 5 mos. | .42 ± .20 |
| | | 2 yrs. | .58 ± .20 |

source: Gordon, et al. 1958. Pediatrics 21:673

---

[10]Therefore, high plasma vitamin E levels occur in hyperlipidemic conditions (hypothyroidism, diabetes, hypercholesterolemia); while low plasma vitamin E levels occur in conditions involving low plasma lipids (abetalipoproteinemia, protein malnutrition, cystic fibrosis).

[11]Rats, horses and chicks transport 70-80% of plasma α-tocopherol with HDL, 18-22% with LDL, and <8% with VLDL. Human females, too, transport α-tocopherol preferentially with HDL; but males transfer most (65%) with LDL, only 24% with HDL, and 8% with VLDL.

[12]Patients with abetalipoproteinemia are notable exceptions. They may show normal erythrocyte tocopherols concentrations even though their serum tocopherols levels are undetectable.

[13]Serum tocopherol concentrations of infants are ca. 25% of those of their mothers. They increase to adequate levels within a few weeks after birth, except in infants with impaired abilities to utilize lipids (e.g., premature infants, biliary atresiacs) which show very low circulating levels of vitamin E.

*cellular uptake*    The mechanisms of cellular uptake of vitamin E from the plasma are poorly understood, but two mechanisms appear to be involved. The first involves receptor-mediated uptake of vitamin E-carrying lipoproteins. Indeed, evidence has been presented that the binding of LDL to specific cell surface receptors must occur to allow the vitamin E to enter cells either by diffusion and/or bulk entrance of lipoprotein-bound lipids[14]. The second involves the lipoprotein lipase-mediated release of lipid from chylomicra and VLDL in the plasma, where their lipid products are transferred into tissues by fatty acid- and lipid-binding proteins.

*tocopherol-*    The intracellular transport of the vitamin, at least in the liver, appears to
*binding*    involve specific ***tocopherol-binding proteins (TBPs)***. Several TBPs have
*proteins*    been discovered: an erythrocyte plasma membrane protein with both high- and low-affinity binding sites[15]; an acidic, none-histone protein associated with the nuclear chromatin; a 30-34 kD protein in liver cytoplasm with high affinity for the tocopherols and slight specificity for *a*-tocopherol. The cytosolic TBP has been found to effect the transfer of vitamin E from the cytoplasm to the endoplasmic reticulum and mitochondria. Its slight binding preference for *RRR-a*-tocopherol over the *SRR*-stereoisomer has been proposed to be the basis for the differences in the tissue retention and biopotency of these stereoisomers[16]. In addition, intracellular vitamin E-binding lipoproteins have been identified in several tissues (liver, heart, brain, intestinal mucosa), although they to do appear to participate in the intracellular transport of tocopherol. Tocopherol has also been found to bind to the interphotoreceptor retinol-binding protein (IRBP), apparently in the same site as retinol, as the latter readily displaces it. This raises the possibility that some of the retinoid-binding proteins may also function in the intracellular transport of vitamin E.

*vitamin E*    In most non-adipose cells, vitamin E is localized almost exclusively in their
*storage:*    membranes. Kinetic studies indicate that such tissues have two pools of
*two pools*    the vitamin: a *'labile'*, rapidly turning over pool; and a *'fixed'*, slowly turning over pool. Apparently, the labile pools predominate in such tissues as plasma and liver, as the tocopherol contents of those tissues are depleted rapidly under conditions of vitamin E deprivation. In contrast, in adipose tissue vitamin E resides predominately in the bulk lipid phase, which appears to be a fixed pool of the vitamin. Thus, it is only slowly mobilized from that tissue with only long-term physiological significance.

---

[14]Fibroblasts from an individual with an hereditary deficiency of LDL-receptors were found to be unable to take up LDL-bound vitamin E at normal rates.

[15]The putative erythrocyte tocopherol receptor has been found to contain 65 Kd and 125 Kd components and does not appear to show specificity for the various isomers of tocopherol.

[16]Neither LDL-receptor nor lipoprotein lipase mechanisms of vitamin E uptake by cells discriminate between these stereoisomers.

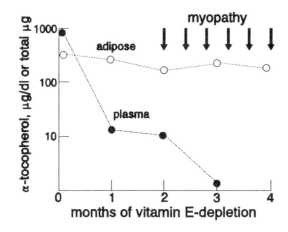

source:  Machlin, et al. 1979. J. Nutr. 109:105-109

Due to the very slow rates of turnover of such "fixed" pools, the amounts of vitamin E in adipose tissue can be nearly normal even in animals showing clinical signs of vitamin E deficiency.  Similarly, persons on a weight-loss program were found to lose triglycerides but not vitamin E from their adipose tissues.  However, circulating tocopherol levels have been found to rise significantly (10-20%) during intensive exercise, and it has been suggested that vitamin E may be mobilized from its "fixed" pools by way of the lipolysis induced under such conditions.  Tissue tocopherol contents tend to be related exponentially to vitamin E intake; unlike most other vitamins, they show no deposition or saturation thresholds.  Thus, tissues vary considerably in tocopherol contents, not consistently related to the amounts or types of lipids present.

Concentrations of $a$-tocopherol in human tissues:

| tissue | $a$-tocopherol | |
|---|---|---|
| | μg/g tissue | μg/g lipid |
| plasma | 9.5 | 1.4 |
| erythrocytes | 2.3 | .5 |
| platelets | 30 | 1.3 |
| adipose | 150 | .2 |
| kidney | 7 | .3 |
| liver | 13 | .3 |
| muscle | 19 | .4 |
| ovary | 11 | .6 |
| uterus | 9 | .7 |
| testis | 40 | 1.0 |
| heart | 20 | .7 |
| adrenal | 132 | .7 |
| hypophysis | 40 | 1.2 |

source:   Machlin, L.J. 1984. Handbook of Vitamins, Marcel Dekker, New York, p. 99.

## METABOLISM OF VITAMIN E

*limited*
*metabolism*

The metabolism of vitamin E is limited and most absorbed tocopherols are transported unchanged to the tissues. The *in vivo* antioxidant function of the vitamin results in its oxidation to **tocopherylquinone**, which proceeds through the semi-stable **tocopheroxyl radical** intermediate. It is important to note that, while the monovalent oxidation of tocopherol to the tocopheroxyl radical is a *reversible* reaction (at least *in vitro*), that further oxidation of the radical intermediate is *unidirectional*. Because, tocopherylquinone has no vitamin E activity, its production represents catabolism and loss of the vitamin from the system. Tocopherylquinone can be partially reduced to **a-tocopherylhydroquinone** which can be conjugated with glucuronic acid and secreted in the bile, thus, making excretion with the feces the major route of elimination of the vitamin. Under conditions of intakes of nutritional levels of vitamin E, less than 1% of the absorbed vitamin is excreted with the urine. The products identified in urine (**a-tocopheronic acid** and **a-tocopheronolactone**)[17] are side-chain oxidation derivatives of tocopherol; they may occur in conjugated form with glucuronic acid. That a large fraction of a-tocopherol can be found in the skin after injection suggests that dermal elimination of the vitamin may also be significant.

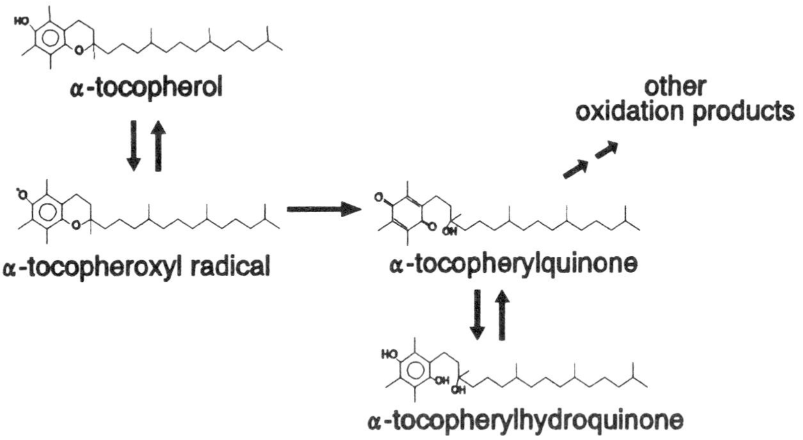

α-tocopherol

other
oxidation products

α-tocopheroxyl radical        α-tocopherylquinone

α-tocopherylhydroquinone

---

[17]These are collectively referred to as *"Simon's metabolites"*, after E.J. Simon who discovered them in the urine of rabbits and humans. There is still some question as to whether these metabolites result from metabolism of the vitamin *in vivo* (e.g., by β-oxidation in the kidney), or whether they may be artifacts resulting from oxidation during their isolation.

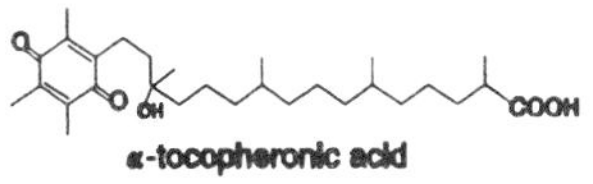

a-tocopheronic acid

a-tocopheronolactone

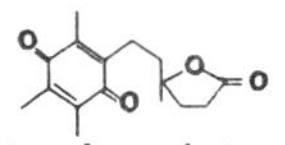

*recycling possible*

It has been proposed that a significant portion of vitamin E may be recycled *in vivo* by reduction of the tocopheroxyl radical back to tocopherol. Several findings have been cited as presumptive evidence for this hypothesis: the very low *in vivo* turnover of *a*-tocopherol; the slow rate of its depletion in vitamin E-deprived animals; the relatively low molar ratio of vitamin E to PUFA (ca. 1:850) in most biological membranes. Two mechanisms have been proposed for the *in vivo* recycling of tocopheroxyl: one with ascorbic acid as the reductant; the other with thiol. Ascorbic acid has been shown *in vitro* to reduce tocopheroxyl to tocopherol, being oxidized to dehydroascorbic acid in the process; however, unless that reaction can occur at the membrane:cytosol interface, it would appear to require a third factor capable of linking the major reactants, which are otherwise compartmentalized within the cell (ascorbic acid in the cytosol, and tocopheroxyl in the membrane). Indeed, studies with experimental animals have not shown significant nutritional *"sparing"* of vitamin E by ascorbic acid. The second mechanism is supported by recent evidence indicating that the reduced form of glutathione (GSH) can reduce membrane-bound tocopheroxyl in the presence of a ***tocopheroxyl "reductase" activity*** found in the endoplasmic reticulum and mito-chondria. That reductase activity may correspond to the heat-labile, GSH-dependent microsomal factor that has been found to inhibit lipid peroxidation in the presence of tocopherol. Thus, it is possible that the recycling of tocopherol may be coupled to the shuttle of electrons between GSH in the soluble phase of the cell and radicals in the membrane, resulting in the quenching (reduction) of the latter.

## METABOLIC FUNCTIONS OF VITAMIN E

*vitamin E as a biological antioxidant*

Although it was earlier debated whether vitamin E functions solely as a lipid antioxidant or whether it may also be required for the function of some other critical but unknown metabolic factor, information presently available indicates that all of its nutritional effects are consistent with its role as a biological antioxidant[18]. In this regard, vitamin E is thought to have basic functional importance in the maintenance of membrane integrity in virtually all cells of the body. Its antioxidant function involves the reduction of free radicals thus protecting against the potentially deleterious reactions of such highly reactive oxidizing species.

*mechanism of lipid peroxidation*

Potentially damaging free radicals (X·) are produced in cells under normal conditions either by homolytic cleavage of a covalent bond (e.g., the formation of a C-centered free radical of a polyunsaturated fatty acid), or

---

[18]An antioxidant is an agent that inhibits oxidation and, thus, prevents such oxidation reactions as the conversion of polyunsaturated fatty acids to fatty hydroperoxides, the conversion of free or protein-bound sulfhydryls to disulfides, etc.

by a univalent oxidation (e.g., metabolism of the herbicide paraquat to its N-centered radical anion species) or reduction (e.g., reduction of $O_2$ to form the superoxide radical $O_2^-$)[19]. The PUFAs of biological membranes are particularly susceptible to attack by free radicals by virtue of their 1,4-pentadiene systems which allow for the abstraction of a complete hydrogen atom (with its electron) from one of the -$CH_2$- groups in the carbon chain, and the consequent generation of a **C-centered free radical** (-C·-). This initial step in lipid peroxidation can be accomplished by hydroxyl radical (OH·) and possibly HOO· (but *not* by $H_2O_2$ nor $O_2^-$). The C-centered radical, being unstable, undergoes molecular rearrangement to form a **conjugated diene**, which is susceptible to attack by molecular oxygen ($O_2$) to yield a **peroxyl radical** (ROO·). Peroxyl radicals are capable of abstracting a hydrogen atom from other PUFAs and, thus, producing a **chain reaction** that can continue until the membrane PUFAs are completely oxidized to hydroperoxides (ROOH).

chain-cleavage products
(e.g., malonyldialdehyde, alkanes)

Fatty acyl hydroperoxides so formed are degraded in the presence of transition metals ($Cu^{++}$, $Fe^{++}$, $Fe^{+++}$), heme and heme proteins (cyto-

---

[19]There appear to be three main sources of free radicals in tissues, all of which give rise to $O_2^-$: normal oxidative metabolism; microsomal cytochrome $P_{450}$ activity; the *respiratory burst* of stimulated phagocytes.

chromes, hemoglobin, myoglobin) to release radicals that can continue the chain reaction of lipid peroxidation[20], as well as other chain-cleavage products, *malonyldialdehyde*[21], *pentane* and *ethane*[22]. This oxidative degradation of membrane phospholipid PUFAs is believed to result in physiochemical changes resulting in membrane dysfunction within the cell[23]. Cellular oxidant injury can also occur without significant lipid peroxidation, by oxidative damage to critical macromolecules (DNA, proteins) and decompartmentalization of $Ca^{++}$.[24]

*vitamin E as a scavenger of free radical*
Because of the reactivity of the phenolic hydrogen on its C-6 hydroxyl group and the ability of the chromanol ring system to stabilize an unpaired electron, vitamin E has antioxidant activity capable of terminating chain reactions among PUFAs in the membranes wherein it resides. This action, termed free radical *"scavenging"*, involves the donation of the phenolic H to a fatty acyl free radical (or $O_2^{.}$) to prevent the attack of that species on other PUFAs. The antioxidant activities of the vitamers E, thus, relate to the leaving ability of their phenolic H. The tocopherols have greatest reactivities toward peroxyl and phenoxyl radicals; when assessed *in vitro* in chemically defined systems, activities are greatest for α-tocopherol[25], with the β- and γ-isomers roughly comparable and greater than the δ-

---

[20]Therefore, a single radical can initiate a chain reaction that may propagate over and over again.

[21]Although malonyldialdehyde (MDA) is a relatively minor product of lipid peroxidation, it has received a great deal of attention in part because of the ease of measuring it colorimetrically using 3-thiobarbituric acid (TBA). In fact, the TBA test has been widely used to assess MDA concentrations as measures of lipid peroxidation. It is important to note that the TBA test is subject to several limitations. Specifically, much of the MDA it detects may not have been present in the original sample, as lipid peroxides are known to decompose to MDA during the heating stage of the test, that reaction being affected by the concentration of Fe-salts.

[22]The volatile alkanes, pentane and ethane, are excreted across the lungs and can be detected in the breath of vitamin E-deficient subjects. Pentane is produced from the oxidative breakdown of ω-6 fatty acids (linoleic acid family); whereas, ethane is produced from the ω-3 fatty acids (linolenic acid family).

[23]Whether lipid peroxidation does, indeed, occur *in vivo* has been surprisingly difficult to determine. Tissues of animals contain little of no evidence of lipid peroxides or their decomposition products. While expired breath contains volatile alkanes that might have originated from the decomposition of fatty acyl hydroperoxides, it is difficult to exclude the possibility of their production by bacteria of the gut or skin. Perhaps the greatest presumptive evidence for *in vivo* lipid peroxidation is that biological systems have evolved redundant mechanisms of antioxidant protection, specifically involving the powerful chain-breaking antioxidant α-tocopherol in the membrane and several other antioxidants (glutathione, cysteine, ascorbate, uric acid, glutathione peroxidase, ceruloplasmin) in the soluble phase. Indeed, it is clear that deficiencies of this antioxidant defense system can greatly impair physiological function.

[24]For example, pulmonary injury by the bipyridinium herbicide paraquat involves lipid peroxidation only as a late stage event, rather than as a cause of it.

[25]The antioxidant activity of α-tocopherol is ca. 200-fold that of the commonly used food antioxidant butylated hydroxytoluene (BHT).

isomer. In the process, vitamin E is itself converted to a semi-stable radical intermediate, the **tocopheroxyl** (or **chromanoxyl**) **radical**. Unlike the free radicals formed from PUFAs, the tocopheroxyl radical is relatively unreactive, thus, stopping the destructive propagative cycle of lipid peroxidation. In fact, tocopheroxyl is sufficiently stable to react with a second peroxyl radical to form inactive, non-radical products including **tocopheryl-quinone**. Because $a$-tocopherol can compete for peroxyl radicals much faster than PUFAs, small amounts of the vitamin are able to effect the anti-oxidant protection of relatively large amounts of the latter.

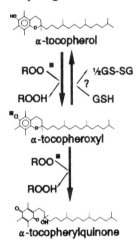

α-tocopherol

α-tocopheroxyl

α-tocopherylquinone

While $a$-tocopherol is clearly the most abundant lipid-soluble chain-breaking antioxidant, the fact that it is typically present at such low amounts relative to the membrane PUFAs it protects suggests that it is both recycled (as discussed above) and highly mobile within the membrane. Recent evidence suggests the presence of two membrane pools of $a$-tocopherol: a highly mobile one and a relatively fixed one. A model that would appear to fit the latter was presented some years ago; it proposed that the vitamin may actually reside in intimate contact with PUFAs by virtue of their complementary three-dimensional structures.

*other factors*  Because it is hydrophobic and, therefore, distributed in membranes, vitamin
*in antioxidant*  E serves as a lipid-soluble biological antioxidant with high specificity for
*defense*  loci of potential lipid peroxidation. However, in its antioxidant function vitamin E is but one of several factors that act in concert to effect antioxidant protection of the cell. That multi-component system includes

vitamin E, which scavenges radicals within the membrane (both blocking the initiation as well as interrupting the propagation of lipid peroxidation), and a group of metalloenzymes which collectively block the initiation of peroxidation from within the soluble phase of the cell. Those enzymes include the **superoxide dismutases**[26], which convert $O_2^-$ to $H_2O_2$, and **catalase**[27] and **glutathione peroxidase**[28], both of which further reduce $H_2O_2$. The aggregate effect of this enzymatic system is to clear $O_2^-$ by reducing it fully to $H_2O$, thus, preventing the generation of other more highly reactive oxygen species (e.g., hydroxyl radical, singlet oxygen) that can act as potent initiators of lipid peroxidation. Glutathione peroxidase can also reduce fatty acyl hydroperoxides to the corresponding fatty alcohols, thus, serving to interrupt the propagation of lipid peroxidation.

That the various components of the cellular antioxidant defense system function cooperatively is evidenced by the nutritional sparing observed particularly for vitamin E and Se in the etiologies of several deficiency diseases (e.g., exudative diathesis in chicks, liver necrosis in rats, white muscle disease in lambs and calves). In those species, nutritional

---

[26]The superoxide dismutases (SODs) are metalloenzymes. The mitochondrial SOD contains Mn at its active center; whereas, the cytosolic SOD contains both Cu and Zn as essential cofactors. Although not found in animals, an Fe-centered SOD has been identified in blue-green algae.

[27]Catalase has an Fe redox center. Because its distribution is almost exclusively limited to the peroxisomes/lysosomes, it is probably not important in antioxidant protection in the cytosol.

[28]Glutathione peroxidase contains Se at its active center and is dependent upon adequate supplies of that element for its synthesis. It uses reducing equivalents from reduced glutathione (GSH) to reduce $H_2O_2$ to water or fatty acyl hydroperoxides to the corresponding fatty alcohols. Its activity, therefore, depends upon a functioning glutathione cycle (i.e., the flavoenzyme glutathione reductase) to regenerate GSH from its oxidized form (GSSG). Its role as an essential component of glutathione peroxidase is the only known biochemical function of Se.

deprivation of either vitamin E *or* Se *alone* is usually asymptomatic; whereas, deficiencies of *both* nutrients are required to produce disease. This phenomenon is thought to follow from the interruption of the cellular antioxidant defense that has been produced.

*protection from oxyradicals*

Factors that increase the production of reactive oxygen (e.g., xenobiotic metabolism, ionizing radiation, exposure to such pro-oxidants as ozone and $NO_2$) can be expected to increase the metabolic demand for antioxidant protection, including the need for vitamin E and the other nutrients involved in this system. Accordingly, vitamin E has been proposed as playing an important role in general health with specific implications regarding protection from conditions thought to involve untoward effects of oxyradicals. For example, because vitamin E-deficiency has been found to increase the susceptibility of experimental animals to the pathological effects of ozone, it has been suggested that vitamin E supplements may protect against harmful effects of chronic exposures to ozone in smog.

Because experimental data suggest a causative role of oxyradicals in *aging* processes[29], it has been suggested that status with respect to vitamin E and other antioxidants may affect and longevity. Free radical events have also been implicated in the etiologies of a number of diseases. Epidemiological studies have indicated that patients with senile *cataracts*, the pathogenesis of which appears to involve oxyradicals, tend to have lower low plasma concentrations of vitamin E (as well as ascorbic acid and carotenoids) than matched controls. The results of a pilot study suggest that the progression of *Parkinson's disease*, a syndrome that has been proposed to involve the formation of oxyradicals *via* endogenous enzymatic oxidation and non-enzymatic autoxidation in monoamine neurons[30], can be retarded by high doses of vitamins E and C.

Vitamin E and other free radical scavengers have been found to affect the functions of mitochondria and sarcoplasmic reticula in animal models of myocardial injury induced by *ischemia-reperfusion*. That injury, which occurs in tissues reperfused after a brief period of ischemia, appears to be due to oxidative stress of re-oxygenation, involving the production of oxyradicals. The phenomenon has been demonstrated for several tissues

---

[29]For example, mammalian life spans tend to correlate directly with tissue concentrations of specific antioxidants and inversely with oxidative damage to DNA. It has been suggested that oxyradicals may be a cause of improper gene regulation, thus, affecting aging and longevity. Alternatively, it has also been suggested that, by affecting *"peroxide tone"* (i.e., the net presence of oxyradicals within the cell), particularly the presence of lipid peroxides, antioxidant status may influence the dioxygenation reactions of cyclooxygenase and lipoxygenase to modulate arachidonic acid metabolism and prostaglandin synthesis. Such effects are thought to be associated with aging processes, as the concentration of prostaglandin $E_2$ in the brain is known to decline with age; in mice, that decline has been shown to be reduced by supplemental vitamin E.

[30]This is the *"endogenous toxin"* hypothesis. The etiology of Parkinson's disease is unknown; however, this and other hypotheses have been offered. These include viral encephalitis, intra-uterine influenza, hereditary factors, nutrient deprivation *in utero*, and other endogenous toxins.

(heart, brain, skin, intestine and pancreas) and has relevance to the preservation of organs for transplantation. A disorder that appears to involve natural ischemia-reperfusion injury in *intraventricular hemorrhage*[31] of the premature infant. The results of a recent randomized clinical trial clearly demonstrate that vitamin E supplements (given by intramuscular injection) can be very effective in protecting premature infants against intraventricular hemorrhage. In disorders of this type, it is thought that vitamin E may act as a radical scavenger to protect against the oxidative stress associated with ischemia-reperfusion.

Vitamin E has frequently proven effective as a therapeutic measure in several disorders of humans, even though it may not be directly involved in their etiologies. These include hemolytic *anemia of prematurity*, some hereditary *muscular dystrophies*, *angina pectoris*, *intermittent claudication*[32], and *chronic hemolysis* in patients with glucose-6-phosphate dehydrogenase deficiency. In veterinary practice, vitamin E (most frequently administered with Se) has had reported efficacy in the treatment of several disorders including *"tying up"* in horses, and postpartum *placental retention* in cows. Formerly, vitamin E was thought to protect against retinopathy of prematurity[33]; however, a recent controlled clinical trial showed that its use failed to reduce the prevalence of the syndrome.

Because chemical carcinogenesis is thought to involve the electrophilic attack of radicals with DNA, it would seem reasonable to expect that antioxidants such as vitamin E may protect against *cancer* by acting as protective reductants. That a product of lipid peroxidation, *malonyldialdehyde*, has been found to increase tumor production in certain animal models further strengthens an hypothesis for a role of vitamin E status in cancer risk. While the results of several epidemiological studies have supported that hypothesis (showing inverse relationships of plasma $\alpha$-tocopherol levels and risk to tumors of breast, lung, stomach, pancreas and urogenital tract), those of studies with experimental animals model have been inconsistent in detecting anti-carcinogenic effects of the vitamin.

---

[31] Hemorrhage in an around the lateral ventricles of the brain occurs in ca. 40% of infants born prior to 33 weeks of gestation.

[32] nocturnal leg cramps.

[33] formerly, *"retrolental fibroplasia"*

## EXTREMES IN VITAMIN E INTAKE

*deficiency*    Vitamin E deficiency can result from insufficient dietary intake or impaired absorption of the vitamin. Several other dietary factors affect the need for vitamin E. Two are most important in this regard: Se and PUFAs. Selenium spares the need for vitamin E; accordingly, animals fed low-Se diets generally require more vitamin E than animals fed the same diets supplemented with an available source of Se. In contrast, the dietary intake of PUFAs *directly* affects the need for vitamin E; animals fed high-PUFA diets require more vitamin E than those fed low-PUFA ones[34]. Other factors that can be expected to increase vitamin E needs are deficiencies of S-containing amino acids[35]; deficiencies of Cu, Zn and/or Mn[36]; and deficiency of riboflavin[37]. Alternatively, vitamin E can be replaced by several lipid-soluble synthetic antioxidants[38] (e.g. BHT[39], BHA[40], DPPD[41]) and, to some extent, by vitamin C[42].

Conditions involving the ***malabsorption of lipids*** can also lead to vitamin E deficiency. Such conditions include those resultant of loss of pancreatic exocrine function (e.g., pancreatitis, pancreatic tumor, nutritional pancreatic

---

[34]Various researchers have suggested values for the incremental effects of dietary PUFA level on the nutritional requirement for vitamin E in the range of .18-.60 mg $\alpha$-tocopherol per g PUFA. Although the upper end of that range is frequently cited as a guideline for estimating vitamin E needs, it is fair to state that there is no consensus among experts in the field as to the quantitation of this obviously important relationship.

[35]Cysteine, which can be synthesized *via* transsulfuration from methionine, is needed for the synthesis of glutathione, i.e., the substrate for the Se-dependent glutathione peroxidase.

[36]These are essential cofactors of the superoxide dismutases.

[37]Riboflavin is required for the synthesis of FAD, the coenzyme for glutathione reductase which is required for regeneration of reduced glutathione *via* the so-called *'glutathione cycle'*.

[38]The fact that vitamin E can be replaced by a variety of antioxidants was a point of debate concerning the status of the nutrient as a vitamin. It should be noted that, while such replacement can occur, the effective levels of other antioxidants are considerably greater (e.g., two orders of magnitude) than those of $\alpha$-tocopherol. Therefore, it is now generally agreed that, while the metabolic role of vitamin E is that of an antioxidant which can be fulfilled by other reductants, tocopherol performs this function with high biological specificity and is, therefore, appropriately considered a vitamin.

[39]butylated hydroxytoluene.

[40]butylated hydroxyanisole.

[41]N,N'-diphenyl-*p*-phenylenediamine.

[42]The sparing effect of vitamin C may involve its function in the reductive recycling of tocopherol.

atrophy in severe Se-deficiency), those involving a luminal deficiency of bile (e.g., biliary stasis due to mycotoxicosis, biliary atresia), and those due to defects in lipoprotein metabolism (e.g., abetalipoproteinemia[43]). Premature infants, which typically have impaired ability to utilize dietary fats, are also at risk to vitamin E deficiency.

Signs of vitamin E deficiency:

| organ system | sign | responds to | | |
|---|---|---|---|---|
| | | vitamin E | Se | antioxidants |
| general | loss of appetite | + | + | + |
| | reduced growth | + | + | + |
| dermatologic | none | | | |
| muscular | myopathies | | | |
| | striated muscles[a] | + | + | |
| | cardiac muscle[b] | + | | |
| | smooth muscle[c] | + | + | |
| skeletal | none | | | |
| vital organs | liver necrosis[d] | + | + | |
| | renal degeneration[d] | + | | + |
| nervous system | encephalomalacia[e] | + | | + |
| | areflexia, ataxia[f] | + | | |
| reproduction | fetal death[g] | + | + | + |
| | testicular degen.[h] | + | + | |
| ocular | cataract[i] | + | | |
| | retinopathy[j] | +? | | |
| vascular | anemia[j,k] | + | | |
| | RBC hemolysis[l] | + | | |
| | exudative diathesis[e] | + | + | |
| | intraventricular hemorrhage[j] | + | | |

[a]Nutritional muscular dystrophies (*"white muscle"* diseases) of chicks, rats, guinea pigs, rabbits, dogs, monkeys, minks, sheep, goats and calves.   [b]*"Mulberry heart"* disease of pigs.   [c]Gizzard myopathy of turkeys and ducks.   [d]In rats, mice and pigs.   [e]In chicks.   [f]In abetalipoproteinemic humans.   [g]In rats, cattle and sheep. [h]In chickens, rats, rabbits, hamsters, dogs, pigs and monkeys.   [i]Reported only in rats.   [j]Low vitamin E status is suspect in this condition in premature human infants.   [k]In monkeys, pigs and humans.   [l]In chicks, rats, rabbits and humans.

The clinical manifestations of vitamin E deficiency vary considerably between species. In general, however, the targets are the *neuromuscular*[44], *vascular* and *reproductive systems*. The various signs of vitamin E deficiency are believed to be manifestations of membrane

---

[43]Humans with this rare hereditary disorder are unable to produce apoprotein B, an essential component of chylomicra, VLDL and LDL. The absence of these particles from the serum prevents the absorption of vitamin E due to the inability to transport it into the lymphatics. These patients show generalized lipid malabsorption with steatorrhea and have undetectable serum vitamin E levels.

[44]The skeletal myopathies of vitamin E-deficient animals entail lesions predominantly involving type I fibers.

dysfunction resultant of the oxidative degradation of polyunsaturated membrane phospholipids and/or the disruption of other critical cellular processes[45]. Many deficiency syndromes (e.g., encephalomalacia in the chick, intraventricular hemorrhage in the premature human infant, and at least some myopathies) appear to involve local cellular anoxia resulting from primary lesions of the vascular system. Others (e.g., retrolental fibroplasia in the premature human infant[46]) appear to involve the lack to protection from oxidative stress. It has also been proposed that some effects (e.g., impaired immune cell functions) may involve loss of control of the oxidative metabolism of arachidonic acid in its conversion to leukotrienes; vitamin E is known to inhibit the 5'-lipoxygenase in that pathway.

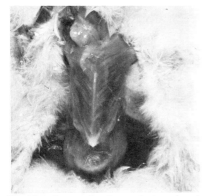

Nutritional muscular dystrophy in a vitamin E-deficient chick; Zenker's degeneration of *m. pectorales* gives a striated appearance.

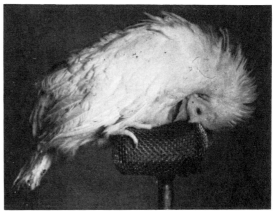

Encephalomalacia in a vitamin E-deficient chick.

*hyper-vitaminosis*    Vitamin E is **one of the least toxic of the vitamins**. Animals and humans appear to be able to tolerate rather high levels (i.e., at least two orders of magnitude above nutritional requirements, e.g., 1000-2000 IU/kg diet) of the vitamin without untoward effects.[47]

---

[45] It is interesting to note a situation in which vitamin E-deficiency would appear advantageous: The efficacy of the antimalarial drug derived from Chinese traditional medicine, 'qinghaosu' (artemisinin), is enhanced by deprivation of vitamin E. The drug, an endoperoxide, is thought to act against the Plasmodial parasite by generating free radicals *in vivo*. Thus, depriving the patient of vitamin E appears to limit the parasite's access to the protective antioxidant.

[46] The pathogenesis of this condition involves exposure to a hyperoxic environment during neonatal oxygen therapy. Retrolental fibroplasia can affect as many as 11% of infants with birth weights below 1500 g, resulting in blindness of ca. one-quarter of them.

[47] The $LD_{50}$ values of all-*rac*-$\alpha$-tocopherol or all-*rac*-$\alpha$-tocopheryl acetate for rats, mice and rabbits are >2 g/kg body weight.

At very high doses, however, vitamin E can produce signs indicative of antagonism of the function of the other fat-soluble vitamins.   Thus, hypervitaminotic E animals have been found to show impaired bone mineralization, reduced hepatic storage of vitamin A, and coagulopathies. In each case, these signs could be corrected with increased dietary supplements of the appropriate vitamin (i.e., vitamins D, A and K, respectively) and the antagonism seemed to be based at the level of absorption.   Isolated reports of negative effects in human subjects consuming up to 1000 IU vitamin E per day included headache, fatigue, nausea, double vision, muscular weakness, mild creatinuria and gastro-intestinal distress.

Potentially deleterious metabolic effects of high-level vitamin E status include inhibitions of *retinyl ester hydrolase* and *vitamin K-dependent carboxylations*.   The former effect has been demonstrated in animals where it results in impaired ability to mobilize vitamin A from hepatic stores. Evidence for the latter effect is still circumstantial, i.e., patients given megadoses of vitamin E (e.g. 1200 IU/day) showed prolonged blood clotting times due to hypoprothrombinemia.   This effect may only be of concern with regard to patients on anti-coagulant therapy; indeed, it may have therapeutic utility.   Although the metabolic basis of the effect is not clear, it is thought to involve tocopherylquinone which, bearing structural similarities to vitamin K, may act as an inhibitor of vitamin K metabolism.

Massive doses (e.g., 30-300 times required levels) of vitamin E have also been reported to enhance atherogenesis in cholesterol-fed rabbits and DNA-adduct formation in the rat.   The significance of these reports is presently unclear.

## CASE STUDY

| | |
|---|---|
| *Instructions:* | *Review the following case report paying special attention to the diagnostic indicators upon which the treatments were based.   Then answer the questions that follow.* |

*case 1*     At birth, a male infant with **acidosis**[48] and **hemolytic anemia**[49] was diagnosed as having **glutathione (GSH) synthetase**[50] deficiency associated with **5-keto-prolinuria**[51] ; he was treated symptomatically. During his second year, he experienced six episodes of bacterial **otitis media**[52]. His white cell counts fell to 3,000-4,000 cells per $\mu l$ during two of these infections with notable losses of **polymorphonuclear leukocytes**[53] **(PMNs)**. Between infections, the child had normal white and differential cell counts, and PMNs were obtained for study.

Functional studies of PMNs showed the following results:

| parameter | finding |
|---|---|
| GSH synthetase activity | 10% of normal |
| phagocytosis of *Staphylococcus aureus* | less than normal |
| iodination of phagocytized zymosan | |
| particles | much less than normal |
| $H_2O_2$ production during phagocytosis | well above normal |

The child was then treated daily with 30 IU of all-*rac*-*a*-tocopheryl acetate per kg body weight (ca. 400 IU/day).  His plasma vitamin E concentration rose from 0.34 mg/dl (normal for infants) to 1.03 mg/dl.  After three months of treatment, the same studies of his PMNs were performed.

---

[48] the condition of reduced alkali reserve.

[49] reduced number of erythrocytes per unit blood volume, resulting from their destruction.

[50] This is the rate-limiting enzyme in the pathway of the biosynthesis of glutathione (GSH), a tripeptide of glycine, cysteine and glutamic acid, and the most abundant cellular thiol compound.  The oxidized form is a dimer joined by a disulfide bridge between the cysteinyl residues (GSSG).

[51] This is the condition of abnormally high urinary concentrations of 5-ketoproline, the intermediate in the pathway of GSH biosynthesis (the *'γ-glutamyl cycle'*).

[52] inflammation of the middle ear.

[53] The PMN is a type of white blood cell important in disease resistance which functions by phagocytizing bacteria and other foreign particles.

Although there were no changes in the activity of *GSH peroxidase*[54] or the concentration of GSH (which remained near 25% of normal during this study) in his plasma, the production of $H_2O_2$ by his PMNs had declined to normal levels, the iodination of proteins during phagocytosis had increased, and the bactericidal activity toward *S. aureus* had increased to the control level. Before his vitamin E therapy, electron microscopy of his neutrophils had revealed defective cytoskeletal structure, with more than the usual number of *microtubules*[55] seen at rest and a disappearance of microtubules seen during phagocytosis. This ultrastructural defect was corrected after vitamin E treatment.

*case 2*    A 23-year-old woman with a 10-year history of neurologic disease was admitted complaining of severe ataxia[56], titubation of the head[57], and loss of proprioceptive sense in her extremities.[58] Her past history revealed that she had experienced difficulty walking and was unsteady at age 10 years; there was no family history of ataxia, malabsorption or neurologic disease. At 18 years of age, she had been hospitalized for her neurologic complaints; at that time, she had been below the 5th percentile for both height and weight. Her examination had revealed normal higher intellectual function, speech and cranial nerve function; but her limbs had been found hypotonic[59] with preservation of strength and moderately severe ataxia. Her deep tendon reflexes were absent, plantar responses were abnormal, vibrational sense was absent below the wrists and iliac crests, and joint position sense was defective at the fingers and toes. Laboratory findings at that time had been negative, i.e., she showed no indications of hepatic or renal dysfunction. No etiologic diagnosis was made. Two years later, when she was 20 years old, the patient was re-evaluated. By that time, her gait had deteriorated and her proprioceptive loss had become more severe.

Over the next three years, her symptoms worsened and, by age 23 years, she had trouble walking unassisted. Still, she showed no sensory, visual, bladder, respiratory or cardiac signs and ate a normal and nutritious diet.

---

[54] an enzyme that catalyzes the reduction of hydroperoxides (including $H_2O_2$) with the concomitant oxidation of glutathione (2GSH converted to GSSG).

[55] a subcellular organelle.

[56] loss of muscular coordination.

[57] unsteadiness

[58] senses of position, etc., originating from the arms and legs.

[59] having abnormally low tension.

Her only gastrointestinal complaint was of constipation, with bowel movements only once per week.  Nerve conduction tests revealed that the action potentials of both her sensory and motor nerves, recorded from the median and ulnar nerves, were normal.  Electromyography of the biceps, vastas medialis and tibialis anterior muscles was normal.  However, her cervical and cortical somatosensory-evoked responses to median nerve stimulation were abnormal: there was no peripheral delay and the nature of the response was abnormal.  Further, no consistent cortical responses could be recorded after stimulation of the tibial nerve at the ankle.  These findings were interpreted as indicating **spinocerebellar disease** characterized by delayed sensory conduction in the posterior columns.

Routine screening tests failed to detect $a$-tocopherol in her plasma, although she showed elevated circulating levels of cholesterol (448 mg/dl vs. normal: 150-240 mg/dl) and triglycerides (184 mg/dl vs. normal: 50-150 mg/dl).  Her plasma concentrations of 25-(OH)-$D_3$, retinol and vitamin K-dependent clotting factors were in normal ranges.  Tests of lipid malabsorption showed no abnormality.  Her glucose tolerance and pancreatic function (assessed after injections of cholecystokinin and secretin) were also normal.

The patient was given 2 g $a$-tocopheryl acetate with an ordinary meal; her plasma $a$-tocopherol level, which had been non-detectable before the dose, was in the subnormal range 2 hours later and she showed a relatively flat absorption[60] curve.  She was given the same large dose of the vitamin daily for 2 weeks at which time her plasma $a$-tocopherol concentration was 24 $\mu$g/ml.  When her daily dose was reduced to 800 mg $a$-tocopheryl acetate per day for 10 weeks, her plasma level was 1.2 mg/dl, i.e., in the normal range.  During this time, she showed marked clinical improvement.

---

Questions:    i.      What *two* inborn metabolic errors were apparent in the first patient?

ii.     What sign/symptom indicated a vitamin E-related disorder in each case?

iii.    Why are PMNs useful for studying protection from oxidative stress, as in the first case?

iv.     What inborn metabolic error might you suspect that led to vitamin E deficiency in the second patient?

---

[60] i.e., plasma $a$-tocopherol concentration vs. time

## Study Questions and Exercises:

i.      Construct a *concept map* illustrating the nutritional interrelationships of vitamin E and other nutrients.

ii.     Construct a *'decision tree'* for the *diagnosis* of vitamin E deficiency in a human or animal.

iii.    What *features* of the *chemical structure* of vitamin E relate to its *nutritional activity*?

iv.     How might *vitamin E utilization* be affected by a diet high in polyunsaturated fat? of a fat-free diet?  of a Se-deficient diet?

v.      What kinds of *prooxidants* might you expect people or animals to encounter daily?

vi.     How can nutritional deficiencies of *vitamin E* and *Se* be distinguished?

## Recommended Reading:

Anonymous. 1983. Biology of Vitamin E, CIBA Found. Symp., Pitman, London. 260 pp.

Bendrich, A. and L.J. Machlin. 1988. Safety of oral intake of vitamin E. Am. J. Clin. Nutr. 48:612-619.

Bieri, J.G. 1990. Vitamin E, Chapter 13 in Present Knowledge in Nutrition, 6th edition, (M. Brown, ed.), Internat. Life Sci. Inst.-Nutr. Found., Washington, D.C., pp. 117-121.

Bjørneboe, A., G.E. Bjørneboe and C.A. Drevon. 1990. Absorption, transport and distribution of vitamin E. J. Nutr. 120:233-242.

Burton, G.W. and M.G. Trabor. 1990. Vitamin E: antioxidant activity, biokinetics and bioavailability. Ann. Rev. Nutr. 10:357-382.

Diplock, A.T. 1991. Antioxidant nutrients and disease prevention: an overview. Am. J. Clin. Nutr. 53:189S-193S.

Diplock, A.T. 1985. Vitamin E, Chapter 3 in Fat-Soluble Vitamins. Their Biochemistry and Applications (A.T. Diplock, ed.), Technomic Publ. Co., Basel, pp. 154-224.

Friedrich, W. 1988. Vitamins. Walter de Gruyter, New York, pp. 217-283.

Machlin, L.J. 1991. Vitamin E. Chapter 3 in Handbook of Vitamins, 2nd ed. (L.J. Machlin, ed.), Marcel Dekker, New York, pp. 99-144.

Machlin, L.J. (ed.). 1980. Vitamin E. A Comprehensive Treatise. Marcel Dekker, New York, 660 pp.

Mergens, W.J. and H.N. Bhagavan. 1989. $\alpha$-Tocopherols (vitamin E). Chapter 12 in Nutrition and Cancer Prevention, Investigating the Role of Micronutrients (T.E. Moon and M.S. Micozzi, eds.), Marcel Dekker, New York, pp. 305-340.

Pryor, W.A. 1991. Can vitamin E protect humans against the pathological effects of ozone in smog? Am. J. Clin. Nutr. 53:702-722.

Thurnham, D.I. 1990. Antioxidants and prooxidants in malnourished populations. Proc. Nutr. Soc. 49:247-259.

# CHAPTER 8   *VITAMIN K*

*". . . little progress in elucidating the role of vitamin K in the synthesis of the clotting factors was made until the mid-1960s [when it was found] that prothrombin was formed from a liver precursor protein [by a] vitamin K-dependent step. . . . These studies culminated in 1974 with the demonstration that prothrombin contained a number of residues of a previously unidentified amino acid . . . [and that vitamin K functions] as a cofactor for an enzyme that carboxylates peptide-bound glutamyl residues and converts them to γ-carboxyglutamyl residues."*

J.W. Suttie

## Anchoring Concepts:

| | |
|---|---|
| i. | Vitamin K is the generic descriptor for 2-methyl-1,4-naphthoquinone and all its derivatives exhibiting qualitatively the anti-hemorrhagic activity of phylloquinone. |
| ii. | The vitamers K are side-chain homologues; each is hydrophobic and, thus, insoluble in such aqueous environments as plasma, interstitial fluids and cytoplasm. |
| iii. | The 1,4-naphthoquinone ring system of vitamin K renders it susceptible to metabolic reduction. |
| iv. | Deficiencies of vitamin K have a narrow clinical spectrum: hemorrhagic disorders. |

## Learning Objectives:

| | |
|---|---|
| i. | To understand the nature of the various *sources* of vitamin K. |
| ii. | To understand the means of *absorption* and *transport* of the vitamers K. |
| iii. | To understand the *metabolic functions* of vitamin K in the biosynthesis of plasma clotting factors and other Ca-binding proteins. |
| iv. | To understand the *physiologic implications* of impaired vitamin K function. |

*Vocabulary:*

atherocalcin
γ-carboxyglutamate
coagulopathy
coprophagy
coumarins
dicoumarol
dysprothrombinemia
extrinsic clotting system
factor II
factor VII
factor IX
factor X
fibrin
hemorrhage
hydroxy vitamin K
hypoprothrombinemia
intrinsic clotting system
menadione
menadione sodium bisulfite complex

menadione pyridinol bisulfite
menaquinone
naphthoquinone
osteocalcin
phylloquinone
protein C
protein M
protein S
protein Z
Stuart factor
superoxide
thrombin
thromboplastin
vitamin K-dependent carboxylase
vitamin K epoxide
vitamin K hydroquinone
vitamin K oxide
warfarin
zymogen

# SOURCES OF VITAMIN K

*distribution in foods*

There are two natural sources of vitamin K. ***Green plants*** synthesize the ***phylloquinones***; phylloquinone[1] is a normal component of chloroplasts. ***Bacteria*** (including those of the normal intestinal microflora) and some spore-forming ***actinomycetes*** synthesize the ***menaquinones***.  The predominant vitamers of the menaquinone series contain 6-10 isoprenoid units; however, vitamers with as many as 13 isoprenoid groups have been identified. ***Menadione***[2], the formal parent compound of the menaquinone series, does not occur naturally but is a common ***synthetic*** form.  The synthetic menadione forms a water-soluble sodium bisulfite addition product, ***menadione sodium bisulfite***, the practical utility of which is limited by its instability in complex matrices such as feeds.  However, in the presence of excess sodium bisulfite, it crystallizes as a complex with an additional mole of sodium bisulfite (i.e., ***menadione sodium bisulfite complex***) which has greater stability and, therefore, is used widely as a supplement to poultry feeds.  A third water-soluble compound is ***menadione pyridinol bisulfite*** (MPB), a salt formed by the addition of dimethyl-pyridinol.

*biopotency of vitamers*

The relative biopotencies of the various vitamers K differs according to the route of administration.  Studies using restoration of normal clotting in the vitamin K-deficient chick have shown that, when administered orally, phylloquinone or menaquinone homologues with 3-5 isoprenoid groups had greater activities than those with longer side-chains.  The difference in biopotency appears to relate to the relatively poor absorption of the long-chain vitamers.  In fact, studies with the vitamin K-deficient rat showed that the long-chain homologues (especially MK-9) had the greatest activities when administered intracardially.  Of the three synthetic forms, some studies indicate MPB to be somewhat more effective in chick diets; however, each is generally regarded to be comparable in biopotency to phylloquinone.

*dietary sources*

Green leafy vegetables tend to be rich in vitamin K, while fruits and grains are poor sources.  The vitamin K activities of meats and dairy products tend to be moderate.  Unfortunately, data for the vitamin K contents of foods are limited by the lack of good analytical methods.  Nevertheless, it is clear that, because dietary needs for vitamin K are low, most foods contribute significantly to those needs[3].

---

[1] 2-methyl-3-phytyl-1,4-naphthoquinone.

[2] 2-methyl-1,4-naphthoquinone.

[3] In fact, it is difficult to formulate an otherwise normal diet that does not contain ca. 100 $\mu$g of the vitamin.

Vitamin K contents of common foods:

| food | vitamin K, $\mu$g/100 g | food | vitamin K, $\mu$g/100g |
|---|---|---|---|
| *vegetables* | | *fruits* | |
| asparagus | 39 | apples | 4[*] |
| beans, mung | 33 | bananas | .5 |
| beans, snap | 28 | cranberries | 1.4 |
| beets | 5 | oranges | 1.3 |
| broccoli | 154 | peaches | 3 |
| cabbage | 149 | strawberries | 14 |
| carrots | 13 | | |
| cauliflower | 191 | *meats* | |
| chick peas | 48 | beef | .6 |
| corn | 4 | chicken | .01 |
| cucumbers | 5 | beef liver | 104 |
| kale | 275 | chicken liver | 80 |
| tomatoes | 48 | pork liver | 88 |
| lettuce | 113 | | |
| peas | 28 | *dairy products and eggs* | |
| potatoes | .5 | milk, cow's | 4 |
| spinach | 266 | eggs | 50 |
| sweet potatoes | 4 | egg yolk | 149 |
| | | | |
| *oils* | | *grains* | |
| canola (rapeseed) | 830 | oats | 63 |
| corn | 5 | rice | .05 |
| olive | 58 | wheat | 20 |
| peanut | 2 | wheat bran | 83 |
| soybean | 200 | wheat germ | 39 |
| source: USDA data, 1990 | | [*]almost 90% in the skin (peeling) | |

*intestinal microbial synthesis*

Microbial synthesis of vitamin K[4] in the intestine appears to have nutritional significance in most animal species. This is indicated by observations that germ-free animals have greater dietary requirements for the vitamin than animals with normal intestinal microfloras, and that prevention of coprophagy is necessary to produce vitamin K deficiency in some species (e.g., chicks, rats). The human gut contains substantial amounts of menaquinones of bacterial origin. The nutritional significance of this source of the vitamin is not clear, as the extent of absorption of those forms from the large intestine is not established[5].

---

[4]Bacteria and plants synthesize the aromatic ring system of vitamin K from shikimic acid. The ultimate synthesis of the menaquinones in bacteria proceeds through 1,4-dihydroxy-2-naphthoic acid (*not* menadione), which is prenylated, decarboxylated and, then, methylated.

[5]It appears that menaquinones produced by the gut microflora are absorbed across the large intestine at least to a limited extent, as the liver normally contains a significant amount of those forms of vitamin K.

## ABSORPTION OF VITAMIN K

*micellar*
*solubilization*

The vitamers K are absorbed from the intestine into the lymphatic (in mammals) or portal (in birds, fishes and reptiles) circulation by processes that first require that these hydrophobic substances be dispersed in the aqueous lumen of the gut *via* the formation of mixed micelles in which they are dissolved. Vitamin K absorption, therefore, depends on normal pancreatic and biliary function. Conditions resulting in impaired luminal micelle formation (e.g., dietary mineral oil, pancreatic exocrine dysfunction, bile stasis), therefore, impair the enteric absorption of vitamin K. It can be expected that any diet will contain a mixture of menaquinones and phylloquinones. In general such mixtures appear to be absorbed with efficiencies in the range of 40-70%; however, these vitamers are absorbed *via* different mechanisms.

*active*
*transport of*
*phylloquinone*

Studies of the uptake of vitamin K by everted gut sacs of the rat show that phylloquinone is absorbed by an ***energy-dependent process*** from the proximal small intestine. The process is not affected by menaquinones or menadione; it is inhibited by the addition of short- and medium-chain fatty acids to the micellar medium.

*other vitamers*
*absorbed by*
*diffusion*

In contrast, the menaquinones and menadione are absorbed strictly *via* non-carrier-mediated ***passive diffusion***, the rates of which are affected by the micellar contents of lipids and bile salts. This kind of passive absorption has been found to occur in the distal part of the small intestine as well as in the colon. Thus, non-coprophagous[6] animals appear to profit from the bacterial synthesis of vitamin K in their lower guts by being able to absorb the vitamin from that location[7].

---

[6]Coprophagy is the ingestion of excrement. This behavior is common in many species, exposing them to nutrients such as vitamin K produced by the microbial flora of their lower guts. Coprophagy can be easily prevented in some species (e.g., chicks) by housing them on raised wire floors; it is very difficult to prevent in others (e.g., rats) without the use of such devices as tail cups.

[7]Humans appear to be able to utilize menaquinones produced by their lower gut microflora. Indirect evidence for this is that hypoprothrombinemia is rare *except* among patients given antibiotics, even when vitamin K-free purified diets have been used.

## TRANSPORT OF VITAMIN K

*absorbed*        Upon absorption, vitamin K associates with chylomicra whereby it is trans-
*vitamin K*       ported to the liver.  Vitamin K is rapidly taken up by the liver, but it has a
*transferred to*  relatively short half-life there (ca. 17 hrs.) and it is transferred to VLDL and
*lipoproteins*    LDL which carry it in the plasma.  No specific carriers have been identified
                  for any of the vitamers K.  Plasma levels of phylloquinone are correlated
                  with those of triglycerides and $\alpha$-tocopherol; those of healthy humans are
                  in the range of .1-.7 ng/ml.

*tissue*          When administered as either phylloquinone or menaquinone, vitamin K is
*distribution*    rapidly taken up by the liver.  In contrast, little menadione is taken up by
                  that organ; instead, it is distributed widely to other tissues.   Hepatic
                  storage of vitamin K has little long-term significance, as the vitamin is
                  rapidly removed from that organ and rapidly excreted.  The vitamin is
                  found at low levels in many organs; several tend to concentrate it: adrenal
                  glands, lungs, bone marrow, kidneys, lymph nodes.  The transplacental
                  movement of vitamin K is poor; the vitamin is frequently not detectable in
                  the cord blood from mothers with normal plasma levels[8].

                  The tissues of most animals ingesting plant materials contain phyllo-
                  quinones as well as menaquinones with 6-13 isoprenoid units in their side-
                  chains.  That tissues show such mixtures of vitamers K even when the sole
                  dietary form is vitamin MK-4, indicates that much of vitamin K in the tissues
                  normally has an intestinal bacterial origin.  In each organ, vitamin K is
                  found localized primarily in cellular membranes (endoplasmic reticulum,
                  mitochondria).   Under conditions of low vitamin K intake, the vitamin
                  appears to be depleted from membranes more slowly than from cytosol.

                  Vitamers K Occurring in Livers of Several Animal Species:

| vitamer | human | cow | horse | dog | pig |
|---------|-------|-----|-------|-----|-----|
| K-1   | + + + | +     | + + + |       | +     |
| MK-4  |       |       |       |       | +     |
| MK-6  |       |       |       | +     |       |
| MK-7  | + + + |       |       | +     |       |
| MK-8  | +     |       |       | + + + | + + + |
| MK-9  | +     |       |       | + + + | + + + |
| MK-10 | +     | + + + |       | + + + | + + + |
| MK-11 | +     | + + + |       | +     |       |
| MK-12 |       | + + + |       | +     |       |
| MK-13 |       |       |       | +     |       |

---

[8]For this reason, newborn infants are susceptible to hemorrhage.  Further, because human milk contains
less vitamin K than cow's milk, infants who receive only their mother's milk are more susceptible to hemorrhage
than those who drink cow's milk.

# METABOLISM OF VITAMIN K

side-chain
modification

That tissues contain menaquinones when the dietary source of vitamin K was phylloquinone was once taken as evidence for the metabolic de-alkylation of the phylloquinone side chain (converting it to menadione) followed by its re-alkylation to the menaquinones.  That conversion, however, does not occur unless phylloquinone is administered orally. Therefore, it appears that the de-alkylation involved in that conversion occurs as the result of metabolism of the vitamin by gut microbes.  The alkylation of menadione (either from a practical feed supplement or produced from microbial degradation of phylloquinone) does occur *in vivo*. This step has been demonstrated in chick liver homogenates where it was found to use geranyl pyrophosphate, farnesyl pyrophosphate or geranyl-geranyl pyrophosphate as alkyl donors in a reaction inhibitable by $O_2$ or Warfarin[9].  The main product of the alkylation of menadione is MK-4.

degradation
excretion

Menadione is rapidly metabolized and excreted, leaving only a relatively minor portion to be converted to MK-4.  It is excreted primarily in the urine (e.g., ca. 70% of a physiological dose may be lost within 24 hrs.) as the phosphate, sulfate or glucuronide of menadiol.  It is also excreted in the bile as the glucuronide conjugate.

The catabolism of phylloquinone and the menaquinones is much slower than that of menadione.  Little is known about menaquinone metabolism, but it is likely that extensive side-chain conversion occurs.  Phylloquinone has been shown to undergo oxidative shortening of the side chain to 5- or 7-carbon carboxylic acids, and it is thought that other more extensively degraded metabolites are also formed.  The primary route of excretion of these metabolites is the feces, which contain glucuronic acid conjugates excreted via the bile.

vitamin K
epoxide

The vitamin K naphthoquinone ring can be altered by an hepatic micro-somal enzyme system to yield the 2,3-epoxide, which is called *vitamin K epoxide* or *vitamin K oxide*.  This ring-altered metabolite comprises ca. 10% of the total vitamin K in the liver of the normal rat, and can be the predominant form in the livers of rats treated with Warfarin or other coumarin anti-coagulants.  One other ring-altered metabolite has been

---

[9] 4-hydroxy-3-(3-oxo-1-phenylbutyl)-2H-1-benzopyran-2-one. Synthesized by Link's group at the University of Wisconsin (and named for the Wisconsin Alumni Research Foundation), this analog of the naturally occurring hemorrhagic factor dicoumarol is a potent vitamin K antagonist.

Warfarin

dicoumarol

identified: 3-hydroxy-2,3-dihydrophylloquinone, also called *"hydroxy vitamin K"*. Both vitamin K epoxide and hydroxy vitamin K are thought to be degraded metabolically before excretion. That these may have different routes of degradation is suggested by the finding that Warfarin treatment greatly increases the excretion of phylloquinone metabolites in the urine while decreasing the amounts of metabolites in the feces.

phylloquinone-2,3-epoxide                     hydroxyphylloquinone

## *METABOLIC FUNCTIONS OF VITAMIN K*

*vitamin K-dependent GLA-containing proteins*

Vitamin K functions in the post-translational carboxylation of specific glutamate residues to *γ-carboxyglutamate (Gla)* residues[10] in at least a dozen proteins which are, therefore, referred to as being *"vitamin K-dependent"*. Among these are the four clotting factors originally identified as being vitamin K-dependent: *prothrombin [factor II]* and *factors VII, IX and X*. More recently four other vitamin K-dependent proteins have been identified in plasma (i.e., *proteins C, S, Z and M*). In addition, a major protein of the bone matrix, *osteocalcin*, has been found to be vitamin K-dependent. Several other Gla-containing proteins have also been identified but not as well characterized as these.

*vitamin K-dependent carboxylase*

Vitamin K is the cofactor of a specific microsomal carboxylase that catalyzes the γ-carboxylation of peptide-bound glutamic acid residues. This *vitamin K-dependent carboxylase* is found predominantly in liver but also in several other organs[11]. In the reduced form, vitamin K provides reducing equivalents for the reaction, thus, undergoing oxidation to vitamin K-2,3-epoxide. This is coupled to the formation of a carbanion at the γ-position of a peptide-bound Glu residue; that is followed by carboxylation

---

[10] This unusual amino acid was discovered in investigations of the molecular basis of abnormal clotting in vitamin K deficiency. While it had been known that vitamin K deficiency and 4-hydroxycoumarin anti-coagulants each caused hypoprothrombinemia, studies in the early 1970s revealed the presence, in each condition, of a protein that was antigenically similar to prothrombin but which did not bind $Ca^{++}$ and, therefore, was not functional. Studies of the prothrombin $Ca^{++}$-binding sites revealed them to have Gla residues; whereas, these were replaced by glutamate (Glu) residues in the abnormal prothrombin. Subsequently, Gla residues were found in each of the other vitamin K-dependent clotting factors, as well as in several other $Ca^{++}$-binding proteins in other tissues.

[11] e.g., lung, spleen, kidney, bone, placenta, skin.

in a step that does not involve vitamin K.  The enzyme requires reduced vitamin K (*vitamin K hydroquinone*), $CO_2$ as the carboxyl precursor, and $O_2$[12].  It is frequently referred to as the *vitamin K carboxylase/epoxidase* to indicate the coupling of the $\gamma$-carboxylation step with the conversion of vitamin K to the 2,3-epoxide.   Normally, this coupling is tight; however, under conditions of low $CO_2$ levels or in the absence of peptidyl-Glu, the epoxidation of the vitamin proceeds without concomitant carboxylation[13].

Liver microsomes also contain a dithiol-dependent *vitamin K epoxide reductase* and at least two *quinone reductases*, one of which is also dependent upon dithiol. These enzymes catalyze, in two steps, the regeneration of the fully reduced vitamin K: first, by reducing the epoxide to the quinone form and, then, reducing the quinone to the active dihydroxy form. These dithiol-dependent enzymes are inhibited by the coumarin-type anticoagulants; their inhibition blocks the recycling of the vitamin between its oxidized and reduced forms, and results in the accumulation of vitamin K-2,3-epoxide with concomitant loss of $\gamma$-carboxylation of the vitamin K-dependent proteins due to the loss of the dihydroquinone[14].  Nevethess, reduction of vitamin K quinone occurs in anti-coagulant-treated individuals. This is due to the presence of another quinone reductase which uses

---

[12]The *in vitro* activity of the carboxylase is stimulated almost four-fold by pyridoxal phosphate when the substrate was a pentapeptide. It is doubtful whether that co-factor is important *in vivo*, as no stimulation was observed in the carboxylation of endogenous microsomal proteins.

[13]This activity is referred to as the *"vitamin K epoxidase"*.

[14]Resistance to Warfarin, widely used for years as a rodenticide, has been observed in rats and humans. It appears to involve a mutant form of the vitamin K-epoxide reductase which is not sensitive to the coumarin. The vitamin $K_1$ analog, 2-chloro-3-phytyl-1,4-naphthoquinone (chloro-K), is a very effective inhibitor in Warfarin-resistant rats.

NAD(P)H as a source of reducing equivalents; in contrast to the dithiol-dependent enzyme, it is relatively insensitive to coumarin-inhibition[15].

Three groups of GLA-containing proteins have been identified:

| | |
|---|---|
| i. | **phospholipid-binding proteins** - Found only in plasma, these bind negatively charged phospholipids via $Ca^{++}$ held by Gla residues. These include four **clotting factors** (*II*-prothrombin, **VII**, **IX** and **X**) and two *coagulation-inhibiting proteins* (**factors** C and S). |
| ii. | **Ca salt-binding proteins** - Found exclusively in calcified matrices, these are thought to be involved in the regulation of calcification. These include **osteocalcin** in bone, a similar protein in dentine, **atherocalcin** in atherosclerotic tissue, and a **Gla-protein** in renal stones. |
| iii. | **less well characterized Gla-proteins**, e.g., **Gla-protein Z** of sperm and plasma. |

*vitamin K-proteins in plasma*

The eight vitamin K-dependent proteins in plasma have homologous amino acid sequences in the first 40 positions; all require $Ca^{++}$ for activity. Protein C inhibits coagulation; and, stimulated by protein S, it promotes fibrinolysis.

Characteristics of the Vitamin K-Dependent Plasma Proteins:

| parameter | II° | VII | IX | X | C | M | S | Z |
|---|---|---|---|---|---|---|---|---|
| level, $\mu g/ml$ | 100 | 1 | 3 | 20 | 10 | < 1 | 1 | < 1 |
| MW, kD | 72 | 46 | 55 | 55 | 57 | 50 | 69 | 55 |
| % carbohydrate | 8 | 13 | 26 | 13 | 8 | + | + | + |
| chains | 1 | 1 | 1 | 2 | 2 | 1 | 1 | 1 |
| Gla residues | 10 | 10 | 12 | 12 | 11 | + | 10 | 13 |

°prothrombin

The four classical (long-known) clotting factors (II, VII, IX and X) are components of a complex system of proteins that function to prevent hemorrhage and lead to thrombus formation. The protein components of this system circulate as **zymogens**, i.e., inactive precursors of the functional forms each of which is a serine protease that participates in a cascade of proteolytic activation[16] of a series of factors ultimately leading to the conversion of a soluble protein, fibrinogen, to an insoluble one, the

---

[15]This enzyme, called *"diaphorase"*, is a flavoprotein.

[16]Each of the conversions of vitamin K-dependent factors in this cascade involve the $Ca^{++}$-mediated association of the active protein, its substrate and another protein factor with a phospholipid surface.

fibrin clot. The key step in this system is the activation of **factor X** [17], which can occur by the actions of either **factor IX** [18] (which itself is activated by **plasma thromboplastin** acting as the result of a contact with a foreign surface) in what is called the **"intrinsic system"**, or **factor VII** [19] (which itself is activated by **tissue thromboplastin** released as the result of injury) in what is called the **"extrinsic system"**. In each case, the activation of a zymogen factor involves the proteolytic removal of a short polypeptide. Once so activated, factor X, binding $Ca^{++}$ and phospholipid, catalyzes the activation of **prothrombin (factor II)** to its active form, **thrombin (factor IIa)**. It is thrombin which catalyzes the proteolytic change in **fibrinogen** that renders it insoluble (as **fibrin**) for clot formation.

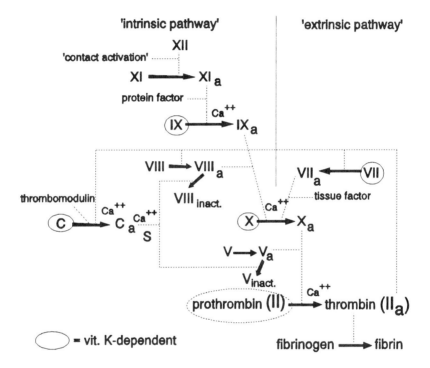

**Protein C** functions in this system in an anti-coagulant role. It is activated by thrombin (factor IIa) in the presence of an endothelial cell protein, **thrombomodulin**. It acts in a complex with **protein S** by partially hydrolyzing the activated factors V and VIII, thus, inactivating them. That this function is vital is evidenced by the fact that patients with inherited deficiency of factor C are at high risk for thromboses. Protein S is found in

---

[17] also called **Stuart factor**.

[18] also called **Christmas factor**, or **plasma thromboplastin component**.

[19] also called **proconvertin**.

the plasma both in the free form and in association with a component of complement, suggesting that it may also have some role in regulation of the latter. The physiological functions of proteins M and Z are not known.

*vitamin K-dependent proteins in calcified matrices*

The best characterized vitamin K-dependent protein of calcified tissues is **osteocalcin**, a low molecular weight (ca. 5.7 kD) protein found chiefly in rapidly growing regions of bones. Osteocalcin shows no apparent homology with the vitamin K-dependent plasma proteins; however, it is very homologous between various species. It contains three Gla residues in a 49 amino acid segment; it binds $Ca^{++}$ weakly, that binding serving to maintain its secondary structure. Osteocalcin is believed to function in the regulation of the incorporation of calcium phosphates into bone. It is synthesized by osteoblasts and is the second most abundant protein[20] in the bone matrix, comprising ca. 2% of total bone protein and 10-20% of non-collagen protein. Its synthesis is inhibited by warfarin treatment, and is stimulated (at least *in vitro*) by 1,25-$(OH)_2$-vitamin $D_3$. Osteocalcin is synthesized in bone and is secreted into the plasma; greatest circulating levels of the protein are found in young children and patients with certain bone diseases involving increased bone resorption/mineralization).

Plasma osteocalcin concentrations in humans:

| group | osteocalcin, ng/ml |
|---|---|
| children | 10-40[a] |
| adults | 4-8 |
| women, 60-69 yrs. | 7 |
| women, 80-89 yrs. | 8 |
| Paget's disease patients | 39 |
| secondary hyperparathyroidism patients | 47 |
| osteopenia patients | 9 |

[a]Highest levels observed in patients at 10-15 yrs. of age.

The functions of the other Gla-containing proteins are even less clear. It is presumed that the one isolated from rat dentine has some role in dental calcification, but that remains to be established. Because the Gla-protein **atherocalcin** was discovered in calcified atherosclerotic tissue, it has been suggested that arterial vitamin K-dependent γ-glutamyl carboxylase (which is found in the walls of arteries but not veins) may be involved in the development of atherosclerosis. A renal Gla-protein that is inhibited by PTH and vitamin $D_3$ has been described; it is thought to have some role in the transport/excretion of $Ca^{++}$ in the kidney. Other Gla-proteins have been reported in sperm, urine, hepatic mitochondria, shark skeletal cartilage, and snake venom. Therefore, it is clear that vitamin K functions widely in physiological systems beyond those involved in blood clotting.

---

[20]Collagen is the most abundant protein in bone.

# EXTREMES IN VITAMIN K INTAKE

*deficiency*    Vitamin K deficiency is rare among humans and most other animal species, the important exception being the rapidly growing chick raised in a wire-floored cage.  This is due to the wide occurrence of vitamin K in plant and animal foods and to the significant microbial synthesis of the vitamin that occurs in the intestines of most animals[21].  In fact, for many species including humans, the intestinal synthesis of vitamin K appears to meet normal needs.  The most frequent causes of vitamin K deficiency, thus, are factors that involve or cause lipid malabsorption (e.g., diseases of the gastro-intestinal tract, biliary stasis, liver disease, cystic fibrosis, celiac disease, ascaris infection), factors that interfere with the microbial synthesis of vitamin K (e.g., the neonate with a relatively sterile gastro-intestinal tract; patients treated with antibiotics), and factors that interfere with the *in vivo* metabolism of the vitamin (e.g., treatment with 4-hydroxycoumarins).

Neonates are at special risk to vitamin K deficiency for several reasons:

| | |
|---|---|
| i. | *Placental transport of the vitamin is poor*, e.g., serum vitamin K levels of neonates are typically about half those of their mothers. |
| ii. | The neonatal *intestine is sterile* for the first few days of life, thus not providing an enteric microbial source of the vitamin. |
| iii. | *Hepatic biosynthesis of the clotting factors is inadequate* in the young infant, e.g., the plasm prothrombin concentrations of fetuses and infants are typically one-quarter those of their mothers. |
| iv. | *Human milk is an inadequate source of vitamin K*, e.g., the frequency of vitamin K-responsive hemorrhagic disease in one month-old infants is 1/4000 overall, but 1/1700 among breast-fed infants. |

*Hemorrhagic disease of the newborn* can affect infants as old as 3-4 months.  It is more common among breast-fed infants than among those fed formulated diets[22].  It involves intracranial hemorrhage and has high associated rates of death (ca. 27%) and central nervous system damage (ca. 47%).  For this reason, it is a common practice in many countries to treat all infants at birth with parenterally administered vitamin K (2-5 $\mu$g).

Humans and other animals can experience impaired vitamin K utilization as the result of treatment with certain types of drugs.  These include warfarin and other 4-hydroxycoumarin anti-coagulants, and large doses of

---

[21] Species with short gastro-intestinal tracts and very short intestinal transit times (e.g., ca. 8 hrs. in the chick) less than the generation times of many bacteria, do not have well colonized guts.  Thus, being unable to harbor vitamin K-producing bacteria, they depend of their diet as the source of their vitamin K.

[22] The frequency of the disease among one-month-old infants is 1/4000 overall, but 1/1700 among breast-fed infants.

salicylates, which inhibit the redox cycling of the vitamin. In each case, high doses of vitamin K are generally effective in normalizing clotting mechanisms. Sulfonamides and broad-spectrum antibiotic drugs can virtually sterilize the lumen of the intestine, thus, removing an important source of vitamin K for most animals. Therefore, patients on antibiotic therapy can be at high risk to vitamin K deficiency[23]. In addition, cephalosporin antibiotics can inhibit the vitamin K-dependent carboxylase. Poultry are particularly sensitive to dietary deprivation of vitamin K when they are raised on wire floors and, thus, not exposed to their feces. For this reason, the chick is the animal model of choice for the basic study of vitamin K.

The predominant clinical sign of vitamin K deficiency is *hemorrhage* which, in severe cases can lead to a *fatal anemia*. The blood shows *prolonged clotting time* and *hypoprothrombinemia*. Several congenital disorders of vitamin K-dependent proteins have been identified in human patients: at least a dozen forms of *congenital dysprothrombinemia*, at least three variants of *factor VII*, a congenital deficiency of *protein C*. Patients with these disorders show coagulopathies; none respond to high doses of vitamin K.

Signs of vitamin K deficiency:

| organ system | sign |
| --- | --- |
| general | |
| growth | decrease |
| dermatologic | hemorrhage |
| muscular | hemorrhage |
| gastro-intestinal | hemorrhage |
| vascular | |
| erythrocytes | anemia |
| platelets | decreased clotting |

*hyper-vitaminosis*

Phylloquinone exhibits no adverse effects when administered to animals in massive doses by any route. The menaquinones are similarly thought to have negligible toxicity. Menadione, however, can be toxic, producing fatal anemia, hyperbilirubinemia and severe jaundice. The intoxicating doses appear to be at least three orders of magnitude above those levels required for normal physiological function. At such high levels, the basis of menadione toxicity appears to be oxidative stress: menadione undergoes monovalent reduction to the semiquinone radical which, in the presence of $O_2$, is re-oxidized to the quinone resulting in the formation of the superoxide radical anion. In addition, high levels of menadione are known to react with free sulfhydryl groups, thus, depleting GSH.

---

[23]This can be exacerbated by inanition. Because vitamin K is rapidly depleted from tissues, periods of reduced food intake, such as may occur post-surgically, can produce vitamin K deficiency in patients with reduced intestinal microbial synthesis of the vitamin.

## CASE STUDY

| | |
|---|---|
| *Instructions:* | *Review the following case report, paying special attention to the diagnostic indicators upon which the treatments were based. Then answer the questions that follow.* |

*case 1*

A 60-year-old woman involved in an automobile accident sustained injuries to the head and compound fractures of both legs. She was admitted to the hospital where she was treated for acute trauma. Her recovery was slow, and for the next four months she was drowsy and reluctant to eat. Her diet consisted mainly of orange and glucose drinks with a multi-vitamin supplement that contained no vitamin K. Then, her compound fractures became infected and she was treated with a combination of antibiotics (penicillin, gentamicin, tetracycline and co-trimoxazole). Then, she developed intermittent diarrhea, which was treated with codeine phosphate. After a month, all antibiotics were stopped and 46 days later (six months after the injury) she experienced bleeding from her urethra. At that time other signs were also noted: *bruising* of the limbs, *bleeding gums*, *generalized purpura*[24]. The clinical diagnosis was *scurvy* until it was learned that the patient was taking 25 mg ascorbic acid per day *via* her daily vitamin supplement.

Laboratory results:

| parameter | patient | normal range |
|---|---|---|
| Hb | 9.0 g/dl | 12-16 g/dl |
| mean RBC volume | 79 fl | 80-100 fl |
| white cells | $6.3 \times 10^9$/l | $5-10 \times 10^9$/l |
| platelets | $320 \times 10^9$/l | $150-300 \times 10^9$/l |
| plasma Fe | 22 µg/dl | 72-180 µg/dl |
| total Fe-binding capacity | 123 µg/dl | 246-375 µg/dl |
| Ca | 7.6 mg/dl | 8.4-10.4 mg/dl |
| inorganic P | 2.4 mg/dl | 2.4-4.3 mg/dl |
| folate | 1.6 ng/ml | 3-20 ng/ml |
| vitamin $B_{12}$ | 110 ng/l | 150-1000 ng/l |
| prothrombin time | 273 sec. | 13 sec. (control) |
| thrombin time | 10 sec. | 10 sec. (control) |

When her abnormal prothrombin time was noted, specific coagulation assays were performed. These showed that the activities of each of the vitamin K-dependent factors (factors II, VII, IX and X) was <1% of the normal level and that the activity of factor V was 76% of normal. A xylose tolerance test performed with a single oral dose of 5 g xylose showed tolerance within normal limits. A stool culture showed normal fecal flora. The patient was then given phylloquinone (10 mg i.v. daily for 3 days), and showed a complete recovery of all coagulation factor activities to normal.

---

[24] subcutaneous hemorrhages.

She was given a high-protein/high-energy diet supplemented with $FeSO_4$ and, for a week, daily oral doses of 10 mg phylloquinone. Her diarrhea subsided, her wounds healed and she returned to normal health.

case 2      A 55-year-old man with arteriosclerotic heart disease and type IV hyperlipo-proteinemia was admitted to the hospital with a hemorrhagic syndrome. Six months earlier, he had suffered a myocardial infarction[25] complicated by pulmonary embolism[26] for which he was treated with heparin[27] followed by warfarin. Two months earlier, he had been admitted for a cardiac arrhythmia at which time his physical examination was normal and chest radiograph showed no abnormalities, but his electrocardiogram showed first-degree atrioventricular block[28] with frequent premature ventricular contractions. At that time, he was taking 5 mg warfarin per day.

Laboratory findings two months prior to admission:

| parameter | patient | normal |
|---|---|---|
| prothrombin time | 16.6 sec | 12.7 sec |
| plasma triglycerides | 801 mg/dl | 20-150 mg/dl |
| serum cholesterol | 324 mg/dl | 150-250 mg/dl |

(Blood count, blood urea-N, blood bilirubin and urinalysis were all normal.)

He was treated with warfarin (5 mg/day), digoxin[29], diphenylhydantoin[30], furosemide[31], potassium chloride[32] and clofibrate[33]. Within a month, quinidine gluconate[34] was substituted for diphenylhydantoin because the

---

[25] dysfunction due to necrotic changes resulting from an obstruction of a coronary artery.

[26] obstruction or occlusion of a blood vessel by a transported clot.

[27] a highly sulfated mucopolysaccharide with specific anticoagulant properties.

[28] impairment of normal conduction between the atria and ventricles.

[29] a cardiotonic

[30] a cardiac depressant (and anticonvulsant)

[31] a diuretic

[32] i.e., to correct for the loss of $K^+$ induced by the diuretic.

[33] an antihyperlipoproteinemic

[34] a cardiac depressant (antiarrhythmic)

patient showed persistent premature ventricular beats, but that drug was discontinued because of diarrhea and procainamide[34] was used instead. At that time, his prothrombin time was 31.5 sec, and his warfarin dose was reduced first to half the original dose and then to one-quarter of that level.

At the time of the present admission, the patient appeared well-nourished, but had ecchymoses[35] on his arms, abdomen and pubic area. He had been constipated with hematuria[36] for the preceding two days. His physical examination was unremarkable except for occasional premature beats, and his laboratory findings were similar to those observed on his previous admission with the exception that his prothrombin time had increased to 36.6 sec. In questioning the patient, it was learned that he had been taking orally as much as 1.2 mg all-*rac*-*a*-tocopheryl acetate each day for the preceding two months.

Both his warfarin and vitamin E treatments were discontinued, and two days later his prothrombin time had dropped to 24.9 sec and his ecchymoses began to clear. The patient consented to participate in a clinical trial of vitamin E (800 mg all-*rac*-*a*-tocopheryl acetate per day) in this standard regimen of warfarin and clofibrate.

Effect of vitamin E on the activities of the patient's coagulation factors

| activity | initial value | + Vit. E (6 wks) | - Vit. E (1 wk) | normal range |
|---|---|---|---|---|
| factor II (prothrombin)[a] | 11 | 7 | 21 | 60-150 |
| factor VII[a] | 27 | 16 | 20 | 50-150 |
| factor IX[a] | 30 | 14 | 23 | 50-150 |
| factor X[a] | 15 | 10 | - | 50-150 |
| prothrombin time, sec | 20.7 | 29.2 | 22.3 | 11.0-12.5 |

[a]Values are % of normal means.

---

Questions:  i.  What signs indicated vitamin K-related problems in each case?

ii.  What factors probably contributed to the vitamin K deficiency of the patient in case 1? Why was phylloquinone chosen over menadione for treating that patient?

iii.  What factors may have contributed to the coagulopathy of the patient in case 2? What might be the basis of the effect of high levels of vitamin E seen in that case?

---

[35]Ecchymoses are purplish patches of the skin caused by extravasation of blood; they differ from the smaller petechiae only in size.

[36]the condition of blood in the urine.

## Study Questions and Exercises:

i.   Construct a *concept map* illustrating the ways in which vitamin K affects blood coagulation.

ii.  Construct a *'decision tree'* for the diagnosis of vitamin K deficiency in a human or animal.

iii. What *features* of the *chemical structure* of vitamin K relate to its *metabolic function*?

iv.  What relevance to their vitamin K nutrition would you expect of the rearing of experimental animals in a *germ-free* environment or fed a *fat-free diet*?

v.   How does the *concept* of a *coenzyme* relate to vitamin K?

## Recommended Reading:

Flodin, N.W. 1988. Vitamin K, Chapter 4, *in* Pharmacology of Micronutrients, Alan R. Liss, New York, pp. 93-102.

Friedrich, W. 1988. Vitamins. Walter de Gruyter, New York, pp. 285-338.

Furie, B. and B.C. Furie. 1990. Molecular basis of vitamin K-dependent carboxylation. Blood 75:1753-1762.

Olson, R.E. 1984. The function and metabolism of vitamin K. Nutr. Rev. 4:281-337.

Price, P.A. 1985. Vitamin K-dependent formation of bone GLA protein (osteocalcin) and its function. Vit. Horm. 42:65-108.

Suttie, J.W. 1988. Vitamin K-dependent carboxylation of glutamyl residues in proteins. BioFactors 1:55-60.

Suttie, J.W. 1991. Vitamin K, Chapter 4, *in* Handbook of Vitamins, 2nd edition (L.J. Machlin, ed.). Marcel Dekker, New York, pp. 145-194.

# CHAPTER 9  *VITAMIN C*

*"I still had a gram or so of hexuronic acid. I gave it to [Svirbely] to test for vitaminic activity. I told him that I expected he would find it identical with vitamin C. I always had a strong hunch that this was so but never had tested it. I was not acquainted with animal tests in this field and the whole problem was, for me, too glamorous, and vitamins were, to my mind, theoretically uninteresting. 'Vitamin' means that one has to eat it. What one has to eat is the first concern of the chef, not the scientist. Anyway, Svirbely tested hexuronic acid . . . after one month the result was evident: hexuronic acid was vitamin C."*

A. Szent-Györgyi

## Anchoring Concepts:

*i.*     Vitamin C is the generic descriptor for all compounds exhibiting qualitatively the biological activity of ascorbic acid.

*ii.*    Vitamin C-active compounds are hydrophilic and have an oxidizable/-reducible 2,3-enediol grouping.

*iii.*    Deficiencies of vitamin C are manifest as connective tissue lesions (e.g., capillary fragility, hemorrhage, muscular weakness).

## Learning Objectives:

*i.*    To understand the nature of the various *sources* of vitamin C.

*ii.*    To understand the means of vitamin C *synthesis* by most species.

*iii.*    To understand the means of *enteric absorption* and *transport* of vitamin C.

*iv.*    To understand the *functions* of vitamin C in connective tissue metabolism, in drug and steroid metabolism and in mineral utilization.

*v.*    To understand the physiologic implications of *low* and *high* intakes of vitamin C.

## Vocabulary:

albumin
antioxidant
ascorbic acid
L-ascorbic acid 2-sulfate
ascorbyl free radical
carnitine
cholesterol 7$\alpha$-hydroxylase
collagen
dehydroascorbic acid
dehydroascorbic acid reductase
dopamine-$\beta$-monooxygenase
elastin
glucuronic acid pathway
guinea pig
L-gulonolactone oxidase
histamine
homogentisate 1,2-dioxygenase
hydroxylysine
4-hydroxyphenylpyruvate
hydroxyproline

hypoascorbemia
Indian fruit bat
insulin
iron
lysyl oxidase
Moeller-Barlow disease
monodehydroascorbic acid
monodehydroascorbic acid reductase
oxalic acid
peptidylglycine $\alpha$-amidating monooxygenase
petechiae
prolyl oxidase
pro-oxidant
red-vented bulbul
L-saccharoascorbic acid
scurvy
systemic conditioning
tropoelastin
tyrosine
vitamin C

# SOURCES OF VITAMIN C

*distribution*
*in foods*

Vitamin C is widely distributed in both plants and animals, occurring as both *ascorbic acid* and *dehydroascorbic acid*, the two species in probable equilibrium.  Fruits, vegetables[1], and organ meats (e.g., liver and kidney) are generally the best sources; only small amounts are found in muscle meats.  Plants synthesize L-ascorbic acid from carbohydrates; most seeds do not contain ascorbic acid, but start to synthesize it upon sprouting.  Some plants accumulate high levels of the vitamin (e.g., fresh tea leaves, some berries, guava, rose hips).  For practical reasons, citrus fruits are good daily sources of vitamin C, as they are generally eaten raw and are, therefore, not subjected to cooking procedures that can destroy vitamin C.

Vitamin C contents of some uncooked foods:

| food | vitamin C mg/100g | food | vitamin C mg/100g |
|------|------|------|------|
| fruits | | vegetables | |
| apple | 10-30 | asparagus | 15-30 |
| banana | 10 | bean | 10-30 |
| cherry | 10 | broccoli | 90-150 |
| grapefruit | 40 | cabbage | 30-60 |
| guava | 300 | carrot | 5-10 |
| hawthorne berries | 160-800 | cauliflower | 60-80 |
| melons | 13-33 | celery | 10 |
| orange, lemon | 50 | collard greens | 100-150 |
| peach | 7-14 | corn | 12 |
| raspberry | 18-25 | kale | 120-180 |
| rose hips | 1000 | leek | 15-30 |
| strawberry | 40-90 | oat, wheat | 0 |
| tangerine | 30 | onion | 10-30 |
| | | pea | 10-30 |
| | | parsley | 170 |
| animal products | | pepper | 125-200 |
| meats | 0-2 | potato | 10-30 |
| liver, kidney | 10-40 | rhubarb | 10 |
| milk, cow | 1-2 | rice | 0 |
| milk, human | 3-6 | spinach | 50-90 |

*stability*
*in foods*

The vitamin C contents of most foods decrease dramatically during storage due to the aggregate effects of several processes by which the vitamin can be destroyed.  Ascorbic acid is susceptible to oxidation to dehydroascorbic acid which is quickly and irreversibly degraded further by hydrolytic opening of the lactone ring.  These reactions occur in the presence of $O_2$, even traces of metal ions, and are enhanced by heat and conditions of neutral to alkaline pH.  It is also reduced by exposure to oxidases in plant tissues.  Therefore, substantial losses of vitamin C can

---

[1] Historically, the potato was the best source of vitamin C in North America and Europe.

occur during storage[2] and are enhanced greatly during cooking[3]. Losses in cooking are usually greater with such methods as boiling, as the stability of ascorbic acid is much less in aqueous solution. Alternatively, quick heating methods can protect food vitamin C by inactivating oxidases.

Vitamin C losses from foods stored for 2 days:

| food | % lost at 4°C | % lost at 20°C |
|---|---|---|
| beans | 33 | 53 |
| cauliflower | 8 | 26 |
| lettuce | 36 | 42 |
| parsley | 13 | 70 |
| peas | 10 | 36 |
| spinach | 32 | 80 |
| spinach (winter) | 7 | 22 |

*biosynthesis of ascorbic acid*

In addition to probably all green plants, most higher animals species can synthesize vitamin C *via* the ***glucuronic acid pathway*** from glucose. The enzymes of this pathway are localized in the kidneys of amphibians, reptiles and the more primitive orders of birds, but they occur in the livers of higher birds and mammals[4]. The transfer of ascorbic acid synthesis from the kidney to the larger liver has been interpreted as an evolutionary adaptation that provided increased synthetic capacity of the larger organ to meet the increased needs associated with homeothermy.

The biosynthesis of ascorbic acid is inhibited by deficiencies of vitamins A and E and biotin, but is stimulated by certain drugs (e.g., barbiturates, aminopyrine, antipyrine, chlorobutanol) and by certain carcinogens (e.g., 3-methylcholanthrene, benzo-*a*-pyrene). The stimulation of synthesis that occurs due to exposure to xenobiotic compounds appears to be due to a general induction of the enzymes of the glucuronic acid pathway which produces glucuronic acid for conjugating foreign compounds as a means of their detoxification[5].

---

[2] e.g., Stored potatoes lost 50% of their vitamin C within 5 months, and 65% within 8 months of harvest. Apples and cabbage stored for winter lost 50% and 40%, respectively, of their original vitamin C contents.

[3] e.g., Potatoes can lose 40% of their vitamin C content by boiling.

[4] Egg-laying mammals synthesize ascorbic acid only in their kidneys, and many marsupials use both their liver and kidneys for this purpose.

[5] Because ascorbic acid synthesis and excretion are increased by exposure to xenobiotic inducers of hepatic, cytochrome $P_{450}$-dependent mixed-function oxidases (MFOs), it has been suggested that urinary ascorbic acid concentration may be useful as a non-invasive screening parameter of MFO status.

Estimated rates of ascorbic acid biosynthesis in several species:

| species | synthetic rate (mg/kg body weight) | $T_{1/2}$, days | turnover, %/day |
|---|---|---|---|
| mouse | 125 | 1.4 | 50 |
| golden hamster | 20 | 2.7 | 26 |
| rat | 25 | 2.6 | 26 |
| rabbit | 5 | 3.9 | 18 |
| guinea pig | 0 | 3.8 | 18 |
| human | 0 | 10-20 | 3 |

*enzyme deficiency causes dietary need for ascorbic acid*    The inability to perform this synthesis occurs only in invertebrates, most fish[6] and a few species of birds (e.g., *red-vented bulbul*) and mammals (*humans, other primates, guinea pigs, Indian fruit bat*)[7]. In each case, the inability to synthesize the vitamin appears to result from the congenital absence of the last enzyme in the biosynthetic pathway, *L-gulonolactone oxidase*[8,9,10]. This microsomal flavoenzyme catalyzes the oxidation of

---

[6]While some fish appear to be able to synthesize ascorbic acid, only the carp and Australian lungfish appear to be able to do so at rates sufficient to meet their physiologic needs.

[7]A mutant strain (ODS-od/od) of rat (derived from the Wistar strain) that does not synthesize ascorbic acid has been identified. It has been said that there are individual humans and guinea pigs that can perform this synthesis.

[8]This has been established for primates, guinea pigs and fruit bats; whether the loss of this enzyme activity is the basis of the inabilities of other species to synthesize ascorbic acid is speculative.

[9]Injection of the enzyme plus its substrate, L-gulonolactone, prevented scurvy in guinea pigs.

L-gulonolactone to L-2-ketogulonolactone, which spontaneously isomerizes to form L-ascorbic acid. It is the loss of this single enzyme that renders ascorbic acid, an otherwise normal metabolite, a vitamin. It is apparent that even the species capable of producing this key enzyme may not express it early in development. For example, the fetal rat has been found incapable of ascorbic acid biosynthesis until the 16th day of gestation; this developmental lag in the expression of this pathway may account for the perinatal declines in tissue ascorbic acid concentrations that have been observed experimentally.

## ABSORPTION OF VITAMIN C

*active uptake in species with dietary needs; passive uptake in others*
Species that cannot synthesize ascorbic acid (e.g., humans, guinea pigs) absorb the vitamin by a saturable, carrier-mediated active transport mechanism that is dependent on $Na^+$ and is inhibited by aspirin[11]. This means of uptake appears to be particularly important at low intakes of the vitamin; however, uptake by passive diffusion also occurs and is likely important at higher vitamin C intakes. Species that can synthesize ascorbic acid do not have such systems; they absorb it strictly by passive diffusion. In either case, the efficiency of absorption of physiological doses (e.g., $\leq 180$ mg per day for a human adult) of vitamin C is high, e.g., 80-90%. In humans, the efficiency of absorption declines markedly at vitamin C doses greater than ca. 1 g[12].

---

[10] Therefore, scurvy can correctly be considered a congenital metabolic disease *"hypoascorbemia"*.

[11] e.g., a 900 mg dose of aspirin blocked the expected rises in plasma, leucocyte and urinary levels of ascorbic acid due to a simultaneous dose of 500 mg vitamin C in humans.

[12] The efficiency of vitamin C absorption declined from ca. 75% of a 1 g dose, to ca. 40% of a 3 g dose and ca. 24% of a 5 g dose; net absorption plateaued at 1-1.2 g at doses of at least 3 g.

# TRANSPORT OF VITAMIN C

bound to
albumin

Vitamin C is transported in the plasma in association with the protein albumin. The reduced form (ascorbic acid) of the vitamin normally predominates.

cellular uptake
necessitates
reduction

Under physiological conditions, vitamin C exists as the monoanion, ascorbate, which cannot cross most membranes readily. In the cases of erythrocytes, lymphocytes and neutrophils, the cellular uptake of vitamin C involves *dehydroascorbic acid*, which appears to enter *via* a membrane transport system, as evidenced by the fact that extracellular discrimination between the D- and L-isomers has been demonstrated[13]. Once it is taken into the cell, dehydroascorbic acid is quickly reduced to ascorbic acid by an intracellular enzyme *dehydroascorbic acid reductase*, which uses *reduced glutathione* (GSH) as the source of reducing equivalents. *Insulin* has been show to promote the cellular uptake of dehydroascorbic acid, and glucose to inhibit it. Thus, diabetic patients can have abnormally high plasma levels of dehydroascorbic acid[14]. Ascorbic acid is resorbed with specificity by the kidney *via* a $Na^+$-dependent, active transport system.

tissue
distribution

Vitamin C is concentrated in many vital organs with active metabolism. Some tissues (e.g., peripheral mononuclear leukocytes) can accumulate concentrations as great as several millimolar. This is accomplished *via* specific transport systems. Facilitated transport has been demonstrated in nervous tissue, and both low- and high-affinity membrane transporters have been identified in neutrophils. At high rates of intake, accumulation proceeds according to zero-order kinetics; at saturation levels, dehydroascorbic acid comprises about 60% of the total amount of the vitamin in tissues. Tissue levels are decreased by virtually all forms of stress, which also stimulates the biosynthesis of the vitamin in those animals able to do so[15]. The concentration of ascorbic acid in the adrenal is very high (72-168 mg/100 g in the cow); approximately one-third of the vitamin is concentrated in the reduced form at the site of catecholamine formation in that organ[16] from which it is released with newly synthesized cortico-

---

[13]Studies with cultured cells have shown that D-isoascorbic acid has only 20-30% of the activity in stimulating collagen production of L-ascorbic acid. The basis of this difference involved the much slower cellular uptake of the D-form, as, once inside the cell, both vitamers behaved almost identically.

[14]In fact, it is thought that the impaired cellular uptake of vitamin C, due to competition with glucose, may be one of the causes of pathology in diabetes.

[15]The ascorbic acid content of brown adipose tissue of rats has been found to increase by ca. 60% due to cold stress.

[16]the chroffamin tissue.

steroids in response to stress[17]. The ascorbic acid concentration of brain tissue also tends to be high (5-28 mg/100 g), the greatest concentrations are found in regions that are also rich in catecholamines. Brain ascorbic acid levels are only late to be affected by dietary deprivation of vitamin C in those animals unable to synthesize the vitamin. The eye also contains a relatively large amount of ascorbic acid, where it is thought to protect from oxidation critical sulfhydryl groups of proteins[18]. Blood cells contain a substantial fraction of the ascorbic acid in the blood; of these, leukocytes have particular diagnostic value, as their ascorbic acid concentrations, which are independent of plasma concentration[19], reflect the levels found in the tissues[20]. There is no stable reserve of vitamin C; excesses are quickly excreted. At saturation, the total body pool of the human has been estimated to be 1.5-5 g[21] the major fractions being found in the liver and muscles by virtue of their relatively large masses.

Ascorbic acid concentrations in human tissues:

| tissue | ascorbic acid mg/100g |
|---|---|
| adrenals | 30-40 |
| pituitary | 40-50 |
| liver | 10-16 |
| thymus | 10-15 |
| lungs | 7 |
| kidneys | 5-15 |
| heart | 5-15 |
| muscle | 3- 4 |
| brain | 3-15 |
| pancreas | 10-15 |
| lens | 25-31 |
| plasma | .4- 1 |

[17] *via* the adrenocorticotrophic hormone (ACTH).

[18] Lenses of cataract patients have lower lens ascorbic acid concentrations (e.g., 0-5.5 mg/100 g) than those of healthy patients (e.g., 30 mg/100 g).

[19] A continuously low plasma ascorbic acid level (<0.1 mg/dl) can lead to scurvy. In humans, a plasma level of 0.4-1.4 mg/dl corresponds to a daily intake of ca. 40 mg vitamin C; higher levels indicate saturation.

[20] Leukocyte ascorbic acid concentrations are usually greater in women than men and normally decrease with age and in some diseases.

[21] The first signs of scurvy are not seen until this reserve is depleted to 300-400 mg.

# METABOLISM OF VITAMIN C

*oxidation*

Ascorbic acid is oxidized *in vivo* via two successive losses of single electrons.  The first monovalent oxidation results in the formation of the *L-ascorbyl free radical*,[22] which forms a reversible electrochemical couple with ascorbic acid but which can be further oxidized irreversibly to *dehydro-L-ascorbic acid*.

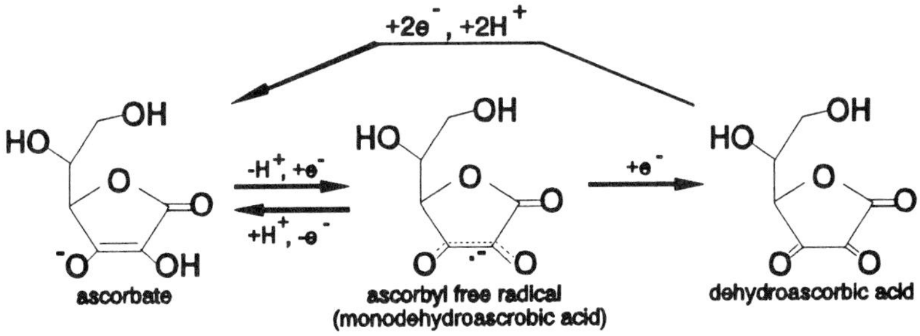

$$+2e^-, +2H^+$$

ascorbate            ascorbyl free radical
(monodehydroascrobic acid)            dehydroascorbic acid

Subsequent irreversible hydrolysis of dehydroascorbic acid yields 2,3-diketo-L-gulonic acid which undergoes either decarboxylation to $CO_2$ and 5-C fragments (xylose, xylonic acid, lyxonic acid), or oxidation to *oxalic acid* and 4-C fragments (e.g., threonic acid).  In addition, the formation of *L-ascorbic acid 2-sulfate* from ascorbic acid in humans and fishes, and the oxidation of the ascorbic acid C-6 to *L-saccharoascorbic acid* has been demonstrated in monkeys.

Animal species vary in their routes of disposition of dehydroascorbic acid.  Guinea pigs and rats degrade it to $CO_2$[23], which is lost across the lungs.  Humans, however, normally degrade only a very small amount *via* that route[24], excreting the vitamin primarily as various urinary metabolites (e.g., 20-25% ascorbic acid and dehydroascorbic acid, ca. 20% as diketo-

---

[22] also called *"monodehydroascorbic acid"*.

[23] The C-1 of ascorbic acid is the main source of $CO_2$ derived from the vitamin, while C-1 and C2 are the precursors of oxalic acid.

[24] Degradation by this path in increased greatly in some diseases and can then account for nearly half of ascorbic acid loss.

gulonic acid, 40-45% as oxalate[25] , with only very small amounts of ascorbate 2-sulfate). When blood ascorbic acid concentrations exceed 1.2-1.8 mg/dl (when tissue saturation is reached), virtually all ascorbic acid is excreted in the urine.

ascorbic acid regeneration
Ascorbic acid can be regenerated from dehydroascorbic acid by **dehydro ascorbic acid reductase**. That enzyme is thought to use reduced glutathione (GSH) as a source of reducing equivalents (thus, functioning as *glutathione dehydrogenase*), but recent studies have demonstrated in the colonic mucosa of the rat another form of the enzyme that uses NADPH as a hydrogen donor[26].

# METABOLIC FUNCTIONS OF VITAMIN C

varied roles
In its various known metabolic functions, vitamin C as ascorbic acid serves as a classical enzyme cofactor (e.g., at the active site of hydroxylating enzymes), as a protective agent (e.g., of hydroxylases in collagen biosynthesis) and as ascorbyl radical in reactions with transition metal ions. Each of these functions of the vitamin appear to involve its redox properties.

electron transport
Because of its reversible monovalent oxidation to the ascorbyl radical, ascorbic acid can serve as a biochemical redox system. As such, it is involved in many electron transport reactions including those involved in the synthesis of collagen, the degradation of 4-hydroxyphenylpyruvate[27], the synthesis of norepinephrine[28], and the desaturation of fatty acids. In

---

[25] The excretion of oxalate as a degradation product of ascorbic acid is relevant to the putative increased risk of renal stone formation among individuals consuming large amounts of vitamin C. It is estimated that, of the oxalate excreted daily (e.g., 30-40 mg) by humans consuming physiological amounts of vitamin C, 35-50% comes from ascorbic acid degradation (the balance coming from glycine and glyoxylate). Subjects consuming very high doses of vitamin C have been found to have increased urinary oxalates (e.g., the intake of 10 g vitamin C per day for 5 days increased daily urinary oxalate excretion from ca. 50 mg to ca. 87 mg). However, as oxalate excretion is not a useful indicator of risk to renal calculi (e.g., a comparison of 75 patients with renal calculi and 50 healthy controls showed the same average oxalate excretion of ca. 28 mg/day) and, as the contributions of high doses of vitamin C to oxalate formation are rather small, the physiological implications of these effects are unclear.

[26] It is thought that the presence of more than one dehydroascorbic acid reductase may serve to promote a favorable ascorbate redox potential, indirectly preserving other antioxidants (e.g., tocopherol), thus, playing a prominent role in the defense mechanisms of the body. That the NADPH-dependent enzyme is found in the intestinal mucosa suggests that this function may be important in protecting against the many of radical species generated there.

[27] the first product of tyrosine metabolism.

[28] noradrenalin.

many of these functions ascorbate is not required *per se*, i.e., it can be replaced by other reductants (e.g., reduced glutathione, cysteine, tetra-hydrofolate, dithiothreitol, 2-mercaptoethanol); however, ascorbate is the most effective *in vitro*.   In each, ascorbic acid is regenerated as the electron acceptor ascorbyl radical is reduced by either of two microsomal enzymes *monodehydroascorbate reductase* or *ascorbate-cytochrome $b_5$ reductase*, the latter being part of the fatty acid desaturation system.

*collagen synthesis*

The best characterized metabolic role of vitamin C is in the synthesis of *collagen* proteins[29] in which it is involved in the *hydroxylation* of specific *prolyl* and *lysyl* residues of procollagen. These reactions are catalyzed by the enzymes *prolyl hydroxylase* and *lysyl hydroxylase* which require $Fe^{++}$ and ascorbate.   Each is a dioxygenase[30] stoichiometrically linked to the oxidative decarboxylation of 2-ketoglutarate.   It is thought that ascorbate's role in each reaction is to maintain iron in the reduced state ($Fe^{++}$), which dissociates from a critical region (an SH-group) of the active site to reactivate the enzyme after catalysis.   The post-translational hydroxylation of these procollagen amino acid residues are necessary for folding into the triple helical structure that can be secreted by fibroblasts. *Hydroxyproline* residues contribute to the stiffness of the collagen triple helix, and *hydroxylysine* residues bind (*via* their hydroxyl groups) carbohydrates and form intramolecular cross-links that give structural integrity to the collagen mass.   The under-hydroxylation of procollagen, which accumulates[31] and is degraded, appears to be the basis of the pathophysiology of *scurvy*.

Studies have indicated some modest effects of vitamin C deficiency on the hydroxylation of proline in the conversion of the soluble *tropoelastin* to the soluble *elastin*[32].   A component of complement, C1q, resembles collagen in containing hydroxyproline and hydroxylysine.   Curiously, vitamin C deprivation reduces overall complement activity, but does not affect the synthesis of C1q.   A role has been suggested for ascorbate in the synthesis of proteoglycans.

---

[29] Collagens are the major components of skin and connective tissues, the organic substances of bones and teeth, the cornea, and the "ground substance" between cells. Collectively, collagen is the most abundant animal protein, comprising 25-30% of total body protein.

[30] One half of the $O_2$ molecule is incorporated into the peptidyl prolyl (or peptidyl lysyl) residue, and the other half is incorporated into succinate.

[31] Accumulated procollagen also inhibits its own synthesis and mRNA translation.

[32] About 1% of the prolyl residues in elastin are hydroxylated.  This amount can apparently be increased by vitamin C, suggesting that normal elastin may by "under-hydroxylated".

*other*
*hydroxylations*   Ascorbic acid has important roles in several hydroxylases involved in the metabolism of neurotransmitters, steroids, drugs and lipids. It serves as an electron donor for **dopamine-β-monooxygenase**[33], Cu-enzyme located in the chromaffin vesicles[34] of the adrenal medulla and in adrenergic synapses, that hydroxylates dopamine to form the neurotransmitter norepinephrine. In this reaction ascorbate is oxidized to ascorbyl radical (monodehydroascorbate), which is returned to the reduced state by **monodehydroascorbate reductase**.

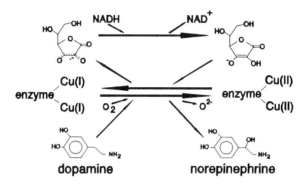

dopamine                    norepinephrine

A similar enzyme has been identified in the hypophyses of rats and cattle. This Cu-dependent enzyme, **peptidyl glycine α-amidating monooxygenase**, catalyzes the α-amidation of peptides and requires ascorbate and $O_2$. It is thought to be involved in the amidation of the C-terminae of physiologically active peptides[35]. That catalase inhibits its activity *in vitro* suggests that $H_2O_2$ is an intermediate in the reaction.

Ascorbic acid is a cofactor of two $Fe^{++}$-containing hydroxylases[36] involved in the synthesis of **carnitine**, which is required for the transport of fatty acids into mitochondria for oxidation to provide energy for the cell. Scorbutic guinea pigs show abnormally low carnitine levels in muscle and heart, and it is thought that the fatigue, lassitude and hypertriglyceridemia observed in scurvy may be due to impaired formation of carnitine.

---

[33]The specific activity of this enzyme has been found to be abnormally low in schizophrenics with anatomical changes in the brain, suggesting impaired norepinephrine- and dopamine-neurotransmission in those patients.

[34]These vesicles accumulate and store chatecholamines in the adrenal medulla; they also contain very high concentrations of ascorbic acid, e.g., 20 mM.

[35]e.g., bombesin (human gastrin-releasing peptide), calcitonin, cholecystokinin, corticotropin-releasing factor, gastrin, growth hormone releasing factor, α- and γ-melanotropin, metorphamide, neuropeptide Y, oxytocin, vasoactive intestinal peptide, vasopressin.

[36]*ε-N-trimethyllysine hydroxylase* and *γ-butyrobetaine hydroxylase*.

*drug and steroid metabolism*

Ascorbic acid is thought to be involved in *microsomal hydroxylation reactions* of drug and steroid metabolism, i.e., those coupled to the microsomal electron transport chain. For example, the activity of *cholesterol 7α-hydroxylase* the hepatic microsomal enzyme involved in the biosynthesis of bile acids, is diminished in the chronically vitamin C-deficient guinea pig and is stimulated by feeding that animal high levels of vitamin C[37]. Epidemiologic studies have detected significant positive correlations of ascorbic acid and HDL-cholesterol in the plasma/serum of free-living humans[38].

The metabolism of drugs and other xenobiotic compounds is similarly affected by ascorbic acid. Vitamin C-deficient guinea pigs showed significant increases in the half-lives of phenobarbital, acetanilide, aniline and antipyrine. Studies in animal models have clearly demonstrated positive correlations between ascorbic acid status, hepatic activity of cytochrome $P_{450}$, and drug metabolism (hydroxylations, demethylations). The activities of mitochondrial and microsomal steroid hydroxylases of the adrenal have been found to be impaired in scorbutic animals in which they respond to vitamin C therapy. In these cases, ascorbic acid appears to function as a protective antioxidant. It is thought that reduced synthesis of corticosteroids accounts for the diminished plasma glucocorticoid responses to stress of vitamin C-deficient animals.

*tyrosine metabolism*

Vitamin C is involved in the oxidative degradation (which normally proceeds completely to $CO_2$ and water) of tyrosine *via* two mixed-function oxidases that are dependent on the presence of ascorbic acid. The first is *4-hydroxyphenylpyruvate oxidase*, which catalyzes the oxidation and decarboxylation of the intermediate of tyrosine degradation, 4-hydroxylphenyl-pyruvic acid, to *homogentisic acid*. The second ascorbate-requiring enzyme catalyzes the next step in tyrosine degradation, *homogentisate 1,2-dioxygenase*. By impairing both reactions, vitamin C-deficiency can result in *tyrosinemia*[39] and the excretion of tyrosine metabolites in the urine; both conditions respond to vitamin C supplements.

*metal ion metabolism*

Ascorbic acid can interact with several metallic elements of nutritional significance. Due to its activity as a reductant, ascorbic acid reduces the toxicities of elements the reduced forms of which are poorly absorbed or

---

[37]Guinea pigs fed 500 mg ascorbic acid per kg of diet showed substantial reductions in plasma (ca. 40%) and liver (ca. 15%) cholesterol concentrations. Human studies have been inconsistent in showing similar effects.

[38]A recent study in a healthy elderly Japanese population found serum ascorbic acid to account for ca. 5% and 11% of the variation in serum HDL-cholesterol concentrations in men and women, respectively.

[39]Temporary tyrosinemia (serum levels >4 mg/dl) occurs frequently in premature infants and involves reduced 4-hydroxyphenylpyruvate dioxygenase activity. Low doses of ascorbic acid usually normalize the condition.

more rapidly excreted (e.g., *Se, Ni, Pb, V* and *Cd*). High dietary levels of the vitamin have been shown to reduce the efficiency of enteric absorption of $Cu^{40}$. In contrast, ascorbic acid can enhance the utilization of physiologic doses of *Se*, increasing the apparent biologic availability of a variety of inorganic and organic forms of that essential nutrient[41].

*enhanced Fe bioavailability*    Ascorbic acid increases the bioavailability of Fe in foods. This effect is associated with increased enteric absorption[42] (which is normally low) of the mineral; it affects both *non-heme-Fe* as well as *heme-Fe*. Its effect on non-heme-Fe involves its reducing the ferric form of the element ($Fe^{+++}$), predominant in the acidic environment of the stomach, to the ferrous from ($Fe^{++}$) and, then, forming a soluble stable chelate that stays in solution in the alkaline environment of the small intestine and is, thus, rather well absorbed. This effect depends on the presence of both ascorbic acid and Fe in the gut at the same time, e.g., the consumption of a vitamin C-containing food with the meal[43]. Ascorbic acid also promotes the utilization of heme-Fe; whereas the basis of this effect is less well understood, it is thought to involve enhanced incorporation of Fe in to the its intracellular storage form, *ferritin*[44]. Studies with cultured cells have shown that ascorbic acid also enhances the stability of ferritin by blocking its degradation through reduced lysosomal autophagy of the protein. Thus, the decline in ferritin and accumulation of *hemosiderin*[45] in scorbutic animals is reversed by ascorbic acid treatment[46].

---

[40] This effect does not appear to be significant at moderate intakes of the vitamin. A study with healthy young men found that intakes up to 605 mg/person/day for three weeks had no effects on Cu absorption or retention, or on serum Cu or ceruloplasmin concentrations (although the oxidase activity of the protein was decreased by 23% in that treatment).

[41] This effect was a surprising finding, as it is known that ascorbic acid can reduce Se-compounds to insoluble forms of little or no biological value. The biochemical mechanism of the stimulation of Se bioavailability by ascorbic acid appears to involve enhanced post-absorptive utilization of Se for the synthesis of selenoproteins perhaps by creating a redox balance of glutathione in favor of its reduced form (GSH).

[42] This effect can be 200-600%.

[43] Thus, the inhibitions of Fe-absorption normally caused by polyphenols, tea, phytate, phytate-containing foods, or calcium phosphate can be overcome with simultaneously administered ascorbic acid.

[44] An soluble, Fe-protein complex found mainly in the liver, spleen, bone marrow, and reticuloendothelial cells. Containing 23% Fe, it is the main storage form of Fe in the body. When its storage capacity is exceeded, Fe accumulates as the insoluble hemosiderin.

[45] A dark yellow, insoluble, granular, iron-storage complex found mainly in the liver, spleen and bone marrow.

[46] The reverse relationship is apparently not significant, i.e., Fe-loading has been found to have no effect on ascorbic acid catabolism in guinea pigs.

*anti-histamine*   Ascorbic acid is involved in ***histamine*** metabolism, acting with $Cu^{++}$ to
*reactions*        inhibit its release and enhance its degradation.  It does so by undergoing
                   oxidation to dehydroascorbic acid with the concomitant rupture of the
                   histamine imidazole ring.  In tissue culture systems, this effect results in
                   reductions of endogenous histamine levels as well as ***histidine decarb-***
                   ***oxylase*** activities, a measure of histamine synthetic capacity.  It is also
                   thought that ascorbic acid may enhance the synthesis of the prostaglandin
                   E-series (over the F-series) members of which mediate histamine sensi-
                   tivity.  Circulating histamine concentration is known to be reduced by high
                   doses of vitamin C, a fact that has been the basis of the therapeutic use
                   of the vitamin to protect against histamine-induced anaphylactic shock.
                   Further, blood histamine concentrations are elevated in several
                   complications of pregnancy that are associated with marginal ascorbic acid
                   status:  pre-eclampsia[47], abruption[48] and prematurity.  Because blood
                   histamine and ascorbic acid concentrations were negatively correlated in
                   women in pre-term labor, it has been suggested that the combined effects
                   of marginal vitamin C status and reduced plasma histaminase may result
                   in the marked elevations of blood histamine levels seen in those conditions.

*immune*           Ascorbic acid has been found to affect immune function in several different
*functions*        ways.  It can stimulate the production of interferons, the proteins that
                   protect cells against viral attack.  It can stimulate the positive chemotactic
                   and proliferative responses of neutrophils.  It can protect against free
                   radical-mediated protein inactivation associated with the *'oxidative burst'*[49]
                   of neutrophils.  It can stimulate of the synthesis of humoral thymus factor
                   and antibodies of the IgG and IgM classes.  Some studies have found
                   massive oral doses of the vitamin (10 g/day) to enhance delayed-type
                   hypersensitivity responses in humans, although somewhat lower doses (2
                   g/day) have shown no such effects.

*anti-*            Ascorbic acid C has been observed to reduce the binding of polycyclic
*carcinogenicity*  aromatic carcinogens to DNA[50] and to reduce/delay tumor formation in
                   several animal models.  The vitamin also is a potent inhibitor of nitros-
                   amine-induced carcinogenesis.  Its protective function involves its action

---

[47] the nonconvulsive stage of an acute hypertensive disease of pregnant and puerperal (after childbirth) women.

[48] premature detachment of the placenta.

[49] Neutrophils, when stimulated, take up molecular oxygen ($O_2$) and generate reactive free-radicals and singlet oxygen, which, along with other reactive molecules, can kill bacterial pathogens.  This process, called the *'oxidative burst'* because it can be observed *in vitro* as a rapid consumption of $O_2$, also involves the enzymatic generation of bacteriocidal halogenated molecules *via **myeloperoxidase***.  These killing processes are usually localized in intracellular vacuoles containing the phagocytized bacteria.

[50] Reactions of this type are believed to comprise the molecular basis of carcinogenesis.  These kinds of effect of vitamin C probably involve its function as a free radical scavenger.

as a reducing agent that serves as a nitrite-scavenger *in vivo*. It reduces nitrate (the actual nitrosylating agent of free amines) to NO, thus, blocking the formation of nitrosamines[51]. There is evidence that ascorbic acid, normally secreted in relatively high concentrations in gastric juice[52], is a limiting factor in nitrosation reactions in people. This appears to be particularly true for persons with gastric pathologies that affect secretion. Epidemiological studies of human cancer incidence provide evidence for protective roles of vitamin C against cancers of the esophagus, larynx, oral cavity, pancreas, stomach, rectum and breast[53].

*antioxidant/ prooxidant functions*

Ascorbic acid can act either as an antioxidant or as a prooxidant. Its antioxidant activity is based on its ability to react with free radicals, being first converted to ascorbyl radical which quickly disproportionates to ascorbate and dehydroascorbate. Thus, ascorbic acid can react with the toxic forms of oxygen, the superoxide anion ($O_2^-$) and hydroxyl radical ($OH^-$). This reaction is likely to be of fundamental importance in all aerobic cells, which must defend against the toxicity of the very element depended upon as the terminal electron acceptor for energy production via the respiratory chain enzymes. It is this type of reaction that appears to be the basis of most, if not all, of the essential biological functions of ascorbic acid. One of these is important in extending the antioxidant protection to the hydrophobic regions of cells: ascorbic acid appears to be able to reduce the semi-stable chromanoxyl radical, thus, regenerating the metabolically active form of the lipid antioxidant vitamin E[54].

The antioxidant efficiency of vitamin C is greatest at low concentrations of the vitamin. Under those conditions, the predominant reaction is a radical chain-terminating one of ascorbate ($AH^-$) with a peroxyl radical to yield a hydroperoxide and the ascorbyl radical ($A^-$), which proceeds to reduce a second peroxyl radical and yield the vitamin in its oxidized form, dehydroascorbic acid (A).

---

[51] Vitamin E also has this effect.

[52] The concentration of ascorbic acid in gastric juice have been found often to exceed those in the plasma.

[53] Statistically significant protective effects of dietary vitamin C have been detected in two-thirds of the epidemiologic studies in which a dietary vitamin C index was calculated. In several cases, high vitamin C intake was associated with half the cancer risk associated with low intake. Protective effects have also been detected in a similarly high proportion of studies in which the intake of fruit, but not vitamin C, was assessed.

[54] Evidence for such an effect comes from demonstrations *in vitro* of the reduction by ascorbic acid of the tocopheroxyl radical to tocopherol, as well as from findings in animals that supplemental vitamin C can increase tissue tocopherol concentrations and spare dietary vitamin E.

At low concentrations of the vitamin, two moles of peroxyl radical are reduced for every mole of ascorbate consumed:

$$AH^- + ROO^{\cdot} \longrightarrow A^{\cdot-} + ROO^- \; (\xrightarrow{H^+} ROOH)$$

$$A^{\cdot-} + R'OO^{\cdot} \longrightarrow A \; + R'OO^- \; (\xrightarrow{H^+} R'OOH)$$

At higher vitamin C concentrations, however, a slower radical chain-propagating reaction of ascorbyl radical and molecular oxygen appears to become significant. It yields dehydroascorbic acid and superoxide radical which, in turn, can oxidize ascorbate to return ascorbyl radical:

$$A^{\cdot-} + O_2 \longrightarrow A + O_2^{\cdot-}$$

$$O_2^{\cdot-} + AH^- \longrightarrow HOO^{\cdot} + A^{\cdot-}$$

It is thought that, at high vitamin C concentrations, this two-reaction sequence can develop into a radical chain autoxidation process that consumes ascorbate, thus, *"wasting"* the vitamin. Hence, in aerobic systems, the efficiency of radical-quenching of ascorbate is inversely related to the concentration of the vitamin.

In the presence of metal ions (e.g., $Fe^{+++}$, $Cu^{++}$), high concentrations of vitamin C can also function as a pro-oxidant. It does so by donating a single electron to reduce such ions to forms that, in turn, can react with $O_2$ to form oxygen radicals (the metal ions being re-oxidized in the process). Thus, ascorbate can react with Cu- or Fe-salts and lead to the formation of superoxide radical anion and hydroxyl radical.

## EXTREMES IN VITAMIN C INTAKE

*deficiency*    Acute vitamin C deficiency results in **scurvy** in individuals unable to synthesize the vitamin. In guinea pigs, the syndrome is characterized by intermittent reductions in growth, hematomas (especially of the hind limbs), extremely brittle bones, calcification of bone-cartilage boundaries, and death usually occurring within 25-30 days. In children, the syndrome is called **Moeller-Barlow disease**; it is seen in non-breast-fed infants usually at ca. 6 months of age (when maternally derived stores of vitamin C have been exhausted) and is characterized by widening of bone-cartilage boundaries, particularly of the rib cage and stressed epiphyseal cartilage of the extremities, by severe joint pain and, frequently, by anemia and fever.

*Classical scurvy* is manifest in human adults after 45-80 days of stopping vitamin C consumption[55].   Signs of the disease occur primarily in mesenchymal tissues.   Defects in collagen formation are manifest as impaired wound healing, and to edema and hemorrhage (due to deficient formation of intercellular substance) in the skin, mucous membranes, internal organs and muscles, and weakening of collagenous structures in bone, cartilage, teeth and connective tissues.   Scorbutic individuals may show swollen, bleeding gums with tooth loss; but that condition may signify accompanying periodontal disease.   They also show lethargy, fatigue, rheumatic pains in the legs, muscular atrophy, skin lesions, massive *"sheet"* hematomas in the thighs and ecchymoses[56] and hemorrhages in many organs including the intestines, subperiosteal tissues and eyes.   These features are frequently accompanied by psychological changes:  hysteria, hypochondria and depression.

Ascorbic acid deficiency in at least some species of fishes (salmonids and carp) results in spinal curvature (scoliosis[57] and lordosis[58]), reduced survival, reduced growth rate, anemia and hemorrhaging especially in the fins, tail, muscles and eyes.   Similar signs have been reported in vitamin C-deficient shrimp and eels.   Guinea pigs that are deprived of vitamin C show reduced feed intake and growth, anemia, hemorrhages, abnormalities of epiphyseal bone growth, altered dentin and gingivitis.

*Mild vitamin C deficiency*[59] results in several non-specific *"pre-scorbutic"* signs/symptoms including lassitude, fatigue, anorexia, muscular weakness and increased susceptibility to infection.   In the guinea pig, such conditions also result in hypertriglyceridemia, hypercholesterolemia and decreased vitamin E concentrations in liver and lungs.   Epidemiologic data indicate significant associations of low plasma ascorbic acid concentration with

---

[55]Clinical signs/symptoms of scurvy in humans are manifest when the total body pool of vitamin C is reduced to less than ca. 300 mg, from its normal level of ca. 1500 mg.  At that low level, patients show plasma vitamin C levels of .13-.25 mg/dl (normal levels are .8-1.4 mg/dl).

[56]bluish patches caused by extravasation of blood into the skin (a "black and blue" spot); similar to petechiae except for their larger size.

[57]lateral curvature of the spine

[58]anteroposterior curvature of the spine

[59]in humans, plasma vitamin C level less than ca. .75 mg/dl and total body vitamin C pool less than ca. 600 mg.

increased risk to ischemic heart disease or hypertension in humans[60]. Marginal vitamin C deficiency can be caused by low dietary intakes, as well as by a variety of factors that increase ascorbate turnover in the body (e.g., smoking[61], stress, chronic disease, diabetes). In addition, elderly people typically show total body vitamin C pools of reduced size, perhaps due to reduced enteric absorption and increased turnover.

Signs of Vitamin C Deficiency:

| organ system | signs |
|---|---|
| general | |
|   appetite | decrease |
|   growth | decrease |
|   immunity | decrease |
|   heat resistance | decrease |
| muscular | skeletal muscle atrophy |
| vascular | |
|   vessels | increased capillary fragility, hemorrhage |
| nervous | tenderness |

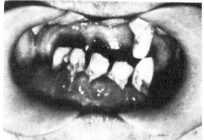

Scurvy in a middle-aged man. Note: swollen, bleeding gums and tooth loss. Courtesy J. Marks, Cambridge University.

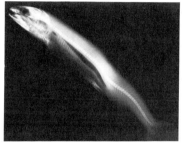

Radiograph of a vitamin C-deficient trout showing lordosis; courtesy of G.L. Rumsey, Tunnison Laboratory of Fish Nutrition, USDI.

*high-level intake*   Despite the fact that tissue saturation of vitamin C occurs in humans at intakes of 100-150 mg/day, higher intakes can result in elevated concentrations of the vitamin in extracellular fluids (plasma, connective tissue fluid, humors of the eye) where pharmacologic action of this antioxidant vitamin may be possible. Further, vitamin C intakes greater than those required to

---

[60] Both effects may indicate relationships of antioxidant status to these diseases, as each is also associated with relatively low status with respect to vitamin E and/or Se. In the case of hypertension, a recent placebo-controlled, double-blind study showed that vitamin C supplements (1 g/day for 3 mos.) significantly reduced systolic and diastolic pressures in borderline hypertensive subjects with normal serum ascorbic acid levels.

[61] The ascorbic acid concentrations of serum and urine of smokers tend to be ca. 0.2 mg/dl less than those of non-smokers; these effects have been observed even after correcting for vitamin C intake, which was found to be ca. 53 mg/day less in smokers. Further, smokers have been found to have lower rates of vitamin C turnover of ca. 100 mg/day *vs.* those of non-smokers of ca. 60 mg/day. It has been estimated that smokers require 52-68 mg vitamin C per day more than non-smokers to attain comparable plasma ascorbic acid levels.

prevent scurvy have been found to promote the bioavailability of dietary iron and, particularly, to counteract the negative effects of dietary fiber on the utilization of that essential mineral. Thus, gram-size doses of vitamin C have been advocated for the prophylaxis/ treatment of several conditions including the common cold, *herpes labialis*[62], general immune support, cardiovascular diseases, hypercholesterolemia, hypertension, hypertriglyceridemia, diabetes[63] and some types of cancer[64].

Most of the clinical studies in which supranutritional doses of vitamin C have been found to be of some benefit have compared treated subjects with controls who did not have tissue-saturation with respect to the vitamin. Such studies, therefore, cannot indicate whether the effects of the vitamin C treatments were due simply to effecting tissue saturation, or to pharmacologic actions of the vitamin in extracellular fluids. Thus, while there appear to be benefits associated with increasing vitamin C intakes to levels that effect tissue saturation, the evidence in support of benefits of vitamin C doses above that level is not clear. The most widely publicized use of so-called *"megadoses"* of vitamin C are in prophylaxis and treatment of the common cold, a use advocated by Dr. Irwin Stone and the Nobel laureate[65] Linus Pauling. In the nearly 20 years since their proposal of a protective effect of gram-doses of vitamin C against colds in humans, many controlled clinical studies have been conducted to test that hypothesis. In general, most results have indicated only small positive effects in reducing the incidence, shortening the duration and ameliorating the symptoms of the common cold. It has been suggested that, in at least some cases, these apparent benefits may have been *"placebo effects"*.

*hyper-*
*vitaminosis*
The reported benefits of gram doses of vitamin C have led to widespread ingestion of vitamin C supplements in many western countries, thus raising issues of the safety of such practices. Specifically, it has been proposed that megadoses of vitamin C may increase oxalate production and, thus, increase the formation of renal stones, competitively inhibit the renal reabsorption of uric acid, enhance the destruction of vitamin $B_{12}$ in the gut, enhance the enteric absorption of non-heme-Fe (thus, leading to Fe-overload), have mutagenic effects, and increase ascorbate catabolism that

---

[62]*herpes* type I: cold sores.

[63]It is thought that long-term high plasma ascorbate concentrations may be able to overcome to some degree the competitive inhibition of transport of ascorbic acid into insulin-sensitive tissues by high blood glucose levels, and possibly to allow a reduction of insulin dosage by potentiating the action of the hormone.

[64]Dietary vitamin C appears to be able to inhibit, at least partially, gastric nitrosation of proline (and, presumably, other amines), thus, reducing nitrosamine formation and the gastric cancer that it can produce.

[65]Professor Pauling received the Nobel Prize in Chemistry in 1954 and a second Nobel Prize for Peace in 1962.

would persist after returning to lower intakes of the vitamin. Present knowledge indicates that most, if not all, of these concerns are not warranted.

Perhaps the greatest concern associated with high intakes of vitamin C has to do with increased oxalate production. In humans, unlike other animals, oxalate is a major metabolite of ascorbic acid, which accounts for 35-50% of the 35-40 mg of oxalate excreted in the urine each day[66]. The health concern, therefore, is that increases in vitamin C intake may lead to increased oxalate production and, thus, to increase risk to the formation of urinary calculi. Although metabolic studies indicate that the turnover of ascorbic acid is limited and that high intakes of vitamin C, therefore, should not greatly affect oxalate production, clinical studies have revealed slight oxaluria in patients given daily multiple-gram doses of vitamin C. Whether this effect actually constitutes an increased risk to the formation of renal calculi is not clear, however, as its magnitude is low (within normal variation)[67]. Nevertheless, prudence dictates the avoidance of megadoses of vitamin C for individuals with a history of forming renal stones, particularly in view of the fact that a few individuals have been found to excrete considerable amounts of oxalate after doses of the vitamin that do not affect oxalate excretion by most people.

Concerns that uricosuria might be induced by megadoses of vitamin C are based upon speculation that, because both ascorbic acid and uric acid are reabsorbed by the renal tubules by saturable processes, a common transport system may be involved and, thus, high levels of ascorbic acid may competitively inhibit uric acid reabsorption. Studies with healthy subjects have shown that multi-gram doses of ascorbic acid do not affect serum or urinary uric acid concentrations. The results of studies with hyperuricemic subjects including those with clinical signs of gout, are less clear; but, in aggregate, they do not provide a basis for this concern.

In the 1970s, it was claimed that high levels of ascorbic acid added to test meals that were held warm for 30 min resulted in the destruction (presumed to occur by chemical reduction) of food vitamin $B_{12}$, thus raising the concern that megadoses of vitamin C may antagonize the utilization of that important vitamin. More recent studies have not supported that claim; in fact, the only form of vitamin $B_{12}$ that is sensitive to reduction and subsequent destruction by ascorbic acid is aquocobalamin, which is not a major form of the vitamin in foods. Further, the results of a recent study indicate that high doses of vitamin C can, in fact, partially protect rats from

---

[66] The balance of urinary oxalate comes mainly from the degradation of glycine (ca. 40% of the total); but some also can come from the diet (5-10%).

[67] e.g., subjects given five doses of either 1 or 2 g of ascorbic acid daily (i.e., doses of 5 or 10 g/day) excreted oxalate in their urine at only slightly higher levels (35-45 mg/day or 57-67 mg/day, respectively) than those of subjects consuming 200 mg vitamin C per day who excreted 20-30 mg oxalate per day.

vitamin $B_{12}$ deficiency[68]. The results of several clinical investigations have shown clearly that high doses of vitamin C do not affect vitamin $B_{12}$ status.

That ascorbic acid can enhance the enteric absorption of dietary Fe has led some to express concern that megadoses of vitamin C may lead to progressive Fe accumulation in Fe-replete individuals (*"iron storage disease"*). Such an effect is not to be expected, however, as optimal Fe absorption is effected with rather low doses of vitamin (25-50 mg ascorbic acid per meal). Nevertheless, patients with hemochromatosis or other forms of excess Fe accumulation should avoid taking vitamin C supplements with their meals.

Persistent, enhanced ascorbic acid catabolism after prolonged intake of large amounts of vitamin C (so-called *"systemic conditioning"*) has been proposed, based on uncontrolled observations of a few individuals and what is now widely regarded as erroneous interpretations of experimental results[69]. Controlled studies have not consistently demonstrated such effects. Kinetic studies in humans indicate that high-doses of ascorbic acid are mostly degraded to $CO_2$ by microbial microbes, with major portions also excreted intact in the urine. While such results would appear to refute the prospect of induced catabolism, a recent well controlled study with guinea pigs found plasma ascorbic acid levels to drop transiently in some animals removed from high-level vitamin C treatments; the authors attributed that finding to *"systemic conditioning"*.

The suggestion that ascorbic acid might be mutagenic comes from studies with cultured cells which show a dependence on $Cu^{++}$ for such effects (the vitamin is not intrinsically mutagenic), which apparently involve the production of reactive oxygen radicals. No evidence of mutagenic effects *in vivo* has been produced; that probably indicates that the antioxidant defenses[70] of the cell effectively handle oxidative stresses of that type.

The only consistent deleterious effects of vitamin C megadoses in humans are gastro-intestinal disturbances and diarrhea. Little information is available on vitamin C toxicity in animals, although acute $LD_{50}$ values for most species and routes of administration appear to be at least several grams per kg of body weight. A single study showed mink to be very sensitive to hypervitaminosis C; with daily intakes of 100-200 mg ascorbic acid, pregnant females developed anemia and had reduced litter sizes.

---

[68]Rats given ascorbic acid (6 g/l in the drinking water) showed greater hepatic vitamin $B_{12}$ levels and lower urinary methylmalonic acid excretion, both indicators of enhanced vitamin $B_{12}$ status, than controls.

[69]e.g., enhanced $^{14}CO_2$ excretion from guinea pigs with larger body pools of ascorbic acid taken as evidence of greater catabolism.

[70]vitamin E, glutathione, Se-dependent glutathione peroxidase, catalase, superoxide dismutase.

## CASE STUDY

*Instructions:*     *Review each of the following case reports, paying special attention to the diagnostic indicators upon which the treatments were based.  Then answer the questions that follow.*

*case 1*     A 26-year-old man volunteered for a 258-day experiment of ascorbic acid metabolism.  He was 184 cm tall and weighed 84.1 kg.  His medical history, physical examination, vital signs and past diet history revealed a healthy individual with no irregularities.  During the experiment, his temperature, pulse and respiration rates were recorded 4 times daily, and his blood pressure was measured twice daily.  He was examined by an internist daily; periodically he was examined by an ophthalmologist, and had chest radiograms and electrocardiograms made.  Twenty-four-hour collections of urine and feces were made daily for determining urinary and fecal N and for the radioactive assay of ascorbic acid.  Samples of expired air were collected for the measurement of radioactivity.

The subject was fed a control diet consisting of soy-based products.  The diet provided 2.5 mg ascorbic acid per day, which was supplemented by a daily capsule containing an additional 75 mg ascorbic acid.  The subject's body vitamin C pool was labeled with L-ascorbate-1-$^{14}$C one week prior to initiating vitamin C depletion; it was calculated to be 1500 mg.  Beginning on day 14, the diet was changed to a liquid formula containing no vitamin C, as ascertained by actual analysis.  This diet, based on vitamin-free casein, provided 3300 kcal and supplied protein, fat and carbohydrate as 15%, 40% and 45% of total calories, respectively.  It was fed from days 14-104 during which time the subject developed signs of scurvy.  Ascorbic acid was not detectable in his urine after 30 days of depletion.  He showed *petechiae* on the 45th day, when his vitamin C pool was 150 mg and his plasma level was 0.19 mg/dl.  Spontaneous *ecchymoses* occurred over days 36-103; these were followed by *coiled hairs*, *gum changes*, *hyperkeratosis*[71], *congested follicles* and the *Sjögren sicca syndrome*[72], *dry mouth* and *enlarged parotid salivary glands*.  The subject developed *joint pains* on the 68th day and *joint effusions*[73] shortly thereafter, when his vitamin C pool was 100 mg and his plasma ascorbic acid level was less than 0.16 mg/dl.  He also had the unusual complication of a *bilateral femoral neuropathy*, which began on the 71st day when his vitamin C pool was 80 mg and his plasma ascorbic acid level

---

[71] a mouth disease with clinical characteristics usually of variously sized and shaped, grayish white, flat, adherent patches; having diffuse borders, and a smooth surface with no papillary projections, fissures, erosions or ulcerations.

[72] dry eyes due to reduction in tears, i.e., keratoconjunctivitis.

[73] the escape of fluid from the blood vessels or lymphatics into the joint capsule.

was 0.15 mg/dl. This, accompanied the joint effusions, was attributed to hemorrhage into the sheaths of both femoral nerves. On the 80th day, he experienced a rapid *increase in weight*, from 81 to 84 kg, showed with *dyspnea*[74] on exertion and *swelling of the legs*. At this time, his vitamin C pool was 40 mg and his plasma level was 0.15 mg/dl.

Beginning on day 105, the subject was put on a vitamin C-repletion regimen involving daily doses of 4 mg ascorbic acid. Immediately following this treatment, the *edema* worsened, urinary output dropped to 340 ml/day and weight increased to 86.6 kg on day 109. There was no evidence of pulmonary congestion or cardiac failure. The ascorbic acid-repletion dose was increased to 6.5 mg/day on day 111. His edema persisted for 4 days, at which time he had a profound *diuresis* with complete disappearance of the edema by day 133 at which time his weight was 77.2 kg (he lost 9.4 kg of extracellular fluid). From days 101 to 133, his body ascorbic acid pool increased from 33 to 128 mg. The subject was given 6.5 mg ascorbic acid per day from day 133 to 227. During this time, all his scorbutic manifestations disappeared, and his plasma ascorbic acid fluctuated between 0.10-0.25 mg/dl. His body pool was restored slowly to an excess of 300 mg. On day 228, he received 600 mg/day ascorbic acid, which rapidly repleted his body pool. At the end of the study, his weight was 81 kg and he was discharged from the metabolic ward in excellent health.

case 2:    A 72-year-old man was admitted to the hospital with symptoms of increasing *anorexia*, *epigastric discomfort* unrelated to meals and non-radiating *precordial* [75] *pain*. During the year before admission, he had become increasingly weak and easily *fatigued*, and had lost nearly 13 kg in weight. Six weeks prior to admission, he began to have sudden attacks of severe substernal pain followed by cough and *dyspnea*, and one month before admission, he had a small *hematemesis*[76] and had noted bright red *blood in his stools*. He had been living alone and his diet during the past year had consisted chiefly of bread and milk with various soups. For a considerable period, he had noted easy *bruising* of his skin. His past health had been good except for occasional *seizures*; these began two years prior to admission and involved loss of consciousness, spasmodic twitching of the limbs and incontinence preceded by abdominal discomfort.

Physical examination upon admission revealed a thin, *depressed, lethargic* man with a rather gray complexion and numerous *petechiae* over the arms, legs and trunk. His blood pressure was 140/80, his pulse was 68,

---

[74]subjective difficulty or distress in breathing, frequently rapid breathing.

[75]relating to the diaphragm and anterior surface of the lower part of the thorax.

[76]vomiting of blood.

his respiration was 19, and his temperature was 98.8°F.  Examination of his head and neck showed an edentulous[77] mouth, foul breath, ulcerated palate and retracted gums without hemorrhage.  He had a large *ecchymosis* (15 cm in diameter) on his right thigh.  Neurological examination was negative.

Laboratory findings:

| parameter | patient | normal range |
|---|---|---|
| Hb | 13.2 g/dl | 15-18 g/dl |
| WBC | 8,000/$\mu$l | 5,000-9,000/$\mu$l |
| platelets | 140,000/$\mu$l | 150,000-300,000/$\mu$l |
| clotting time | 5.75 min | 5-15 min |
| blood urea | 48 mg/dl | 10-20 mg/dl |
| serum protein | 7 g/dl | 6-8 g/dl |
| serum albumin | 3.9 g/dl | 3.5-5.5 g/dl |
| serum ascorbic acid | <0.1 mg/dl | 0.4-1.0 mg/dl |

His heart was not enlarged and there were no heart murmurs; but, his electrocardiogram showed changes typical of an old myocardial infarction[78].  His chest radiograms showed emphysematous[79] and atheromatous[80] changes.  His urine contained occasional pus cells with moderate growth of *E. coli*; no abnormal bacilli were seen in the sputum.  Sigmoidoscopy revealed no lesions in the distal 25 cm of the bowel.  Because of his anorexia, epigastric discomfort, weight loss and hematemesis, further investigation of the gastro-intestinal tract was made using a barium bolus; this revealed a mass and ulcer crater in the pre-pyloric area of the stomach suggesting a gastric neoplasm.  A laparotomy[81] was planned.  The tentative diagnoses were anterior myocardial infarction, suspected cancer of the stomach, epilepsy, and hemorrhagic diathesis[82] (probably scurvy).  Accordingly, the patient was given a high protein diet and ascorbic acid (1 g/day for two weeks, then 150 mg/day for a month).

---

[77] toothless.

[78] necrotic changes resulting from obstruction of an end artery.

[79] Emphysema involves dilation of the pulmonary air vesicles, usually due to atrophy of the septa between the alveoli.

[80] Atheroma refers to the focal deposit or degenerative accumulation of soft, pasty, acellular, lipid-containing material frequently found in intimal and subintimal plaques in arteriosclerosis (also called atherosclerosis).

[81] a surgical procedure involving incision through the abdominal wall.

[82] any of several syndromes showing a tendency to spontaneous hemorrhage, resulting from weakness of the blood vessels and/or a clotting defect.

The patient showed marked improvement following ascorbic acid treatment. He no longer showed an air of lassitude; he gained weight and began to relish his meals. His skin hemorrhages rapidly decreased and no new ones appeared. Three weeks after admission, blood disappeared from his feces. At that time, his epilepsy was satisfactorily controlled using phenobarbital, his liver function tests and blood chemistry were normal.

Laboratory findings after ascorbic acid treatment:

| parameter | patient |
|---|---|
| blood urea | 28 mg/dl |
| serum protein | 6.3 g/dl |
| serum albumin | 3.9 g/dl |
| serum ascorbic acid | 1.0 mg/dl |

A second radiological examination, conducted one month after ascorbic acid treatment, indicated a normal pylorus; this was confirmed by gastroscopy. A biopsy of the previously involved area showed only a natural glandular pattern, with hemorrhage of the superficial layer of the gastric mucosa. The patient was discharged after 8 wks. of hospitalization and was well when seen later in the out-patient clinic. The gastric lesion did not recur. It was concluded that what had appeared to be a pre-pyloric tumor and ulcer had actually been a bleeding site with a hematoma[83].

Questions:   i.   What thresholds are suggested by the results of the first case study for total body ascorbic acid pool size and plasma ascorbic acid concentration associated with freedom from signs of scurvy?

ii.   Compute the rate of reduction in ascorbic acid body pool size from the observations on the subject of the first case. Was it linear throughout the study?

iii.   What signs/symptoms did the patient in the second case show that indicated a problem related to vitamin C status?

[83] a localized mass of extravasated blood, usually clotted.

## Study Questions and Exercises:

i.      Construct a **concept map** illustrating the relationship of the chemical properties and physiological functions of vitamin C.

ii.     Construct a **'decision tree'** for the diagnosis of vitamin C deficiency in humans.

iii.    What **health complications** might you expect to be shown by scorbutic individuals?

## Recommended Reading:

Block, G. 1991. Vitamin C and cancer prevention: the epidemiological evidence. Am. J. Clin. Nutr. 53:270S-282S.

Chalmers, T.C. 1975. Effects of Ascorbic Acid on the Common Cold: An Evaluation of the Evidence. Am. J. Med. 58:532-536.

England, S. and S. Seifter. 1986. The Biochemical Functions of Ascorbic Acid. Ann. Rev. Nutr. 6:365-406.

Flodin, N.W. 1988. Pharmacology of Micronutrients. Alan R. Liss, Inc., pp. 201-244.

Friedrich, W. 1988. Vitamins. Walter de Gruyter, New York, pp. 929-1001.

Levine, M. and K. Morita. 1985. Ascorbic acid in endocrine systems. Vit.Horm.42:1-64.

Moser, U. and A. Bendich. 1991. Vitamin C, Chapter 5 in Handbook of Vitamins, 2nd. ed. (L. Machlin, ed.), Marcel Dekker, New York, pp. 195-232.

Pauling, L. 1970. Vitamin C and the Common Cold. W.H. Freeman and Company, San Francisco, 122 pp.

Rivers, J.M. 1989. Safety of High-Level Vitamin C Ingestion in Elevated Dosages of Vitamins (P. Walter, H. Stähelin and G. Brubacher, eds.), Hans Huber Publications, Lewiston, N.Y. pp. 95-102.

Sauberlich, H.E. 1990. Ascorbic Acid, Chapter 15 in Present Knowledge in Nutrition, 6th edition (M. Brown, ed.), Int. Life Sci. Inst.-Nutr. Found., Washington, D.C., pp. 132-141.

# CHAPTER 10    THIAMIN

*"There is present in rice polishings a substance different from protein and salts, which is indispensable to health and the lack of which causes nutritional polyneuritis."*                    C. Eijkman and C. Grijns

## Anchoring Concepts:

*i.*     Thiamin is the trivial designation of a specific compound, 3-(4-amino-2-methylpyrimidin-5-methyl)-5-(2-hydroxyethyl)-4-methylthiazolium, which is sometimes also called vitamin $B_1$.

*ii.*    Thiamin is hydrophilic and its protonated form has a quaternary nitrogen center in the thiazole ring.

*iii.*   Deficiencies of thiamin are manifest chiefly as neuromuscular disorders.

## Learning Objectives:

*i.*     To understand the chief natural *sources* of thiamin.

*ii.*    To understand the means of *absorption* and *transport* of thiamin.

*iii.*   To understand the *biochemical function* of thiamin as a co-enzyme and the relationship of that function to the physiological activities of the vitamin.

*iv.*    To understand the physiologic implications of *low thiamin status*.

251

## Vocabulary:

acute pernicious beri-beri
alcohol
anorexia
ataxia
ATPase
beri-beri
bradycardia
cardiac beri-beri
cardiac hypertrophy
Chastak paralysis
cocarboxylase
confabulation
*"dry"* beri-beri
dyspnea
encephalopathy
hexose monophosphate shunt
$\alpha$-ketoglutarate dehydrogenase
nystagmus
ophthalmoplegia
opisthotonos
pentose phosphate pathway
perseveration
phosphorylase
polioencephalomalacia
polyneuritis

pyrimidine ring
pyrithiamin
pyruvate decarboxylase
pyruvate dehydrogenase
*"shoshin"* beri-beri
*"star-gazing"*
sulfites
tachycardia
TBP
thiamin disulfide
thiaminase
thiamin diphosphate
thiamin diphosphate phosphotransferase
thiamin monophosphate
thiamin monophosphatase
thiamin pyrophosphate
thiamin pyrophosphatase
thiamin pyrophosphokinase
thiazole ring
thiochrome
transketolase
vitamin $B_1$
Wernicke-Korsakoff syndrome
*"wet"* beri-beri

## SOURCES OF THIAMIN

*distribution*     In foods derived from plants, thiamin occurs predominantly as free thiamine.
*in foods*         In contrast, thiamin occurs in animal tissues almost entirely (95-98%) in
                   phosphorylated forms (thiamin mono-, di- and tri-phosphates) the predomi-
                   nant form (80-85%) being the co-enzyme *thiamin di-phosphate*[1].

Thiamin contents of foods:

| food | thiamin mg/100g | food | thiamin mg/100g |
|---|---|---|---|
| grains | | fruits | |
| cornmeal | .20 | apples | .04 |
| oatmeal | .55 | apricots | .03 |
| rice, brown | .29 | bananas | .05 |
| rice, white | .07 | grapes | .05 |
| rice, white, cooked | .02 | oranges | .10 |
| rye, whole-grain | .30 | pears | .02 |
| rye, degerminated | .19 | pineapples | .08 |
| wheat, whole-grain | .55 | | |
| wheat, white | .06 | meats | |
| | | beef | .08 |
| vegetables | | duck | .10 |
| asparagus | .18 | pork | 1.10 |
| beans, green | .07 | pork, cured ham | .74 |
| broccoli | .10 | veal | .18 |
| cabbage | .05 | trout | .09 |
| carrots | .06 | salmon | .17 |
| cauliflower | .11 | heart, veal | .60 |
| kale | .16 | liver, beef | .30 |
| peas, green | .32 | liver, pork | .43 |
| potatoes | .11 | | |
| tomatoes | .06 | dairy products and eggs | |
| | | cheese | .02-.06 |
| other | | milk | .04 |
| brewer's yeast | 15.6 | eggs | .12 |
| human milk | .01 | | |

Thiamin is widely distributed in foods, but most contain only low concentrations of the vitamin. The richest sources are yeasts (e.g., dried brewer's
and baker's yeasts) and liver (especially pork liver); however, cereal grains
comprise the most important dietary sources of the vitamin in most human
diets[2].  Whole grains are typically rich in thiamin; however, the vitamin is

---

[1] Thiamin diphosphate is also called **thiamin pyrophosphate (TPP)**.

[2] Sauberlich has estimated that, in the national food supply of the United States, thiamin was contributed
mostly by grains and grain products (41% of total thiamin intake), followed by meat products (27%), vegetables
(12%), dairy products (8%), legumes (5%), fruit (4%) and eggs (2%).

distributed unevenly in grain tissues[3], such that milling and refining yield products with very low thiamin contents.

*stability in foods*

Thiamin is susceptible to destruction by several factors including neutral and alkaline conditions, heat, oxidation and ionizing radiation. It is stable at low pH (pH<7), but decomposes when heated, particularly under non-acidic conditions[4]. Protein-bound thiamin, found in animal tissues, is more stable to such losses. Thiamin is stable during frozen storage; substantial losses occur during thawing, however, mainly due to removal *via* drip fluid.

Thiamin losses in food processing:

| procedure | food | loss, % |
|---|---|---|
| convection cooking | meats | 25-85 |
| baking | bread | 5-35 |
| heating with water | vegetables | 0-60 |
| pasteurization | milk | 9-20 |
| spray-drying | milk | ca. 10 |
| canning | milk | ca. 40 |
| room temp. storage | fruits, vegetables | 0-20 |

*thiamin antagonists*

Thiamin in foods can be destroyed by **sulfites** added in processing and by **thiamin-degrading enzymes (thiaminases)** and other **anti-thiamin compounds** that may occur naturally. Many cases of thiamin deficiency have been found to be related to the ingestion of food containing such thiamin antagonists[5]. Sulfites react with thiamin to cleave its methylene bridge between the pyrimidine and thiazole rings; the reaction is slow at high pH, but is rapid in neutral and acidic conditions. Thiamin-destroying enzymes occur in a variety of natural products. These are heat labile, but can be effective antagonists of the vitamin when consumed without heat treatment. Heat-stable thiamin antagonists occur in several plants (e.g., ferns, tea, betel nut). These include o- and p-hydroxy **polyphenols** (e.g., caffeic acid,

---

[3] The greatest concentrations of thiamin in grains are typically found in the scutellum (the thin layer between the germ and the endosperm) and the germ. The endosperm (the starchy interior) is quite low in the vitamin. Therefore, milling to degerminate grain which, because it removes the highly unsaturated oils associated with the germ, yields a product that will not rancidify and, thus, has a longer storage life, also yields a product of substantially reduced thiamin content.

[4] Therefore, the practice of adding sodium bicarbonate to peas or beans for retention of their color in cooking or canning results in large losses of thiamin.

[5] Perhaps the best known of these is the condition referred to as "Chastak paralysis", which was a neurological disorder in commercially raised foxes fed a diet containing raw carp. The syndrome, named for the fox producer, was found to be a manifestation of thiamine deficiency brought on by a thiaminase present in fish gut tissue. Cooking the fish prior to feeding them to Mr. Chastak's foxes did not produce the syndrome, apparently by heat-denaturing the intestinal thiaminase.

chlorogenic acid, tannic acid)[6], which react with thiamin to oxidize the thiazole ring to yield the non-absorbable form *thiamin disulfide*. In addition, some *flavonoids* (quercetin, rutin) have been reported to antagonize thiamin, and *hemin*[7] in animal tissues is thought to bind the vitamin.

Two types of *thiaminases* have been found:

| type | present in | mechanism |
|------|-----------|-----------|
| I | fresh fish, shellfish, ferns, some bacteria | displaces pyrimidine methylene group with a nitrogenous base or SH-compound, to eliminate the thiazole ring |
| II | certain bacteria | hydrolytic cleavage of methylene-thiazole-N bond to yield the pyrimidine and thiazole moieties |

# ABSORPTION OF THIAMIN

*two means of uptake*
Thiamin is absorbed by an *active, carrier-mediated* process at low concentrations in the intestinal lumen ($<2\ \mu M$); but, at higher concentrations (e.g., a 2.5 mg dose for a human), it is also absorbed by *passive diffusion*. The active transport mechanism is greatest in the proximal regions of the small intestine (jejunum and ileum); therefore, thiamin produced by the lower gut microflora is not utilized by non-coprophagous animals. The cells of the intestinal mucosa have a *thiamin pyrophosphokinase* activity, with a $K_m$ of the same order as that of the carrier-mediated absorption process; however, it is not clear whether that enzyme is linked to the active absorption of the vitamin[8]. While most of the thiamin present in the intestinal mucosa is in phosphorylated form, thiamin arriving on the serosal side of the intestine is largely in the free (non-phosphorylated) form. Therefore, the uptake of thiamin by the mucosal cell may be coupled in some way to its phosphorylation/dephosphorylation; evidence indicates that the serosal discharge of thiamin by those cells is dependent on a *$Na^+$-dependent ATPase* on that side of the cell[9]. Because adrenalectomized rats have been found to absorb thiamin poorly, it is thought that enteric absorption of the vitamin may also be subject to control by corticosteroid hormones.

---

[6]These and related compounds are found in blueberries, red currents, red beets, brussels sprouts, red cabbage, betel nuts, coffee and tea.

[7]ferriprotoporphyrin, the non-protein, $Fe^{+++}$-containing portion of hemoglobin

[8]Both processes follow Michaelis-Menton kinetics, with half-maximal rates at 0.1-0.4 $\mu M$ concentrations of thiamin. This finding led to the assumption that the two processes may be closely associated.

[9]The ingestion of alcohol can inhibit the enteric absorption of thiamin. That parenterally administered alcohol can also inhibit thiamin utilization suggests that the basis of the antagonism may be in the absorption process itself, probably at the level of the $Na^+$-dependent ATPase, which is known to be inhibited by alcohol.

## TRANSPORT OF THIAMIN

*bound both to*  Most of the thiamin in serum is bound to protein, chiefly albumin.  It
*albumin and*   appears, however, that thiamin is taken up by cells of the blood and other
*a specific*    tissues by both passive diffusion and active transport. Thus, ca. 90% of the
*carrier*       total thiamin in blood (typically, 5-12 $\mu g/dl$) is present in the cell fraction
                with erythrocyte thiamin comprising ca. 90% of that fraction[10].  A specific
                binding protein, ***thiamin-binding protein (TBP)***[11] has been identified in rat
                serum[12].  It is believed that TBP is a specific, hormonally regulated carrier
                protein that is essential for the distribution of thiamin to critical tissues.

*cellular uptake*  The uptake of thiamin by cells appears to proceed by the same processes
*both by carrier*  as the enteric absorption of the vitamin, that is, active transport at low con-
*and diffusion*    centrations and passive diffusion at higher concentrations.

*tissue*        In animal tissues, thiamin occurs predominately as its ***phosphate esters***
*distribution*  most of which is bound to proteins.  Plasma, milk and cerebrospinal fluid
                (and probably all extracellular fluids) contain only free (unesterified) thiamin
                and thiamin monophosphate (TMP), suggesting that the free and mono-
                phosphorylated forms of the vitamin can cross the cell membrane, but that
                TPP and TPPP cannot.  Tissue levels of thiamin vary within and between
                species with *no appreciable storage in any tissue*[13].  In general, the
                thiamin contents of human tissue tend to be less than those of analogous
                tissues in other species, while those of porcine tissues tend to be greater.

---

[10]Several children who died of SIDS (*"sudden infant death syndrome"*) have been found to have extraordin-
arily high plasma thiamin concentrations, e.g., five-fold those of infants who died of other diseases. The physiological basis of this effect is unknown, although thiamin deficiency is not thought to be a cause of death in SIDS.

[11]TBP has a molecular weight of ca. 38 kD. It binds one mole of free thiamin per mole and forms a 1:1
complex with the riboflavin-binding protein. Like the latter, TBP appears to be regulated by estrogens (i.e., it
is inducible in male or ovariectomized rats by parenterally administered estrogen).

[12]TBP has also been identified in rat liver and hen's eggs (in both the yolk and albumen).

[13]Thiamin concentrations are generally greatest in the heart (.28-.79 mg/100 g), kidneys (.24-.58 mg/100
g), liver (.20-.76 mg/100 g) and brain (.14-.44 mg/100 g), and are retained longest in the brain.

# METABOLISM OF THIAMIN

*role of phos-* | Thiamin is phosphorylated in the tissues to the di- and tri-phosphate esters
*phorylation* | by **thiamin phosphokinase** and **thiamin diphosphate phosphokinase**, respectively, each of which uses ATP as the phosphate donor. Each of these esters is catabolized by a **phosphorylase**, one of which (thiamin pyrophosphate phosphorylase)[14] yields the mono-phosphorylated product **thiamin monophosphate (TMP)**.

*urinary* | All thiamin in excess of that which binds in tissues is rapidly excreted[15]
*excretion* | in the urine, chiefly as **free thiamin** and **thiamin mono-phosphate**, but also in small amounts as the **diphosphate ester** and **other metabolites** (e.g., thiochrome, thiamin disulfide and some 20 other metabolites a half-dozen of which are of quantitative importance[16]) most of which retain the pyrimidine-thiazole ring-linkage. The latter metabolites account for increasing proportions of total thiamin excretion as thiamin status declines.

---

[14]TPP-phosphorylase is present mainly in the intestinal mucosa. It is also found in the brain where its discrete localization in the Golgi apparatus makes it useful as an enzyme marker for that subcellular organelle.

[15]The half-life of thiamin in humans has been estimated to be 9.5-18.5 days.

[16]These include:    2-methyl-4-amino-5-pyrimidine carboxylic acid
4-methylthiazole-5-acetic acid
2-methyl-4-amino-5-hydroxymethylpyrimidine
5-(2-hydroxyethyl)-4-methylthiazole
3-(2'-methyl-4-amino-5'-pyrimidinylmethyl-4-methylthiazole-5-acetic acid
2-methyl-4-amino-5-formylaminomethylpyrimidine

## METABOLIC FUNCTIONS OF THIAMIN

co-
carboxylase

The metabolically functional form of thiamin is its diphosphate ester, **thiamin pyrophosphate (TPP)**, which is also called *"cocarboxylase"*. Several enzymes use TPP as an essential cofactor for the cleavage of the C-C bond of $a$-ketoacids (e.g., pyruvate) to yield products subsequently transferred to an acceptor. In each case, TPP serves as a classical coenzyme, binding covalently to the holoenzyme. Each TPP-dependent enzyme also requires $Mg^{++}$ or some other divalent cation for activity.

The **general mechanism of the coenzyme action** of TPP involves its deprotonation to form a carbanion at C-2 of the thiazole ring, which reacts with the polarized 2-carbonyl group of the substrate (an $a$-ketoacid or $a$-ketosugar) to form a covalent bond. This bond formation results in the labilization of certain C-C bonds to release $CO_2$, with the remaining adduct reacting either by protonation to give an *"active aldehyde"* addition product (e.g., decarboxylases), by direct oxidation with suitable electron acceptors to yield a high-energy 2-acyl product, by reaction with oxidized lipoic acid to yield an acyldihydrolipoate product (e.g., oxidases or dehydrogenases) or by addition to an aldehyde carbonyl to yield a new ketol (e.g., transketolase). In higher animals, the decarboxylation is oxidative (producing a carboxylic acid); these involve the transfer of the aldehyde from TPP to lipoic acid (forming a 6-$S$-acylated dihydrolipoic acid and free TPP) from which it is transferred to coenzyme A[17].

Several effective *thiamin antagonists* are analogues of the vitamin that differ from it with respect to the chemical structure of the thiazole ring. Some involve substitutions on either the pyrimidine or thiazole rings[18]; loss of catalytic activity occurs with any change that disturb the peculiar environment of the thiazole ring system, which is required to make the C-2 reactive. Most have hydroxyethyl groupings, which allow them to compete for phosphorylation (*via* thiamin pyrophosphorylase) with the vitamin. In addition, a large group of synthetic thiamin-antagonists with anti-coccidial activity have a thiamin-like pyrimidine ring combined through a methylene

---

[17] Coenzyme A is the metabolically active form of the vitamin **pantothenic acid.**

[18]

thiamin          2-methylthiamin          oxythiamin          pyrithiamin bridge to a quaternary N of a pyridine ring[19,20]. These, not having an hydroxyethyl group, cannot be phosphorylated. They inhibit the carrier-mediated cellular uptake of thiamin.

*α-ketoacid dehydro-genases*

In animals, TPP functions in the oxidative decarboxylation of α-ketoacids by serving as an essential cofactor in multi-enzyme **α-ketoacid dehydro-genase complexes**. There are three classes of this type of TPP-dependent enzyme, each with a different optimal activity.

TPP-dependent α-ketoacid dehydrogenases:

| | |
|---|---|
| i. | **pyruvate dehydrogenase**, converting pyruvate to acetyl-CoA; |
| ii. | **α-ketoglutarate dehydrogenase**, converting α-ketoglutarate to succinyl CoA; |
| iii. | **branched-chain α-ketoacid dehydrogenase**, converting branched-chain α-keto-acids to the corresponding acyl-CoAs. |

Each of these complexes is composed of a **decarboxylase** (which binds TPP), a **core enzyme** (which binds lipoic acid), and a **flavoprotein dihydrolipoamide dehydrogenase** (which regenerates lipoamide). In addition, each contains one or more regulatory components[21].

*transketolase*

Thiamin functions in the form of TPP as an essential cofactor for **transketolase**[22] which catalyzes the cleavage of a C-C bond in α-keto-sugars (xylulose 5-phosphate, sedoheptulose 7-phosphate, fructose 6-

---

19

amprolium

[20] The amprolium-type thiamin antagonists are valuable in the protection of young poultry from coccidial infections. Their anti-coccidial activities are, in fact, due to their functions as thiamin antagonists. They resemble pyrithiamin in that they have a pyrimidine ring combined by a methylene bridge to a quaternary N of a pyridine ring; but, having no hydroxyethyl group, they are not substrates for thiamin pyrophosphokinase. Therefore, they do not inhibit the TPP-dependent enzymes. Instead, they inhibit the cellular uptake of thiamin. At low doses, this inhibition affects chiefly thiamin transport by enteric coccidia, but at higher doses it can affect the enteric absorption of the vitamin, producing clinical thiamin deficiency.

[21] In the case of pyruvate dehydrogenase, the regulatory components are a kinase and a phosphatase. These are active in regulating the activity of the enzyme complex by interconversion between the active non-phosphorylated and the inactive phosphorylated forms.

[22] Transketolase isolated from cultured fibroblasts from patients with Wernicke-Korsakoff syndrome was found to have an abnormally low binding affinity for TPP ($K_m = 195 \mu M$ vs. $K_m = 16 \mu M$ for control subjects). That this difference persisted after many passages in tissue culture indicates an hereditary defect in this enzyme in these patients.

phosphate, D-xylulose, D-fructose), transferring the resulting 2-C fragment[23] to an aldose[24] acceptor. Transketolase functions at two steps in the **hexose monophosphate shunt** for the oxidation of glucose[25]. Although the synthesis of the enzyme is not affected by thiamin status, its catalytic activity depends on its binding TPP. In subjects adequately nourished with respect to thiamin, that binding is at least 85% of saturation, while in thiamin-deficiency the percentage of transketolase bound to TPP is much less. This phenomenon is exploited in the clinical assessment of thiamin status; the increase, upon addition of exogenous TPP, in the activity of erythrocyte transketolase in vitro can be used to determine the percentage TPP-saturation of the enzyme and, hence, thiamin status[26].

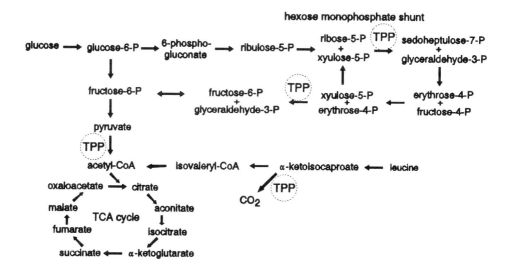

*other TPP-enzymes in microbes*

Several other TPP-dependent enzymes have been identified in micro-organisms. These include a pyruvate decarboxylase in yeast, and a pyruvate dehydrogenase in *E. coli*. Each is different in both size and molecular mechanism from the analogous enzyme mentioned above.

---

[23] the so-called *'active glycoaldehyde'*.

[24] a sugar aldehyde.

[25] This pathway, also called the *'pentose pathway'*, is an important alternate to the glycolysis-Krebs cycle pathway, especially for the production of pentoses for RNA and DNA synthesis and NADPH for the biosynthesis of fatty acids, etc.

[26] The percentage stimulation in erythrocyte transketolase activity by the addition of TPP is called the transketolase *'activity coefficient'*. Subjects with activity coefficients < 1.15 are considered to be at low risk to thiamin deficiency, while those with activity coefficients of 1.15-1.25 or > 1.25 are considered to be a moderate and high risk, respectively.

*nervous*
*function*

It is clear that thiamin has a vital role in nerve function, although the biochemical nature of that role is still unclear. That thiamin is required by nervous tissue is evidenced by the localization of signs of thiamin deprivation which are mainly neurologic. Further, thiamin has been identified in mammalian brain, in synaptosomal membranes and in cholinergic nerves. Studies have shown that brain thiamin concentrations tend to be resistant to change by dietary thiamin deprivation or parenteral thiamin administration, a finding suggesting homeostasis of the vitamin in that organ. Nervous stimulation by either electrical or chemical means has been found to result in the release of thiamin (as free thiamin and the mono-phosphate ester) that is associated with the dephosphorylation of its higher phosphate esters (thiamin di- and tri-phosphates). The antagonist *pyrithiamin*[27] can displace thiamin from nervous tissue and to change the electrical activity of the tissue. Irradiation with UV light at wavelengths absorbed by thiamin destroys the electrical potential of nerve fibers in a manner corrected by thiamin treatment, suggesting a direct function of thiamin in nervous tissue.

Because the oxidative decarboxylation of pyruvate and $\alpha$-ketoglutarate are essential steps in energy production *via* the Krebs cycle, which plays an important role in the energy metabolism of the brain, it has been suggested that the neurological signs of thiamin deficiency may be due to failure of this system by the absence of sufficient amounts of its essential cofactor, TPP. However, several experiments have indicated that the depressions of pyruvate and $\alpha$-ketoglutarate dehydrogenase activities that occur in thiamin-deficient animals are not of sufficient magnitude to produce the neurological dysfunction associated with the deficiency. Nevertheless, it has also been found that the metabolic flux though the alternative pathway, the so-called "$\gamma$-aminobutyric acid (GABA) shunt" is considerably increased in the brains of thiamin-deficient individuals, suggesting that, in addition to its role in the synthesis of that neurotransmitter (GABA), it may also serve to yield energy under conditions of thiamin-deprivation. Transketolase has also been found to be highly responsive to thiamin-deprivation; however, it is not clear whether the pentose phosphate pathway is important in brain metabolism. It has also been suggested that thiamin may be involved in the synthesis of myelin, but the fact that the turnover of myelin is much slower (its half-time is 4-5 days) than the response of thiamin therapy (full recovery within 24 hrs.) does not appear to support that possibility.

Therefore, it has been proposed that thiamin has another function, that is, a non-metabolic role related to nerve transmission. Currently, two hypothesis for such a role have been presented: that thiamin has a catalytic activity in the mechanism of $Na^+$ permeability; that thiamin, probably as TPP, is involved in maintaining the fixed negative charge on the inner surface of the membrane.

---

[27]Pyrithiamin is an analog of thiamin that consists of a pyridine moiety replacing the thiazole ring.

## EXTREMES IN THIAMIN INTAKE

*deficiency*       Thiamin deficiency in humans and animals is characterized by three general types of signs/symptoms: *anorexia*[28] and attendant weight loss, *cardiac involvement* and *neurologic involvement*. Thiamin-deficient subjects typically show increased plasma concentrations of *pyruvate*, *lactate* and to a lesser extent *α-ketoglutarate* (especially after a glucose meal), as well as decreased activities of erythrocyte *transketolase*.

*animals:*        Thiamin-deficiency in animals leads to the triad of signs indicated above.
*polyneuritis*    The most remarkable sign in most species is *anorexia*, which is so severe and more specific than any associated with other nutrient deficiencies (apart from that of sodium) that it is a useful diagnostic indicator for thiamin deficiency. Other signs of thiamin deficiency are secondary effects of reduced total feed intake: *weight loss*, *impaired efficiency of feed utilization*, *weakness*, *hypothermia*. The appearance of anorexia correlates with the loss of transketolase activity and precedes changes in pyruvate or α-ketoglutarate dehydrogenase activities.

Animals also show *neurologic dysfunction* due to thiamin deficiency, especially birds, which show a tetanic retraction of the head called *opisthotonos* and "*star-gazing*"[29]. Other species generally show *ataxia* and *incoordination* which progresses to *convulsions* and *death*. These conditions are generally referred to as *polyneuritis*.

Most species, but especially dogs and pigs, show *cardiac hypertrophy*[30] in thiamin deficiency, with slowing of the heart rate[31] and signs of congestive heart failure including *labored breathing* and *edema*. Some species also show *diarrhea* and *achlorhydria* (rodents), *gastro-intestinal hemorrhage* (pigs), *infertility* (chickens[32]), high *neonatal mortality* (pigs), and *impaired learning* (cats).

The rumen microflora are important sources of thiamin for ruminant species. Nevertheless, thiamin-deficiency can occur in ruminants if their microbial yield of the vitamin is impaired. Such cases have occurred due

---

[28] loss of appetite.

[29] This sign occurs in young mammals, but it is not usual.

[30] enlargement

[31] bradycardia

[32] Thiamin deficiency impairs the fertility of both roosters (via testicular degeneration) and hens (via impaired oviductal atrophy).

either to depressed thiamin synthesis (e.g., due to a change in diet which disturbs rumen fermentation), to enhanced thiamin degradation (e.g., due to an alteration in the microbial population which increases total thiaminase activity[33]), or to the consumption of thiamin-antagonists (e.g., due to feeding on bracken fern or the use of excess amprolium).   The clinical manifestation of thiamin deficiency in young ruminants is the neurologic syndrome called *polioencephalomalacia*[34], a potentially fatal condition involving inflammation of brain gray matter and presenting as *opisthotonus*; it readily responds to thiamin treatment[35].

*humans:*
*beri-beri*

The classical syndrome resulting from thiamin deficiency in humans is *beri-beri*.  This disease is prevalent in southeast Asia, where polished rice is the dietary staple.  The general symptoms of beri-beri are *anorexia*, *cardiac enlargement*, *lassitude*, *muscular weakness* (with resulting *ataxia*), *paresthesia*[36], *loss of knee and ankle jerk responses* (with subsequent *foot and wrist droop*), and *dyspnea on exertion*.

Beri-beri occurs in three clincial types:

| | |
|---|---|
| *i.* | *"dry"* or *neuritic* beri-beri |
| *ii.* | *"wet"* or *edematous* beri-beri |
| *iii.* | *infantile* or *acute* beri-beri |

*Dry beri-beri* occurs primarily in adults; it is characterized by atrophy of the legs with accompanying peripheral neuritis.  It usually does not have cardiac involvement.  *Wet beri-beri* involves, as its prominent sign, cardiac hypertrophy[37] and edema; in severe cases, heart failure is the outcome[38].  The onset of this form of beri-beri can vary from chronic to

---

[33]Increased ruminal degradation of thiamin is usually associated with the presence of certain microbial species, including *Bacteroides thiaminolyticus*, *Clostridium sporogenes*, *Megasphaera elsdenii* and *Streptococcus bovis*.  Of these, *B. thiaminolyticus* appears to be of greatest pathogenic importance, as appears to occur routinely in the ruminal contents and feces of all cases of polioencephalomalacia.

[34]cerebrocortical necrosis

[35]Polioencephalomalacia is thought to be a disease of thiamin deficiency that is induced by thiaminases such as those synthesized by rumen bacteria or present in certain plants.  Affected animals are listless and have uncoordinated movements; they develop progressive blindness and convulsions.  The disease is ultimately fatal, but responds dramatically to thiamin.

[36]an abnormal spontaneous sensation, such as burning, pricking, numbness, etc.

[37]In contrast to thiamin-deficient animals, which show *bradycardia* (slow heart beat), beri-beri patients show *tachycardia* (rapid heart rate, >100 beats/min).

[38]Wet beri-beri is also called *"cardiac beri-beri"*.

acute, in which case it is called *"shoshin beri-beri"*[39] and is characterized by greatly elevated lactic acid concentrations in the blood. *Infantile beri-beri* occurs in breast-fed infants of thiamin-deficient mothers, most frequently at 2-6 mos. of age. It has a rapid onset, with death due to heart failure, usually within a few hours. Affected infants are anorexic and milk is regurgitated; they may have vomiting, diarrhea, cyanosis, tachycardia and convulsions. Their mothers may show no signs of thiamin deficiency.

*Wernicke-Korsakoff syndrome*

Due to the fortification of rice with thiamin, frank thiamin deficiency is rare in industrialized countries but continues to be prevalent in countries without such fortification programs. Nevertheless, *subclinical thiamin insufficiency* appears to occur in industrialized countries. When such conditions are associated with excessive alcohol consumption[40], they produce an encephalopathy called the *Wernicke-Korsakoff syndrome*[41]. The signs of this syndrome range from mild confusion to coma; they include *ophthalmoplegia*[42] with lateral or vertical *nystagmus*[43], cerebellar *ataxia*, *psychosis*, *confabulation*[44] and severely *impaired retentive memory and cognitive function*. Patients with the syndrome have been found to have a high incidence of an apparently inherited abnormal transketolase which has an abnormally low binding affinity for TPP. In most cases, it appears that this low affinity can be overcome by using high intramuscular doses of thiamin, to which most affected patients respond. Some patients fail to respond to such treatment; it has been suggested that they may have another aberrant transketolase (or other TPP-dependent enzyme) that cannot bind TPP at all.

---

[39] Shoshin beri-beri is also called *"acute pernicious beri-beri"*.

[40] Excessive alcohol intake appears to be antagonistic to adequate thiamin status in three ways. First, the diets of alcoholics are frequently low in thiamin, a large percentage of the daily energy intake being displaced by nutrient-deficient alcoholic beverages. Second, the metabolic demands for TPP and, thus, for thiamin, are increased by the consumption of a diet rich in carbohydrates (i.e., alcohol) as a primary source of energy. Third, alcohol can inhibit the intestinal ATPase involved in the enteric absorption (and, probably, the cellular uptake) of thiamin.

[41] This is also called **Wernicke's encephalopathy**.

[42] paralysis of one or more of the motor nerves of the eye.

[43] rhythmical oscillation of the eyeballs, either horizontally, rotary or vertically.

[44] readiness to answer any question fluently with no regard whatever to facts.

Signs of thiamin deficiency:

| organ system | signs |
|---|---|
| general | |
| appetite | severe decrease |
| growth | decrease |
| dermatologic | edema |
| muscular | cardiomyopathy, bradycardia, heart failure |
| | weakness |
| gastro-intestinal | inflammation, ulcer |
| vital organs | hepatic steatosis |
| nervous | peripheral neuropathy |
| | opisthotonos |

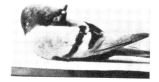

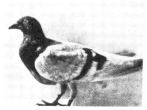

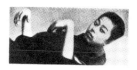

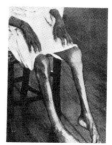

Opisthotonus in a thiamin-deficient pigeon before (t.); and after thiamin treatment (b.); courtesy Cambridge Univ. Press.

Neurologic signs of beri-beri; courtesy Cambridge Univ. Press.

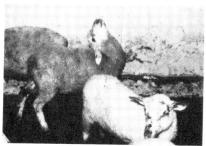

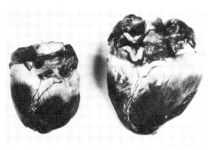

Opisthotonus in a thiamin-deficient sheep; courtesy M. Hidiroglou, Agricultural Canada, Ottawa, Ontario, Canada.

Hearts from normal (l.) and thiamin-deficient (r.) pigs; courtesy T. Cunha.

*hyper-*
*vitaminosis*    Little information is available concerning the toxic potential of thiamin for livestock or humans. Most of the published information pertains to the toxicity of the vitamin administered in the form of thiamin hydrochloride. From those studies it is clear that at least that form can be fatal, apparently by suppressing the respiratory center, at levels approximately 1000-fold those required to prevent signs of thiamin deficiency. Such doses of the vitamin to animals produce curare[45]-like signs, suggestive of blocked nerve transmission: restlessness, epileptiform convulsions, cyanosis and dyspnea. In humans, parenteral doses of thiamin at 100-fold the recommended intake have been found to produce headache, convulsions, weakness, paralysis, cardiac arrythmia and allergic reactions.

# CASE STUDY

*Instructions:*    *Review each of the following case reports, paying special attention to the diagnostic indicators upon which the treatments were based. Then answer the questions that follow.*

*case 1*    A 35-year-old man with a history of high alcohol intake for 18 yrs. was admitted to the hospital complaining of massive swelling and shortness of breath on exertion. For several months, he had subsisted almost entirely on beer and whiskey, taking no solid food. He was grossly edematous, slightly jaundiced and showed transient cyanosis[46] of the lips and nail beds. His heart showed gallop rhythm[47]. His left pleural cavity contained fluid. His liver was enlarged with notable ascites[48]. He had a course tremor of the hands and reduced tendon reflexes. His electrocardiogram showed sinus tachycardia[49]. His radiogram showed pulmonary edema and cardiac enlargement. He was evaluated by cardiac catheterization.

---

[45] Curare is an extract of various plants (e.g., *Strychnos toxifera, S. castelraei, S. crevauxii, Chondodendron tomentosum*). Practically inert when administered orally, when administered intravenously or intramuscularly it is a powerful muscle relaxant which exerts its effect by blocking nerve impulses at the myoneural junction. Curare is used experimentally and clinically to produce muscular relaxation during surgery. Originally it was used as an arrow poison by indigenous hunters of South America to kill prey by inducing paralysis of the respiratory muscles.

[46] Dark bluish discoloration of the skin due to deficient oxygenation of the blood in the lungs or abnormally reduced flow of blood through the capillaries.

[47] triple cadence to the heart sounds at rates of $\geq 100$ beats/min, indicative of serious myocardial disease

[48] accumulation of serous fluid

[49] rapid beating of the heart ($\geq 100$ beats/min) originating in the sinus node

Results:

| parameter | patient | normal value |
|---|---|---|
| systemic arterial pressure, mm Hg | 100/55 | 120/80 |
| systemic venous pressure, cm $H_2O$ | 300 | <140 |
| pulmonary artery pressure, mm Hg | 64/36 | <30/<13 |
| right ventricular pressure, mm Hg | 65/17 | <30/<5 |
| $O_2$ consumption, ml/min | 259 | |
| peripheral blood $O_2$, ml/l | 148 | 170-210 |
| pulmonary arterial blood $O_2$, ml/l | 126 | 100-160 |
| cardiac output, l/min | 11.8 | 5-7 |
| blood hemoglobin, g/dl | 11.0 | 14-19 |
| cyanide circulation time, sec. | 12 | 20 |
| femoral arterial pyruvate, mg/dl | 1.5 | 0.8 |
| femoral arterial lactate, mg/dl | 14.1 | 4.7 |
| femoral arterial glucose, mg/dl | 86 | 74 |

The patient was given thiamin intravenously (10 mg every 6 hrs.) for several days. Improvement was evident by 48 hours and continued for two weeks. Thirty days later, he was free of edema, dyspnea and cardio-megaly. Cardiac catheterization at that time showed that his blood, systemic venous and all intracardiac pressures, as well as cardiac output had all returned to normal.

case 2    Fibroblasts were cultured from skin biopsies from four patients with *Wernicke-Korsakoff* syndrome and from four healthy control subjects. The properties of *transketolase* were studied. The first patient was a 50-year-old woman with a history of chronic alcoholism. She had been admitted to the hospital with *disorientation, nystagmus, sixth-nerve weakness*[50], *ataxia* and *malnutrition*. Treatment with intravenous thiamin and large oral doses of multi-vitamins had improved her neurologic signs over a few months, but her mental state had deteriorated. She was read-mitted with *disorientation* in both place and time, *impaired short-term memory, nystagmus, ataxia* and signs of *peripheral neuropathy*. She was treated with parenteral thiamin and enteral B-vitamins with thiamin; this had improved her general health but had not affected her mental status. The second patient, a 48-year-old man with a 20-year history of *chronic alcoholism*, was admitted in a severe confusional state. He was *disori-ented*, had severe *impairment of recent memory, confabulation, persev-eration*[51], *delusions, nystagmus* and *ataxia*. Treatment with thiamin and B-vitamins had improved his behavior, without affecting his memory.

---

[50] the 6th cranial nerve, *nervus abducens*, the small motor nerve to the lateral rectus muscle of the eye.

[51] the constant repetition of a meaningless word or phrase.

Characteristics of transketolase from Wernicke-Korsakoff patients:

| parameter | patients | controls |
|---|---|---|
| $V_{max}$, nmoles/min/mg protein | $27 \pm 3$ | $17 \pm 1$ |
| $K_m$, $\mu M$ TPP | $195 \pm 31$ | $16 \pm 2$ |

These results show that the affinity of transketolase for its co-enzyme (TPP) in Wernicke-Korsakoff patients was less, by an order of magnitude, than that of controls. Further, this biochemical abnormality persisted in fibroblasts cultured for >20 generations in media containing excess thiamin and no ethanol. The characteristics of pyruvate and $\alpha$-ketoglutarate dehydrogenases were similar in fibroblasts from patients and controls.

Questions:     i.       What factors would appear to have contributed to the thiamin deficiencies of these patients?

               ii.      What defect in cardiac energy metabolism would appear to be the basis of the high-output cardiac failure observed in the first case?

               iii.     What evidence suggests that the transketolase abnormality of these patients was hereditary?   Would you expect such patients to be more or less susceptible to thiamin deprivation?  Explain.

## Study Questions and Exercises:

i.  Construct a schematic map of *intermediary metabolism* showing the enzymatic steps in which TPP is known to function as a co-enzyme.

ii.  Construct a *'decision tree'* for the diagnosis of thiamin deficiency in humans or animals.

iii.  How does the *chemical structure* of thiamin relate to its *biochemical function*?

iv.  What parameters might you measure to assess the *thiamin status* of a human or animal?

v.  Construct a *concept map* illustrating the possible interrelationships of excessive alcohol intake and thiamin status.

## Recommended Reading:

Brown, M. 1990. Thiamin, Chapter 16 *in* Present Knowledge in Nutrition, 6th ed. (M. Brown, ed.), Int. Life Sci. Inst.-Nutr. Found., Washington, D.C., pp. 142-145.

Flodin, N.W. 1988. Pharmacology of Micronutrients. Alan R. Liss, Inc., New York, pp. 103-116.

Friedrich, W. 1988. Vitamins. Walter de Gruyter, New York. pp. 339-401.

Gubler, C.J. 1991. Thiamin, Chapter 6 *in* Handbook of Vitamins, 2nd ed. (L.J. Machlin, ed.), Marcel Dekker, New York. pp. 233-281.

Harmeyer, J., and U. Kollenkirchen. 1989. Thiamin and Niacin in Ruminant Nutrition. Nutr. Res. Rev. 2:201-225.

Sable, H.Z. and C.J. Gubler (eds.) 1982. Thiamin: Twenty Years of Progress. Ann. N.Y. Acad. Sci. vol. 378, 470 pp.

# CHAPTER 11  *RIBOFLAVIN*

*"In retrospect – the discovery of riboflavin may be considered a scientific windfall. It opened the way to the unraveling of the truly complex vitamin B$_2$-complex. Perhaps even more significantly, it bridged the gap between an essential constituent and cell enzymes and cellular metabolism. Today, with the general acceptance of this idea, it is not considered surprising that water-soluble vitamins represent essential parts of enzyme systems."*

P. György

## Anchoring Concepts:

*i.*      Riboflavin is the trivial designation of a specific compound, 7,8-dimethyl-10-(1'-D-ribityl)-isoalloxazine, sometimes also called vitamin B$_2$.

*ii.*      Riboflavin is a yellow, hydrophilic, tri-cyclic molecule that is usually phosphorylated (to FMN and FAD) in biological systems.

*iii.*      Deficiencies of riboflavin are manifest chiefly as dermal and neural disorders.

## Learning Objectives:

*i.*      To understand the chief natural *sources* of riboflavin.

*ii.*      To understand the means of enteric *absorption* and *transport* of riboflavin.

*iii.*      To understand the *biochemical function* of riboflavin as a component of key redox co-enzymes, and the relationship of that function to the physiological activities of the vitamin.

*iv.*      To understand the physiologic implications of *low riboflavin status*.

## Vocabulary:

acyl-CoA dehydrogenase
adrenodoxin reductase
alkaline phosphatase
amino acid oxidases
cheilosis
curled-toe paralysis
dehydrogenase
erythrocyte glutathione reductase
ETF
FAD
FAD-phyrophosphorylase
FAD-synthetase
flavin
flavokinase
flavoprotein
FMN
FMN-phosphatase
geographic tongue
glossitis
L-gulonolactone oxidase

hypoplastic anemia
leukopenia
lumichrome
monoamine oxidase
NADH-cytochrome $P_{450}$ reductase
NADH dehydrogenase
normocytic anemia
ovoflavin
oxidase
reticulocytopenia
RfBPs
riboflavin-5'-phosphate
riboflavinuria
stomatitis
subclinical deficiency
succinate dehydrogenase
thrombocytopenia
thyroxine
ubiquinone reductase
vitamin $B_2$

# *SOURCES OF RIBOFLAVIN*

*distribution in foods*

Riboflavin is widely distributed in foods, where it is present almost exclusively bound to proteins mainly in the form of *flavin mononucleotide (FMN)* and *flavin adenine dinucleotide (FAD)*[1,2]. Rapidly growing, green, leafy vegetables are rich in the vitamin; however, meats and dairy products are the most important contributors of riboflavin to American diets, with milk products providing about one-half of the total intake of the vitamin[3].

Riboflavin contents of foods:

| food | riboflavin mg/100g | food | riboflavin mg/100g |
|---|---|---|---|
| dairy products | | vegetables | |
| milk | .17 | asparagus | .18 |
| yogurt | .16 | broccoli | .20 |
| cheese, American | .43 | cabbage | .06 |
| cheese, cheddar | .46 | carrots | .06 |
| cheese, cottage | .28 | cauliflower | .08 |
| ice cream | .21 | corn | .06 |
| | | lima beans | .10 |
| meats | | potatoes | .04 |
| liver, beef | 3.50 | spinach | .14 |
| beef | .24 | tomatoes | .04 |
| chicken | .19 | | |
| lamb | .22 | fruits | |
| pork | .27 | apples | .01 |
| ham, cured | .19 | bananas | .04 |
| | | oranges | .03 |
| cereals | | peaches | .04 |
| wheat, whole grain | .11 | strawberries | .07 |
| rye | .08 | | |
| oat meal | .02 | other | |
| rice | .01 | eggs | .30 |

*stability*

Riboflavin is stable to heat; therefore, most means of heat-sterilization, canning and cooking do not affect the riboflavin contents of foods. Exposure to light (e.g., sun-drying, sunlight exposure of milk in glass bottles, cooking in a open pot) can result in substantial losses, as the

---

[1] Notable exceptions are milk and eggs which contain appreciable amount of free riboflavin.

[2] It should be noted that, strictly speaking, FMN is not a nucleotide nor is FAD a dinucleotide because each is a D-ribityl derivative; nevertheless, these names have been accepted.

[3] It is estimated that milk and milk products contribute ca. 50% of the riboflavin in the American diet, with meats, eggs and legumes contributing a total of ca. 25%, and fruits and vegetables each contributing ca. 10%.

vitamin is, however, very sensitive to destruction by light[4]. Also, because riboflavin is water-soluble, it leaches into water used in cooking and the drippings of meats. As riboflavin in cereal grains is located primarily in the germ and bran, the milling of such materials[5], which removes those tissues, results in considerable losses in their contents of the vitamin.

*bio-*
*availability*      In general, riboflavin from animal products is absorbed with greater efficiency than that from plant-derived foods, that is, riboflavin in animal products tends to have a greater bioavailability than that in plant products. This appears to be due to the presence of flavin complexes in plants are more stable to digestion (less digestible) than those of animal tissues.


## *ABSORPTION OF RIBOFLAVIN*


*active transport*  Riboflavin is absorbed in the free form by means of a specific, saturable,
*of free*          *active transport* system located in the proximal small intestine. Absorption
*riboflavin*       is enhanced by bile salts[6].

*hydrolysis of*    Because riboflavin occurs in most foods as protein complexes of the co-
*coenzyme*         enzyme forms FMN and FAD, the utilization of the vitamin in foods depends
*forms*            upon their hydrolytic conversion to free riboflavin. This occurs by the proteolytic activity of the intestinal lumen, which releases the riboflavin coenzymes from their protein complexes, and the subsequent hydrolytic activities of several brush border phosphatases that liberate riboflavin in free form. These include the relatively non-specific *alkaline phosphatase*[7], as well as *FAD-pyrophosphatase* (which converts FAD to FMN) and *FMN-phosphatase* (which converts FMN to free riboflavin).

---

[4]Irradiation of food results in the production of reactive free radical species of oxygen (e.g., superoxide radical anion, hydroxyl radical) that react with riboflavin to destroy it. Thus, exposure of milk in glass bottles to sunlight can result in the destruction of more than one-half of its riboflavin within a day. The short exposure of meat to sterilizing quantities of γ-radiation destroys 10-15% of its riboflavin content.

[5]About half of the riboflavin in whole-grain rice, and more than a third of that of whole wheat, is lost when these grains are milled. Thus, it is the practice in many countries to enrich refined wheat products with several vitamins including riboflavin, which results in their actually containing *more* riboflavin than the parent grains (e.g., 0.20 mg/100g *vs.* 0.11 mg/100g). However, rice is usually *not* enriched with riboflavin to avoid coloring the product yellow by this intensely colored vitamin. Parboiled ('*converted*') rice, contains most of the riboflavin of the parent grain, as the steam-processing of whole brown rice before milling this product drives vitamins originally present in the germ and aleurone layers into the endosperm where they are retained.

[6]Children with biliary atresia (a congenital condition involving the absence or pathological closure of the bile duct) show reduced riboflavin absorption.

[7]Alkaline phosphatase appears to have the greatest hydrolytic capacity of the brush border phosphatases.

*absorption*
*linked to phos-*
*phorylation*

Although it is the free form of riboflavin that is transported into the intestinal mucosal cell, much of that form is quickly trapped at that site by phosphorylation to FMN. This is accomplished by *flavokinase*, using ATP. Thus, riboflavin enters the portal circulation as both the free vitamin and FMN.

## TRANSPORT OF RIBOFLAVIN

*protein-binding*

Riboflavin is transported in the plasma as both free riboflavin and FMN, both of which are bound in appreciable amounts (e.g., about half of the free riboflavin and 80% of FMN) to plasma proteins. These include the *globulins* and *fibrinogen*; but the most important protein in this regard is *albumin*. These proteins bind riboflavin and FMN weakly by hydrogen bonding; the vitamin can be displaced readily by boric acid[8] or several drugs[9] which, thus, inhibit transport of the vitamin to peripheral tissues.

*specific*
*binding*
*proteins*

In addition, specific *riboflavin-binding proteins* (*RfBPs*) have been identified in plasma of the laying hen, the pregnant cow and pregnant mice and rats. The plasma RfBP of the hen has been well characterized; it is synthesized in the liver, apparently under the stimulus of estrogen, as it is not found in the immature female but can be induced by treatment with estrogens. It is a 32 kD phosphogylcoprotein with a single binding site for riboflavin. It appears to be one of three products of a single gene which are variously modified post-translationally to yield the RfBPs in egg white and yolk. The hen plasma RfBP is antigenically similar to the serum RfBPs of pregnant mice and rats. Each protein is believed to function in the transplacental/transovarian movement of riboflavin.

*tissue*
*distribution*

Riboflavin is transported into cells in its free form. However, in the tissues, riboflavin is converted to the coenzyme form, predominantly as *FMN* (60-95% of total flavins) but also as *FAD* (5-22% of total flavins in most tissues but ca. 37% in kidney), both of which are found almost exclusively bound to specific *flavoproteins*. The greatest concentrations of the vitamin are found in the liver, kidney and heart. In most tissues, free riboflavin comprises <2% of the total flavins. Significant amounts of free riboflavin

---

[8]In fact, the feeding of boric acid to humans and rats has been shown to produce riboflavinuria and precipitate riboflavin deficiency. In addition, some effects of boric acid toxicity can be overcome by feeding riboflavin.

[9]e.g., ouabain, theophylline, penicillin

are found only in the retina, the urine and cow's milk[10], where it is loosely bound to casein. Although the riboflavin content of the brain is not great, the turnover of the vitamin in that tissue is high and the concentration of the vitamin is relatively resistant to gross changes in riboflavin nutriture. These findings suggest a homeostasis mechanism for regulating the ribo-flavin content of the brain; such a mechanism has been proposed for the *plexus chorioidei*[11] in which riboflavin transport has been found to be inhibited by several of its catabolic products and analogues. It has been estimated that the total body reserve of riboflavin in the adult human is equivalent to the metabolic demands for 2-6 weeks.

Tissue RfBPs have been identified in the liver, egg albumen[12] and egg yolk of the laying hen. Each is similar to the plasma RfBP[13] in that species, differing only in the nature of their carbohydrate[14] contents[15]. An hereditary abnormality in the chicken results in the production of defective RfBPs (in plasma as well as liver and egg). Affected hens show *riboflavinuria* and produce eggs with about half the normal amount of riboflavin and embryos that fail to develop[16].

---

[10] It should be noted that cow's milk differs from human milk in both the amount and form of riboflavin. Cow's milk typically contains 1160-2020 $\mu$g riboflavin per liter, which (like the milk of most other mammals studied) is present mostly as the free vitamin. In contrast, human milk typically contains 120-485 $\mu$g riboflavin per liter (depending on the riboflavin intakes of the mother), which is present mainly as FAD and FMN.

[11] the anatomical site of the blood-cerebral spinal fluid barrier

[12] This is the flavoprotein formerly called *'ovoflavin'*. Comprising nearly 1% of the total protein in egg white, it is the most abundant of any vitamin-binding protein. Unlike the plasma RfBP which is normally saturated with its ligand, the egg white RfBP is normally less than half-saturated with riboflavin, even when hens are fed diets high in the vitamin. Still, its bound riboflavin is responsible for the faint yellow tinge of egg albumen.

[13] It appears that the plasma RfBP, produced and secreted by the liver in response to estrogens, is the precursor to these other binding proteins found in tissues.

[14] primarily in their contents of sialic acid

[15] It is interesting to note that egg white RfBP forms a 1:1 complex with the thiamin-binding protein (TBP) from the same source.

[16] Embryos from hens that are homozygous recessive for the mutant *rd* allele die of riboflavin deficiency at about the 13th day of incubation. They can be rescued by injecting riboflavin or FMN into the eggs.

## METABOLISM OF RIBOFLAVIN

*conversion to*    After it is taken up by the cell, free riboflavin is converted to its coenzyme
*coenzyme*    forms. The first step in this process is an ATP-dependent phosphorylation
*forms*    to yield ***riboflavin-5′-phosphate***, also called ***flavin mononucleotide***
***(FMN)***. This occurs in the cytoplasm of most cells and is catalyzed by the
enzyme ***flavokinase***[17]. Most of the FMN is then converted to the other
coenzyme ***flavin adenine dinucleotide (FAD)*** by ***FAD-pyrophosphory-***
***lase***[18]. Both steps appear to be regulated by thyroid hormones.

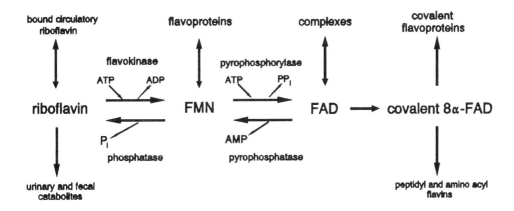

In tissues, most riboflavin occurs as non-covalently linked FAD in functional
***flavoproteins***. This includes associations *via* H-bonding with purines[19],
phenols and indoles (e.g., to peptidyl tryptophan in RfBPs). In addition,
some essential enzymes contain FAD attached covalently. Linkages of this
type involve the riboflavin 8-methyl group, which can form a methylene
bridge to the peptide histidyl imidazole function (e.g., in succinic
dehydrogenase and sarcosine oxidase), or to the thioether function of a
former cysteinyl residue (e.g., in monoamine oxidase)[20].

---

[17]Also called ***riboflavin kinase***, the activity of this enzyme is regulated by ***thyroxine***, which stimulates its synthesis. Therefore, hypothyroidism is associated with reduced flavokinase activity and, accordingly, reduced tissue levels of FMN and FAD. Hyperthyroidism, in contrast, results in increased flavokinase activity, although tissue levels of FMN and FAD, which appear to be regulated *via* degradation, do not rise.

[18]Also called ***FAD synthetase***, the activity of this enzyme, too, appears to be increased by ***thyroxine***.

[19]In FAD, the riboflavin and adenine moieties are predominantly (85%) hydrogen-bonded in an intramolecular complex.

[20]Another type of linkage involving the 8-methyl group, i.e., a thiohemiacetal linkage, is found in a microbial FAD-containing cytochrome.

*catabolism of*    Flavins that are bound to proteins are resistant to degradation; however,
*FAD and FMN*    when those proteins are saturated with flavins, the unbound forms are
subject to catabolism. Both FAD and FMN are catabolized by intracellular
enzymes in ways directly analogous to the breakdown of these forms in
foods during their absorption across the intestinal mucosal cell. Thus, FAD
is converted to FMN by ***FAD-pyrophosphatase*** (releasing AMP), and FMN
is degraded to free riboflavin by ***FMN-phosphatases***. Both FAD and FMN
are split to yield free riboflavin by ***alkaline phosphatase***.

*catabolism of*    The degradation of riboflavin *per se* involves initially its hydroxylation at the
*riboflavin*    7*a*- and 8*a*-positions of the isoalloxazine ring by hepatic microsomal cytochrome $P_{450}$-dependent processes. It is thought that catabolism proceeds
by the oxidation and then removal of the methyl groups. The liver, in at
least some species, has the ability to form riboflavin *a*-glycosides.

*excretion*    Riboflavin is rapidly excreted primarily in the urine[21,22] where it is present
primarily as free riboflavin[23]. Much smaller amounts, as 7*a*- and 8*a*-
hydroxyriboflavin, riboflavinyl-*a*-D-glucoside, lumichrome[24] and 10-formyl-
methylflavin are also found. Small amounts of riboflavin degradation
products are found in the feces (<5% of an oral dose); as only ca. 1% of
an oral dose of the vitamin is excreted in the bile by humans, most fecal
metabolites are thought to be mostly of gut microbial origin. Little, if any,
riboflavin is oxidized to $CO_2$[25]. Because riboflavin is rapidly excreted,
dietary needs are determined by excretion, not metabolism, of the vitamin.

---

[21]Studies in the rat show riboflavin to be turned over with a half-life of ca. 16 days in adequately nourished animals and much longer in riboflavin-deficient animals.

[22]In a riboflavin-adequate human adult, nearly all of a large oral dose of the vitamin will be excreted, the urine showing a peak within ca. 2 hrs.

[23]In normal human adults, the urinary excretion of riboflavin is ca. 200 $\mu$g/24 hr; whereas, riboflavin-deficient individuals may excrete only 40-70 $\mu$g/24 hrs. Riboflavin excretion at <27 $\mu$g/mg creatinine is generally considered to indicate riboflavin deficiency in adults; however, this parameter tends to reflect current intake of the vitamin rather than total flavin stores.

[24]7,8-Dimthylalloxazine, an irradiation product of riboflavin believed also to be produced by intestinal microbes.

[25]Rats have been found to oxidize less than 1% of an oral dose of the vitamin.

# METABOLIC FUNCTIONS OF RIBOFLAVIN

*coenzyme*
*functions*

Riboflavin functions metabolically as the essential component of the coenzymes **FMN** and **FAD**, which act as intermediaries in transfers of electrons in biological oxidation-reduction reactions.   More than one hundred enzymes are known to bind FAD or FMN in animal and microbial systems. These enzymes, called **flavoproteins** or **flavoenzymes**, include **oxidases**, which function aerobically, and **dehydrogenases**, which function anaerobically.  Some involve one-electron transfers, while others involve two-electron transfers.  This versatility allows flavoproteins to serve as switching sites between obligate two-electron donors (e.g., NADH, succinate) and obligate one-electron acceptors (e.g., Fe-S proteins, heme proteins).   Flavoproteins serve this function by undergoing reduction through two single-electron transfer steps involving a **riboflavinyl radical** or **semiquinone** intermediate (with the unpaired electron localized at N-5). Because the radical intermediate can react with molecular oxygen, flavoproteins can also serve as cofactors in the two-electron reduction of $O_2$ to $H_2O$, and in the four-electron activation and cleavage of $O_2$ in monooxygenase reactions.

riboflavin          riboflavinyl radical          fully reduced riboflavin

Collectively, the flavoproteins show great versatility in accepting and transferring one or two electrons with a range of potentials.  This feature owes to the variation in the angle between the two planes of the isoalloxazine ring system (intersecting at N-5 and N-10), which is modified by specific protein binding.   The flavin-containing dehydrogenases or reductases (their reduced forms) react slowly with molecular oxygen, in contrast to the fast reactions of the flavin-containing oxidases and monooxygenases.  In the former reactions, hydroperoxide derivatives of the flavoprotein are cleaved to yield superoxide anion ($O_2^-$), but in the latter a heterolytic cleavage of the hydroperoxide group occurs to yield the peroxide ion ($OOH^-$).  Many flavoproteins contain a metal (e.g., Fe, Mo, Zn), and the combination of flavin and metal ion is often involved in the adjustments of these enzymes in transfers between single- and double-electron donors.  In some flavoproteins, the means for multiple-electron transfers is provided by the presence of multiple flavins as well as metals.

*metabolic*   A large group of enzymes involved in biological oxidations and reductions,
*roles*       the flavoproteins are essential for the metabolism of **carbohydrates**, **amino
              acids** and **lipids**. Some are also essential for the activation of the vitamins
              **pyridoxine** and **folate** to their respective coenzyme forms.

Important flavoproteins of animals:

| flavoprotein | flavin | metabolic function |
|---|---|---|
| **1-electron transfers** | | |
| mitochondrial electron-trans-flavoprotein (ETF) | FAD | e⁻ acceptor for acyl-CoA-, branched-chain acyl-CoA-, glutaryl-CoA-, sarcosine- and dimethylglycine- dehydrogenases; links primary flavoprotein dehydrogenases with respiratory chain *via* ETF-ubiquinone reductase |
| ubiquinone reductase | FAD | 1-e⁻ transfer from ETF and coenzyme Q of respiratory chain |
| NADH-cytochrome $P_{450}$ reductase[a] | FMN | 1-e⁻ transfer from FMN to cytochrome $P_{450}$ (mono-oxygenase) |
| **pyridine-linked dehydrogenases** | | |
| NADH-cytochrome $P_{450}$ reductase[a] | FAD | 2-e⁻ transfer from NADPH to FAD |
| adrenodoxin reductase | FAD | 2-e⁻ transfer from NADPH to adrenodoxin[b] in steroid hydroxylation by adrenal cortex |
| NADH dehydrogenase | FMN | 2-e⁻ transfer from NADPH to FMN, then, to ubiquinone[c] |
| **non-pyridine nucleotide-dependent dehydrogenases** | | |
| succinate dehydrogenase | FAD | transfer reducing equivalents from succinate to ubiquinone, yielding fumarate |
| acyl-CoA dehydrogenases | FAD | 2-e⁻ transfer from substrate to flavin, in oxidation of the N-methyl groups of choline and sarcosine |
| **pyridine nucleotide oxidoreductases** | | |
| glutathione reductase | FAD | reduces GSSG to GSH using NADPH |
| lipoamide dehydrogenase[d] | FAD | oxidizes dihydrolipoamide to lipoamide using NAD⁺ |
| **reactions of reduced flavoproteins with oxygen** | | |
| D-amino acid oxidase | FAD | dehydrogenation of D-amino acid substrates to imino-acids, which are hydrolyzed to α-ketoacids |
| L-amino acid oxidase | FMN | dehydrogenation of L-amino acid substrates to imino-acids, which are hydrolyzed to α-ketoacids |
| monoamine oxidase | FAD | dehydration of biogenic amines[e] to corresponding imines with transfer of H to $O_2$, forming $H_2O_2$ |
| xanthine oxidase | FAD | oxidation of hypoxanthine and xanthine to uric acid with formation of $H_2O_2$ |
| L-gulonolactone oxidase | FAD | oxidation of L-gulonolactone to ascorbic acid |
| **flavoprotein monooxygenase** | | |
| microsomal flavoprotein monooxygenase | FAD | oxidation of N-, S-, Se- and I-centers of various substrates in drug metabolism |

[a]A component of microsomal cytochrome $P_{450}$, it contains one molecule each of FAD and FMN.
[b]An Fe-S protein.
[c]Also has NADH-ubiquinone reductase activity, reductively releasing Fe from ferritin.
[d]A component of the pyruvate dehydrogenase and α-ketoglutarate dehydrogenase complexes.
[e]e.g., serotonin, noradrenalin, benzylamine.

## EXTREMES IN RIBOFLAVIN INTAKE

*deficiency*     Many tissues are affected by riboflavin deficiency.  Therefore, deprivation
of the vitamin causes such general signs in animals as *loss of appetite*,
*impaired growth* and *reduced efficiency of feed utilization*, all of which
constitute significant costs in animal agriculture.  In addition, both animals
and humans show specific *epithelial lesions* and *nervous disorders*.
These manifestations are accompanied by abnormally low activities of a
variety of flavoenzymes.  The most rapid and dramatic of these are shown
by loss of *erythrocyte glutathione reductase* activity, making that enzyme
a useful marker for riboflavin status[26].  Substantial losses also occur in the
activities of *flavokinase* and *FAD-synthetase*; thus, the *biosynthesis of
flavoproteins is lost* in under conditions of riboflavin deprivation.  Thus,
riboflavin-deficiency results in impairments in the metabolism of energy,
amino acids and lipids.   These metabolic impairments are manifest
morphologically as arrays of both general and specific signs/symptoms.

*deficiency*       Riboflavin deficiency in animals is potentially fatal.   In addition to the
*disorders in*    general signs already mentioned, animals show other signs that vary with
*animals*         the species.    Riboflavin-deficient rodents show dermatologic signs
(*alopecia, seborrheic inflammation*[27], moderate *epidermal hyperkeratosis*[28] with *atrophy of sebaceous glands*), and a generally ragged
appearance. *Red, swollen lips* and *abnormal papillae of the tongue* are
seen.   Ocular signs may also be seen (*blepharitis*[29], *conjunctivitis*[30],
and *corneal opacity*).  Feeding a high-fat diet can increase the severity of
deficiency signs; high-fat-fed rats showed *anestrus*, multiple *fetal skeletal
abnormalities* (shortening of the mandible, fusion of ribs, cleft palate,
deformed digits and limbs), *paralysis of the hind limbs* (degeneration of
the myelin sheaths of the sciatic nerves[31]), *hydrocephalus*[32], *ocular*

---

[26]Estimation of the degree of saturation of erythrocyte glutathione reductase (*EGR*) by FAD has proven
extremely useful to assess riboflavin status, in a manner analogous to the use of erythrocyte transketolase
saturation by TPP to assess thiamin status (*see* p. 266).  Studies have shown that *in vitro* EGR activities of
normal, riboflavin-adequate individuals is stimulated ≤20% by the addition of exogenous FAD.  Individuals
showing activity coefficients (native EGR activity/EGR activity with added FAD) of 20-30% and >30% are
considered to be at moderate and high risk, respectively, to riboflavin deficiency.

[27]involving excess oiliness due to excess activity of the sebaceous glands

[28]hypertrophy of the horny layer of the epidermis

[29]inflammation of the eyelids

[30]inflammation of the mucous membrane covering the anterior surface of the eyeball

[31]the nerve situated in the thigh

*lesions*, *cardiac malformations* and *hydronephrosis*[33].

The riboflavin-deficient chick also experiences myelin degeneration of nerves, affecting the *sciatic nerve* in particular. This results in the inability to extend the digits, the syndrome called *"curled-toe paralysis"*. In hens, the deficiency is involves reductions of both egg production and embryonic survival (decreased hatchability of fertile eggs). Riboflavin-deficient turkeys show severe dermatitis. The deficiency is rapidly fatal in ducks.

Riboflavin-deficient dogs are *weak* and *ataxic*. They show *dermatitis* (chest, abdomen, inner thighs, axillae and scrotum) and *hypoplastic anemia*[34] with fatty infiltration of the bone marrow. They can have *bradycardia* and *sinus arrythmia*[35] with *respiratory failure*. *Corneal opacity* has been reported. The deficiency can be fatal, with *collapse* and *coma*. Swine fed a riboflavin-deficient diet grow slowly and develop a *scaly dermatitis* with *alopecia*. They can show *corneal opacity*, *cataracts*, *adrenal hemorrhages*, *fatty degeneration of the kidney*, *inflammation of the mucous membranes of the gastrointestinal tract*, and *nerve degeneration*. In severe cases, deficient individuals can *collapse* and *die*.

Riboflavin deficiency in the newborn calf[36] is manifest as *redness of the buccal mucosa*[37], angular *stomatitis*[38], *alopecia*, *diarrhea*, *excessive tearing and salivation*, and *inanition*. Signs of riboflavin deficiency appear to develop rather slowly in Rhesus monkeys. The first signs seen are *weight loss* (6-8 weeks), followed by *dermatologic changes* in the mouth, face, legs and hands and a *normocytic hypochromic anemia*[39] (2-6

---

[32](...continued)

[32]a condition involving the excessive accumulation of fluid in the cerebral ventricles, dilating these cavities and, in severe cases, thinning the brain and causing a separation of the cranial bones

[33]dilation of one or both kidneys due to obstructed urine flow

[34]progressive non-regenerative anemia resulting from depressed, inadequate functioning of the bone marrow

[35]irregular heart beat, with the heart under control of its normal pacemaker, the sinus (S-A) node

[36]Ruminants do not normally require a dietary source of riboflavin, as the bacteria in their rumens synthesize the vitamin in adequate amounts. However, newborn calves and lambs, whose rumen microflora is not yet established, require riboflavin in their diets. This is normally supplied by their mothers' milk or by supplements in their milk-replacer formula diets.

[37]the mucosa of the cheek

[38]lesions in the corners of the mouth

[39]anemia involving erythrocytes of normal size but low hemoglobin content

months) and, ultimately, by *collapse* and *death* with *fatty degeneration of the liver*.   Similar signs have been produced in baboons made riboflavin-deficient for experimental purposes.

*deficiency signs in humans*

Uncomplicated riboflavin deficiency is manifest in humans only after 3-4 months of deprivation of the vitamin.  Signs include *cheilosis*[40], angular *stomatitis*, *glossitis*[41], *hyperemia*[42] and *edema*[43] of the oral mucosa, *seborrheic dermatitis* around the nose and mouth and scrotum/vulva, a normocytic, *normochromic anemia* with *reticulocytopenia*[44], *leuko-penia*[45] and *thrombocytopenia*[46].    Riboflavin-deficient Humans also experience neurological dysfunction involving *peripheral neuropathy* of the extremities characterized by hyperesthesia[47], coldness and pain, as well as decreased sensitivity to touch, temperature, vibration and position.

*sub-clinical deficiency*

Although clinical signs of riboflavin deficiency are rarely seen in the industrialized world, *sub-clinical riboflavin deficiency* (that is, the condition wherein a subject's intake of the vitamin may be sufficient to prevent clinical signs but not to keep the flavoproteins saturated for optimal metabolism) is not uncommon[48].   Sub-clinical riboflavin deficiency in children may result in subnormal growth.  That riboflavin deficiency has been shown to enhance cellular resistance to *malaria*[49] may indicate a beneficial aspect to sub-clinical deficiency of the vitamin.

---

[40] lesions of the lips

[41] inflammation of the tongue. This can involve disappearance of filiform papillae and enlargement of fungiform papillae with the tongue color changing to a deep red.  Subjects with this condition, called '*geographical tongue*', have soreness of the tongue and loss of taste sensation.

[42] increased amount of blood present

[43] accumulation of excessive fluid in the tissue

[44] abnormally low number of immature red blood cells in the circulating blood

[45] abnormally low number of white blood cells in the circulating blood ($<$5,000/ml)

[46] abnormally low number of platelets in the circulating blood

[47] excessive sensibility to touch, pain, etc.

[48] One study found that nearly 27% of a group of lower socio-economic status urban American teenagers showed sub-clinical riboflavin deficiency.

[49] The mechanism of this effect is still unclear.  One hypothesis is that the deficiency my predispose erythrocytes to oxidative stress, causing hemolysis and death of the parasite.

Signs of riboflavin deficiency:

| organ system | signs |
|---|---|
| general | |
| appetite | decrease |
| growth | decrease |
| dermatologic | cheilosis, stomatitis |
| muscular | weakness |
| gastro-intestinal | inflammation, ulcer |
| skeletal | deformities |
| vital organs | hepatic steatosis |
| vascular | |
| erythrocytes | anemia |
| nervous | ataxia, paralysis |
| reproductive | |
| male | sterility |
| female | decreased egg production |
| fetal | malformations, death |
| ocular | |
| retinal | photophobia |
| corneal | decreased vascularization |

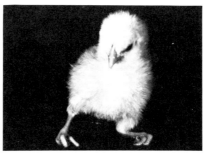 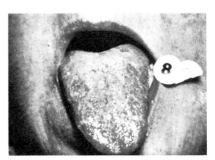

"*Curled-toe paralysis*" in a riboflavin-deficient chick.

"*Geographical tongue*" in riboflavin deficiency; courtesy Cambridge University Press.

*factors contributing to deficiency*  **Inadequate diet** is the most important cause of riboflavin deficiency. Frequently, this involves the low consumption of milk[50], which is the most important source of the vitamin available in most diets. In industrialized countries, riboflavin deficiency occurs most frequently among **alcoholics**, whose dietary practices are often faulty, leading to this and other deficiencies. In addition, high intakes of alcohol appear to antagonize the utilization of FAD from foods. **Phototherapy** given to infants with hyper-bilirubinemia often leads to riboflavin deficiency (by photo-destruction of

---

[50] The same study mentioned in fn #47, found a strongly inverse correlation between milk consumption and riboflavin status. Youths consuming at least 3 cups of milk per day were least likely to be riboflavin-deficient, while those consuming less than a cup of milk per week were most likely to be deficient.

the vitamin)[51] if such therapy does not also include the administration of riboflavin[52].  Although earlier studies purported to show reduced riboflavin status among some women using oral contraceptive agents, more recent critical studies have failed to detect any such interaction.  Patients on diuretics or undergoing hemodialysis experience enhanced loss of riboflavin (as well as other water-soluble vitamins).

hyper-        The toxicity of riboflavin is *very low* and, thus, problems of hypervitaminosis
vitaminosis   are not expected.  Probably because it is not well absorbed, high oral doses of riboflavin are essentially non-toxic[53].  The vitamin is somewhat more toxic when administered parenterally[54].

# CASE STUDY

Instructions:    *Review the following summary of a research report, paying special attention to the diagnostic indicators upon which the treatments were based.  Then, answer the questions that follow.*

case         An experiment was conducted to determine the basis of protection by riboflavin deficiency against malarial infection.  An animal model, which previously showed such protection against *Plasmodium berghei*, was used.  It involved depleting three-week-old male rats of riboflavin by feeding them a sucrose-based purified diet containing <1 mg of riboflavin per kg.  A control group was pair-fed[55] the same basal diet supplemented with 8.5

---

[51] Phototherapy can be an effective treatment for infants with mild hyperbilirubinemia; however, the mechanism by which it leads to the degradation of bilirubin (to soluble substances that can be excreted) necessarily leads also to the destruction of riboflavin.  It is the photo-activation of riboflavin in the patient's plasma that generates singlet oxygen which reacts with bilirubin.  Thus, plasma riboflavin levels of such patients have been found to drop as the result of phototherapy.  Riboflavin supplementation prevents such a drop and has been shown to enhance bilirubin destruction.

[52] e.g., 0.5 mg riboflavin sodium phosphate per kg body weight per day

[53] Oral riboflavin as great as 2-10 g/kg body weight produced no adverse effects in dogs and rats.

[54] The $LD_{50}$ values for the rat given riboflavin by the intraperitoneal, subcutaneous and oral routes have been estimated to be 0.56 g/kg, 5 g/kg and >10 g/kg, respectively.

[55] Pair-feeding is a method of controlling for the effects of reduced food intake that may be secondary to the independent experimental variable (e.g., a nutrient deficiency).  It involves the matching of one animal from the experimental treatment group with one of similar body weight from the control group, and the feeding of the latter individual a measured amount of feed equivalent to the amount of feed consumed by the former individual on the previous day.  In experiments of more than a few days duration, this approach normalizes the feed intake of both the experimental and control groups.

mg riboflavin per kg[56].   At six weeks of age, several biochemical
characteristics of erythrocytes (RBCs) were measured:  reduced glutathione levels, activities of antioxidant enzymes, stabilities of erythrocytes to
hemolysis (measured by incubating 0.5% suspensions of RBCs with pro-
oxidants [500 $\mu$m $H_2O_2$ or 2.5 $\mu$M ferriprotoporphyrin IX] or in a hypotonic
medium [151 mosmol] for 1 hr at 37°C. Oxidative damage was assessed
by measuring $H_2O_2$-induced production of malonyldialdehyde (MDA).
Other studies with this and similar animal models have shown that the
riboflavin-deficient group, when infected with the parasite, *grows better*
and shows *lighter parasitemia* than pair-fed controls.

Results of biochemical studies of erythrocytes:

| parameter | riboflavin deficient | control | P value |
|---|---|---|---|
| reticulocytes, % total RBCs | 1.50 ± 0.29 | 1.26 ± 0.37 | n.s. |
| hemoglobin, g/dl blood | 14.7 ± 0.6 | 14.9 ± 0.3 | n.s. |
| GSH, mmoles/g Hb | 7.97 ± 2.89 | 6.19 ± 2.52 | <0.001 |
| glutathione reductase, mU*/mg prot. | 42 ± 6 | 124 ± 16 | <0.001 |
| glutathione reductase activity coeffic. | 2.37 ± 0.19 | 1.20 ± 0.08 | <0.01 |
| glutathione peroxidase, mU*/g Hb | 918 ± 70 | 944 ± 62 | n.s. |
| in vitro hemolysis, % | | | |
|   $H_2O_2$-induced | 32 ± 9 | 55 ± 9 | <0.05 |
|   hypotonicity | 69 ± 4 | 53 ± 7 | <0.01 |
|   ferriprotoporphyrin IX | 42 ± 3 | 29 ± 4 | <0.001 |
| MDA, nmoles/g HB | | | |
|   before incubation | 25.5 ± 3.8 | 25.9 ± 3.4 | n.s. |
|   incubated with $H_2O_2$ | 34.8 ± 1.2 | 42.7 ± 1.8 | <0.01 |

*1 mU = 1 nmole NADPH oxidized per min

Questions:   i.      What *dependent variables* did the investigators measure to
                     confirm that riboflavin deficiency had been produced in their
                     experimental animals?

             ii.     Propose an *hypothesis* to explain the apparently discrepant
                     results regarding the effects of riboflavin deficiency on erythrocyte
                     stability.

             iii.    Propose an *hypothesis* for the protective effect of riboflavin
                     deficiency against malarial infection. What *other nutrients* might
                     you expect to influence susceptibility to this erythrocyte-attacking
                     parasite?

---

[56]This level is ca. three times the amount normally required by the rat.

## Study Questions and Exercises:

i.      **Diagram** the several general areas of metabolism in which FAD- and FMN-dependent enzymes are involved.

ii.     Construct a **'decision tree'** for the diagnosis of riboflavin deficiency in humans or an animal species.

iii.    What **key feature** of the chemistry of riboflavin relates to its biochemical functions in flavoproteins?

iv.     What **parameters** might you measure to **assess the riboflavin status** of a human or animal?

## Recommended Reading:

Cooperman, J.M. and R. Lopez. 1991. Riboflavin, Chapter 7 *in*, Handbook of Vitamins, 2nd ed. (L.J. Machlin, ed.), Marcel Dekker, New York. pp. 283-310.

Flodin, N.W. 1988. Pharmacology of Micronutrients. Alan R. Liss., Inc., New York, pp. 117-127.

Friedrich, W. 1988. Vitamins. Walter de Gruyter, New York. pp. 403-471.

McCormick, D.B. 1990. Riboflavin, Chapter 17 in Present Knowledge in Nutrition, 6th ed. (M. Brown, ed.), Int. Life Sci. Inst.-Nutr. Found., Washington, D.C., pp. 146-154.

White, H.B. and A.J. Merrill, Jr. 1988. Riboflavin-binding proteins. Ann. Rev. Nutr. 8: 279-299.

# CHAPTER 12    *NIACIN*

*"So far as they have been studied, the foodstuffs that appear to be good sources of the black tongue preventive also appear to be good sources of the pellagra preventive. . . .  Considering the available evidence as a whole, it would seem highly probable, if not certain, that experimental black tongue and pellagra are essentially identical conditions and, thus, that the preventive of black tongue is identical with the pellagra preventive, or factor P-P.  On the basis of the indications afforded by the test in the dog, liver, salmon and egg yolk are recommended for use in the treatment and prevention of pellagra in humans."*    J. Goldberger

## Anchoring Concepts:

i.    Niacin is the generic descriptor for pyridine 3-carboxylic acid and derivatives exhibiting qualitatively the biological activity of nicotinamide.

ii.   The two major forms of niacin, nicotinic acid and nicotinamide, are active metabolically as the pyridine nucleotide co-enzymes NAD(H) and NADP(H).

iii.  Deficiencies of niacin are manifest as dermatologic, gastro-intestinal and neurologic changes and can be fatal.

## Learning Objectives:

i.    To understand the chief natural *sources* of niacin.

ii.   To understand the means of enteric *absorption* and *transport* of niacin.

iii.  To understand the *biochemical function* of niacin as a component of co-enzymes of a variety of metabolically important redox reactions, and the relationship of that function to the physiological activities of the vitamin.

iv.   To understand the factors that can effect *low niacin status*, and the physiological implications of that condition.

## Vocabulary:

α-amino-β-carboxymuconic-ε-semialdehyde
anthranilic acid
black tongue disease
Casal's collar
flushing
formylase
formylkynurenine
Hartnup disease
3-hydroxyanthranilic acid
3-hydroxyanthranilic acid oxidase
3-hydroxykynurenine
kynurenic acid
kynurenine
kynurenine-3-hydroxylase
leucine
1-methyl nicotinamide
1-methyl nicotinic acid
1-methyl-6-pyridone 3-carboxamide
NAD(H)
NAD kinase
NAD synthetase
NADP(H)

NAD(P)$^+$ glycohydrolase
nicotinate phorphoribosyltransferase
nicotinamide
nicotinamide methylase
nicotinamide riboside
nicotinic acid
pellagra
perosis
phosphodiesterase
picolinic acid
picolinic acid carboxylase
pyridine nucleotide
pyridoxal phosphate
quinolinic acid
schizophrenia
transaminase
transhydrogenase
trigonelline
tryptophan
tryptophan pyrrolase
xanthurenic acid

## SOURCES OF NIACIN

*distribution*
*in foods*
Niacin occurs in greatest quantities in brewers' yeasts and meats, but significant amounts are also found in many other foods. The vitamin is distributed unevenly in grains, being present mostly in the bran fractions. Niacin occurs predominantly in bound forms, e.g., in plants mostly as protein-bound *nicotinic acid* (*NA*) and in animal tissues mostly as *nicotinamide* (*NAm*) in *nicotinamide adenine dinucleotide* (*NAD*) and *nicotinamide adenine dinucleotide phosphate* (*NADP*).

Niacin contents of foods:

| food | niacin mg/100g | food | niacin mg/100g |
|---|---|---|---|
| dairy products | | vegetables | |
| milk | .2 | asparagus | 1.5 |
| yogurt | .1 | beans | .5-2.4 |
| cheeses | 1.2 | broccoli | .9 |
| | | brussels sprouts | .9 |
| meats | | cabbage | .3 |
| beef | 4.6 | carrots | .6 |
| chicken | 4.7-14.7 | cauliflower | .7 |
| lamb | 4.5 | celery | .3 |
| pork | .8-5.6 | corn | 1.7 |
| turkey | 8.0 | kale | 2.1 |
| calf heart | 7.5 | lentils | 2.0 |
| calf kidney | 6.4 | onions | .2 |
| herring | 3.6 | peas | .9-25.0 |
| cod | 2.2 | peppers | 1.7-4.4 |
| flounder | 2.5 | potatoes | 1.5 |
| haddock | 3.0 | soy beans | 1.4 |
| tuna | 13.3 | spinach | .6 |
| | | tomatoes | .7 |
| cereals | | | |
| barley | 3.1 | fruits | |
| buckwheat | 4.4 | apples | .6 |
| cornmeal | 1.4-2.9 | bananas | .7 |
| rice, polished | 1.6 | grapefruit | .2 |
| rice, unpolished | 4.7 | oranges | .4 |
| rye | .9-1.6 | peaches | 1.0 |
| wheat, whole grain | 3.4-6.5 | strawberries | .6 |
| wheat bran | 8.6-33.4 | most nuts | .6-1.8 |
| | | peanuts | 17.2 |
| other | | | |
| eggs | .1 | | |
| mushrooms | 4.2 | | |
| yeast | 50.1 | | |

*stability*
Niacin in foods is ***very stable*** to storage and to normal means of food preparation and cooking (e.g., moist heat).

*bio-*
*availability*

Niacin is found in many types of foods in forms from which it is not released upon digestion, thereby, rendering it unavailable to the eater. In grains, niacin is present in covalently bound complexes with small peptides and carbohydrates, collectively referred to as *"niacytin"*[1]. The esterified niacin in these complexes is not normally available; however, its bioavailability can be improved substantially by treatment with base to effect the alkaline hydrolysis of those esters[2]. In other foods, niacin is present as a methylated derivative (1-methylnicotinic acid, also called *trigonelline*) that functions as a plant hormone but is also not biologically available to animals. This form, however, is heat-labile and can be converted to NA by heating[3].

*bio-*
*synthesis*

A substantial amount of niacin can be synthesized from the indispensable amino acid *tryptophan*, although the apparent efficiency of that process is relatively low in most species (in humans, ca. 60 mg tryptophan produce 1 mg equivalent of niacin). Therefore, the nutritional adequacy of diets with respect to niacin involves not only the level of the preformed vitamin, but also that of its potential amino acid precursor.

The contents of niacin-equivalents in several foods:

| food | pre-formed niacin mg/1000 kcal | tryptophan mg/1000 kcal | niacin equivalents* mg/1000 kcal |
|---|---|---|---|
| cow's milk | 1.21 | 673 | 12.4 |
| human milk | 2.46 | 443 | 9.84 |
| beef | 2.47 | 1280 | 23.80 |
| eggs (whole) | 0.60 | 1150 | 19.80 |
| pork | 1.15 | 61 | 2.17 |
| wheat flour | 2.48 | 297 | 7.43 |
| corn meal | 4.97 | 106 | 6.74 |
| corn grits | 1.83 | 70 | 3.00 |
| rice | 4.52 | 290 | 9.35 |

*based on a conversion efficiency of 60:1 for humans

---

[1] A polysaccharide extracted from wheat bran has been found to contain more than 1% nicotinic acid bound via an ester linkage to glucose in a complex also containing arabinose, galactose and xylose.

[2] Thus, it has long been a tradition in Central American cuisine to soak corn in lime-water prior to the preparation of tortillas. This practice effectively renders available the niacin in that staple grain and appears to be responsible for effective protection against pellagra in that part of the world.

[3] Thus, the roasting of coffee beans effectively removes the methyl group from trigonelline, increasing the nicotinic acid content of that food from 20 to 500 mg/kg. This practice, too, appears to have contributed to the rarity of pellagra in the maize-eating cultures of South and Central America.

## ABSORPTION OF NIACIN

*digestion of*
*NAD/NADP*

The predominant forms of niacin in most animal-derived foods, NAD(H) and NADP(H), appear to be digested to release *NAm* in which form the vitamin is absorbed. Both co-enzyme forms can be degraded by the intestinal mucosal enzyme *NAD(P)$^+$ glycohydrolase*, which cleaves the pyridine nucleotides into NAm and ADP-ribose. NAD can be cleaved at the pyrophosphate bond to yield *nicotinamide mononucleotide* (*NMN*) and 5'-AMP, or by a *phosphodiesterase* to yield *nicotinamide riboside* (*NR*) and ADP. The dephosphorylation of NMN also yields NR which can be converted to NAm by either hydrolysis (yielding ribose) or phosphorylation yielding ribose-1-phosphate. The cleavage of NAm to free NA appears to be accomplished by intestinal microorganisms and is believed to be of quantitative importance in niacin absorption.

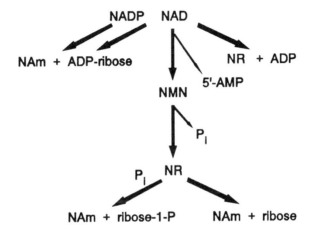

*facilitated*
*diffusion*

Studies using everted intestinal sacs prepared from rats have demonstrated that both NA and NAm are absorbed at low concentrations via a Na$^+$-dependent, carrier-mediated facilitated diffusion[4], but that the rate of diffusion of NA is about half that of NAm. At high concentrations, however, each is absorbed *via* passive diffusion. Therefore, at pharmacologic concentrations the vitamin is absorbed nearly completely[5]. The presence or absence of food in the gut appears to have no effect on niacin absorption. Because NR is not found in plasma, it appears not to be absorbed *per se*, but first converted to NAm.

---

[4] Both forms of the vitamin are absorbed across the human buccal mucosa by the same mechanism.

[5] In humans at steady-state consuming 3 g nicotinic acid per day, 85% of the vitamin was excreted in the urine.

## TRANSPORT OF NIACIN

*free*
*in plasma*

Niacin is transported in the plasma as both NA and NAm in unbound forms. Each is taken up by most peripheral tissues by passive diffusion; however, some tissues have transport systems that facilitate niacin uptake. These include the uptake of NA by the anion-transport system of erythrocytes, by a $Na^+$-dependent, saturable transport system of renal tubules[6] and by energy-dependent transport systems in the brain[6,7].

*tissue*
*storage*

Niacin is retained in tissues that take it up as NA and/or NAm by being trapped by conversion to the *pyridine nucleotides*, *NAD(H)* and *NADP(H)*. By far the greater amount is found as NAD(H) most of which, in contrast to NADP(H), is found in the oxidized form ($NAD^+$).

Pyridine nucleotide contents of various organs of rats:

| organ | NAD$^+$ mg/kg | NADH mg/kg | NADP$^+$ mg/kg | NADPH mg/kg |
|---|---|---|---|---|
| liver | 370 | 204 | 6 | 205 |
| heart | 299 | 184 | 4 | 33 |
| kidney | 223 | 212 | 3 | 54 |
| brain | 133 | 88 | <2 | 8 |
| thymus | 116 | 35 | <2 | 12 |
| lung | 108 | 52 | 9 | 18 |
| pancreas | 80 | 78 | <2 | 12 |
| testes | 80 | 71 | <2 | 6 |
| blood | 55 | 36 | 5 | 3 |

source: Offermanns et al, 1984. Kirk-Othmer Encycl. Chem. Technol. 24:59.

---

[6] This has been demonstrated in the rabbit.

[7] The site of the blood-cerebrospinal fluid barrier, the choroid plexus, appears to have separate systems for the accumulation/release of NA and NAm. In addition, brain cells also have a high-affinity transport system for NAm. These two levels of control effect the homeostasis of niacin in the brain, with NAm but not NA entering readily.

## METABOLISM OF NIACIN

*biosynthesis*     All animal species (including humans) appear to be capable, to varying degrees, of the *de novo* synthesis of the metabolically active forms of niacin, NAD(H) and NADP(H), from **quinolinic acid**, a metabolite of the indispensable amino acid **tryptophan**.    This conversion involves the oxidative cleavage of the tryptophan pyrrole ring[8] and the removal of the resulting formyl group[9] to form **kynurenine**, which is then ring-hydroxylated to yield **3-hydroxykynurenine (3-OH-Ky)**[10].

---

[8] **Tryptophan pyrrolase** converts tryptophan to N-formylkynurenine.

[9] This step is catalyzed by a **formylase**.

[10] This step is catalyzed by the FAD-dependent enzyme **kynurenine-3-hydroxylase**.

The latter intermediate can be deaminated to yield **xanthurenic acid** [11], which is excreted in the urine, or its side chain can be cleaved of the amino acid alanine to yield **3-hydroxyanthranilic acid (3-OH-AA)**[12]. That intermediate (3-OH-AA) is oxidatively ring-opened by an $Fe^{++}$-dependent dioxygenase[13] to yield the semi-stable **α-amino-β-carboxymuconic-ε-semialdehyde (ACS)**, which is a branch-point intermediate in the pathway as it can either be converted to **NMN** or catabolized to niacin-inactive products. Catabolism of ACS can be effected by both non-enzymatically via spontaneous cyclization and decarboxylation to yield picolinic acid, or enzymatically by **picolinic acid carboxylase (PAC)** which decarboxylates it to yield **α-aminomuconic-ε-semialdehyde**, which is then reduced and further decarboxylated ultimately to yield **acetyl CoA**. Alternatively, ACS can spontaneously cyclize to form **quinolinic acid (QA)** (with dehydration but not decarboxylation), which can be phosphoribosylated (in a step involving decarboxylation) to yield **NMN**[14]. That form is phospho-adenylated to form **NAD**[15].

*three sources*
*of NAD(P)(H)*
Therefore, the metabolically active forms of niacin, the pyridine nucleotides NAD(H) and NADP(H), are synthesized from three precursors: nicotinic acid, nicotinamide and tryptophan. Whereas nicotinic acid and nicotin-amide are formal intermediates in the biosynthesis of NAD from tryptophan, that step (quinolinate phosphoribosyltransferase) actually leads *directly* to NAD via NMN. Both nicotinic acid and nicotinamide are converted to NAD by the same pathway after the latter is deamidated to yield nicotinic acid[16]. Nicotinic acid is then phosphoribosylated[17], adenylated[18] and

---

[11] This is catalyzed by a **pyridoxal phosphate-dependent transaminase** (a Zn-activated enzyme) that can also use as substrate kynurenine, yielding in the latter case another urinary metabolite, **kynurenic acid**.

[12] This step is catalyzed by the **pyridoxal phosphate-dependent** enzyme **kynureninase**, which can also use as substrate the upstream intermediate **kynurenine** to produce the urinary metabolite **anthranilic acid**.

[13] This step is catalyzed by **3-hydroxyanthranilic acid oxygenase**.

[14] This step is catalyzed by **quinolate phosphoribosyltransferase**.

[15] This step is catalyzed by **NAD synthetase**.

[16] As the nicotinamide deamidase activities of animal tissues are very low, this step is thought to be carried out by the intestinal microflora.

[17] This step is catalyzed by **nicotinate phosphoribosyltransferase**.

[18] This step is catalyzed by **deamido-NAD pyrophosphorylase**.

amidated[19] to yield NAD, which can be phosphorylated[20] to yield NADP.

Although the various tissues of the body are each apparently capable of synthesizing their own pyridine nucleotides, there is clearly an exchange between the tissues that occurs primarily at the level of nicotinamide which is rapidly transported between tissues. In the rat, nicotinic acid appears to be the most important precursor of these coenzymes in the liver, kidneys, brain and erythrocytes; but in the testes and ovaries nicotinamide appears to be a better precursor.

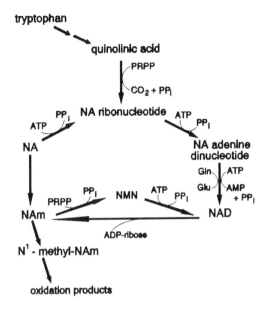

3-HAAO, PAC activities determine conversion efficiency

In general, the conversion of tryptophan to NAD is a fairly inefficient process. Humans appear normally to convert 60 mg tryptophan to 1 mg niacin[21]; this ratio is also wide for the chick (45:1) and the rat (50:1). Higher niacin-biosynthetic efficiencies are associated with *high* activities of 3-HAAO (enhancing production of ACS, the branch-point intermediate in the pathway), and *low* activities of PAC (removing that intermediate). Thus, the ratio of the hepatic activities of 3-HAAO:PAC and, in particular, the hepatic activity of PAC vary greatly between animal species and are inversely correlated with their dietary requirements for preformed niacin.

---

[19] This step is catalyzed by **NAD synthetase**.

[20] This step is catalyzed by an ATP-dependent **NAD kinase**.

[21] This conversion efficiency improves under conditions of niacin deficiency, e.g., humans are estimated to be able to use nearly 3% of dietary tryptophan for niacin biosynthesis, thus, being able to satisfy two-thirds of their requirement for the vitamin from the metabolism of this amino acid.

Relationship of 3-HAAO:PAC ratio and dietary niacin requirement:

| animal | 3-HAAO:PAC | niacin requirement[a] (mg/kg diet) |
|---|---|---|
| rat | 273 | 0 |
| chick, low-niacin requirement strain | 48 | 5 |
| chick, high-niacin requirement strain | 27 | 15 |
| duck | 5.3 | 40 |
| cat | 5 | 45 |
| brook trout, lake trout | 2.5 | 88 |
| turkey | 1.6 | 70 |
| rainbow trout, Atlantic salmon | 1.3 | 88 |
| coho salmon | 3.4 | 175 |

[a]animals fed tryptophan

source: Poston and Combs, 1980. Proc. Soc. Exp. Biol. Med. 163:452.

Hepatic picolinic acid carboxylase (PAC) activities in animals:

| animal | PAC activity IU/g |
|---|---|
| cat | 50,000 |
| lizard | 29,640 |
| duck | 17,330 |
| frog | 13,730 |
| turkey | 9,230 |
| cow | 8,300 |
| pig | 7,120 |
| pigeon | 6,950 |
| chicken, high-niacin requirement strain | 5,380 |
| chicken, low-niacin requirement strain | 3,200 |
| rabbit | 4,270 |
| mouse | 4,200 |
| guinea pig | 3,940 |
| human | 3,180 |
| hamster | 3,140 |
| rat | 1,570 |

source: DiLorenzo, R.N. 1972, Ph.D. thesis, Cornell Univ., Ithaca, NY

*role of vitamin B$_6$ in tryptophan niacin conversion*

It should also be noted that ***pyridoxal phosphate-dependent enzymes*** are involved at four points in the tryptophan-niacin pathway: two ***transaminases*** (which catalyze the conversions of kynurenine to kynurenic acid and of 3-hydroxykynurenine to xanthurenic acid) and ***kynureninase*** (which catalyzes the conversion of kynurenine to anthranilic acid as well as that of 3-hydroxykynurenine to 3-hydroxyanthranilic acid). Thus, the conversion efficiency of tryptophan to niacin is reduced under conditions of pyridoxine deficiency. Despite the dependence of each on the active form of pyridoxine (pyridoxal phosphate), only the latter is affected by deficiency of that vitamin. The affinity of kynureninase for pyridoxal phosphate, as measured by its $K_m$[22], is ca. $10^{-3}$M; whereas those for transaminases are

---

[22]Michaelis constant; in this case, the concentration of pyridoxal phosphate necessary to support half-maximal enzyme activity

typically on the order of $10^{-8}$M. Accordingly, the deprivation of pyridoxal phosphate that occurs in pyridoxine deficiency reduces kynureninase activity in most cases without affecting the activities of the transaminases which themselves require only $10^{-5}$ as much of the cofactor. Thus, pyridoxine deficiency impairs the overall conversion of tryptophan to niacin by blocking the production of 3-hydroxyanthranilic acid[23]. It does not, however, block the excretion of the urinary metabolites kynurenic acid and xanthurenic acid. This phenomenon has been exploited for the assessment of pyridoxine status by monitoring the urinary excretion of xanthurenic acid after a tryptophan load.

catabolism

The pyridine nucleotides are catabolized in animals by hydrolytic cleavage of their two β-glycosidic bonds, primarily the one at the nicotinamide moiety, by **NAD(P)$^+$ glycohydrolase**. Nicotinamide so released can be deamidated to form nicotinic acid in which form it can be re-converted to NAD. Alternatively, it can be methylated (mainly in the liver) by **nicotinamide methylase** to yield 1-methylnicotinamide[24,25], which can be oxidized to a variety of products that are excreted in the urine.

excretion

Niacin is excreted as a variety of water-soluble metabolites in the urine. At typical levels of intake of the vitamin, the major urinary metabolites are **1-methylnicotinamide**[26] and its oxidation product **1-methyl-6-pyridone 3-carboxamide**. Under such conditions, intact nicotinic acid and nicotinamide, as well as other oxidation products[27], are also excreted, but in much smaller amounts. At high rates of niacin intake, the vitamin is excreted predominantly (65-85% of total) in unchanged form. At all rates of intake, however, nicotinamide tends to be excreted as its metabolites

---

[23] It has also been suggested that the deficiency of Zn, an essential cofactor of **pyridoxal kinase** (see Chapter 13), may also impair tryptophan-niacin conversion by reducing the production of pyridoxal phosphate.

[24] Nicotinamide methylase activity is very low in fetal rat liver, increasing only in mature animals or in animals in which hepatocyte proliferation has been stimulated (e.g., after partial hepatectomy or treatment with thioacetamide). Such increases in enzyme activity are accompanied by drops in tissue NAD concentrations, as 1-methylnicotinamide reduces NAD synthesis either by inhibiting NAD synthetase and/or stimulating NAD(P)$^+$ glycohydrolase. Thus, it is thought that nicotinamide methylase and its product may be involved in the control of hepatocyte proliferation.

[25] Nicotinic acid appears not to be methylated by animals. Trigonellin (1-methylnicotinic acid) does appear, however, in the urine of coffee drinkers due to its presence in that food.

[26] Humans normally excrete daily up to 30 mg of total niacin metabolites of which 7-10 mg are 1-methylnicotinamide.

[27] Most mammals excrete several metabolites: nicotinamide 1-oxide, 1-methyl-4-pyridone-3-carboxamide, 1-methyl-6-pyridone-3-carboxamide, 6-hydroxynicotinamide and 6-hydroxynicotinic acid; some species also excrete nicotinic acid/nicotinamide-conjugates of ornithine (2,5-dinicotinyl ornithine by birds only) or glycine (nicotinuric acid by rabbits, guinea pigs, sheep, goats and calves).

more extensively than is nicotinic acid. Further, the biological turnover of each vitamer is determined primarily by its rate of excretion; thus, at high intakes, the half-life of nicotinamide is shorter than that of nicotinic acid.

## METABOLIC FUNCTIONS OF NIACIN

*co-enzyme functions*

Niacin functions metabolically as the essential component of the enzyme co-substrates **NAD(H)**[28] and **NADP(H)**[29]. The most central electron transport carriers of cells, each acts as an intermediate in most of the H-transfers in metabolism, including more than 200 reactions in the metabolism of **carbohydrates**, **fatty acids** and **amino acids**. The H-transport by the pyridine nucleotides are two-electron transfers in which the hydride ion (H⁻) serves as a carrier for both electrons. The transfer is stereo-specific, involving C-4 of the pyridine ring[30]. The reactions catalyzed by the pyridine nucleotide-dependent dehydrogenases occur by the abstraction of the proton from the alcoholic hydroxyl group of the donor substrate, and the transfer of hydride ion from the same C-atom to the C-4 of nicotinamide. In many cases, this reaction is coupled to a further reaction, such as phosphorylation or decarboxylation.

*metabolic roles*

Despite their similarities of mechanism and structure[31], NAD(H) and NADP(H) have quite different metabolic roles and most dehydrogenases have specificity for one or the other[32]. In the reactions involving NAD(H), its oxidized form $NAD^+$ usually serves as a hydrogen acceptor, forming NADH which, in turn, functions as a hydrogen donor to the respiratory chain for ATP production. These reactions include those of intracellular respiration, and NADP also serves as a co-dehydrogenase in the oxidation

---

[28] historically known as "coenzyme I", or **diphosphopyridine nucleotide (DPN)**

[29] Historically known as "coenzyme II", or **triphosphopyridine nucleotide (TPN)**

[30] The two H atoms at C-4 of NADH and NADPH are not equivalent; each is stereospecifically transferred by the enzymes to the corresponding substrates. In recognition of this phenomenon, the pyridine nucleotide-dependent enzymes are classified according to the side of the dihydropyridine ring to which each transfers H, i.e., Class A and Class B. In general, stereospecificity is independent of the nature of the substrate and the source of the enzyme and few regularities are apparent except that dehydrogenases with phosphorylated substrates tend to be B-stereospecific, while those with small (i.e., no more than three C atoms) non-phosphorylated substrates tend to be A-stereospecific.

[31] e.g., each contains adenosine, which appears to serve as a hydrophobic "anchor"

[32] A small number of dehydrogenases can use either NAD(H) or NADP(H).

of physiological fuels[33]. In the reactions involving NADP(H), the reduced form NADPH[34] usually serves as a source of reducing equivalents for biosynthetic reactions, many of which also involve flavoproteins[35]. These reactions involve reductive biosyntheses, such as those of fatty acids and steroids. In addition, NADP also serves as a co-dehydrogenase for the oxidation of glucose 6-phosphate in the pentose phosphate pathway.

Some important pyridine nucleotide-dependent enzymes of animals:

| enzyme | pyridine nucleotide |
|---|---|
| carbohydrate metabolism | |
| 3-phosphoglyceraldehyde dehydrogenase | NAD(H) |
| glucose-6-phosphate dehydrogenase | NADP(H) |
| 6-phosphogluconate dehydrogenase | NADP(H) |
| lactate dehydrogenase | NAD(H) |
| alcohol dehydrogenase | NAD(H) |
| | |
| lipid metabolism | |
| α-glycerophosphate dehydrogenase | NAD(H) |
| β-hydroxyacyl CoA dehydrogenase | NAD(H) |
| 3-ketoacyl ACP reductase | NADP(H) |
| enoyl-ACP reductase | NADP(H) |
| 3-hydroxy-3-methylglutaryl-CoA reductase | NADP(H) |
| | |
| amino acid metabolism | |
| glutamate dehydrogenase | NAD(H)/NADP(H) |
| | |
| other | |
| glutathione reductase | NADP(H) |
| dihydrofolate reductase | NADP(H) |
| thioredoxin-NADP reductase | NADP(H) |
| 4-hydroxybenzoate hydroxylase | NADP(H) |
| NADH dehydrogenase/NADH-ubiquinone | |
|   reductase complex | NAD(H) |
| NADPH-cytochrome $P_{450}$ reductase | NADP(H) |

*in glucose tolerance factor*    Niacin has been identified as part of the chromium-containing *"glucose tolerance factor"* of yeast, which enhances the response to insulin. Its role, if any, in that factor is not clear, as free niacin has not similar effect.

---

[33] e.g., glyceraldehyde 3-phosphate, lactate, alcohol, 3-hydroxybutyrate, pyruvate, and α-ketoglutarate dehydrogenases

[34] The NADP$^+$/NADPH couple is largely reduced in animal cells, owing to the *transhydrogenase* activity that catalyzes the energy-dependent exchange of hydride between the pyridine nucleotides coupled to proton transport across the mitochondrial membrane in which it resides (the so-called *"redox-driven proton pump"*).

[35] The first step in most biological redox reactions is the reduction of a flavoprotein by NADPH.

## EXTREMES IN NIACIN INTAKE

deficiency          Because a substantial amount of niacin can be synthesized from
tryptophan, nutritional status with respect to niacin involves not only the
level of intake of the preformed vitamin, but also that of its potential amino
acid precursor. Accordingly, clinical manifestation of niacin deficiency
evidences an unbalanced diet concerning both of these essential nutrients
and, frequently, pyridoxine. Thus, the occurrence of pellagra, as well as
niacin-deficiency diseases in animals, is properly viewed as the result of a
multi-factorial dietary deficiency rather than of insufficient intake of niacin
per se[36]. In addition to tryptophan and pyridoxine[37] supplies being
important determinants of niacin status, it has been suggested that excess
intakes of the branched chain amino acid *leucine* may antagonize niacin
synthesis and/or utilization and, thus, also may be a precipitating factor in
the etiology of pellagra. Excess leucine has been shown to inhibit the
production of quinolinic acid from tryptophan by isolated rat hepatocytes;
however, the magnitude of this effect is small in comparison to the $K_m$ of
quinolinate phosphoribosyl-transferase for quinolinate, indicating that
excess leucine (and/or its metabolites) is unlikely to affect the rate of NAD-
biosynthesis by the liver. Some studies with intact animals (rats) have
produced results supporting the view that excess leucine can impair the
synthesis of NAD from tryptophan (either by inhibiting the enzymatic
conversion itself, or the cellular uptake of the amino acid); however, others
have yielded negative results in this regard. Therefore, the role that high
leucine intakes may have in the etiology of pellagra is not clear at present.

General signs of niacin deficiency - *"four Ds"*:

| | |
|---|---|
| Dermatitis | Delirium |
| Diarrhea | Death |

deficiency          Niacin deficiency in humans results in changes in the *skin*, *gastrointestinal*
sign in humans *tract*, and *nervous system*. The dermatologic changes which are usually
most prominent, being called *"pellagra"*, are most pronounced in the parts

---

[36]The knowledge that supports this view provides answers for some long-troubling questions about the
etiology of pellagra: *Why does milk, which contains little niacin, prevent pellagra? Why does rice, which contains
less niacin than corn, not produce pellagra?*

[37]Zinc, which is required by the enzyme *pyridoxal phosphokinase*, is also related to the function of pyridoxine in this system. Alcoholics, who are typically of low Zn-status, have been shown to excrete high levels
of the niacin metabolites 1-methyl 6-pyridone 3-carboxamide and 1-methylnicotinamide. The excretion of these
metabolites was increased by Zn-supplementation, presumably due to increased pyridoxal phosphokinase activities and the consequent activation of pyridoxine to the form (pyridoxal phosphate) that facilitates tryptophan-
niacin conversion. It has also been suggested that Zn deficiency may reduce the availability of tryptophan for
niacin biosynthesis by enhancing its oxidation, as has been shown for several other amino acids.

of the skin that are exposed to sunlight (face, neck[38], backs of the hands and forearms).  In some patients, lesions resemble early sunburn; in chronic cases the symmetric lesions feature *cracking, desquamation*[39], *hyperkeratosis* and *hyperpigmentation*.  Lesions of the gastro-intestinal tract include *angular stomatitis, cheilosis, glossitis* as well as alterations of the buccal mucosa, tongue, esophagus, stomach (resulting in *achlor-hydria*[40]) and intestine (resulting in *diarrhea*)[41].  Pellagra almost always involves *anemia*[42].  Early neurological symptoms associated with pellagra include *anxiety, depression* and *fatigue*[43]; later symptoms include depression, apathy, headache, dizziness, irritability and tremors.

*hereditary disorders of niacin metabolism*

Two hereditary disorders of humans involve impaired niacin function and are successfully treated with high doses of niacin:  *schizophrenia* and *Hartnup disease*.  Schizophrenia appears to be a NAD-deficiency disease involving a failure to provide sufficient amounts of that pyridine nucleotide to critical areas of the brain.  Affected individuals apparently oxidize nicotinamide more readily than do healthy persons, as they excrete greater amounts of *1-methyl-6-pyridone 3-carboxamide* than do healthy controls.  As the excretion of this methylated product is increased by treatment with methylated hallucinogens (e.g., methylated indoles) and is decreased by treatment with tranquilizers, if has been suggested that the high endo-genous production of methylated hallucinogenic substances[44] in schizo-phrenics results in a depletion of nicotinamide (*via* its methylation and excretion) resulting in a substrate-limitation on NAD synthesis.  Indeed, schizophrenics respond to high oral doses (e.g., 1 g per day) of nicotinic acid[45].  Patients with a rare familial disorder involving the malabsorption

---

[38] This is referred to as *"Casal's collar"*.

[39] the shedding of the epidermis in scales

[40] the absence of hydrochloric acid from the gastric juice, usually due to gastric parietal cell dysfunction

[41] Many of these gastro-intestinal changes also occur in schizophrenia.

[42] The anemia associated with pellagra is of the macro- or normocytic, hypochromic types.

[43] Many of these symptoms also occur in schizophrenia.

[44] e.g., methylated derivatives of norepinephrine, dopamine and epinephrine such as the so-called *"pink factor"* (3,4-dimethoxyphenylethylamine).

[45] It is also likely that, at such high doses of nicotinic acid, the enhanced metabolic production of nicotinamide will further increase NAD(H) levels (by retarding its turnover), as the latter vitamer can inhibit NADase, the activity of which is high in brain.

of tryptophan (and other amino acids), Hartnup disease[46], also respond to treatment with nicotinic acid. That hereditary disease is characterized by hyperaminoaciduria[47], a pellagra-like skin rash (precipitated by psychological stress, sunlight or fever) and neurological changes including attacks of ataxia and psychiatric disorders ranging from emotional instability to delirium. Patients appear to have abnormally low capacities to convert tryptophan to niacin, which appears to result from reduced enteric absorption and renal reabsorption of monoamino monocarboxylic acids (including tryptophan). In these patients, non-reabsorbed tryptophan appears to be degraded by microbial tryptophanase to pyruvate and indole, the latter of which is reabsorbed from the intestine and is neurotoxic.

*deficiency*
*disorders*
*in animals*

Niacin deficiency in animals is characterized by a variety of species-specific signs that are usually accompanied by loss of appetite, poor growth and reduced efficiency of feed utilization. Pigs and ducks are particularly sensitive to niacin deficiency. Pigs show diarrhea, anemia and degenerative changes in the intestinal mucosa and nervous tissue[48]; ducks show severely bowed and weakened legs and diarrhea. Niacin-deficient dogs show necrotic degeneration of the tongue with changes of the buccal mucosa and severe diarrhea[49]. Rodents show alopecia and nerve cell histopathology. Chickens show inflammation of the upper gastro-intestinal tract, dermatitis of the legs, reduced feather growth and perosis[50].

It has been thought that ruminants are not susceptible to niacin deficiency, owing to the synthesis of the vitamin by their rumen microflora. While that appears to be true for most ruminant species, recent evidence indicates that fattening beef cattle and some high-producing dairy cows can benefit from niacin supplements. That ruminal synthesis of the vitamin may not meet the nutritition needs of the host would appear most likely in circumstances wherein rumen fermentation is altered to enhance energy utilization, with associated reductions in rumen microbial growth.

---

[46] The disease was named for the first case, described in 1951, involving a boy thought to have pellagra. Since that time some 50 proved cases involving 28 families have been described.

[47] the presence of abnormally high concentrations of amino acids in the urine

[48] The syndrome is called *"pig pellagra"*.

[49] *"black tongue disease"*

[50] inflammation and misalignment of the tibiotarsal joint (*"hock"*) in severe cases involving slippage of the Achilles tendon from its condyles, causing crippling due to inability to extend the lower leg

Signs of Niacin Deficiency:

| organ system | signs |
|---|---|
| general | |
|   appetite | decrease |
|   growth | decrease |
| dermatologic | dermatitis, photosensitization |
| gastro-intestinal | inflammation, diarrhea, glossitis |
| skeletal | perosis |
| vascular | |
|   erythrocytes | anemia |
| nervous | ataxia, dementia |

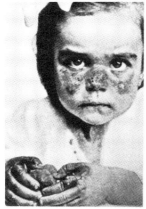

Pellagra: affected child with facial *"butterfly wing"*; courtesy Cambridge University Press.

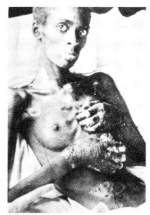

Pellagra: affected woman with *"pellagra glove"*; courtesy Cambridge University Press.

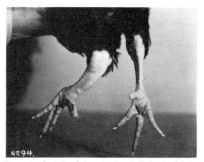

Perosis (left leg) in niacin-deficient chick.

*pharmacologic uses*　　High doses of niacin have been used in treating humans for their pharmacologic effects. Daily oral doses of several grams of nicotinic acid can *be hypocholesterolemic* and *hypotriglyceridemic* by lowering the concentrations of the low-density (LDL) and very-low-density (VLDL) lipoproteins. In addition, treatment with nicotinic acid *increased plasma high-density (HDL) lipoprotein-associated cholesterol*. These effects, in aggregate, are associated with reduced risk to atherosclerosis and provide the basis of current interest in nicotinic acid in the prophylaxis of coronary artery disease. Recent reviews of the clinical use of high doses of nicotinic acid show it to be among the most useful drugs for the treatment of hypercholesterolemia and for the prevention of coronary disease[51].

Nicotinamide has been used successfully with tryptophan in the treatment of clinical *depression*, enhancing the effect of tryptophan in supporting brain serotonin levels. Nicotinamide, which reduces the urinary excretion of tryptophan metabolites in patients treated with the amino acid, appears to block the tryptophan-niacin pathway and thus increase the availability of tryptophan for the synthesis of serotonin, which effect is anti-depressive. Nicotinic acid has also been used with humans as a *vasodilator* and as an agent to stimulate tooth eruption, to increase gastric juice flow and to increase intestinal motility.

*hyper-vitaminosis*　　In general, the toxicity of niacin is *low* (non-ruminant animals can tolerate oral exposures of at least 10-20 fold their normal requirements for the vitamin). There are, however, side effects that are seen in the clinical use of high doses of the vitamin for humans. These include *flushing*, an *itching urticaria*[52] and severe *gastrointestinal discomfort* (heartburn, nausea, vomiting, rarely diarrhea). In some patients, high doses have caused *altered glucose tolerance, hyperuricemia*[53] and, rarely, transient elevations in the plasma activities of liver enzymes (without associated hepatic dysfunction). It has been suggested that niacin toxicity results from the depletion of methyl groups as the result of the metabolism of the vitamin in high doses. The toxic potential of nicotinamide appears to be greater than that of nicotinic acid, probably by a factor of four.

---

[51] A retrospective evaluation of results from the US Coronary Drug Project showed nicotinic acid treatment to have reduced lethal coronary events resulting in highly significant reduction of mortality from all causes by 11% (vs. a placebo).

[52] hives

[53] Nicotinic acid can inhibit uricase, thereby depressing intestinal microbial uricolysis.

## CASE STUDY

Instructions: *Review the following report, paying special attention to the responses to the experimental treatments. Then, answer the questions that follow.*

case        Fourteen patients with **alcoholic pellagra** and 7 healthy controls, all aged 21-45 years, were studied in the metabolic unit of the hospital. None had severe hepatic dysfunction on the basis of medical history, clinical examination and routine laboratory tests. The nutritional status of each subject was evaluated at the beginning of the study by clinical examination, anthropometric measurements (body mass index [BMI = wt./ht.$^2$], triceps skin-fold thickness, arm and muscle circumference), biochemical tests (24-hr. urinary creatinine, serum albumin, total Fe-binding capacity [TIBC]) and 24-hour recalls of food consumption. Results indicated that, before admission, the patients' with alcoholic pellagra consumed a daily average of 270 g ethanol. Each showed signs of protein-calorie malnutrition (reduced BMI, skinfold thickness, arm and muscle circumference, serum albumin and TIBC). In addition, their plasma Zn concentrations were significantly lower than those of controls, although their urinary Zn concentrations were not different from the control group.

The pellagra patients were assigned to one of two experimental treatment groups and the healthy controls to another (3 treatments, each with n = 7). During the 7-day study, each group received enteral diets prepared from 10% crystalline amino acids (adequate amounts of each except tryptophan) and 85% sucrose, which supplied daily amounts of 0.8 g protein/kg body wt. and 200 kcal/g N. In addition, each patient was given weekly by vein 500 ml of an essential fatty acid emulsion as well as a vitamin-mineral supplement. The diets were administered by intubation directly to the mid-portion of the duodenum. The control diet was supplemented with trypto-phan and the vitamin-mineral supplement contained both niacin and Zn. The diets of the each group of pellagra patients contained no tryptophan and neither did their vitamin supplement contain niacin. One group of pellagra patients received supplemental Zn (220 mg ZnSO$_4$) while the other did not. Several biochemical measurements were made at the beginning of the experiment and, again, after 4 days.

Results:

| subject group | parameter | initial value | day 4 value |
|---|---|---|---|
| healthy controls | plasma Zn, $\mu$moles/l | 14.2 ± 1.5 | 16.0 ± 2.2 |
| | plasma tryptophan, mmoles/l | 50.8 ± 12.5 | 74.3 ± 18.5 |
| | urine Zn, $\mu$moles/d | 7.34 ± 1.38 | 9.18 ± 2.91 |
| | urine 6-pyridone[a], $\mu$moles/d | 70 ± 22 | 640 ± 235 |
| | urine CH$_3$-NAm[b], $\mu$moles/d | 78 ± 32 | 143 ± 48 |
| pellagra patients | plasma Zn, $\mu$moles/l | 9.9 ± 1.1 | 9.6 ± 2.0 |
| | plasma tryptophan, mmoles/l | 33.3 ± 15.3 | 29.5 ± 6.1 |
| | urine Zn, $\mu$moles/d | 9.79 ± 3.06 | 11.93 ± 10.55 |
| | urine 6-pyridone[a], $\mu$moles/d | 16 ± 10 | 19 ± 12 |
| | urine CH$_3$-NAm[b], $\mu$moles/d | 6 ± 3 | 9 ± 6 |
| pellagra patients fed Zn | plasma Zn, $\mu$moles/l | 9.8 ± 1.0 | 15.8 ± 3.2 |
| | plasma tryptophan, mmoles/l | 37.3 ± 17.8 | 23.7 ± 7.6 |
| | urine Zn, $\mu$moles/d | 9.80 ± 3.10 | 24.02 ± 8.11 |
| | urine 6-pyridone[a], $\mu$moles/d | 16 ± 11 | 55 ± 18 |
| | urine CH$_3$-NAm[b], $\mu$moles/d | 6 ± 3 | 33 ± 20 |

[a] 1-methyl-6-pyridone-3-carboxamide
[b] 1-methylnicotinamide

Each of the biochemical measurements was repeated after 7 days of treatment. In most cases, the results showed the same effects but of greater magnitudes.

*Questions:*

i. What signs support the diagnosis of protein-calorie malnutrition in these alcoholic patients with pellagra?

ii. Propose an hypothesis for the mechanism of action of Zn in producing the responses that were observed in these patients with alcoholic pellagra. Outline an experiment (using either pellagra patients or a suitable animal model) to test that hypothesis.

iii. List the probable contributing factors to the pellagra observed in these patients.

## Study Questions and Exercises:

i.      **Diagram** the several general areas of metabolism in which NAD(H)- and NADP(H)-dependent enzymes are involved.

ii.     In general, how do the pyridine nucleotides **interact** with the flavoproteins in metabolism?  What is the **fundamental metabolic significance** of this interrelationship?

ii.     Construct a **"decision tree"** for the diagnosis of niacin deficiency in humans or an animal species.

iii.    What **key feature** of the chemistry of nicotinamide relates to its biochemical functions as an enzyme co-substrate?

iv.     What parameters might you use to **assess niacin status** of a human or animal?

## Recommended Reading:

Flodin, N.W. 1988. Pharmacology of Micronutrients. Alan R. Liss., Inc., New York, pp. 129-138.

Friedrich, W. 1988. Vitamins.  Walter de Gruyter, New York. pp. 473-542.

Harmeyer, J., and U. Kollenkirchen. 1989. Thiamin and Niacin in Ruminant Nutrition. Nutr. Res. Rev. 2:201-225.

Henderson, L.M. 1983. Niacin.  Ann. Rev. Nutr. 3:289-297.

Jacob, R.A., and M.E. Swendseid. 1990. Niacin, Chapter 19 in Present Knowledge in Nutrition, 6th edition (M. Brown, ed.), Int. Life Sci. Inst.-Nutr. Found., Washington, D.C., pp. 163-169.

van Eys, J. 1991. Nicotinic acid, Chapter 8 in Handbook of Vitamins (L.J. Machlin, ed.), Marcel Dekker, New York, pp. 311-340.

# CHAPTER 13    *VITAMIN B₆*

*"Had we been able to afford monel metal or stainless steel cages, we would have missed xanthurenic acid."*                    S. Lepkovsky

## Anchoring Concepts:

| | |
|---|---|
| i. | Vitamin B₆ is the generic descriptor for all 3-hydroxy-2-methylpyridine derivatives exhibiting qualitatively the biological activity of pyridoxine (3-hydroxy-4,5-*bis*[hydroxymethyl]-2-methylpyridine). |
| ii. | The metabolically active form of vitamin B₆ is pyridoxal phosphate, which functions as a co-enzyme for reactions involving amino acids. |
| iii. | Deficiencies of vitamin B₆ are manifest as dermatologic, circulatory and neurologic changes. |

## Learning Objectives:

| | |
|---|---|
| i. | To understand the chief natural *sources* of vitamin B₆. |
| ii. | To understand the means of *absorption* and *transport* of vitamin B₆. |
| iii. | To understand the *biochemical function* of vitamin B₆ as a co-enzyme of a variety of reactions in the metabolism of amino acids, and the relationship of that function to the physiological activities of the vitamin. |
| iv. | To understand the physiological implications of *low vitamin B₆ status*. |

*Vocabulary:*

| | |
|---|---|
| acrodynia | pyridoxal dehydrogenase |
| aldehyde oxidase | pyridoxal kinase |
| alkaline phosphatase | pyridoxal oxidase |
| cystathionuria | pyridoxal phosphate |
| decarboxylases | pyridoxamine |
| epinephrine | pyridoxamine phosphate |
| GABA | 4-pyridoxic acid |
| glycogen phosphorylase | pyridoxine |
| hemoglobin | pyridoxol |
| homocysteinuria | racemases |
| histamine | Schiff base |
| isonicotinic hydrazide | schizophrenia |
| kynureninase | serotonin |
| methionine load | sideroblastic anemia |
| norepinephrine | steroid hormone receptor complex |
| phosphorylases | transaminases |
| premenstrual syndrome | tryptophan load |
| pyridoxal | xanthurenic acid |

## *SOURCES OF VITAMIN B$_6$*

*distribution in foods*

Vitamin B$_6$ is widely distributed in foods, occurring in greatest concentrations in meats, whole-grain products (especially wheat), vegetables and nuts. A large portion of the vitamin B$_6$ in many foods is present bound to proteins[1] as well as to non-proteins (e.g., as glycosides such as 5'-O-[$\beta$-D-glucopyranosyl]pyridoxine in grains). In the cereal grains, vitamin B$_6$ is concentrated primarily in the germ and aleuronic layer; thus, refining of grains in the production of flours, which removes much of these fractions, results in substantial reductions in vitamin B$_6$ content. White bread, therefore, is a poor source of vitamin B$_6$ unless it is fortified. The chemical forms of vitamin B$_6$ tend to vary among foods of plant and animal origin; plant tissues contain mostly *pyridoxine* (the free alcohol form, pyridoxol), while animal tissues contain mostly *pyridoxal* and *pyridoxamine*.

*stability*

Vitamin B$_6$ in foods is stable under acidic conditions, but unstable under neutral and alkaline conditions, particularly when exposed to heat or light. Of the several vitamers, pyridoxine is far more stable than either pyridoxal or pyridoxamine. Therefore, the cooking losses of vitamin B$_6$ tend to be highly variable (0-40%), with plant-derived foods (which contain mostly pyridoxine) losing little if any of the vitamin and animal products (which contain mostly pyridoxal and pyridoxamine) losing substantial amounts[2]. The storage losses of naturally occurring vitamin B$_6$ from many foods and feedstuffs, although they occur at slower rates, can also be substantial (25-50% within a year). Because it is particularly stable, *pyridoxine hydrochloride* is used for food fortification and in multi-vitamin supplements.

*bio-availability*

Much of the vitamin B$_6$ in foods is not biologically available, occurring in complexed forms (e.g., pyridoxal-5-$\beta$-D-glycosides), which are poorly digested. In addition, the vitamin can condense with peptide lysyl and/or cysteinyl residues during food processing, cooking or digestion, to reduce the utilization of the vitamin. An example is wheat bran, which not only contains vitamin B$_6$ in largely unavailable form(s) but also can reduce the availability of the vitamin from other foods consumed at the same time[3]. Because plants generally contain complexed forms of pyridoxine, bioavailability of the vitamin in meats tends to be greater than in plant materials.

---

[1] Much of the protein-binding of vitamin B$_6$ in foods involves the binding of the vitamin *via* the $\epsilon$-amino group of lysyl residues and the sulfhydryl group of cysteinyl residues.

[2] For example, milk can lose 30-70% of its inherent vitamin B$_6$ upon drying, while pyridoxine added to the milk is retained.

[3] Due to the poor availability of vitamin B$_6$ from the bran fraction of the grain, the bioavailability of the vitamin from whole-wheat bread is less than that of pyridoxine-fortified white bread.

Vitamin B$_6$ contents of foods:

| food | vitamin B$_6$ mg/100g | food | vitamin B$_6$ mg/100g |
|---|---|---|---|
| dairy products | | vegetables | |
| milk | .04 | asparagus | .15 |
| yogurt | .05 | beans | .08-.18 |
| cheeses | .04-.08 | broccoli | .17 |
| meats | | brussels sprouts | .18 |
| beef | .33 | cabbage | .16 |
| chicken | .33-.68 | carrots | .15 |
| lamb | .28 | cauliflower | .21 |
| pork | .35 | celery | .06 |
| ham | .32 | corn | .20 |
| calf liver | .84 | onions | .13 |
| herring | .37 | peas | .16 |
| haddock | .18 | potatoes | .25 |
| tuna | .43 | spinach | .28 |
| oysters | .05 | fruits | |
| shrimp | .10 | apples | .03 |
| cereals | | grapefruit | .03 |
| corn meal | .20 | oranges | .06 |
| rice, polished | .17 | peaches | .02 |
| rice, unpolished | .55 | strawberries | .06 |
| wheat, whole | .29 | tomatoes | .10 |
| other | | peanuts | .40 |
| eggs | .19 | pecans | .18 |
| human colostrum | .001-.002 | walnuts | .73 |
| human milk | .010-.025 | | |

# ABSORPTION OF VITAMIN B$_6$

*diffusion linked to phosphorylation*

The various forms of vitamin B$_6$ are freely absorbed *via **passive diffusion*** primarily in the jejunum and ileum[4]. The capacity for absorption is, therefore, very large; animals have been found to be able to absorb the vitamin at 2-3 orders of magnitude greater than their physiological needs demand. The driving forces of vitamin B$_6$ absorption appear to be the ***phosphorylation*** and ***protein-binding*** which occur in the intestinal mucosa and blood. ***Dephosphorylation*** of pyridoxal phosphate and pyridoxamine phosphate is catalyzed by a membrane-bound ***alkaline phosphatase*** during the absorption of those vitamers. Those products, and the non-phosphorylated vitamers that are absorbed directly, are phosphorylated in the jejunal mucosa by a ***pyridoxal kinase***. Phosphorylated pyridoxine and pyridoxamine are then oxidized to the common form, ***pyridoxal phosphate***.

[4] Although the microflora of the colon synthesize vitamin B$_6$, it is not absorbed there and non-coprophagous animals derive no benefit from this microbial source of the vitamin. In contrast, ruminant species benefit from their rumen microflora which produces vitamin B$_6$, in adequate amounts to meet their needs, ahead of the loci of its enteric absorption.

# TRANSPORT OF VITAMIN B$_6$

*protein-binding*  The predominant form of vitamin B$_6$ in the blood is ***pyridoxal phosphate*** which, like the smaller amount of free pyridoxal, is tightly bound to proteins (primarily ***albumin*** in the plasma and ***hemoglobin*** in erythrocytes[5]) *via* ***Schiff-base*** linkages[6].  Pyridoxal more readily crosses cell membranes than pyridoxal phosphate; thus, it appears to be the form taken up by the tissues, suggesting roles of phosphatases in uptake of the vitamin.

*phosphor-*   After being taken into the cell, the vitamin is again phosphorylated by
*ylation*    ***pyridoxal kinase*** to yield the predominant tissue form, ***pyridoxal phos-phate***.  Small quantities of vitamin B$_6$ are stored in the body[7], mainly as ***pyridoxal phosphate*** but also as ***pyridoxamine phosphate***; greatest levels are found in the liver, brain, kidney, spleen and muscle, where it is found bound to various proteins[8,9].  Vitamin B$_6$ is found in the blood largely as pyridoxal phosphate, most of which is derived from the liver after metabolism by hepatic flavoenzymes.

Concentrations (nM) of vitamers B$_6$ in the plasma of several species:

| species | PalP | Pal | Pol | Pam | PamP | P ac. |
|---------|------|-----|-----|-----|------|-------|
| pig     | 29   | 139 | 167 | -   | -    | 139   |
| human   | 62   | 13  | 33  | 6   | <3   | 40    |
| calf    | 308  | 96  | 50  | -   | 9    | 91    |
| sheep   | 626  | 57  | 43  | -   | 466  | 318   |
| dog     | 417  | 268 | 66  | -   | 65   | 109   |
| cat     | 2443 | 139 | 93  | 44  | 271  | 17    |
| [Pyridox-al (Pal), -al P (PalP), -ol (Pol), -amine (Pam), -amine P (PamP), -ic acid (P ac.)] | | | | | | |

---

[5] Vitamin B$_6$ binds *via* the amino group of the N-terminal valine residue of the hemoglobin $\alpha$-chain.  This binding, like that of pyridoxine and pyridoxamine, is twice as strong as that to albumin, appearing to drive uptake by erythrocytes, which normally contain more than six times more vitamin than the plasma.

[6] ***Schiff bases*** are condensation products of aldehydes and ketones with primary amines; they are stable if there is at least one aryl group on either the N or the C that are linked.  Vitamin B$_6$ forms Schiff-base linkages with proteins by the bonding of the keto-C of pyridoxal phosphate to a peptidyl amino group.  The vitamin also forms a Schiff-base linkage with the amino acid substrates of the enzymes for which it functions as a co-enzyme by the bonding of the amino-N of pyridoxal phosphate and the $\alpha$-C of the substrate.

[7] The total body store of vitamin B$_6$ in humans is 40-150 mg, i.e., 20-75 days' needs.

[8] In muscle, pyridoxal phosphate is bound mostly to ***glycogen phosphorylase***; in other tissues it is bound to various enzymes with which it has co-enzyme functions.

[9] It is thought that the protein-binding of pyridoxal phosphate in the tissues serves to protect it from hydrolysis as well as to provide storage of the vitamin.

## METABOLISM OF VITAMIN B$_6$

interconversion   The vitamers B$_6$ are readily interconverted metabolically by reactions involv-
of vitamers       ing *phosphorylation/dephosphorylation*, *oxidation/reduction* and *amina-
                  tion/deamination*. Because the non-phosphorylated vitamers cross mem-
                  branes more readily than their phosphorylated analogues, phosphorylation
                  appears to be an important means of retaining the vitamin intracellularly.
                  The hepatic enzyme *pyridoxal kinase*[10,11,12] phosphorylates pyridoxine,
                  pyridoxal and pyridoxamine, yielding the corresponding phosphates which
                  are dephosphorylated by *alkaline phosphatases*[13] in many tissues (e.g.,
                  liver, brain and intestine). The reduced form (pyridoxine or pyridoxol
                  phosphate) can be oxidized by *pyridoxal dehydrogenase* to yield pyridoxal
                  or pyridoxal phosphate either of which can be aminated by *transaminases*.

[10] Erythrocyte pyridoxal kinase activity in black Americans has been reported to be about half of that of white Americans, although lymphocytes, granulocytes and cultured skin fibroblasts showed no such differences. This difference suggests that the retention of vitamin B$_6$ by erythrocytes, which appears to depend upon the phosphorylation, may be lower in blacks.

[11] Pyridoxal kinase requires, as a substrate, a Zn-ATP complex the formation of which is facilitated by Zn-metallothionine. It has, thus, been suggested that Zn-metallothionine may be important in the regulation of vitamin B$_6$ metabolism.

[12] Pyridoxal kinase is inhibited by the anti-asthmatic drug theophylline. That short-term theophylline therapy induced biochemical signs of vitamin B$_6$ deficiency appears to result from this inhibition *in vivo*.

[13] The conversion of pyridoxine to pyridoxal phosphate is impaired in alcoholics due to the stimulatory effect on alkaline phosphatase (hence, on the dephosphorylation of pyridoxal phosphate) of the metabolite of ethanol, acetaldehyde.

The limiting enzyme in vitamin B$_6$ metabolism appears to be *pyridoxal phosphate oxidase*, which requires flavin mononucleotide (FMN). Therefore, deprivation of *riboflavin* may reduce the conversion of pyridoxine and pyridoxamine to the active coenzyme pyridoxal phosphate.

The liver is the central organ for vitamin B$_6$ metabolism, containing all of the enzymes involved in its interconversions. The major forms of the vitamin in that organ are *pyridoxal phosphate* and *pyridoxamine phosphate* which are maintained at fairly constant intracellular concentrations in endogenous pools that are not readily accessible to newly formed molecules of those species. The latter, instead, comprise a second pool that is readily mobilized for metabolic conversion (mostly to pyridoxal phosphate, pyridoxal and pyridoxic acid) and release to the blood.

*catabolism*    The binding of pyridoxal phosphate to albumin protects the coenzyme from degradation in the circulation. In the liver, it is dephosphorylated and oxidized probably by the FAD-dependent *aldehyde (pyridoxal) oxidase* as well as the NAD-dependent *aldehyde dehydrogenase* to yield *4-pyridoxic acid*. Pyridoxic acid lacks biological activity; it appears to be an end product of metabolism, as it is quantitatively recovered in the urine of individuals given it parenterally.

*excretion*    The products of vitamin B$_6$ metabolism are excreted in the urine, the major one being *4-pyridoxic acid*[14,15]. In addition, small amounts of pyridoxal, pyridoxamine and pyridoxine and their phosphates, as well as the lactone of pyridoxic acid and a ureido-pyridoxyl complex[16] are also excreted when high doses of the vitamin have been given[17]. However, 4-pyridoxic acid is not detectable in the urine of vitamin B$_6$-deficient subjects, making it useful in the clinical assessment of vitamin B$_6$ status[18,19].

---

[14] It is estimated that 40-50% of vitamin B$_6$ consumed is oxidized to 4-pyridoxic acid.

[15] In the rat, the urinary excretion of 4-pyridoxic acid increases with age in parallel with increases in the hepatic activities of pyridoxal oxidase and pyridoxal dehydrogenase.

[16] This is formed by the reaction of an amino group of urea with an hydroxyl group of the hemiacetal form of the aldehyde in position 4 of pyridoxal.

[17] For example, humans given 100 mg pyridoxal excreted ca. 60 mg 4-pyridoxic acid and ca. 2 mg pyridoxal over the next 24 hrs.

[18] In humans, excretion of less than 0.5 mg/day (men) or 0.4 mg/day (women) is considered indicative of inadequate intake of the vitamin. Typical excretion of total vitamin B$_6$ by adequately nourished humans is 1.2-2.4 mg/day. Of that amount, 0.5-1.2 mg (men) or 0.4-1.1 mg (women) is in the form of 4-pyridoxic acid.

[19] Although no explanation has been offered for the correlation, it is of interest that excretion of relatively low amounts (<.81 mg/24 hrs) of 4-pyridoxic acid is associated with increased risk to relapse after mastectomy.

# METABOLIC FUNCTIONS OF VITAMIN $B_6$

*mechanism of action*

The metabolically active form of vitamin $B_6$ is ***pyridoxal phosphate*** which serves as a coenzyme of numerous enzymes most of which are involved in the metabolism of amino acids. The largest group of the vitamin $B_6$-dependent enzymes are the ***transaminases*** most of which use $\alpha$-ketoglutarate as the amino group acceptor. Other pyridoxal phosphate-dependent enzymes include ***decarboxylases***, ***racemases*** and enzymes that catalyze amino acid ***side-chain alterations***. In addition to these functions in amino acid metabolism, pyridoxal phosphate also serves as a coenzyme for the ***phosphorylases*** and as a ***modulator of protein structure*** (e.g., steroid hormone receptor complexes, hemoglobin, other enzymes).

The binding of pyridoxal phosphate to its various apoenzymes always occurs by the formation of a ***Schiff base*** between the keto-C of the coenzyme and the $\epsilon$-amino group of a specific lysyl residue of the apoenzyme. Thus, vitamin $B_6$-dependent enzymes tend to have structural similarities in the coenzyme-binding region. The mechanisms of the reactions catalyzed by the vitamin $B_6$-dependent enzymes also tend to be similar. Each involves the binding of an $\alpha$-C of an $\alpha$-amino acid substrate to the pyridine-N of pyridoxal phosphate. The delocalization of the electrons from the $\alpha$-C by the action of the protonated pyridine-N as an "*electron sink*" results in the conversion of the former to a carbanion at the $\alpha$-C and the labilization of its bonds. This results in the heterolytic cleavage of one of the three bonds to the $\alpha$-C. The particular bond to be cleaved is determined by the particular pyridoxal phosphate-dependent enzyme; each involves the loss of the cationic ligand of an amino acid.

Reactions of pyridoxal phosphate-dependent enzymes:

| bond cleaved | type of reaction |
|---|---|
| $a$-C-COOH | decarboxylation |
| $a$-C-R group | reversible interconversion |
| $a$-C-H | transamination, racemization, elimination, replacement |

*metabolic roles*

Vitamin B$_6$ is widely involved in metabolism. Pyridoxal phosphate is involved in practically all reactions involved in *amino acid metabolism* and (*via* the transaminases) is involved in both their biosynthesis as well as their catabolism[20,21]. Pyridoxal phosphate-dependent enzymes function in the biosynthesis of the neurotransmitters *serotonin* (tryptophan decarboxylase), *epinephrine* and *norepinephrine* (tyrosine carboxylase), and an important source of energy for the brain, *γ-aminobutyric acid (GABA)* (glutamate decarboxylase)[22], and of the vasodilator and gastric secretagogue *histamine* (histidine decarboxylase). Vitamin B$_6$ is required for the *tryptophan-niacin conversion* (kynureninase), and the synthesis of *porphyrin* precursors to heme (δ-aminolevulenic acid synthase).

In addition, vitamin B$_6$ is required for the utilization of *glycogen* to release glucose by serving as a coenzyme of *glycogen phosphorylase* in which it is bound (as pyridoxal phosphate) *via* a Schiff-base linkage to a peptidyl lysine residue. Unlike the other pyridoxal phosphate enzymes, it is not clear whether the vitamin serves directly in catalysis or whether it has a structural role, e.g., as an allosteric effector of catalysis. That it is essential for enzymatic activity is clear; the shift of the enzyme from its inactive form to its active form involves an increase in the binding (2-4 moles per mole of enzyme) of the coenzyme. This role accounts for over half of the vitamin B$_6$ in the body, due to the abundance of both muscle and glycogen phosphorylase (5% of soluble muscle protein). Pyridoxal phosphate also appears to have a role as a modulator of *steroid hormone receptors*. Pyridoxal phosphate has been shown to inhibit the induction of hepatic tyrosine aminotransferase by glucocorticoids, probably by forming Schiff-base linkages to the DNA-binding site of the receptor-steroid complex, to inhibit the binding to DNA and displace the complex from the nucleus.

---

[20] The only amino acids that are *not* substrates for pyridoxal phosphate-dependent transaminases are threonine, lysine, proline and hydroxyproline.

[21] The response of erythrocyte aspartate aminotransferase (EAAT) to *in vitro* additions of pyridoxal phosphate has been used as a biochemical parameter of vitamin B$_6$ status, after the manner of erythrocyte transketolase and glutathione reductase activity coefficients for assessing thiamin and riboflavin status, respectively. However, EAAT activity coefficients can be affected by factors unrelated to vitamin B$_6$ status (e.g., intake of protein and alcohol, differences in body protein turnover, certain drugs, genetic polymorphism of the enzyme), which can compromise its use without careful controls.

[22] It has been shown *in vitro* that pyridoxal phosphate can inhibit the binding of GABA to brain synaptic membranes.

Important pyridoxal phosphate-dependent enzymes of animals:

| type of reaction | enzyme |
|---|---|
| decarboxylations | aspartate 1-decarboxylase |
| | glutamate decarboxylase |
| | ornithine decarboxylase |
| | aromatic amino acid decarboxylase |
| | histidine decarboxylase |
| | |
| R-group interconversions | serine hydroxymethyltransferase |
| | $\delta$-aminolevulinic acid synthase |
| | |
| transaminations | aspartate aminotransferase |
| | alanine aminotransferase |
| | $\gamma$-aminobutyrate aminotransferase |
| | cysteine aminotransferase |
| | tyrosine aminotransferase |
| | leucine aminotransferase |
| | ornithine aminotransferase |
| | glutamine aminotransferase |
| | branched-chain amino acid aminotransferase |
| | serine-pyruvate amino transferase |
| | aromatic amino acid transferase |
| | histidine aminotransferase |
| | |
| racemization | cystathionine $\beta$-synthase |
| | |
| $\alpha,\beta$-elimination | serine dehydratase |
| | |
| $\gamma$-elimination | cystathionine $\gamma$-lyase |
| | kynureninase |

The binding of pyridoxal and pyridoxal phosphate to hemoglobin[23] enhances the $O_2$-binding capacity of that protein and inhibits sickling in sickle-cell hemoglobin. The catalytic properties of other enzymes are also affected (some stimulated[24], others inhibited[25]) by interactions with pyridoxal phosphate (usually *via* valine, histidine or lysine residues), suggesting that vitamin $B_6$ status may have effects beyond those involving its classical coenzyme function. Such effects may be involved in the putative involvement of vitamin $B_6$ in lipid metabolism[26].

---

[23] Pyridoxal phosphate binds at two sites on the $\beta$-chains, i.e., the N-terminal valine and lysine-82 residues; whereas pyridoxal binds at the N-terminal valine residues of the $\alpha$-chains.

[24] e.g., thymidylate synthase, vitamin K-dependent carboxylase/epoxidase

[25] e.g., glucose-6-phosphate dehydrogenase, glycerol-3-phosphate dehydrogenase, ribulose bisphosphate carboxylase, ribosomal peptidyltransferase

[26] This is suggested by the fact that vitamin $B_6$-deficient animals frequently show signs consistent with lesions of lipid metabolism, e.g., decreased carcass fat, hepatic steatosis, dermatitis, arteriosclerosis, hypertriglyceridemia and hypercholesterolemia.

# EXTREMES IN VITAMIN B$_6$ INTAKE

*deficiency*    Severe deficiency of vitamin B$_6$ results in dermatologic and neurologic changes in most species. Less obvious are the metabolic lesions associated with insufficient activities of the coenzyme pyridoxal phosphate. The most prominent metabolic lesion in vitamin B$_6$-deficiency is *impaired tryptophan-niacin conversion*. That process involves the pyridoxal phosphate-dependent enzyme *kynureninase* in the removal of an alanyl residue from 3-hydroxykynurenine in metabolism of tryptophan to the branch-point intermediate α-amino-β-carboxymuconic-ε-semialdehyde[27]. In addition, kynureninase catalyzes the analogous reaction (removal of alanine) using the non-hydroxylated kynurenine as substrate and yielding the non-hydroxylated analogue of 3-hydroxykynurenine, anthranilic acid. Vitamin B$_6$-dependent transaminases are also able to metabolize kynurenine and 3-hydroxykynurenine, yielding kynurenic and xanthurenic acids, respectively. However, because the transaminases have much greater binding affinities for pyridoxal phosphate than kynureninase[28], vitamin B$_6$ deprivation usually reduces the latter activity preferentially to the former ones. The result is a blockage in the tryptophan-niacin pathway with an accumulation of 3-hydroxykynurenine which continues to be transaminated, resulting in increased production of xanthurenic acid. Vitamin B$_6$ deficiency, therefore, impairs the metabolic conversion of tryptophan to niacin, diverting it instead to xanthurenic acid, which appears in the urine[29]. This phenomenon is exploited in the assessment of vitamin B$_6$ status: deficiency is indicated by urinary excretion of xanthurenic acid after a *tryptophan load*.

Vitamin B$_6$ deficiency also results in *impaired transsulfuration of methionine to cysteine*, as that pathway involves two pyridoxal phosphate enzymes (*cystathionine synthase* and *cystathionase*). Because the activities of these enzymes are reduced in vitamin B$_6$ deficiency, affected individuals show homocysteinuria (due to the impaired conversion to cystathionine) and cystathionuria (due to the impaired cleavage of cystathionine

---

[27] see p. 302

[28] The Michaelis constants ($K_m$) for the transaminases are on the order of $10^{-8}$ M; whereas, that for kynureninase is on the order of $10^{-3}$ M.

[29] Xanthurenic acid was discovered quite unexpectedly by Lepkovsky at the University of California who sought to elucidate the nature of rat "adermin" during the Great Depression. Prof. Lepkovsky wrote of his surprise in finding that the urine voided by his vitamin B6-deficient rats was green, while that of his controls was the normal yellow color. In pursuing this observation, he found that urine from deficient animals was normally colored as it was voided, but that it turned green only upon exposure to the rusty dropping pans their limited budget had forced them to use. Thus, he recognized that vitamin B$_6$-deficient rats excreted an unidentified metabolite that reacted with an iron salt to form a green derivative. This small event, which might have been missed by someone "too busy" to observe the experimental animals, resulted in Lepkovsky's identifying the metabolite as xanthurenic acid and discovering the role of vitamin B$_6$ in tryptophan-niacin conversion. His message: "The investigator has to do more than sit at his desk, outline experiments and examine data."

to cysteine and $\alpha$-ketobutyrate). These conditions can be exacerbated for diagnostic purposes by the use of an oral *methionine load*.

*deficiency*
*syndromes in*
*animals*

Vitamin $B_6$ deficiency in animals is generally manifest as symmetrical scaling dermatitis. In rodents, the condition is called *"acrodynia"* and is characterized by *hyperkeratotic*[30] and *acanthotic*[31] *lesions* on the tail, paws, face and upper thorax, as well as by *muscular weakness, hyperirritability, anemia, hepatic steatosis*[32], *increased urinary oxalate excretion, insulin insufficiency*[33] and *poor growth*. Neurological signs include *convulsive seizures* (epileptiform-type) that can be fatal[34]. Reproductive disorders include *infertility, fetal malformations*[35] and *reduced fetal survival*. Some reports indicate effects on blood cholesterol levels and immunity. That tissue carnitine levels are depressed in vitamin $B_6$-deficient animals has been cited as evidence of a role of the vitamin in carnitine synthesis.

Similar changes are observed in vitamin $B_6$-deficient individuals of other species. Chickens and turkeys show *reduced appetite* and *poor growth, dermatitis*, marked *anemia, convulsions, reduced egg production* and *low fertility*. Pigs show *paralysis of the hind limbs, dermatitis, reduced feed intake* and *poor growth*. Monkeys show increased incidence of *dental caries* and altered cholesterol metabolism with *arteriosclerotic lesions*. Ruminants are rarely affected by vitamin $B_6$ deficiency, as their rumen microflora appear to satisfy their needs for the vitamin. Exceptions are *lambs* and *calves* which, before their rumen microfloras are established, are susceptible to dietary deprivation of vitamin $B_6$, showing many dermatologic and neurologic changes observed in non-ruminant species.

*deficiency*
*in humans*

Vitamin $B_6$-deficient humans exhibit symptoms all of which can be quickly corrected by administration of the vitamin: *weakness, sleeplessness,*

---

[30] involving hypertrophy of the horny layer of the epidermis

[31] involving an increase in the prickle cell layer of the epidermis

[32] This can be precipitated by feeding a vitamin $B_6$-deficient diet rich in protein.

[33] This is believed to be due to reduced pancreatic synthesis of the hormone.

[34] Nervous dysfunction is believed to be due to nerve tissue deficiencies of $\gamma$-aminoisobutyric acid (GABA) resulting from decreased activities of the pyridoxal phosphate-dependent *glutamate decarboxylase*. The seizures of vitamin $B_6$-deficient animals can be controlled by administering either the vitamin or GABA.

[35] e.g., omphalocele (protrusion of the omentum or intestine through the umbilicus), exencephaly (defective skull formation with the brain partially outside of the cranial cavity), cleft palate, micrognathia (impaired growth of the jaw), splenic hypoplasia

*nervous disorders* (peripheral neuropathies), *cheilosis*[36], *glossitis*[37], *stomatitis*[32], and *impaired cell-mediated immunity*.  In addition, studies with volunteers fed a vitamin B$_6$-free diet or a vitamin B$_6$ antagonist[38] have shown elevated urinary xanthurenic acid concentrations[39] and increased susceptibility to infection.

Signs of vitamin B$_6$ deficiency:

| organ system | signs |
| --- | --- |
| general | |
| appetite | decrease |
| growth | decrease |
| dermatologic | acrodynia, cheilosis, stomatitis, glossitis |
| muscular | weakness |
| skeletal | dental caries |
| vital organs | hepatic steatosis |
| vascular | |
| vessels | arteriosclerosis |
| erythrocytes | anemia |
| nervous | paralysis, convulsions, peripheral neuropathy |
| reproductive | |
| female | decreased egg production |
| fetal | malformations, death |

*congenital disorders*

Several rare familial disorders of vitamin B$_6$ metabolism have been identified.  Each involves a deficiency of a pyridoxal phosphate-dependent enzyme.  Many, but not all, respond to massive doses of vitamin B$_6$.  Affected individuals generally do not show gross signs of vitamin B$_6$ deficiency but, instead, may be mentally retarded.

Congenital disorders of vitamin B$_6$-dependent metabolism:

| disorder | enzyme deficiency | clinical manifestations |
| --- | --- | --- |
| homocysteinuria* | cystathionine β-synthase | dislocation of lenses, thromboses, malformation of skeletal and connective tissue, mental retardation |
| cystathionuria | cystathionine γ-lyase | mental retardation |
| GABA deficiency | glutamate decarboxylase | neuropathies |
| sideroblastic anemia | δ-aminolevulinate synthase | anemia, cystathionuria, xanthurenic aciduria |
| *Another form is caused by impaired vitamin B$_{12}$-dependent methionine synthesis | | |

---

[36] The lesion is morphologically indistinguishable from that produced by riboflavin deficiency.

[37] The lesion is morphologically indistinguishable from that produced by niacin deficiency.

[38] e.g., 4'-deoxypyridoxine

[39] After tryptophan-loading, vitamin B$_6$-deficient subjects also had elevated urinary concentrations of kynurenine, 3-hydroxykynurenine, kynurenic acid, acetylkynurenine and quinolinic acid.

*pharmacologic uses*  Vitamin B$_6$ is used at supranutritional doses for the therapy of a variety of human disorders. Dosage as great as 200 mg/day (usually as pyridoxine HCl) have been found effective in stimulating hematopoiesis ($\delta$-aminolevulenic acid synthase) in patients with ***sideroblastic anemia***. Complexes of pyridoxal which chelate Fe (e.g., the isonicotinyl and benzoyl hydrazones) are effective in stimulating the excretion of that mineral in patients with ***Fe-storage disease***. High doses (e.g., 400 mg/day) reduce hyperoxaluria and, thus, the formation of ***renal oxalate stones***. The vitamin is used (at 3-5 mg/kg body weight) to counteract the toxic side effect of the anti-tuberculin drug ***isonicotinic hydrazide***[40], which produces a peripheral neuropathy[41] similar to that caused by vitamin B$_6$ deficiency. It is also recommended after the administration of other ***anti-B$_6$ drugs*** (penicillamine and 6-azauridine). Vitamin B$_6$ is recommended (.1-1 g/day alone or in combination with tryptophan or Mg) for the treatment of ***schizophrenia***, and to reduce the incidence of ***seizures in alcoholics***. It is recommended for the treatment of ***Herpes gestationis*** (at 400-4000 mg/day).

Pyridoxine has been reported to be effective in the treatment of ***carpal tunnel syndrome***[42] (100-300 mg/day), ***"Chinese restaurant" syndrome***[43] (50 mg/day) and, for some patients, ***premenstrual syndrome***[44] (40-500 mg/day); however, these effects have not been evaluated in double-blind, controlled clinical trials.

*hyper-vitaminosis*  The toxicity of vitamin B$_6$ appears to be relatively low, although high acute doses of the vitamin (several grams per kg body weight) have been shown to ***sensory neuronopathy*** marked by changes in gait and peripheral sensation. The primary target, thus, appears to be the peripheral nervous system; although massive doses of the vitamin have produced convulsions in rats, central nervous abnormalities have not been reported frequently in humans. The potential for toxicity resulting from the therapeutic or pharmacologic uses of the vitamin for human disorders (which rarely

---

[40] isoniazid

[41] Isoniazid is believed to inhibit pyridoxal phosphate-dependent glutamate-decarboxylase and $\gamma$-aminobutyrate aminotransferase (which produce and degrade GABA, respectively) in nerve tissue.

[42] This is a disorder involving pain and paresthesia of the hand caused by compression of the medial nerve by the transverse ligaments of the wrist. The idiopathic form is caused by a primary vitamin B$_6$ deficiency (identifiable by reduced activity of erythrocyte glutamate oxaloacetate transaminase) which leads to edematous changes to and proliferation of the synovia leading to compression of the nerve in the carpal tunnel.

[43] This involves headache, sensation of heat, altered heartbeat, nausea and tightness of the neck induced by oral intake of monosodium glutamate.

[44] This syndrome occurs in some women 2-3 days before their menstrual flows; it involves tension of the breasts, pain of the lumbar region, thirst, headache, nervous irritability, pelvic congestion, peripheral edema and, usually, nausea and vomiting.

exceed 50 mg/day) must be considered small. Reports of persons taking massive doses of the vitamin (>2 g/day) indicate that the earliest detectable signs were ataxia and loss of small motor control. Many of the signs of vitamin B$_6$ toxicity resemble those of vitamin B$_6$ deficiency; it has been proposed that the metabolic basis of each condition involves the tissue-level depletion of pyridoxal phosphate.

In doses of 10-25 mg, vitamin B$_6$ increases the conversion of L-dopa to dopamine[45] which, unlike its precursor, is unable to cross the blood-brain barrier. The vitamin can, thus, interfere with L-dopa in the management of Parkinson's disease; it should not be administered to persons taking L-dopa without the concomitant administration of a decarboxylase inhibitor.

# CASE STUDY

*Instructions:*     *Review the following case reports, paying special attention to the diagnostic indicators upon which the treatments were based. Then, answer the questions that follow.*

*case 1*     A 16-year-old boy was admitted with ***dislocated lenses*** and ***mental retardation***. Four years earlier, an ophthalmologist had found dislocation of the lenses. On the present occasion, he was thin and blond-headed, with ectopia lentis[46], an anterior thoracic deformity (*pectus excavatum*[47]) and normal vital signs. His palate was narrow with crowding of his teeth. He had mild scoliosis[48] and genu valgum[49], which caused him to walk with a toe-in, *"Chaplin-like"* gait. His neurological examination was within normal limits. Upon radiography, his spine appeared osteoporotic. His performance on the Stanford-Binet Intelligence Scale gave him a development quotient of 60. His hematology, blood glucose and blood urea-N values all within normal limits. His plasma ***homocystine*** level (undetectable in normal patients) was 4.5 mg/dl, and his blood ***methionine*** level was ten-fold normal; the levels of all other amino acids in his blood were within normal limits. Both homocystine and methionine were increased in

---

[45] It has been claimed that, *via* its effect on dopamine, vitamin B$_6$ can inhibit the release of prolactin, thus, inhibiting lactation in nursing mothers. Though this proposal is still highly disputed, their is no evidence that daily doses of less than ca. 10 mg of the vitamin (in multivitamin preparations) has any such effect on lactation.

[46] dislocated lenses

[47] funnel breast

[48] lateral curvature of the spine

[49] knock-knee

his urine, which also contained traces of **S-adenosylhomocystine**.

The patient was given oral **pyridoxine HCl** in an ascending dose regimen. Doses up to 150 mg/day were without effect but, after the dose had been increased to 325 mg/day for 200 days, his plasma and urinary homocystine and methionine levels decreased to normal. These changes were accompanied by a striking change in his hair pigmentation: dark hair grew out from the scalp (the cystine content of the dark hair was nearly double that of the blond hair, 1.5 vs. 0.8 $\mu$Eq/mg). On maintenance doses of pyridoxine, he attained relatively normal function, although the connective tissue changes were irreversible.

*case 2*    A 27-year-old woman had experienced increasing difficulty in walking. Some 2 years earlier, she had been told that vitamin $B_6$ prevented premenstrual edema and she began taking 500 mg/day of **pyridoxine HCl**. After a year, she had increased her intake of the vitamin to 5 g/day. During the period of this increased vitamin $B_6$ intake, she noticed that flexing her neck produced a tingling sensation down her neck and to her legs and soles of her feet[50]. During the 4 months immediately prior to this examination, she had become progressively unsteady when walking, particularly in the dark. Finally, she had become unable to walk without the assistance of a cane. She had also noticed difficulty in handling small objects, and changes in the feeling of her lips and tongue; although she reported no other positive sensory symptoms and was not aware of any weaknesses. Her gait was broad-based and stamping, and she was not able to walk at all with her eyes closed. Her muscle strength was normal, but all of her limb reflexes were absent. Her sensations of touch, temperature, pin-prick, vibration and joint position were severely impaired in both the upper and lower limbs. She showed a mild subjective alteration of touch-pressure and pin-prick sensation over her cheeks and lips, but not over her forehead. Laboratory findings showed the spinal fluid and other clinical tests to be normal. Electrophysiologic studies revealed that no sensory-nerve action potentials could be elicited in her arms and legs, but that motor-nerve conduction was normal.

The patient was suspected of having vitamin $B_6$ intoxication and was asked to stop taking that vitamin. Two months after withdrawal, she reported some improvement and a gain in sensation. By 7 months, she could walk steadily without a cane and could stand with her eyes closed. Neurologic examination at that time revealed that, although her strength was normal, her tendon reflexes were absent. Her feet still had severe loss of vibration sensation, despite definite improvements in the senses of joint-position, touch, temperature and pin-prick. Electrophysiologic examination revealed that her sensory nerve responses were still absent.

---

[50]Lhermitte's sign

Questions:   i.   Propose an *hypothesis* consistent with the findings in *case 1* for the congenital metabolic lesion experienced by that patient.

   ii.   Would you expect supplements of methionine and/or cystine to have been effective in treating the patient in *case 1*? Defend your answer.

   iii.   If the toxicity of pyridoxine involves its competition, at high levels, with pyridoxal phosphate for enzyme binding sites[51], which enzymes would you propose as potentially being affected in the condition described in *case 2*? Provide a rationale for each of the candidate enzymes on your list.

## *Study Questions and Exercises:*

i.   *Diagram* schematically the several steps in amino acid metabolism in which pyridoxal phosphate-dependent enzymes are involved.

ii.   Construct a *'decision tree'* for the diagnosis of vitamin $B_6$ deficiency in humans or an animal species.

iii.   What *key feature* of the chemistry of vitamin $B_6$ relates to its biochemical functions as a coenzyme?

iv.   What parameters might you measure to *assess vitamin $B_6$ status* of a human or animal?

v.   What factors might be expected to affect the *dietary need* for vitamin $B_6$?

---

[51]While this type of mechanism may sound reasonable, it is strictly speculative at this time as the mechanism of pyridoxine toxicity is not elucidated.

## Recommended Reading:

Bossler, K.H. 1988. Megavitamin Therapy with Pyridoxine. Int. J. Vit. Nutr. Res. 58:105-118.

Committee on Dietary Allowances, Food and Nutrition Board, Nat. Res. Council. 1978. Human Vitamin $B_6$ Requirements. Nat. Acad. Sci., Washington, D.C., 293 pp.

Dakshinamurti, K. (ed.). 1990. Vitamin $B_6$. Ann. N.Y. Acad. Sci., New York, vol. 585, 570 pp.

Flodin, N.W. 1988. Pharmacology of Micronutrients. A.R. Liss, New York, pp. 136-160.

Friedrich, W. 1988. Vitamins. Walter de Gruyter, New York. pp. 545-618.

Ink, S.L. and L.M. Henderson. 1984. Vitamin $B_6$ Metabolism. Ann. Rev. Nutr.4:455-470.

Leklem, J.E. 1991. Vitamin $B_6$, Chapter 9 *in* Handbook of Vitamins, 2nd. Ed. (L.J. Machlin, ed.), Marcel Dekker, New York. pp. 341-392.

Leklem, J.E. 1990. Vitamin B-6: a status report. J. Nutr. 120:1503-1507.

Leklem, J.E. and R.D. Reynolds (eds.) 1981. Methods in Vitamin B-6 Nutrition: Analysis and Status Assessment. Plenum Press, New York, 401 pp.

Merrill, Jr., A.H., and F.S. Burnham. 1990. Vitamin B-6, Chapter 18 *in* Present Knowledge in Nutrition, 6th ed. (M. Brown, ed.), Int. Life Sci. Inst.-Nutr. Found., Washington, D.C., pp. 155-162.

Merrill, Jr., A.H. and J. M. Henderson. 1987. Diseases Associated with Defects in Vitamin $B_6$ Metabolism or Utilization. Ann. Rev. Nutr. 7:137-156.

Tryfiates, G.P. (ed.) 1980. Vitamin $B_6$ Metabolism and Role in Growth. Food & Nutrition Press, Westport, Conn., 377 pp.

# CHAPTER 14    *BIOTIN*

*"We started with a bushel of corn, and at the end of the purification process, when the solution was evaporated in a small beaker, nothing could be seen, yet this solution of "nothing" greatly stimulated growth (of propionic acid bacteria).  We now know that the factor was biotin, which is one of the most effective of all vitamins."*        H.G. Wood

---

## Anchoring Concepts:

| | |
|---|---|
| *i.* | Biotin is the trivial designation of the compound hexahydro-2-oxo-1*H*-thieno-[3,4-d]imidazole-4-pentoic acid. |
| *ii.* | Biotin functions metabolically as a coenzyme for carboxylase to which it is bound by the C-2 of its thiophene ring via an amide bond to the $\epsilon$-amino group of a peptidyl lysine residue. |
| *iii.* | Deficiencies of biotin are manifest predominantly as dermatologic lesions. |

## Learning Objectives:

| | |
|---|---|
| *i.* | To understand the chief natural *sources* of biotin. |
| *ii.* | To understand the means of *absorption* and *transport* of biotin. |
| *iii.* | To understand the *biochemical function* of biotin as a component of co-enzymes of metabolically important carboxylation reactions. |
| *iv.* | To understand the *metabolic bases of biotin-responsive disorders*, including those related to dietary deprivation of the vitamin and those involving inherited metabolic lesions. |

329

*Vocabulary:*

| | |
|---|---|
| acetyl CoA carboxylase | FLKS |
| achromatrichia | holocarboxylase |
| acrodynia | kangaroo gait |
| alopecia | 3-methylcrotonyl CoA carboxylase |
| apocarboxylase | multiple carboxylase deficiencies |
| avidin | propionyl CoA carboxylase |
| biocytin | pyruvate carboxylase |
| biotin-binding proteins | SIDS |
| biotin holoenzyme sythetase | spectacle eye |
| biotinidase | streptavidin |
| biotinyl 5'-adenylate | transcarboxylase |
| egg white injury | |

# SOURCES OF BIOTIN

| | |
|---|---|
| *distribution in foods* | Biotin is widely distributed in foods and feedstuffs, but mostly in very low concentrations.  Only a couple of foods (royal jelly[1] and brewer's yeast) contain biotin in large amounts.  Milk, liver, egg (egg yolk) and a few vegetables are the most important natural sources of the vitamin in human nutrition; the oilseed meals, alfalfa meal and dried yeasts are the most important natural sources of the vitamin for the feeding of non-ruminant animals.  The biotin contents of foods and feedstuffs can be highly variable[2]; for the cereal grains at least, it is influenced by such factors as plant variety, season and yield (endosperm/pericarp ratio). |
| *stability* | Biotin is unstable to oxidizing conditions and, therefore, is destroyed by heat, especially under conditions that support simultaneous lipid peroxidation[3].  Therefore, such processing techniques as the canning of foods and the heat curing and solvent extraction of feedstuffs can result in substantial losses of biotin.  These losses can be reduced by the use of an antioxidant (e.g., vitamin C, vitamin E, BHT, BHA). |
| *bio-availability* | The nutritional availability of biotin to animals varies considerably among different foods and feedstuffs and can be very low.  This appears to be due to differential susceptibilities to digestion of the biotin-protein linkages in which the vitamin is found in natural products.  Those linkages involve the formation of covalent bonds between the carboxyl group of the biotin side-chain with free amino groups of proteins[4].  The utilization of biotin bound in such forms thus depends upon the hydrolytic digestion of the proteins and/or the hydrolysis of the amide bonds.  In general, less than one-half of the biotin present in feedstuffs is biologically available.  Although all of the biotin in corn is available, only 20-30% of that in most other grains and none in wheat is available.  Biotin in meat products also tends to be very |

---

[1] Royal jelly is a substance produced by the labial glands of "worker" honey bees and has been found to contain over 400 $\mu$g/100 g. Female honey bee larvae that are fed royal jelly develop reproductive ability as "queens"; whereas, those fed a mixture of honey and pollen fail to develop reproductive ability and become "workers".  Though the active factor in royal jelly has not been identified, it appears to be associated with the lipid fraction of that material (one known component, 10-hydroxy-$\Delta^2$-decenoic acid, has been suggested).  It is interesting to speculate about the apparent survival value to the honey bee colony of biotin as a component of this unique food which is necessary for the sexual development of the female.

[2] In one study the biotin contents of multiple samples of corn and meat meal were found to be 56-115 $\mu$g/kg (n=59) and 17-323 $\mu$g/kg (n=62), respectively.

[3] About 96% of the pure vitamin added to a feed was destroyed within 24 hrs after the addition of partially peroxidized linolenic acid.

[4] The formation of such amide linkages is the means by which biotin binds to the enzymes for which it serves as an essential prosthetic group.  In the cases of the biotinyl enzymes, however, the linkage involves the $\epsilon$-amino group of a peptidyl lysine residue; that form (i.e., biotinyl lysine) is referred to as "*biocytin*".

low. Biotin bioavailability can be determined experimentally by either of two bioassays: healing of skin lesions in avidin-fed rats; support of growth and maintenance of pyruvate carboxylase activity in chicks.

Biotin contents of foods:

| food | biotin µg/100g | food | biotin µg/100g |
|---|---|---|---|
| dairy products | | vegetables | |
| milk | 2 | asparagus | 2 |
| cheeses | 3-5 | brussels sprouts | .4 |
| meats | | cabbage | 2 |
| beef | 3 | carrots | 3 |
| chicken | 11 | cauliflower | 17 |
| pork | 5 | corn | 6 |
| calf kidney | 100 | kale | .5 |
| cereals | | lentils | 13 |
| barley | 14 | onions | 4 |
| cornmeal | 7.9 | peas | 9 |
| oats | 24.6 | potatoes | .1 |
| rye | 8.5 | soy beans | 60 |
| sorghum | 28.8 | spinach | 7 |
| wheat | 10.1 | tomatoes | 4 |
| wheat bran | 36 | fruits | |
| oilseed meals | | apples | 1 |
| rapeseed meal | 98.4 | bananas | 4 |
| soybean meal | 27 | grapefruit | 3 |
| other | | grapes | 2 |
| eggs | 20 | oranges | 1 |
| brewers' yeast | 80 | peaches | 2 |
| alfalfa meal | 54.3 | pears | .1 |
| molasses | 108 | strawberries | 1.1 |
| | | peanuts | 34 |
| | | walnuts | 37 |
| | | watermelons | 4 |

Biotin availability in several feedstuffs:

| feedstuff | total biotin[a] µg/100g | available biotin[b] µg/100g | bioavailability % |
|---|---|---|---|
| barley | 10.9 | 1.2 | 11 |
| corn | 5.0 | 6.5 | 133 |
| wheat | 8.4 | .4 | 5 |
| rapeseed meal | 93.0 | 57.4 | 62 |
| sunflowerseed meal | 119.0 | 41.5 | 35 |
| soybean meal | 25.8 | 27.8 | 108 |

[a]determined by microbiological assay    [b]determined by chick growth assay
source: Whitehead et al., 1982, Brit. J. Nutr. 48:81.

*synthesis by intestinal microflora*

Biotin synthesized by the microflora in the distal intestine can be absorbed and a substantial body of indirect evidence suggests that gut microbial synthesis can contribute significantly to the biotin nutrition of non-ruminant animals. In both rats and humans it has been found that total fecal excretion of biotin (in both urine and feces) exceeds the amount consumed in the diet. In fact, the dietary requirement of the rat for biotin has only been determined under gnotobiotic[5] conditions or with avidin feeding.

# ABSORPTION OF BIOTIN

*liberation from bound forms*  In the digestion of food proteins, protein-bound biotin is released by the hydrolytic action of the intestinal proteases to yield the biotinyllysine adduct, *biocytin*, from which free biotin is liberated by that action of intestinal *biotinidase*[6].

*two types of transport*  Little is known about the mechanism of enteric biotin absorption. Free biotin is absorbed in the proximal small intestine by what appears to be two mechanisms, depending on its lumenal concentration. At low concentrations, it is absorbed by a saturable, *facilitated diffusion* dependent upon $Na^+$. This process has been found to be inhibited by certain anti-convulsant drugs[7] and chronic ethanol exposure. At high concentrations, non-saturable, *simple diffusion* of the vitamin occurs.

*absorption in the distal intestine*  The distal intestine appears to have an important role in the enteric absorption of biotin, which can be present in that region of the gut by virtue of the biosynthesis of the vitamin by intestinal bacteria. Studies with rats have shown that the absorptive capacity of the colon is substantial and that of the cecum is sufficient for the uptake of all bacterially synthesized biotin.

# TRANSPORT OF BIOTIN

*protein-binding likely*  The means by which biotin is transported has not been characterized, although it is thought to involve a specific ligand, e.g., a biotin-binding protein. *Biotin-binding proteins* have been identified in the egg yolks of many species of birds, and a few species of mammals and reptiles. These are believed to function in the transport of the vitamin into the oocyte, as

---

[5] germ-free

[6] biotinamide aminohydrolase

[7] carbamazepine and primidone

their binding to it is weak enough to be reversible[8]. The yolk biotin-binding protein also occurs in the plasma of the laying hen. The only biotin-binding protein in human plasma appears to be **biotinidase**, which has two high-affinity binding sites for the vitamin and, thus, has been proposed to function in its transport. Biotinidase also occurs in human milk, where it may have important functions in the transport of biotin by the mammary gland and/or its utilization by the infant.

*tissue*
*distribution*
Biotin appears to be taken up by cells *via* a specific carrier-mediated process, although that, too, has not been characterized. Appreciable storage of the vitamin appears to occur in the liver, where concentrations of 800-3000 ng/g have been found in various species[9]. Hepatic stores, however, appear to be poorly mobilized during biotin deprivation and, thus, do not show the reductions measurable in plasma under such conditions.

## METABOLISM OF BIOTIN

*linkage to*
*apoenzymes*
Free biotin is attached to its apoenzymes *via* the formation of an amide linkage to the ε-amino group of a specific lysine residue. In each of the four biotin-dependent enzymes, this binding occurs in a region containing the same amino acid sequence (-ALA-MET-biotinylLYS-MET-); it catalyzed by the **biotin holoenzyme synthetases**[10].

*recycling*
*the vitamin*
The normal turnover of the biotin-containing holocarboxylases involves their degradation to yield **biocytin**. The biotinyl-lysine bond is not hydrolyzed by cellular proteases; however, it is cleaved by **biotinidase**[8] to yield free biotin. This step is essential for the re-utilization of biotin, which is accomplished by its re-incorporation into another holoenzyme. Congenital deficiencies of biotinidase have been described. These are characterized by deficiencies of the multiple biotin-dependent carboxylases; in some cases, they can be corrected with pharmacologic doses of the vitamin.

---

[8]The biotin-binding protein of the chicken egg is a glycoprotein with a molecular weight of 74.3 kD and an homologous tetrameric structure each subunit of which binds a biotin molecule. This egg yolk protein is not to be confused with **avidin**, the biotin-binding protein of egg white, which irreversibly binds biotin with an affinity three orders of magnitude greater than that of the yolk protein.

[9]These levels contrast to those of plasma/serum which, in humans and rats, are typically ca. 300 ng/l.

[10]Several holoenzyme synthetases have been characterized in microorganisms; but among animals these have been characterized only in birds. It is presumed, however, that such an enzyme exists in animals including humans which, after all, have biotin bound in the same way in their biotin-dependent carboxylases.

*catabolism*      Little catabolism of biotin seems to occur.  A small fraction is oxidized to biotin D- and L-***sulfoxides***, but the ureido ring system is not otherwise degraded.  The side-chain of a larger portion is metabolized *via* mitochondrial β-oxidation to yield ***bis-nor-biotin*** and its degradation products.

*excretion*      Biotin is rapidly excreted in the urine in the form of *free biotin*, the D- and L-*sulfoxides* and *side-chain products*[11,12,13].

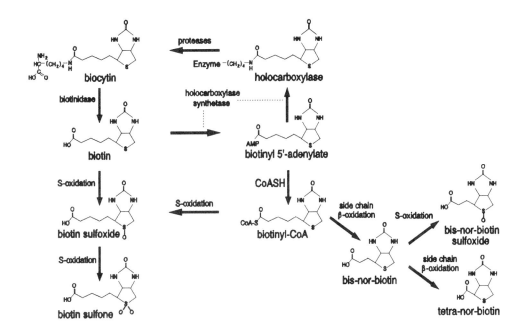

---

[11] The rat was shown to excrete ca. 95% of a single oral dose (5 mg/kg) of the vitamin within 24 hrs.

[12] Although unabsorbed biotin appears in the feces, much fecal biotin is of gut microbial origin and benefits the host.  Thus, at low dietary levels of the vitamin, urinary excretion of biotin can exceed intake.

[13] The urinary excretion of patients with achlorhydria is very low.  It is thought that this reflects impaired release of bound biotin for absorption.

## METABOLIC FUNCTIONS OF BIOTIN

*mechanism*      Biotin functions as a mobile *carboxyl carrier* in *four carboxylase enzymes*
*of action*      of animals and in a number of other carboxylases, transcarboxylases[14]
                 and decarboxylases in microorganisms.  The biotin prosthetic group is
                 linked to each apoenzyme covalently to the $\epsilon$-amino group of a lysyl
                 residue.  The formation of this linkage is catalyzed by *biotin holoenzyme*
                 *synthetases*, in two steps.  The first step involves the activation of the
                 vitamin as *biotinyl 5'-adenylate*; the second step involves the covalent
                 attachment of the vitamin to the apocarboxylase with the release of AMP.

                 The catalytic action of each of the biotin-dependent carboxylases of
                 animals proceed in a non-classic, "two-site", "ping-pong" mechanism, with
                 partial reactions being performed by dissimilar subunits.  The first reaction
                 (*"biotin carboxylase"*) occurs at the *carboxylase sub-site*; it involves the
                 enzymatically carboxylation of biotin using the bicarbonate/ATP system as
                 the carboxyl donor.  The following step (*"carboxyl transferase"*) occurs at
                 the *carboxyl transferase sub-site*; it involves transfer of the carboxyl
                 group from carboxybiotin to the acceptor substrate.  These two sub-sites
                 appear to be spatially separated in each enzyme.  The physiochemical
                 mechanisms proposed for these reactions entail the transfer of biotinyl-$CO_2$
                 between sub-sites *via* movement of the prosthetic group back and forth by
                 virtue of rotation of at least one of the 10 single bonds (probably C2-C6)
                 on the valeryl-lysyl side-chain.

                 Enzyme $-(CH_2)_4-\overset{H}{\underset{}{N}}$

*metabolic*      The biotin-containing carboxylases have important functions in the metab-
*roles*          olism of lipids, glucose, some amino acids and energy.  *Pyruvate carbox-*
                 *ylase*, in conjunction with phosphoenolpyruvate carboxykinase (PEPCK),
                 has a key role in gluconeogenesis:  formation of phosphoenolpyruvate
                 from 3-carbon precursors.  That enzyme also serves to replenish the
                 supply of oxaloacetate in the mitochondria to support the citric acid cycle
                 as well as the formation of citrate for transport to the cytosol for
                 lipogenesis.  *Acetyl CoA carboxylase* catalyzes the first committed step
                 in the synthesis of fatty acids.  *Propionyl CoA carboxylase* catalyzes the
                 oxidation of odd-chain fatty acids produced by the degradation of the
                 branched-chain amino acids as well as methionine and threonine, and by

---

[14]Transcarboxylase is called by those working with it the *"Mickey Mouse Enzyme"*, as the electron
micrograph of the purified bacterial enzyme, with its large single subunit and two smaller subunits flanking to
one side, resembles the head of the famous rodent.

the ruminal and/or gastro-intestinal microflora. The enzyme produces methylmalonyl CoA, which is used for energy and glucose production. The biotin-dependent enzyme *3-methylcrotonyl CoA carboxylase* degrades the ketogenic amino acid, leucine.

Biotin-dependent carboxylases of animals:

| enzyme | location | metabolic function |
|---|---|---|
| pyruvate carboxylase | mitochondria | formation of oxaloacetate from pyruvate; requires acetyl CoA |
| acetyl CoA carboxylase | cytosol | formation of malonyl CoA from acetyl CoA for fatty acid synthesis; requires citrate |
| propionyl CoA carboxylase | mitochondria | formation of methylmalonyl CoA from propionyl CoA produced by catabolism of some amino acids (e.g., isoleucine) and odd-chain fatty acids |
| 3-methylcrotonyl CoA carboxylase | mitochondria | part of the leucine degradation pathway |

# EXTREMES IN BIOTIN INTAKE

deficiency
Because biotin is rather widespread among foods and feedstuffs and is synthesized by the intestinal microflora[15], simple deficiencies of biotin in animals or humans are rare. However, biotin deficiency can be induced by certain antagonists.

"egg white injury"
When, in the mid-1930s, it was found that biotin supplements prevented the dermatitis and alopecia produced in experimental animals by feeding uncooked egg white, the damaging factor was isolated and named *"avidin"*. Avidin is a water-soluble basic glycoprotein secreted by the oviductal cells of birds, reptiles and amphibians and, thus, found in the whites of their eggs[16]. It antagonizes biotin by forming a non-covalent complex with the vitamin[17,18] which is not attacked by the digestive

---

[15] Although it is clear that the gut microflora synthesize biotin, the quantitative importance of this source to the biotin-nutrition of humans and other non-ruminant species is highly speculative.

[16] Avidin has a molecular weight of 67 kD. It is a homologous tetramer each 128 amino acid subunit of which binds a molecule of biotin, probably *via* linkage to a tryptophan residue. The binding of biotin to avidin is the strongest known non-covalent bond in nature. It is thought that biotin functions in the egg as a natural antibiotic.

[17] Avidin binds biotin at a site involving 2-4 tryptophan residues and probably an adjacent lysine.

proteases thus preventing the absorption of biotin[19]. The avidin-biotin complex is unstable to heat; heating to at least 100°C denatures the protein and releases biotin available for absorption[20]. As a tool to produce experimental biotin deficiency, avidin in the form of dried egg white has been very useful[21].

*deficiency*
*syndromes in*
*animals*

Avidin-induced biotin deficiency causes the syndrome originally referred to as *"egg white injury"*. The major lesions appear to involve impairments in lipid metabolism and energy production. In rats and mice, this is characterized by seborrheic *dermatitis* and *alopecia*, a hind limb paralysis that results in *"kangaroo gait"*, and *congenital malformations* (cleft palate, micrognathia[22], micromelia[23]). Fur-bearing animals (mink and fox) show general dermatitis with hyperkeratosis, circumocular alopecia (*"spectacle eye"*), *achromotrichia* of the underfur, and unsteady gait. Pigs and kittens show weight loss, digestive dysfunction, dermatitis, alopecia and brittle claws. Guinea pigs and rabbits show weight loss, alopecia and achromotrichia. Monkeys show severe dermatitis of the face, hands and feet, alopecia and watery eyes with encrusted lids. All species show *depressed activities of the biotin-dependent carboxylases*, which respond rapidly to biotin therapy.

Biotin deficiency can be produced in chicks by dietary deprivation and seems to occur from time to time in practical poultry production, particularly in northern Europe[24]. This results in impaired growth and reduced efficiency of feed utilization, and is characterized by dermatitis (mainly at the corners of the beak). In some instances, death occurs suddenly

---

[18] Two very similar biotin-binding proteins have been identified, both of which show considerable sequence homology at the biotin-binding site with avidin. One, from *Streptomyces avidinii*, is called *"streptavidin"*. The other is an epidermal growth factor homologue found in the purple sea urchin *Stongylocentrotus purpatus*.

[19] It is of interest to note that some cultured mammalian cells (e.g., fibroblasts and HeLa cells) are able to absorb the biotin-avidin complex, using it as a source of the vitamin.

[20] Therefore, while raw egg white is antagonistic to the utilization of biotin, the cooked product is without effect. In reference to the consumption of raw or under-cooked eggs, the avidin antagonism is probably of little consequence as the biotin-binding capacity of avidin in the egg white is roughly comparable to the biotin content of the egg yolk.

[21] Other structural analogues of biotin are also antagonistic to its function: $a$-dehydrobiotin, 5-(2-thienyl)valeric acid, acidomycin, $a$-methylbiotin and $a$-methyldethiobiotin, several of which are antibiotics.

[22] underdevelopment of the jaw (usually the lower jaw)

[23] undergrowth the limbs

[24] In that part of the world, barley and wheat, each of which has little biologically available biotin, are frequently used as major ingredients in poultry diets.

without gross lesions; this condition usually involves hepatic and renal steatosis with hypoglycemia, lethargy, paralysis and hepatomegaly and is, thus, referred to as *"fatty liver and kidney syndrome"* (*"FLKS"*). The etiology of FLKS appears to be complex, involving such other factors as choline, but seems to involve a marginal deficiency of biotin which impairs gluconeogenesis by limiting the activity of pyruvate carboxylase, especially under circumstances of glycogen depletion brought on by stress.

Signs of biotin deficiency:

| organ system | signs |
|---|---|
| appetite | decrease |
| growth | decrease |
| dermatologic | dermatitis, alopecia, achromotrichia |
| skeletal | perosis |
| vital organs | hepatic steatosis, FLKS |

*deficiency signs in humans*

Few cases of biotin deficiency have been reported in humans. Most of these have involved nursing infants whose mothers' milk contained inadequate supplies of the vitamin[25], or patients receiving incomplete parenteral nutrition. One case involved a child fed raw eggs for 6 years. The signs and symptoms included dermatitis, glossitis, anorexia, nausea, depression, hepatic steatosis and hypercholesterolemia. It is thought that marginal biotin status plays a causative role in the etiology of *Sudden Infant Death Syndrome (SIDS)* which occurs in human infants at 2-4 months of age. In many ways, SIDS resembles FLKS in the chick, a marginal biotin status coupled with stress is thought to be an important cause of each disease[26]. The frequency of marginal biotin status (deficiency without clinical manifestation) is not known, but the incidence of low circulating biotin levels has been found to be substantially greater among alcoholics than the general population[27]. Relatively low levels of biotin (*vs.* healthy controls) have also been reported in the plasma or urine of patients with partial gastrectomy or other causes of achlorhydria, burn patients, epileptics[28], elderly individual and athletes.

---

[25]The biotin content of human milk, particularly early in lactation, is often insufficient to meet the demands of infants. Therefore, it is recommended that nursing mothers take a biotin supplement. When this is done, substantial increases in the biotin concentrations of breast milk are observed (e.g., a 3 mg/day supplement increased milk biotin concentrations from 1.2-1.5 $\mu g/dl$ to $>33$ $\mu g/dl$).

[26]Studies have shown that infants who died of SIDS had significantly lower hepatic concentrations of biotin than those of infants who died from unrelated causes.

[27]About 15% of alcoholics has plasma biotin concentrations less than 140 pmoles/l; whereas, only 1% of randomly selected hospital patients had plasma biotin levels that low.

[28]This may be due to anticonvulsant drug therapy, known side effects of which are dermatitis and ataxia. Some anti-convulsants (e.g., carbamazepine and primidone) have been shown to be competitive inhibitors of biotin transport across the intestinal brush border.

*congenital*　　Genetic defects in all of the known biotin enzymes have been identified in
*disorders*　　humans. These are rare, affecting infants and children, and usually having
　　serious consequences. Some, in which the defect involves the absence of
　　a biotin apoenzyme do not respond to supplements of the vitamin and are
　　treated by limiting the production of metabolites upstream of the metabolic
　　lesion through restriction of dietary protein. Other congenital disorders
　　(the multiple carboxylase deficiencies) respond to high doses of biotin.

Congenital disorders of biotin enzymes:

| defect | metabolic basis | physiological effect | treatment |
|---|---|---|---|
| propionyl CoA carb. deficiency | autosomal recessive lack of enzyme[a] | propionate accumulation: acidemia, keto-acidosis, hyperammonemia; high urine citrate, 3-OH-propionate, propionyl glycine<br>*symptoms*[b]: vomiting, lethargy, hypotonia, mental retardation, cramps | restrict protein biotin |
| pyruvate carb. deficiency | autosomal recessive lack of enzyme[c] | changes in energy production, gluconeo-genesis and other pathways<br>*symptoms*: metabolic acidosis (lactate), hypotonia, mental retardation | none |
| 3-methylcrotonyl CoA carb. deficiency | defective enzyme (basis unknown[d]) | high urine 3-$CH_3$-crotonylglycine and and 3-OH-isovaleric acid<br>*symptoms*: cramps | restrict protein |
| acetyl CoA carb. deficiency | lack of enzyme, (basis unknown[e]) | aciduria;<br>*symptoms*: myopathy, neurologic changes | none |
| multiple carb. deficiency, *neonatal type* | autosomal recessive lack of holoenzyme synthase[f] | deficiencies of all biotin-containing holocarboxylases; acidosis and aciduria<br>*symptoms*: vomiting, lethargy, hypotonia | massive doses of biotin |
| multiple carb. deficiency, *juvenile type* | autosomal recessive lack of biotinidase[g] | deficiencies of all biotin-containing holocarboxylases; acidosis and aciduria<br>*symptoms*: skin rash, alopeica, conjunctiv-itis, ataxia, developmental anomalies | massive doses of biotin |

[a]Incidence: 1/350,000　　[b]There is a wide variation in the clinical expression.　　[c]<2 dozen patients described.　　[d]3 confirmed cases.　　[e]1 case described. [f]Involves failure to link biotin to the *apo*-carboxylases to produce active holoenzymes.　[g]Involves failure to release biotin from its bound forms in the holocarboxylases; this reduces use of biotin in foods and blocks endogenous recycling of the vitamin.

*hyper-*　　The toxicity of biotin appears to be very low. No cases have been reported
*vitaminosis*　　of adverse reactions by humans to high levels of the vitamin as are used
　　in treating seborrheic dermatitis in infants, egg white injury or inborn errors
　　or metabolism. Animal studies have revealed few, if any, indications of
　　toxicity, and it is probable that animals including humans can tolerate the
　　vitamin at doses at least an order of magnitude greater than their
　　respective nutritional requirements.

## CASE STUDY

Instructions:   Review the following case report, paying special attention to the diagnostic indicators upon which the treatments were based.   Then, answer the questions that follow.

case   This 12-month-old girl had experienced malrotation[29] and midgut volvulus[30], resulting in extensive infarction[31] of the small and large bowel, at 4 months of age.  Her bowel was resected, after which her clinical course was complicated by failure of the anastomosis[32] to heal, peritoneal infection and intestinal obstruction.  After several subsequent surgeries, she was left with only 30 cm of jejunum, 0.5 cm of ileum and approximately 50% of colon.  By 5 months of age, she had lost 1.5 kg in weight and total parenteral nutrition[33] (TPN) was initiated (providing 125 kcal/kg/day).  By the third month of TPN, she had gained 2.9 kg; thereafter, her energy intake was reduced to 60 kcal/kg/day, which sustained her growth within the normal range.  Soybean oil emulsion[34] was administered parenterally at least twice weekly in amounts that provided 3.9% of total calories as linoleic acid.  Repeated attempts at feeding her orally failed because of vomiting and rapid intestinal transit; therefore, her only source of nutrients was TPN.  She had repeated episodes of sepsis and wound infection; broad spectrum antibiotics were administered virtually continuously from 4-11 months of age.  Multiple enteroenteric and enterocutaneous fistulas[35] were formed; over 8 months, they provided daily fluid losses >500 ml.

During the third month of TPN, an erythematous[36] rash was noted on the

---

[29] failure of normal rotation of the intestinal tract

[30] twisting of the intestine causing obstruction

[31] necrotic changes resulting from obstruction of an end artery

[32] an operative union of two hollow or tubular structures, in this case the divided ends of the intestine

[33] feeding *via* means other than through the alimentary canal, referring particularly to the introduction of nutrients into veins

[34] e.g., Intralipid[R]

[35] passages created between one part of the intestine and another (an enteroenteric fistula) or between the intestine and the skin of the abdomen (an enterocutaneous fistula)

[36] marked by redness of the skin due to inflammation

patient's lower eyelids adjacent to the outer canthi[37]. Over the next 3 months the rash spread, became more exfoliative and exuded clear fluid. New lesions appeared in the angles of the mouth, around the nostrils and in the perineal region[38]. This condition did not respond to topical application of various antibiotics, cortisone and safflower oil.

During the fifth and sixth months of TPN, the patient lost all body hair, developed a waxy pallor, irritability, lethargy and mild hypotonia[39]. That she was not deficient in essential fatty acids was indicated by the finding that her plasma fatty acid triene:tetraene ratio was normal (0.11). During the period from the third to the sixth month, the patient was given parenteral Zn supplements at 7, 30 and 250 times the normal requirement (0.2 mg/day). Her serum Zn concentration increased from 35 to 150 $\mu$g/dl (normal: 50-150 $\mu$g/dl) and, finally, to greater than 2000 $\mu$g/dl without any beneficial effect. Intravenous Zn supplementation was then reduced to 0.4 mg/day. Biotin was determined by a bioassay using *Ochromonas danica*; urinary organic acids were determined by HPLC[40] and GC/MS[41]:

Laboratory results:

| parameter | patient | normal range |
|---|---|---|
| plasma biotin | 135 pg/ml | 215-750 pg/ml |
| urinary biotin excretion | <1 $\mu$g/24 hr | 6-50 $\mu$g/24 hr |
| urinary organic acid excretion: | | |
| methylcitrate | .1 $\mu$mole/mg creatinine | <.01 $\mu$mole/mg creatinine |
| 3-methylcrotonylglycine | .7 $\mu$mole/mg creatinine | <.2 $\mu$mole/mg creatinine |
| 3-hydroxyisovalerate | .35$\mu$mole/mg creatinine | <.2 $\mu$mole/mg creatinine |

Treatment with biotin (10 mg/day) was initiated and, after 1 week, plasma biotin concentration increased to 11,500 pg/ml and organic acid excretion dropped to <0.01 $\mu$mole/mg creatinine. After 7 days of biotin supplementation, the rash had improved strikingly and the irritability had resolved. After 2 weeks of supplementation, new hair growth was noted, waxy pallor of the skin was less pronounced and hypotonia improved. During the next 9 months of biotin therapy, no symptoms and signs of deficiency recurred. The patient's rapid transit time and vomiting did not improve.

---

[37] corners of the eye

[38] the area between the thighs extending from the coccyx to the pubis

[39] a condition of reduced tension of any muscle leading to damage by over-stretching

[40] high-performance liquid-liquid partition chromatography

[41] gas-liquid partition chromatography with mass spectrometric detection

*Questions:*      i.       What signs were first to suggest a problem related to biotin utilization by the patient?

                  ii.      What is the relevance of aciduria to considerations of biotin status?

                  iii.     How were problems involving essential fatty acids and Zn ruled out in the diagnosis of this condition as biotin deficiency?

## Study Questions and Exercises:

i.       ***Diagram*** the areas of metabolism in which biotin-dependent carboxylases are involved.

ii.      Construct a ***"decision tree"*** for the diagnosis of biotin deficiency in humans or an animal species.

iii.     What ***key feature*** of the chemistry of biotin relates to its biochemical function as a carrier of "active" $CO_2$?

iv.      What parameters might you measure to ***assess biotin status*** of a human or animal?

## Recommended Reading:

Bonjour, J.P. 1991. Biotin, Chapter 10 *in* Handbook of Vitamins, 2nd ed. (L.J. Machlin, ed.), Marcel Dekker, New York. pp. 393-427.

Dakshinamurti, K. and H.N. Bhagvan (eds.). 1985. Biotin. Ann. N.Y. Acad. Sci. vol. 447. 441 pp.

Dakshinamurti, K. and J. Chauhan. 1989. Biotin. Vit. Horm. 45:337-384.

Dakshinamurti, K. and J. Chauhan. 1988. Regulation of Biotin Enzymes. Ann. Rev. Nutr. 8:211-233.

Flodin, N.W. 1988. Pharmacology of Micronutrients. Alan R. Liss., Inc., New York, pp. 193-200.

Friedrich, W. 1988. Biotin, Chapter 11 *in* Vitamins. Walter de Gruyter, New York. pp. 753-805.

Mock, D.M. 1990. Biotin, Chapter 22 *in* Present Knowledge in Nutrition, 6th ed. (M. Brown, ed.), Int. Life Sci. Inst.-Nutr. Found., Washington, D.C., pp. 189-207.

# CHAPTER 15   *PANTOTHENIC ACID*

*"A pellagrous-like syndrome in chicks has recently been obtained . . . in an experiment which was originally designed to throw added light upon an unusual type of leg problem occurring in chicks fed semi-synthetic rations. . . . The data obtained in this experiment demonstrate the requirement in another species of the vitamin or vitamins present in autoclaved yeast, occasionally called vitamin B$_2$, vitamin G or the P-P factor, and indicate that the chick may be a more suitable animal than the white rat for delineating the quantities of this vitamin present in feedstuffs."*

L.C. Norris and A.T. Ringrose

---

## Anchoring Concepts:

| | |
|---|---|
| i. | Pantothenic acid is the trivial designation for the compound dihydroxy-$\beta,\beta$-dimethylbutyrl-$\beta$-alanine. |
| ii. | Pantothenic acid is metabolically active as the prosthetic group of coenzyme A (CoA) and the acyl-carrier protein. |
| iii. | Deficiencies of pantothenic acid are manifest as dermal, hepatic, thymic and neurologic changes. |

## Learning Objectives:

| | |
|---|---|
| i. | To understand the chief natural *sources* of pantothenic acid. |
| ii. | To understand the means of *absorption* and *transport* of pantothenic acid. |
| iii. | To understand the *biochemical functions* of pantothenic acid as components of *coenzyme A* and the *acyl-carrier protein*. |
| iv. | To understand the physiological implications of *low pantothenic acid status*. |

## Vocabulary:

acetyl CoA
acyl-carrier protein
acyl-CoA synthase
burning feet syndrome
CoA
dephospho-CoA
dephospho-CoA kinase
fatty acid synthase
malonyl CoA
$w$-methylpantothenic acid
pantothenic acid
pantetheinase

4'-phosphopantetheine
4'-phosphopantetheine adenyl-
    transferase
4'-phosphopantothenic acid
4'-phosphopantothenylcysteine
4'-phosphopantothenylcysteine
    decarboxylase
4'-phosphopantothenylcysteine
    synthase
propionyl CoA
succinyl CoA

# SOURCES OF PANTOTHENIC ACID

*distribution in foods*
As its name implies, pantothenic acid is widely distributed in nature.  It occurs mainly in bound forms (CoA, acyl-carrier protein); therefore, it must be determined in foods and feedstuffs after enzymatic hydrolysis.  The most important food sources of pantothenic acid are meats (liver and heart are particularly rich).  Mushrooms, avocados, broccoli and some yeasts are also rich in the vitamin.  Whole grains are also good sources; however, the vitamin is localized in the outer layers, thus, it is largely removed by milling.  The most important sources of pantothenic acid for animal feeding are rice and wheat brans, alfalfa, peanut meal, molasses, yeasts, and condensed fish solubles.  The richest source of the vitamin in nature is royal jelly[1].

Pantothenic acid contents of foods:

| food | pantothenic acid, mg/100g | food | pantothenic acid, mg/100g |
|---|---|---|---|
| dairy products | | vegetables | |
| milk | .2 | avocado | 1.1 |
| cheeses | .1-.9 | broccoli | 1.2 |
| meats | | cabbage | .1-1.4 |
| beef | .3-2 | carrots | .27 |
| pork | .4-3.1 | cauliflower | 1.0 |
| calf heart | 2.5 | lentils | 1.4 |
| calf kidney | 3.9 | potatoes | .3 |
| chicken liver | 9.7 | soy beans | 1.7 |
| pork liver | 7.0 | tomatoes | .3 |
| cereals | | fruits | |
| cornmeal | .9 | apples | .1 |
| rice, unpolished | 1.1 | bananas | .2 |
| oatmeal | .9 | grapefruits | .3 |
| wheat | 1.0 | oranges | .2 |
| wheat bran | 2.9 | strawberries | .3 |
| barley | 1.1 | walnuts | .7 |
| other | | cashews | 1.3 |
| eggs | 2.9 | peanuts | 2.8 |
| mushrooms | 2.1 | | |
| baker's yeast | 5.3-11 | | |

*stability*
Pantothenic acid in foods and feedstuffs is fairly stable to ordinary means of cooking and storage.  It can, however, be unstable at heat and either alkaline (pH >7) or acid (pH <5) conditions[2].  Appreciable losses (up to 50%) have been reported due to canning and storage of some foods.

---

[1] Royal jelly, the food responsible for the diet-induced reproductive development of the queen honey bee, is also the richest natural source of biotin (see Chapter 14, footnote #1).

[2] Pasteurization of milk, due to its neutral pH, does not affect its content of pantothenic acid.

*bio-*
*availability*     The biologic availability of pantothenic acid from foods and feedstuffs has
                   not been well investigated. The results of one study are available; they
                   indicate that the vitamin in foods has an availability of 40%-60% to humans.


## ABSORPTION OF PANTOTHENIC ACID

*hydrolysis*      Because pantothenic acid occurs in most foods and feedstuffs as CoA and
*of coenzyme*     the acyl-carrier protein (ACP), the utilization of the vitamin in foods depends
*forms*           upon their hydrolytic digestion of these protein complexes to release the
                  free vitamin. Both CoA and ACP are degraded in the lumen of the intestine
                  to release the vitamin as ***4'-phosphopantetheine***. That form is dephos-
                  phorylated to yield ***pantetheine***, which is rapidly converted by the intestinal
                  ***pantetheinase*** to ***pantothenic acid***.

*carrier-*        Pantothenic acid is absorbed by a saturable, $Na^+$-dependent, energy-
*mediated*        requiring process[3]. At high levels, it is also absorbed by simple diffusion
                  throughout the small intestine[4]. The alcohol form, ***panthenol***, which is
                  oxidized to pantothenic acid *in vivo*, appears to be absorbed somewhat
                  faster than the acid form.

---

[3]The intestinal pantothenic acid transporter has been demonstrated in the rat, chick and mouse.

[4]Earlier studies in which unphysiologically high concentrations of the vitamin were employed failed to
detect the carrier-mediated mechanism of its enteric absorption. This led to the conclusion that the vitamin is
absorbed only by simple diffusion.

## TRANSPORT OF PANTOTHENIC ACID

*free in plasma;*   Pantothenic acid is transported in the free acid form in free solution in the
*as CoA in*      plasma. Erythrocytes, which carry most of the vitamin in the blood[5,6],
*blood cells*     contain it predominantly in the form of CoA.

*tissue*           Pantothenic acid is transported into cells in its free acid form by a $Na^+$-
*distribution*   dependent, active process mediated by a specific carrier protein. Upon
cellular uptake, most of the vitamin is converted to CoA, the predominant
form in most tissues. The greatest concentrations of CoA are found in the
liver[7], adrenals, kidneys[8], brain[9], heart and testes.

## METABOLISM OF PANTOTHENIC ACID

*Co A*           All tissues have the ability to synthesize CoA from pantothenic acid of
*biosynthesis*  dietary origin. In each tissue, the rate-limiting step in this process[10] is the
first reaction, which involves phosphorylation of pantothenic acid ***pantothenate kinase*** to yield ***4'-phosphopantothenic acid***. That product is
subsequently condensed with cysteine by ***phosphopantothenylcysteine
synthetase*** to yield ***4'-phosphopantothenylcysteine***[11], the cysteinyl

---

[5] For example, in the human adult, whole blood contains 1120-1960 ng total pantothenic acid per ml; of that, the plasma contains 211-1096 ng/ml.

[6] Blood pantothenic acid levels are generally lower in elderly individuals, e.g., 500-700 ng/ml.

[7] The human liver typically contains ca. 28 mg of total pantothenic acid.

[8] There appear to be two renal mechanisms for regulating the excretion of pantothenic acid: at physiological concentrations of the vitamin in the plasma, pantothenic acid is reabsorbed by active transport; at higher concentrations, tubular secretion of pantothenic acid occurs. Tubular reabsorption appears to be the only mechanism for conserving free pantothenic acid in the plasma.

[9] Pantothenic acid is taken up by a specific transport process in the choroid plexus which, at low concentrations of the vitamin, involves the partial phosphorylation of the vitamin. The cerebrospinal fluid, because it is constantly renewed in the central nervous system, requires a constant supply of pantothenic acid which, as CoA, is involved in the synthesis of the neurotransmitter acetylcholine in brain tissue.

[10] At least in rat liver, all of the enzymes in the CoA biosynthetic pathway are found in the cytosol; the two ATP-requiring enzymes are *also* found in the mitochondria.

[11] It is likely that 4'-phosphopantetheine, produced only in the cytosol, is transported into the mitochondria where it is converted to CoA by the latter enzymes of the biosynthetic pathway that are found in that organelle. That such a precursor serves as a source of mitochondrial CoA is evident, as CoA itself cannot pass the inner mitochondrial membrane.

residue of which is then decarboxylated by *phosphopantothenylcysteine decarboxylase* to yield *4'-phosphopantetheine*. That product is converted to *CoA* by two ATP-requiring steps[12]: *phosphopantetheine adenyltransferase*[13] and *dephospho-CoA kinase*.

The biosynthesis of CoA is inhibited strongly by acetyl CoA, malonyl CoA and propionyl CoA, and more weakly by CoA and long-chain acyl CoAs, all of which appear to act as allosteric effectors of pantothenate kinase. The ethanol metabolite acetaldehyde also inhibits the conversion of

---

[12] Four moles of ATP are required for the biosynthesis of one mole of CoA from a single mole of pantothenic acid.

[13] The reaction is reversible; therefore, at low ATP levels dephospho-CoA can be degraded to yield ATP.

pantothenic acid to CoA, although the mechanism of this effect is not clear[14].

*ACP*
*biosynthesis*

The acyl-carrier protein (ACP) contains a **4'-phosphopantetheine** residue which is transferred to it from CoA by the action of **4'-phosphopante-theine-apoACP transferase**. The prosthetic group is bound to the apo-ACP via linkage at a serinyl residue.

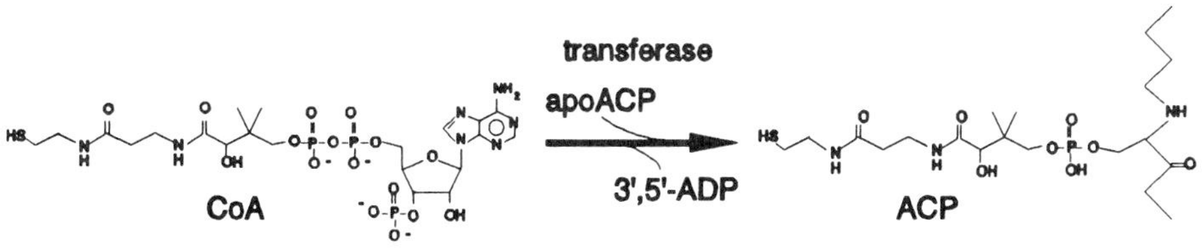

*catabolism of*
*CoA and ACP*

The metabolically active forms of the vitamin (CoA and ACP) are degraded to free pantothenic acid and other metabolites. Although all of these catabolic steps have not been characterized in animals, a **pantetheinase** that cleaves 4'-phosphopantetheine to pantothenic acid and cysteine has been identified in the intestine and its lumen.

*excretion*

Pantothenic acid is excreted mainly in the urine as free **pantothenic acid**[15], as well as some **4'-phosphopantethenate**. An appreciable amount (~15% of daily intake) is oxidized completely and is excreted across the lungs as $CO_2$.

# METABOLIC FUNCTIONS OF PANTOTHENIC ACID

*acyl group*
*transport*

Both CoA and ACP/4'-phosphopantetheine function metabolically as **carriers of acyl groups**. In each case, the linkage with the transported acyl group involves the reactive **sulfhydryl** of the **4'-phosphopantetheinyl prosthetic group**.

*functions*
*of CoA*

Coenzyme A forms high-energy thioester bonds with carboxylic acids. The most important of these is acetic acid, which can come from the metabolism of fatty acids, amino acids or carbohydrates. As acetyl CoA, that

---

[14] Alcoholics have been reported to excrete in their urine large percentages of the pantothenic acid they ingest, a condition corrected upon ethanol withdrawal.

[15] Humans typically excrete in the urine 0.8-8.4 mg pantothenic acid per day.

group (so-called *active acetate*) can enter the TCA cycle[16], can be used for the synthesis of fatty acids[17] or cholesterol, or can be used in acetylations of alcohols, amines and amino acids (e.g., choline, sulfonamides, *p*-aminobenzoate, proteins[18]). Fatty acids must also be *activated* by CoA before they can be incorporated into triglycerides. These reactions involve either the carboxyl group (e.g., formation of acetyl choline, acetylated amino sugars, acetylated sulfonamides[19]) or the methyl group (e.g., condensation with oxaloacetate to yield citrate) of the acyl CoA.

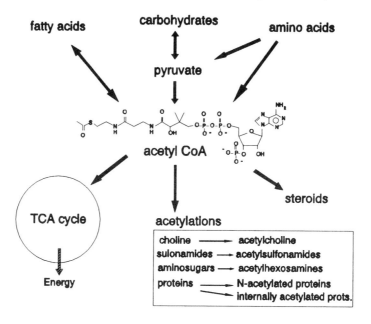

*functions of ACP*     The acyl-carrier protein (ACP) is a component of the *fatty acid synthase* multi-enzyme complex[20] of most species, where it functions to transfer covalently bound intermediates between different active sites with

---

[16] the tricarboxylic acid cycle, often called the *"citric acid cycle"* or the *"Krebs cycle"*

[17] Studies with liver slices *in vitro* have demonstrated a correlation between hepatic CoA content and lipid biosynthetic capacity, suggesting that CoA may be a limiting factor in lipogenesis.

[18] Many CoA-dependent reactions modify protein structure and function *via* acetylations at N-termini or at internal sites (particularly, at the ε-amino groups of lysyl residues).

[19] Coenzyme A was discovered as an essential factor for the acetylation of sulfonamide by the liver and for the acetylation of choline in the brain; hence, *"coenzyme A"* stands for *"coenzyme for acetylations"*.

[20] Fatty acid synthase is the name used to identify the multi-enzyme complex on which the several reactions of fatty acid synthesis (condensations and reductions) occur. The best studied complex is that of *E. coli*; it consists of 7 separate enzymes plus the small (10 kD) protein, ACP.

successive cycles of condensations and reductions[21]. The nature of the fatty acid synthase complex varies considerably among different species; however, in each 4'-phosphopantetheine is the prosthetic group for the binding and transfer of the acyl units during this metabolism. For example, mammalian fatty acid synthase does *not* appear to contain an ACP; instead, it has *non-protein-bound* 4'-phosphopantetheinate.

## EXTREMES IN PANTOTHENIC ACID INTAKE

*deficiency*

Deprivation of pantothenic acid results in metabolic impairments including reduced lipid synthesis and energy production. Signs and symptoms of pantothenic acid deficiency vary among different species; most frequently, they affect the skin, liver, adrenals and nervous system. Due to the wide distribution of the vitamin in nature, dietary deficiencies of pantothenic acid are relatively rare; they are more common in circumstances of inadequate intake of basic foods and vitamins, and are often associated with (and mistakenly diagnosed as) deficiencies of other vitamins.

*antagonists*

Pantothenic acid deficiency has been produced experimentally using purified diets free of the vitamin, or by administering an antagonist. One antagonist is the analogue *ω-methylpantothenic acid*, which has a methyl group in the place of the hydroxymethyl group of the vitamin; this change prevents it from being phosphorylated and inhibits the action of pantothenic acid kinase. Other antagonists include *desthio-CoA*, in which the terminal sulfhydryl of the active metabolite is replaced with an hydroxyl group, and *hopantenate*, in which the 3-carbon β-alanine moiety of the vitamin is replaced with a 4-carbon γ-aminobutyric acid (GABA).

*deficiency syndromes in animals*

Pantothenic acid deficiency in most species results in **reduced growth** and **reduced efficiency of feed utilization**. In rodents, the deficiency results in a **scaly dermatitis, achromotrichia, alopecia**, and **adrenal necrosis**. **Congenital malformations** of offspring of pantothenic acid-deficient dams have been reported. Excess production of porphyrins[22] are excreted in the tears of pantothenic acid-deficient rats in the condition called *"blood-caked whiskers"*. Pantothenic acid-deficient chicks develop *skin lesions at the corners of the mouth, swollen and encrusted eyelids, dermatitis of the entire foot* (with hemorrhagic cracking)[23], *poor feathering, fatty*

---

[21]The 7 functional activities of the fatty acid synthase complex are *acetyltransferase, malonyltransferase, 3-ketoacyl synthase, 3-ketoacyl reductase, 3-hydroxyacyl dehydratase, enoyl reductase* and *thioester hydrolase*.

[22]e.g., protoporphyrin IX

[23]This condition is often confused with that produced by biotin deficiency. Unlike the latter in which lesions are limited to the foot pad, the lesions produced by pantothenic acid deficiency also involve the toes and superior aspect of the foot.

*liver degeneration, thymic necrosis, myelin degeneration of the spinal column with paralysis* and *lethargy*. Chicks produced from deficient hens show high rates of *embryonic and post-hatching mortality*. Pantothenic acid-deficient dogs develop *hepatic steatosis, irritability, cramps, ataxia, convulsions, alopecia* and *death*. Pigs show similar nervous signs, develop *hypertrophy and steatosis of the adrenals, liver and heart*, and show *ovarian atrophy* with *impaired uterine development*.

Marginal deficiency of pantothenic acid in the rat has been found to produce elevated serum levels of triglycerides and free fatty acids. The metabolic basis of this effect is not clear; however, it is possible that it involves a somewhat targeted reduction in cellular CoA concentrations, affecting the deposition of fatty acids in adipocytes (*via* impaired acyl-CoA synthase) but not the hepatic production of triglycerides.

*deficiency signs in humans*

Pantothenic acid deficiency in humans has only been observed in severely malnourished patients and in subjects treated with the antagonist $\omega$-methylpantothenic acid. In cases of the former type, *neurologic signs* (*paresthesia* in the toes and sole of the feet) have been reported[24]. Subjects made deficient in pantothenic acid through the use of $\omega$-methyl-pantothenic acid also develop burning sensations of the feet; in addition, they show *depression, fatigue, insomnia, vomiting*, and *muscular weakness. Changes in glucose tolerance, increased sensitivity to insulin* and *decreased antibody production* have also been reported.

Signs of pantothenic acid deficiency:

| organ system | signs |
|---|---|
| appetite | decrease |
| growth | decrease |
| dermatologic | dermatitis, achromotrichia, alopecia |
| muscular | weakness |
| gastro-intestinal | ulcers |
| vital organs | hepatic steatosis, thymic necrosis, adrenal hypertrophy |
| nervous | ataxia, paralysis |

*hyper-vitaminosis*

The toxicity of pantothenic acid is *negligible*. No adverse reactions have been reported in any species following the ingestion of large doses of the vitamin. Massive doses (e.g., 10 g/day) to humans have not produced reactions more severe than mild intestinal distress and diarrhea. Similarly, no deleterious effects have been identified when the vitamin was administered parenterally or topically. It has been estimated that animals can tolerate without side effects doses of pantothenic acid as great as at least 100 times their respective nutritional requirements for the vitamin.

---

[24]"Burning feet syndrome" was described during World War II in prisoners in Japan and the Philippines who were generally malnourished. That large oral doses of Ca-pantothenate provided some improvement suggested that the syndrome involved, at least in part, deficiency of pantothenic acid.

## CASE STUDY

| Instructions: | Review the following experiment, paying special attention to the independent and dependent variables in the design. Then, answer the questions that follow. |
|---|---|

| experiment | In order to evaluate the possible role of pantothenic acid and ascorbic acid in wound healing, a study was conducted of the effects of these vitamins on the growth of fibroblasts. Human fibroblasts were obtained from neonatal foreskin; they were cultured in a standard medium supplemented with 10% fetal calf serum and antibiotics[25]. The medium contained no ascorbic acid but contained 4 mg/l pantothenic acid. Cells were used between the 3rd and 9th passages. Twenty-four hours before each experiment, the basal medium was replaced by medium supplemented with pantothenic acid (40 mg/l) or pantothenic acid (40 mg/l) plus ascorbic acid (60 mg/l). Cells ($1.5 \times 10^5$) were plated in 3 ml of culture medium in 28 cm$^2$ plastic dishes. After incubation, they were collected by adding trypsin and then scraping; they were counted in a hemocytometer. The synthesis of DNA and protein was estimated by measuring the rates of incorporation of radiolabel from $^3$H-thymidine and $^{14}$C-proline, respectively. Total protein was measured in cells (lysed by sonication and solubilized in 0.5 N NaOH) and in the culture medium. |

Results after 5 days of culture:

| treatment | cells x $10^5$ | $^3$H $10^3$ cpm | $^{14}$C $10^3$ cpm | cell prot. mg/dish | prot. in medium mg/ml |
|---|---|---|---|---|---|
| control | 2.90+.16 | 11.6+0.4 | 1.7+1.0 | 10.0+1.0 | 1.93+.01 |
| + pantothenic ac. | 3.83+.14* | 18.7+0.5* | 2.9+0.1* | 14.5+0.9* | 1.93+.02 |
| + pantothenic ac. and ascorbic acid | 3.74+.19* | 18.1+0.8* | 2.8+0.1* | 8.1+0.9 | 2.11+.01* |

*significantly different from control value, $P < .05$

| Questions: | i. | Why were thymidine and proline selected as carriers of the radiolabels in this experiment? |
|---|---|---|
| | ii. | Why were fibroblasts selected (over some other cell type) for use in this study? |
| | iii. | Assuming that the protein released into the culture medium is largely soluble procollagen, what can be concluded about the effects of pantothenic acid and/or ascorbic acid on collagen synthesis in this system. |
| | iv. | What implications do these results have regarding wound healing? |

---

[25] gentamycin and fungizone

## Study Questions and Exercises:

i.     ***Diagram*** the areas of metabolism in which CoA and ACP (*via* fatty acid synthase) are involved.

ii.    Construct a ***"decision tree"*** for the diagnosis of pantothenic acid deficiency in humans or an animal species.

iii.   What ***key feature*** of the chemistry of pantothenic acid relates to its biochemical functions as a carrier of acyl groups?

iv.    What parameters might you measure to ***assess pantothenic acid status*** of a human or animal?

## Recommended Reading:

Flodin, N.W. 1988. Pharmacology of Micronutrients. Alan R. Liss., Inc., New York, pp. 189-192.

Fox, H.M. 1991. Pantothenic Acid, Chapter 11 *in* Handbook of Vitamins, 2nd ed. (L.J. Machlin, ed.), Marcel Dekker, New York. pp. 429-451.

Friedrich, W. 1988. Vitamins. Walter de Gruyter, New York. pp. 807-835.

Olson, R.E. 1990. Pantothenic Acid, Chapter 23 *in* Present Knowledge in Nutrition, 6th ed. (M. Brown, ed.), Int. Life Sci. Inst.-Nutr. Found., Washington, D.C., pp. 208-211.

Plesofsky-Vig, N. and R. Brambl. 1988. Pantothenic acid and coenzyme A in cellular modification of proteins. Ann. Rev. Nutr. 8:461-482.

# CHAPTER 16    *FOLATE*

*"Using <u>Streptococcus lactis</u> R as a test organism, we have obtained in a highly concentrated and probably nearly pure form an acid nutrilite with interesting physiological properties. Four tons of spinach have been extracted and carried through the first stages of concentration. . . . This acid, or one with similar chemical and physiological properties, occurs in a number of animal tissues of which liver and kidney are the best sources. . . . It is especially abundant in green leaves of many kinds, including grass. Because of this fact, we suggest the name "folic acid" (Latin, <u>folium</u> - leaf). Many commercially canned greens are nearly lacking in the substance."*    H.K. Mitchell, E.S. Snell and R.J. Williams

---

## Anchoring Concepts:

| | |
|---|---|
| i. | Folate is the generic descriptor for folic acid (pteroylmonoglutamic acid) and related compounds exhibiting qualitatively the biological activity of folic acid. That the term *"folates"* refers generally to the compounds in this group, including mono- and poly-glutamates. |
| ii. | Folates are active as co-enzymes in single-carbon metabolism. |
| iii. | Deficiencies of folate are manifest as anemia and dermatologic lesions. |

## Learning Objectives:

| | |
|---|---|
| i. | To understand the chief natural *sources* of folates. |
| ii. | To understand the means of *absorption* and *transport* of the folates. |
| iii. | To understand the *biochemical functions* of the folates as co-enzymes in single-carbon metabolism, and the relationship of that function to the physiological activities of the vitamin. |
| iv. | To understand the metabolic *interrelationship of folate and vitamin $B_{12}$* and its physiological implications. |

## Vocabulary:

acetaminobenzoylglutamate
betaine
cervical paralysis
dihydrofolate reductase
FBPs
$FH_2$
$FH_4$
$FH_4$ formiminotransferase
$FH_4$:glutamate transformylase
folate
folic acid
folyl conjugase
folyl $\beta$-glutamyl hydrolase
folyl polyglutamates
5-formimino $FH_4$
5-formimino $FH_4$ cyclohydrolase
5-formyl $FH_4$
5-formyl $FH_4$ synthetase
homocysteine
leucopenia
macrocytic anemia
megaloblast

5,10-methenyl $FH_4$
5,10-methenyl $FH_4$ cyclohydrase
methionine synthetase
methotrexate
5-methyl $FH_4$
5,10-methylene $FH_4$
5,10-methylene $FH_4$ dehydrogenase
5,10-methylene $FH_4$ reductase
methyl-folate trap
pernicious anemia
pteridine
pterin ring
pteroylglutamic acid
purine
serine hydroxymethyltransferase
single-carbon metabolism
sulfa drugs
tetrahydrofolate reductase
tetrahydrofolic acid
thymidylate
vitamin $B_{12}$

# SOURCES OF FOLATE

*distribution in foods*   Folates (folyl polyglutamates) occur in a wide variety of foods and feed-stuffs of both plant and animal origin. Liver, mushrooms and green leafy vegetables are rich sources of folate in human diets; while oil-seed meals (e.g., soybean meal) and animal by-products are important sources of folate in animal feeds. The folates in foods and feedstuffs are almost exclusively in reduced form, as *polyglutamyl derivatives of tetrahydro-folic acid (FH₄)*. Very little free folate (folyl monoglutamate) is found in foods or feedstuffs.

Folate contents of foods:

| food | folate µg/100g | food | folate µg/100g |
|---|---|---|---|
| dairy products | | vegetables | |
| milk | 5-12 | asparagus | 70-175 |
| cheese | 20 | beans | 70 |
| meats | | broccoli | 180 |
| beef | 5-18 | brussels sprouts | 90-175 |
| beef liver | 140-1070 | cabbage | 15-45 |
| chicken liver | 1810 | cauliflower | 55-120 |
| tuna | 15 | peas | 90 |
| cereals | | soy beans | 360 |
| barley | 15 | spinach | 50-190 |
| corn | 35 | tomatoes | 5-30 |
| rice, polished | 15 | fruits | |
| rice, unpolished | 25 | apples | 5 |
| wheat, whole | 30-55 | bananas | 30 |
| wheat bran | 80 | oranges | 25 |
| other | | | |
| eggs | 70 | | |
| brewer's yeast | 1500 | | |

Analyses of foods have revealed a wide distribution of general types of folate derivatives, the predominant forms being *5-methyl-FH₄* and *10-formyl-FH₄*. The folates found in organ meats (e.g., liver and kidney) are ca. 40% methyl derivatives, while that in milk (and erythrocytes) is exclusively the methyl form. Some plant materials also contain mainly 5-methyl-FH₄ (e.g., lettuce, cabbage, orange juice), but others (e.g., soy-bean) contain relatively little of that form (~15%), the rest occurring as the 5- and 10-formyl derivatives. Most of the folates in cabbage are hexa- and hepta-glutamates, while half of those in soybean are mono-glutamates. More than a third of the folates in orange juice is present as mono-glutamates and nearly half is present as penta-glutamates. Liver and kidney contain mainly penta-glutamates, and ~60% of the folates in milk is mono-glutamate (with only 4-8% each of di- to hepta-glutamates).

*stability*     Most folates in foods and feedstuffs (that is, folates other than folic acid[1] and 5-formyl-FH$_4$) are easily oxidized and, therefore, are unstable to oxidation under aerobic conditions of storage and processing. Under such conditions (especially in the added presence of heat, light and/or metal ions), FH$_4$-derivatives can readily be oxidized to the corresponding derivatives of dihydrofolic acid (FH$_2$) (partially oxidized) or folic acid (fully oxidized)[2], some of which can react further to yield physiologically inactive compounds. Because some folate derivatives of the latter type can support the growth responses of test microorganisms used to measure folates[3], some information in the available literature may overestimate the biologically useful folate contents of foods and/or feedstuffs. Substantial losses in the folate contents of food can occur as the result of leaching in cooking water when boiling[4], as well as to oxidation as described above.

*bio-*          The biological availability of folates is variable among foods (30%-80%, in
*availability*  comparison to folic acid), being generally less well utilized from plant-derived foods than from animal products. The factors affecting the biologic availability of food folates are not well understood, but seem to include iron and vitamin C status. Deficiencies of both of these nutrients in humans is associated with impaired utilization of dietary folate[5,6]. It is thought that the hydrolytic cleavage of the polyglutamyl side-chains of food folates is not normally rate-limiting to their utilization. Folate utilization is reduced, however, under conditions of low pH, which inhibit that enzymatic activity (*"conjugase"*), and by natural *conjugase inhibitors* that are contained in certain foods: cabbage, oranges, yeast, beans (red kidney, pinto, lima,

---

[1] Throughout this text, the term *"folic acid"* is used as the specific trivial name for the compound *pteroylglutamic acid*.

[2] For example, the two predominant folates in fresh foods, *5-methyl-FH$_4$* and *10-formyl-FH$_4$*, are converted to *5-methyl-5,6-FH$_2$* and *10-formylfolic acid*, respectively. For this reason, *5-methyl-5,6-FH$_2$* has been found to account for about half of the folate in most prepared foods. While it can be reduced to the FH$_4$-form (e.g., by ascorbic acid), in the acidity of normal gastric juice it isomerizes to yield *5-methyl-5,8-FH$_2$* which is completely inactive. It is of interest to note that, due to their *gastric anacidosis*, this isomerization does not occur in pernicious anemia patients, who are thus able to utilize the partially oxidized form by absorbing it and subsequently activating it to *5-methyl-FH$_4$*.

[3] *Lactobacillus casei*, *Streptococcus faecium* (formerly, *S. lactis* R and *S. faecalis*, respectively), and *Pediococcus cerevisiae* (formerly, *Leuconostoc citrovorum*) have been used. Of these, *L. casei* responds to the widest spectrum of folates.

[4] Losses of total folates of 22% for asparagus and 84% for cauliflower have been observed.

[5] Some anemic patients respond optimally to oral folate therapy only when they are also given iron.

[6] Patients with scurvy often have megaloblastic anemia apparently due to impaired utilization of folate. In some scorbutic patients, vitamin C has an anti-anemic effect; others require folate to correct the anemia.

navy, soy), lentils and black-eyed peas[7]. The presence of conjugase inhibitors reduces folate availability; for example, this effect appears to be the basis of the low availability of the vitamin (ca. 54%) in orange juice.

Biologic availability of folates in foods:

| food | bioavailability[a] % |
|------|---------------------|
| bananas | 46 |
| eggs | 72 |
| liver (goat) | 70 |
| spinach | 63 |
| tomatoes | 37 |
| brewer's yeast | 10 |

[a]assayed using *L. casei*; results expressed relative to folic acid
source: Babu, S. & S.G. Srikantia. 1976. Am. J. Clin. Nutr. **29**:376.

# ABSORPTION OF FOLATE

*active transport and diffusion*   Dietary folates are absorbed as folic acid (folyl monoglutamate) which is actively transported across the duodenum and jejunum by a $Na^+$-coupled, carrier-mediated process that is stimulated by glucose and shows a pH-maximum at ca. pH 6[8]. A brush-border folate-binding protein (FBP), thought to be involved in this process, has been isolated. Folic acid is also absorbed passively, presumably by diffusion; this mechanism accounts for 20-30% of folate absorption, regardless of folate concentration. It appears that some species (e.g., dogs) can also absorb folyl polyglutamates; however, this does *not* occur in most species. The overall efficiency of folate absorption appears to be ~50% (10%-90%). Malabsorption of the vitamin occurs in diseases affecting the intestinal mucosa.

*folyl conjugase*   Because the majority of food folates occur as reduced polyglutamates, they must be cleaved to the mono- or di-glutamate forms for absorption. This is accomplished by the action of an exocarboxypeptidase *folyl γ-glutamyl hydrolase*, more commonly called *"folyl conjugase"*. Conjugase activity is widely distributed in the mucosa of the proximal small intestine,

---

[7]The conjugase inhibitors in beans and peas reside in the seed coats and are heat-labile.

[8]A *"microclimate hypothesis"* has been proposed for the enteric absorption of folates. It holds that folate absorption is dependent on the pH of the proximal jejunum. According to this hypothesis, the basis of the observation that folate absorption tends to be high in individuals with pancreatic exocrine insufficiency may be due to their low excretion of bicarbonate, hence, they tend not to have intestinal pH >6 under which conditions folate absorption falls off rapidly.

both intracellularly and in association with the brush border[8]. Folyl conjugase activities have also been found in bile, pancreatic juice, kidney, liver, placenta, bone marrow, leukocytes and plasma, although the physiological importance of the activity in these tissues is uncertain. Conjugase activity is reduced by nutritional Zn deficiency, by chronic exposure to alcohol[10], or by exposure to naturally occurring inhibitors in foods. Loss of conjugase activity by either means results in impaired folate absorption.

*limited methylation*  Folic acid taken up by the intestinal mucosal cell is transferred to the plasma mostly without further metabolism. To a limited extent, some is methylated to yield **5-methyl-FH₄**, which is also transferred to the plasma.

## TRANSPORT OF FOLATE

*free in plasma*  Folate is transported to the tissues as monoglutamate derivatives in free solution in the plasma. The predominant form in portal plasma is the reduced form, **tetrahydrofolic acid (FH₄)**. This is taken up by the liver, which releases it to the peripheral plasma after metabolic conversion primarily to **5-methyl-FH₄**, but also to **10-formyl-FH₄**. The concentration of 10-formyl-FH₄ is tightly regulated[11], while that of 5-methyl-FH₄ is not and, thus, varies in response to folate-meals, etc. Thus, folates of dietary origin are absorbed and transported to the liver as FH₄, which is converted to the methylated form and transported to the peripheral tissues.

*cellular uptake*  The cellular uptake of folates occurs exclusively with **monoglutamate derivatives** found in the plasma, as the polyglutamates cannot cross biological membranes. The cellular uptake of folate involves a specific, carrier-mediated process that requires energy and $Na^+$. Within cells, FH₄ is **methylated** to yield 5-methyl-FH₄, which is bound to intracellular macromolecules. Folate is held in cells by conversion to folyl polyglutamates; polyglutamation traps folates inside cells at concentrations one-two orders of magnitude greater than those of extracellular fluids.

---

[9] These appear to be different enzymes. The intracellular enzyme is localized in the lysosomes and has a pH optimum of 4.5; whereas, the brush border enzyme has a pH optimum of 7.5. Although the latter enzyme is present in lower amounts, it appears to be important for the hydrolysis of dietary folylpolyglutamates.

[10] Studies with several animal models have demonstrated that chronic ethanol-feeding can decrease intestinal hydrolysis of folylpolyglutamates and can impair the absorption, transport, cellular release and metabolism of folates. Effects of this nature are thought to contribute to the folate deficiencies frequently observed among chronic alcoholics; however, there are other likely contributing factors, as enterocytes are known to be sensitive to ethanol toxicity, and many of chronic alcoholics can have insufficient dietary intakes of the vitamin.

[11] In humans, the plasma level is held at ca. 80 ng/dl.

*folate-binding*
*proteins*

**Folate-binding proteins (FBPs)** have been identified in plasma, milk and several other tissues (e.g., erythrocytes, leukocytes, intestinal mucosa, kidney, liver, placenta, choroid plexus and urine[12]). Each FBP binds folates non-covalently with high affinity such that the complex does not dissociate under physiological conditions[13]. Low concentrations (e.g., binding <10 ng folic acid per dl) of FBPs have been found in sera of healthy humans; greater concentrations of FBPs have been found in folate-deficient subjects, pregnant women, human milk and leukemic leukocytes. It is hypothesized that the FBPs found in plasma and milk are derived from cellular membranes in which they serve transport functions. This appears to be true in the case of the FBPs in milk[14]; they have been shown to stimulate the enteric absorption of folate from that food. Liver contains two FBPs; one is the enzyme **dimethylglycine dehydrogenase**, the other is the enzyme **sarcosine dehydrogenase**. Each binds reduced folates with much greater affinity (*ca.* 100-fold) that the non-reduced forms. Intestine contains three FBPs of different molecular weight; these are associated with the brush border, the latter two appear to be aggregates of the first.

*tissue*
*distribution*

In humans, the total body content of folate is 5-10 mg, about half of which resides in the liver in the form of **tetra-**, **penta-**, **hexa-** and **hepta-glutamates** of **5-methyl-FH$_4$** and **10-formyl-FH$_4$**[15]. The relative amounts of these two single-C derivatives vary between tissues depending on the rate of cell division. In tissues with rapid cell division (e.g., intestinal mucosa, regenerating liver, carcinoma) relatively low concentrations of 5-methyl-FH$_4$ are found, usually with concomitant elevations in 10-formyl-FH$_4$. In contrast, in tissues with low rates of cell division (e.g., normal liver), 5-methyl-FH$_4$ predominates. It has been suggested that tissue FBPs, which bind polyglutamate forms of the vitamin, may play important roles in stabilizing folates within cells, thus reducing their rates of metabolic turnover and increasing their intracellular retention.

---

[12]Urinary FBP is presumed to be of plasma origin.

[13]Other proteins (e.g., albumin) bind folates non-specifically, forming complexes that dissociate readily.

[14]There are two FBPs in milk. Each is a glycoprotein; one may be a degradation product of the other.

[15]The hepatic reserve of folate should be sufficient to support normal plasma concentrations of the vitamin (>400 ng/dl) for at least 4 weeks. (Signs of megaloblastic anemia are usually not observed within 2-3 months of folate deprivation.) However, some evidence suggests that the release of folate from the liver is independent of nutritional folate status, resulting instead from the deaths of hepatocytes.

## METABOLISM OF FOLATE

*three aspects of folate metabolism*
Folate metabolism consists of reduction of the pterin ring system, reactions of the polyglutamyl side-chain, and acquisition of single-C moieties at certain positions (N-5 or N-10) on the pterin ring.

*ring reduction*
Reduction of the pterin ring from the two non-reduced states, folic acid and dihydrofolic acid ($FH_2$), to the fully reduced form tetrahydrofolic acid ($FH_4$) that is capable of accepting a single-C unit is accomplished by the cytosolic, enzyme ***7,8-dihydrofolate reductase***[16]. This activity is found in high amounts in liver and kidney and in rapidly dividing cells (e.g., tumor). The reductase in inhibited by several important drugs including the cancer chemotherapeutic drug ***methotrexate***[17,18], which appears to exert its anti-tumor action by inhibiting the reductase activity of tumor cells.

**folic acid**                **7,8-dihydrofolic acid**            **5,6,7,8-tetrahydrofolic acid**

*side-chain reactions*
The folyl monoglutamates that are taken up by cells are trapped therein as polyglutamate derivatives that cannot cross cell membranes. This is accomplished by the action of the ATP-dependent ***folyl polyglutamate synthetase***, which links glutamyl residues to the vitamin by peptide bonds involving the γ-carboxyl groups[19]. The enzyme requires prior reduction of folate to $FH_4$ or demethylation of the circulating 5-methyl-$FH_4$ (by vitamin $B_{12}$-dependent methionine synthetase). It is widely distributed at low concentrations in many tissues. That folyl polyglutamate synthetase is

---

[16]Also called ***tetrahydrofolate dehydrogenase***, this 65 kD NADPH-dependent enzyme can reduce folic acid to $FH_2$ and, of greater importance, $FH_2$ to $FH_4$.

[17]4-amino-10-methylfolic acid

[18]Other inhibitors include the anti-malarial drug ***pyrimethamine*** and the anti-bacterial drug ***trimethoprim***.

[19]This enzyme also catalyzes the polyglutamation of the anti-cancer folate-antagonist ***methotrexate***, which enhances its cellular retention. Tumor cells that have greatest capacities to perform this side-chain elongation reaction are particularly sensitive to the cytotoxic effects of the antagonist.

critical in converting the monoglutamyl transport forms of the vitamin to the metabolically active polyglutamyl forms was demonstrated by the discovery of a mutational loss of the synthetase activity, which produced lethal folate deficiency.  Folyl polyglutamates are converted to derivatives of shorter chain-length by cellular conjugases, some of which appear to be Zn-metalloenzymes.

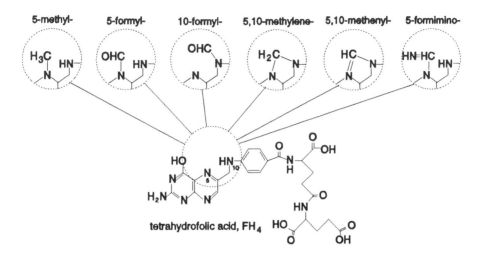

tetrahydrofolic acid, FH$_4$

*acquisition of single-C units*   Folate is metabolically active as a variety of derivatives with single-C units at the oxidation levels of *formate*, *formaldehyde* or *methanol* [20] substituted at the N-5 and/or N-10 positions of the pteridine ring system.  The main source of single-C fragments is *serine hydroxymethyltransferase*, which uses the dispensable amino acid *serine (SER)*[21] as the single-C donor.  Each folyl derivative is a donor of its single-C unit in metabolism[22]; thus, by cycling through the acquisition/loss of single-C units, each derivative transports these species to a variety of metabolic uses.

---

[20] It should be noted that single-carbon at the oxidation level of $CO_2$ *cannot* be transported by folates; such fully oxidized carbon is transported by *biotin* and *thiamin pyrophosphate*.

[21] Serine is biosynthesized from glucose in non-limiting amounts in most cells.

[22] Although the route of its biosynthesis is unknown, eukaryotic cells contain significant amounts of *5-formyl-FH$_4$*.  That folyl derivative, also called *'leucovorin'*, *'folinic acid'* and *'citrovorum factor'*, is used widely to reverse the toxicity of methotrexate and, recently, to potentiate the cytotoxic effects of 5-fluorouracil.

Enzymes involved in the acquisition of single-C units by folates:

| single-C unit | folate derivative | enzymes |
|---|---|---|
| methyl group | 5-methyl-FH$_4$ | 5,10-methylene-FH$_4$ reductase |
| methylene group | 5,10-methylene-FH$_4$ | serine transhydroxymethylase |
| | | 5,10-methylene-FH$_4$ dehydrogenase |
| methenyl group | 5,10-methenyl-FH$_4$ | 5,10-methylene-FH$_4$ dehydrogenase |
| | | 5,10-methenyl-FH$_4$ cyclohydrolase |
| | | 5-formimino-FH$_4$ cyclohydrolase |
| | | 5-formyl-FH$_4$ isomerase |
| formimino group | 5-formimino-FH$_4$ | FH$_4$ formiminotransferase |
| formyl group | 5-formyl-FH$_4$ | FH$_4$:glutamate transformylase |
| | 10-formyl-FH$_4$ | 5,10-methenyl-FH$_4$ cyclohydrolase |
| | | 10-formyl-FH$_4$ synthetase |

*catabolism*    Tissue folates appear to turn over by the cleavage of the polyglutamates at the C-9 and N-10 bonds to liberate the ***pteridine*** and ***p-aminobenzoyl-polyglutamate*** moieties. This cleavage probably results from chemical oxidation of the co-factor both in the intestinal lumen (dietary and entero-hepatically recycled folates) as well as in the tissues. Once formed, p-aminobenzoylpolyglutamate is degraded, presumably by the action of ***folyl conjugase***, and is acetylated to yield ***p-acetaminobenzoylglutamate*** and ***p-acetoaminobenzoate***.

*excretion*    The water-soluble side-chain metabolites ***p-acetaminobenzoylglutamate*** and ***p-acetaminobenzoate*** is excreted in the urine and bile, which also contains ***intact folates***. The total urinary excretion of folates and metabolites is small (e.g., <1% of total body stores). Fecal concentrations of folates are usually rather high; however, they represent mainly folates of intestinal microfloral origin, as enterohepatically circulated folates appear to be absorbed quantitatively.

## *METABOLIC FUNCTIONS OF FOLATE*

*co-enzymes*    The folates function as enzyme co-substrates in many reactions of the met-
*in single-C*    abolism of amino acids and nucleotides. As such, the fully reduced (tetra-
*metabolism*    hydro-) form of each serves as an acceptor or donor of a single-C unit. Collectively, these reaction are referred to as "***single-carbon metabolism***".

The regulation of single-C metabolism is complex. It is effected by the interconversion of oxidation states of the folate intermediates. In mammalian tissues, the $\beta$-C of ***serine*** is the major source of single-C for these aspects of metabolism. That C-fragment is accepted by FH$_4$ to form 5,10-methylene FH$_4$ (by *serine hydroxymethyltransferase*), which has a central role in single-C metabolism. The latter derivative can be used directly for the synthesis of ***thymidylate (dTMP)*** (by *thymidylate* synthetase)[23,24], it can be oxidized to 5,10-methenyl $FH_4$ (by *5,10-methy-lene $FH_4$ dehydrogenase*) for use in the *de novo* synthesis of **purines**, or it can be reduced to 5-methyl-$FH_4$ (by *5,10-methylene $FH_4$ reductase*) for use in the biosynthesis of **methionine**. The result is the **channelling of single-C units** into **methionine, thymidylate** (for DNA synthesis) or **purine** biosynthesis. Because folyl polyglutamates have been found to inhibit a number of the enzymes of single-C metabolism, it has been suggested that variation in their polyglutamate chain lengths (observed in different physio-logical conditions) may play a role in the regulation of single-C metabolism.

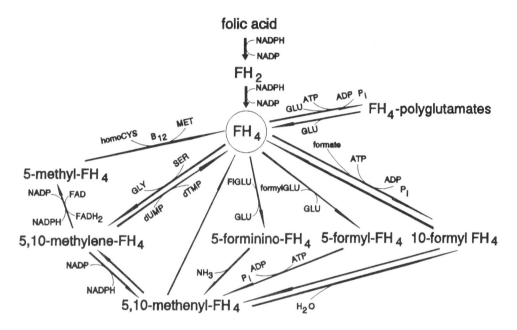

<table>
<tr><td>the<br>"methyl-folate<br>trap"</td><td>The major cycle of single-carbon flux in mammalian tissues appears to be the **serine hydroxymethyltransferase/5,10-methylene-$FH_4$ reductase/ methionine synthetase** cycle in which the **methionine synthetase** reaction is rate-limiting. The committed step (**5,10-methylene-$FH_4$ reductase**) is feedback-inhibited by **S-adenosylmethionine** and product-inhibited by **5-methyl $FH_4$**. Methionine synthetase depends on the transfer of labile methyl groups from 5-methyl-$FH_4$ to vitamin $B_{12}$ which, as methyl-$B_{12}$, serves as the *immediate* methyl-donor for converting **homocysteine**</td></tr>
</table>

[23] This is the sole *de novo* path of thymidylate synthesis. It is also the *only* folate-dependent reaction in which the cofactor serves both as a single-C donor and as a reducing agent.

[24] Thymidylate synthetase is the target of the anti-cancer drug **5-fluorouracil (5-FU)**. The enzyme converts the drug to 5-flurodeoxyuridylate which is incorporated into RNA and also is a suicide inhibitor of the synthetase. Inhibition of the synthetase results in the cellular accumulation of **deoxyuridine triphosphate (dUTP)**, which is normally present at only very low concentrations, and the incorporation of dU into DNA. Having this abnormal base, DNA is enzymatically cleaved at sites containing dU, leading to enhanced DNA breakage.

*(homo-CYS)* to *methionine (MET)*.  Without adequate vitamin $B_{12}$ to accept methyl groups from 5-methyl $FH_4$, that metabolite accumulates at the expense of the other metabolically active folate pools (most notably, $FH_4$).  This is known as the *"methyl-folate trap"*.

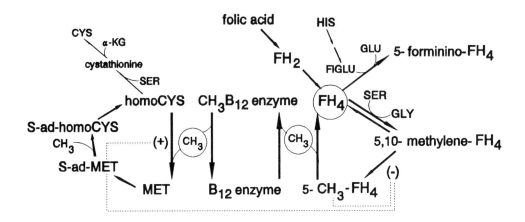

*metabolic roles*

Folates transport formate (as 5,10-methenyl $FH_4$) for *purine synthesis*, and formaldehyde (as 5,10-methylene $FH_4$) for *thymidylate* synthesis from deoxyuridylate for *DNA synthesis*.  As 5,10-methylene-$FH_4$, which is freely interconvertible with 10-formyl-$FH_4$ and 5,10-methenyl-$FH_4$, folates provide labile methyl groups for *methionine synthesis* from homocysteine.

Metabolic roles of folates:

| folate coenzyme | enzyme | metabolic role |
|---|---|---|
| 5,10-methylene-$FH_4$ | serine hydroxymethyl transferase | receipt of a formaldehyde unit in SER catabolism |
|  | thymidylate synthetase | transfers formaldehyde to C-5 of dUMP to form dTMP in pyrimidines |
| 10-formyl-$FH_4$ | 10-formyl-$FH_4$ synthetase | accepts formate from TRY catabolism |
|  | glycinamide ribonucleotide transformylase | donates formate in purine synthesis |
|  | 5-amino-4-imidazolecarboxamide transformylase | donates formate in purine synthesis |
|  | 10-formyl-$FH_4$ dehydrogenase | transfers formate for oxidation to $CO_2$ in HIS catabolism |
| 5-methyl-$FH_4$ | methionine synthetase | provides methyl to convert homoCYS to MET |
| 5-formimino-$FH_4$ | formiminotransferase | accepts formimino group from HIS catabolism |

## EXTREMES IN FOLATE INTAKE

| | |
|---|---|
| *deficiency* | Deficiencies of folate result in impaired biosynthesis of DNA and RNA and, thus, to reduced cell division which is manifest as **anemia** (impaired erythropoiesis), **dermatologic lesions** and **poor growth** in most species. Signs and/or symptoms of folate deficiency are observed among individuals consuming inadequate dietary levels of the vitamin. These effects are exacerbated by physiological conditions that increase folate needs (e.g., **pregnancy, lactation, rapid growth**), by drug treatments that reduce folate utilization (e.g., high levels of **ethanol** [25], **anti-epileptics**[26], **folate antagonists**[27]), by **aging** and by diseases of the intestinal mucosa[28]. |
| *methionine-folate linkage* | Folate utilization is impaired by insufficient supplies of **vitamin B$_{12}$** and/or the indispensable amino acid **methionine (MET)**; therefore, dietary deficiencies of either of those nutrients can produce signs of folate deficiency. Thus, patients with **pernicious anemia**[29] generally have impaired folate utilization and show signs of folate deficiency. The metabolic basis of this effect involves the **methionine synthetase** reaction, which is common to the functions of both folate and vitamin B$_{12}$. Methionine supplements can correct the low circulating folate levels caused by vitamin B$_{12}$ deficiency. The amino acid appears to exert its action *via* **S-adenosylmethionine (S-adMET)**, which *inhibits* **5,10-methylene FH$_4$ reductase** (thus, reducing the *de novo* synthesis of 5-methyl FH$_4$) and *activates* **methionine synthetase**. |
| *relationship with Zn* | Folate utilization can be impaired by depletion of Zn. Dietary Zn deficiency has been found, in humans, to reduce the absorption of folyl polyglutamates (*not* monoglutamates) and, in animals, to reduce liver folates. This is thought to indicate a need for Zn in the enzymes of folate metabolism. |

---

[25] Chronic alcoholics tend to have substantially lower serum folate concentrations than non-alcoholic individuals. Beer-drinkers, however, do not show this effect (they may even show greater serum folate levels), as their beverage is usually a good source of folate.

[26] Examples are **phenytoin** (which increases folate uptake by the central nervous system) and **phenobarbital** (which blocks folate uptake by the CNS). The chronic use of anti-epileptics rarely produces megaloblastic anemia, but will reduce folate concentrations in the serum and erythrocytes.

[27] Examples are **methotrexate** (an anti-cancer drug), **pyrimethamine** (an anti-malarial drug), **trimethoprim** (an anti-bacterial drug) and **aspirin** (an analgesic agent).

[28] Examples include **tropical sprue** (inflammation of the mucous membranes of the alimentary tract) and other types of enteritis that involve malabsorption and, usually, diarrhea.

[29] Pernicious anemia is vitamin B$_{12}$ deficiency resulting from the lack of the **intrinsic factor** required for the enteric absorption of that vitamin (*see* Chapter 17).

Signs of Folate Deficiency:

| organ system | signs |
|---|---|
| general | |
| appetite | decrease |
| growth | decrease |
| dermatologic | alopecia, achromotrichia, dermatitis |
| muscular | weakness |
| gastro-intestinal | inflammation |
| vascular | |
| erythrocytes | macrocytic anemia |
| nervous | depression, neuropathy, paralysis |

*deficiency*
*syndromes*
*animals*

Folate deficiency in animals is generally associated with *poor growth*, *anemia*[30] and dermatologic lesions involving skin and hair/feathers. In chicks, severe *anemia* is one of the earliest signs of the deficiency; it is followed by *leucopenia*[31], *poor growth*, *very poor feathering*, *perosis*, *lethargy* and *reduced feed intake*. Poultry with normally pigmented plumage[32] show *achromotrichia* due to the deficiency. Folate-deficient turkey poults show a spastic type of *cervical paralysis* in which the neck is held rigid[33]. Folate-deficient guinea pigs show *leucopenia* and *depressed growth*. Monkeys show *alopecia*, *dermatitis* and *anemia*. The deficiency is not easily produced in rodents unless a sulfa drug[34] or folate antagonist is fed, in which case *leucopenia* is the main sign[35].

*deficiency*
*signs in*
*humans*

Folate deficiency in humans is characterized by a sequence of signs starting with *nuclear hypersegmentation of circulating polymorphonuclear leukocytes*[36] within about two months of deprivation of the vitamin. This is followed by *megaloblastic anemia* and, then, *general weakness*, *depression* and *polyneuropathy*. In pregnant women, the deficiency can

---

[30]The anemia is of the *macrocytic* (megaloblastic) type, involving abnormally large erythrocyte size (the normal range in humans is 82-92 $\mu^3$) due to the presence of large, nucleated erythrocyte-precursor cells called *megaloblasts*, which are also seen among the hyperplastic erythroid cells in the bone marrow.

[31]Leucopenia is the condition of abnormally *low* numbers of white blood cells in the circulating blood.

[32]Such breeds include the Barred Plymouth Rock, the Rhode Island Red, and the Black Leghorn.

[33]Poults with cervical paralysis may show little or no anemia; the condition is fatal within a couple of days of onset, but responds dramatically (within 15 min.) to parenteral administration of the vitamin.

[34]e.g., sulfanilamide

[35]Although leucopenia was manifest relatively soon after experimental folate depletion, rats kept alive with small doses of folate eventually also develop macrocytic anemia.

[36]These cytological changes are not manifest until well after circulating folate levels drop (by 6-8 weeks).

lead to birth defects or spontaneous abortion. Elderly humans tend to have lower circulating levels of folate, indicating that they may be at increased risk to folate deficiency. While the basis of this finding is not fully elucidated, it appears to involve such age-related factors food habits, that affect intake of the vitamin rather than impairment in folate utilization.

*congenital disorders*

Congenital disorders of folate absorption, transport and metabolism have been identified in humans. These rare conditions have almost always been detected in children, who showed *megaloblastic anemia* and severe *mental retardation*. These disorders have included *congenital folate malabsorption*[37] as well as *deficiencies of folate enzymes* (e.g., 5,10-methylene $FH_4$ reductase, formiminotransferase[38], dihydrofolate reductase[39], 5,10-methenyl $FH_4$ cyclohydrolase[40]). The most common of these disorders is *5,10-methylene $FH_4$ reductase deficiency*. Patients with this autosomal recessive disorder show, in addition to the signs already mentioned, *homocystinuria*, *homocystinemia* and *methionine deficiency* because their enzyme deficiency results in an insufficient production of 5-methyl-$FH_4$ to support methionine biosynthesis by methylation of homocysteine. Some therapeutic success has been reported with the methyl donor betaine or with the combined administration of methionine, folate, pyridoxine and vitamin $B_{12}$.

*effects of high doses in reducing neural tube defects*

It has been suggested that folate supplements may reduce the incidence of *neural tube defects*[41] when given in high doses to women at the time of conception. Two clinical trials conducted in the late 1970s yielded somewhat equivocal results apparently in support of that hypothesis. Recently, a large, well designed, multi-centered trial was conducted by the British Medical Research Council (MRC) to test the hypothesis. It demonstrated clearly that a daily oral dose of 4 mg folic acid significantly reduced the incidence of confirmed neural tube defects among the pregnancies of

---

[37] The five reported cases showed severe megaloblastic anemia at 2-3 months of age and developed mental retardation to varying degrees. The anemia was corrected by high oral or parenteral doses of folate. However, such treatment did not affect the low folate concentration of the cerebrospinal fluid, suggesting an impairment of folate transport as well as absorption.

[38] Only nine cases with this autosomal recessive trait have been reported. Each had elevated serum folate concentration and high urinary excretion of *formiminoglutamate (FIGLU)*.

[39] The few cases reported with this autosomal recessive trait responded only to fully reduced folates ($FH_4$).

[40] Three cases have been reported.

[41] Neural tube defects are the most common severe congenital malformations; they include anencephaly, spina bifida and encephalocele.

women at high risk for such disorders[42]. Questions remain as to whether lower doses of the vitamin may also be effective, whether folate can reduce the incidence of neural tube defects among women *without* previous affected pregnancies, whether such a high level of folate has significant side effects, and as to the mechanism of folate action in reducing the incidence of these birth defects[43].

*hyper-*
*vitaminosis*

No adverse effects of high oral doses of folate have been reported in animals, although parenteral administration of pharmacologic amounts (e.g., 250 mg/kg[44]) has been shown to produce epileptic responses and renal hypertrophy in rats. Inconsistent results have been reported concerning the effects of high folate levels on human epileptics; some have indicated increases in the frequency or severity of seizures and reduced anti-convulsant effectiveness[45], while others have shown no such effects. It has also been suggested that folate may form a non-absorbable complex with Zn, thus, antagonizing the utilization of that essential trace element at high intakes of the vitamin. Studies with animal models have not consistently shown such antagonism; most results indicate that, even at high levels of intake, folate does not affect Zn status.

High doses of folate (e.g., 400 $\mu$g/day intramuscular; 5 mg/day oral) have been shown to *correct the megaloblastic anemia of pernicious anemia* patients. However, because *folate treatment does not affect the neurological lesions* of pernicious anemia or vitamin $B_{12}$ deficiency, concern has been raised that indiscriminate use of large folate supplements may mask those conditions in their early (and more easily treated) stages.

---

[42]The double-blind, randomized clinical trial involved 1817 women, each with a previous affected pregnancy, who were followed in 33 clinics in 7 countries. Each subject was randomly assigned to treatments consisting of a placebo or a multi-vitamin supplement (A, D, C, $B_6$, thiamin, riboflavin and nicotinamide) and/or a placebo or folic acid (4 mg/day) in a complete factorial design and the outcomes of their pregnancies were confirmed. Of a total of 1195 completed pregnancies, 27 had confirmed neural tube defects; these included 21 cases in both groups not receiving folate, but only 6 cases in both folate groups (relative risk = 0.28, 95% C.I.: 0.12-0.71). The multi-vitamin treatment did *not* significantly affect the incidence of neural tube defects. The results were published in 1991 (MRC Vitamin Research Group, Lancet *338:* 131-137).

[43]Two points may be important in considering the role of folate in neural tube defects: *i.* in the MRC trial, 4 mg/day (10-fold of the RDA) reduced significantly *but did not eliminate* neural tube defects; *ii.* serum folate levels of women with affected pregnancies have been found to be comparable to those of women with unaffected pregnancies, as was observed in the MRC trial.

[44]This dose is *ca.* 1000 times the dietary requirement of the rat for folate.

[45]High doses of folate appear to interfere with diphenylhydantoin absorption.

## CASE STUDY

Instructions: Review the following case report, paying special attention to the diagnostic indicators upon which the treatments were based. Then, answer the questions that follow.

case A 15-year-old girl was admitted to the hospital because of progressive *withdrawal, hallucinations, anorexia* and *tremor*. Her early growth and development were normal, and she had done average schoolwork until she was 11 years old, when her family moved to a new area. The next year, she experienced considerable difficulty concentrating and was found to have an IQ of 60. She was placed in a special education program, where she began to fight with other children and have temper tantrums; when punished, she became withdrawn and stopped eating. A year earlier, she had experienced an episode of severe abdominal pain for which no cause could be found, and she was referred to a mental health clinic. Her psychologic examination at that time had revealed inappropriate giggling, poor reality testing and loss of contact with her surroundings. Her verbal and performance IQs were then 46 and 50, respectively. She was treated with thioridazine[46] and, within two weeks, she ate and slept better and was helpful around the house. However, over the succeeding months, while she continued taking thioridazine, her functioning fluctuated and the diagnosis of catatonic schizophrenia was confirmed. Three months before the present admission, she had become progressively withdrawn and drowsy, and needing to be fed, bathed and dressed. She also experienced visual hallucinations, feelings of persecution and night terrors. Upon having a seizure, she was taken to the hospital.

Her physical examination upon admission revealed a tall, thin girl with fixed stare and catatonic posturing, but no neurologic abnormalities. She was mute and withdrawn, incontinent, and appeared to have visual and auditory hallucinations. Her muscle tone varied from normal to diffusely rigid.

On the assumption that her *homocystinuria* was due to *cystathionase deficiency*, she was treated with *pyridoxine HCl* (300 mg/day, orally) for 10 days. Her homocystinuria did not respond; however, her mental status improved and, within 4 days, she was able to conduct some conversation and her hallucinations seemed to decrease. She developed new neurological signs: foot and wrist droop and gradual loss of reflexes. She was then given *folate* (20 mg/day orally) for 14 days because of her low serum folate level. This resulted in a marked decreased in her urinary homocystine and a progressive improvement in intellectual function over the next three months. She remained severely handicapped by her peripheral neuropathy, but she showed no psychotic symptoms. After five months of folate and pyridoxine treatment, she was tranquil and retarded, but showed

---

[46] an anti-schizophrenic drug

no psychotic behavior; she left the hospital against medical advice and without medication.

Laboratory findings:

| parameter | | patient | normal range |
|---|---|---|---|
| *electroencephalogram:* | | diffusely slow | |
| *spinal fluid:* | protein, mg/dl | 42 | 15-45 |
| | cells | none | none |
| *urine:* | homocystine | elevated | |
| | methionine | normal | |
| *serum:* | homocystine | elevated | |
| | methionine | normal | |
| | folate, ng/ml | 3 | 5-21 |
| | vitamin $B_{12}$, pg/ml | 800 | 150-900 |
| *hematology:* | hemoglobin, g/dl | 12.1 | 11.5-14.5 |
| | hematocrit, % | 39.5 | 37-45 |
| | reticulocytes, % | 1 | ~1 |
| *bone marrow:* | | no megaloblastosis | |

The girl was readmitted to the hospital seven months later (a year after her first admission) with a 2-month history of progressive withdrawal, hallucinations, delusions and refusal to eat. The general examination was the same as her first admission, with the exceptions that she had developed hyperreflexia and her peripheral neuropathy had improved slightly. Her mental functioning was at the 2-year-old level. She was incontinent, virtually mute, and had visual and auditory hallucinations. She was diagnosed as having simple schizophrenia of the childhood type. Folate and pyridoxine therapy was started again; it resulted in her decreased homocysteine excretion and gradual improvement in mental performance. After 2 months of therapy in the hospital, she was socializing, free of hallucinations, and able to feed herself and recognize her family. At that time, the activities of several enzymes involved in methionine metabolism were measured in her fibroblasts and liver tissue (obtained by biopsy).

Enzyme activities:

| enzyme | tissue | patient[a] | normal[a] |
|---|---|---|---|
| methionine adenyltransferase | liver | 20.6 | 4.3-14.5 |
| cystathionine-$\beta$-synthetase | fibroblasts | 25.9 | 3.7-65.0 |
| betaine:homocysteine methyltransferase | liver | 26.7 | 1.2-16.0 |
| 5-methyl $FH_4$:homocysteine methyltransferase | fibroblasts | 3.5 | 2.9-7.3 |
| 5,10-methylene $FH_4$ reductase | fibroblasts | 0.5 | 1.0-4.6 |
| | | | [a]enzyme units |

Thereafter, she was maintained on oral folate (10 mg/day). She has been *free* of homocystinuria and psychotic manifestations for several years.

Questions: i. Upon this patient's admission to the hospital, which of her symptoms were consistent with an impairment in a folate-dependent aspect of metabolism?

ii. What finding appeared to counter-indicate an impairment in folate metabolism in this case?

iii. Propose an hypothesis for the metabolic basis of the observed efficacy of oral folate treatment in this case.

## Study Questions and Exercises:

*i.*     ***Diagram*** the metabolic conversions involving folates in single-carbon metabolism.

*ii.*    Construct a *"decision tree"* for the diagnosis of folate deficiency in humans or an animal species.  In particular, outline a way to ***distinguish folate and vitamin B₁₂ deficiencies*** in patients with macrocytic anemia.

*iii.*   What ***key feature*** of the chemistry of folate relates to its biochemical function as a carrier of single-carbon units?

*iv.*    What parameters might you measure to ***assess folate status*** of a human or animal?

## Recommended Reading:

Blau, N. 1988. Inborn errors of pterin metabolism.  Ann. Rev. Nutr. 8:185-209.

Brody, T. 1991.  Folic Acid, Chapter 12 *in* Handbook of Vitamins, 2nd ed. (L.J. Machlin, ed.), Marcel Dekker, New York. pp. 453-489.

Butterworth, Jr., C.E. and T. Tamura. 1989. Folic acid safety and toxicity: a brief review. Am. J. Clin. Nutr. 50:353-358.

Flodin, N.W. 1988. Pharmacology of Micronutrients. Alan R. Liss., Inc., New York, pp. 161-177.

Food and Nutrition Board, National Research Council. 1977. Folic Acid: Biochemistry and Physiology in Relation to the Human Nutritional Requirement.  Nat. Acad. Sci., Washington, D.C., 298 pp.

Friedrich, W. 1988. Vitamins.  Walter de Gruyter, New York. pp. 619-752.

Henderson, G.B. 1990. Folate-binding proteins.  Ann. Rev. Nutr. 10:319-336.

Krumdieck, C.L. 1990. Folic Acid, Chapter 21 *in* Present Knowledge in Nutrition, 6th ed. (M. Brown, ed.), Int. Life Sci. Inst.-Nutr. Found., Washington, D.C., pp. 179-188.

Shane, B. 1989. Foly polyglutamate synthesis and role in the regulation of one-carbon metabolism. Vit. Horm. 45:263-335.

# CHAPTER 17     *VITAMIN B$_{12}$*

*"Patients with Addisonian pernicious anemia have . . . a 'conditioned' defect of nutrition. The nutritional defect in such patients is apparently caused by a failure of a reaction that occurs in the normal individual between a substance in the food (extrinsic factor) and a substance in the normal gastric secretion (intrinsic factor)."*

W.B. Castle and T.H. Hale

---

## Anchoring Concepts:

| | |
|---|---|
| *i.* | Vitamin B$_{12}$ is the generic descriptor for all corrinoids (compounds containing the Co-centered corrin nucleus) exhibiting qualitatively the biological activity of cyanocobalamin. |
| *ii.* | Deficiencies of vitamin B$_{12}$ are manifest as anemia and neurologic changes and can be fatal. |
| *iii.* | The function of vitamin B$_{12}$ in single-C metabolism is interrelated with that of folate. |

## Learning Objectives:

| | |
|---|---|
| *i.* | To understand the chief natural *sources* of vitamin B$_{12}$. |
| *ii.* | To understand the means of enteric *absorption* and *transport* of vitamin B$_{12}$. |
| *iii.* | To understand the *biochemical functions* of vitamin B$_{12}$ as a co-enzyme in the metabolism of propionate and the biosynthesis of methionine. |
| *iv.* | To understand the metabolic *interrelationship of vitamin B$_{12}$ and folate*. |
| *v.* | To understand the factors that can effect *low vitamin B$_{12}$ status*, and the physiological implications of that condition. |

## Vocabulary:

achlorhydria
adenosylcobalamin
anemia
aquocobalamin
cobalamin
cyanocobalamin
gastric parietal cell
haptocorrin
homocysteinuria
IF-receptor
IF-vitamin $B_{12}$ complex
intrinsic factor
leucine mutase
lipotrope
megaloblastic anemia
megaloblastic transformation
methionine synthetase

methylcobalamin
methylfolate trap
methyl-$FH_4$ methyltransferase
methylmalonic acid
methylmalonic acidemia
methylmalonic aciduria
methylmalonyl CoA mutase
pepsin
peripheral neuropathy
pernicious anemia
R-proteins
Schilling test
TC-receptor
transcobalamin
vegan
vitamin $B_{12}$ coenzyme synthetase

# SOURCES OF VITAMIN B$_{12}$

*distribution in*
*foods*

Because the synthesis of vitamin B$_{12}$ is limited almost exclusively to bacteria[1], the vitamin is found only in foods that have been bacterially fermented and those derived from the tissues of animals that have obtained it from their intestinal microflora[2], ingested it either with their diet or coprophagously. Animal tissues that accumulate vitamin B$_{12}$ (e.g., liver[3]) are, therefore, excellent food sources of the vitamin. The richest sources of vitamin B$_{12}$ for animal feeding are animal by-products (e.g., meat and bone meal, fish meal, whey). The naturally occurring vitamin B$_{12}$ in foods is bound in coenzyme form to protein; it is released upon *heating*, gastric *acidification* and/or *proteolysis* (especially by the action of *pepsin*).

Sources of vitamin B$_{12}$ in foods:

| food | vitamin B$_{12}$ μg/100g | food | vitamin B$_{12}$ μg/100g |
|---|---|---|---|
| meats | | fish and sea food | |
| beef | 1.94-3.64 | herring | 4.3 |
| beef brain | 7.83 | salmon | 3.2 |
| beef kidney | 38.3 | trout | 7.8 |
| beef liver | 69-122 | tuna | 2.8 |
| chicken | .32 | clams | 19.1 |
| chicken liver | 24.1 | oysters | 21.2 |
| ham | .8 | lobster | 1.28 |
| pork | .55 | shrimp | 1.9 |
| turkey | .379 | other | |
| dairy products | | eggs, whole | 1.26 |
| milk | .36 | egg whites | .09 |
| cheeses | .36-1.71 | egg yolk | 9.26 |
| yogurt | .06-.62 | | |
| vegetables, grains, fruits | | | |
| *none* contain vitamin B$_{12}$ | | | |

*stability*

Vitamin B$_{12}$ is very stable in both crystalline form and aqueous solution.

---

[1] Until recently, it was thought that cobalamins were synthesized *only* by bacteria (*not* by animals, plants, yeasts and most fungi). Some studies have indicated, however, that under certain conditions, some plants (e.g., peas, beans) may also be able to synthesize small amounts of the vitamin. That notwithstanding, foods derived from those plant have negligible importance as sources of vitamin B$_{12}$ for animals or humans.

[2] The synthesis of vitamin B$_{12}$ by long-gutted animals depends on an adequate supply of Co, which must be ingested in the diet. If the supply of Co is sufficient, the rumen microbial synthesis of vitamin B$_{12}$ in ruminants is substantial. For that reason, not only do those species have no needs for pre-formed vitamin B$_{12}$ in the diet, but their tissues tend to contain appreciably more of the vitamin than those of non-ruminant species.

[3] Vitamin B$_{12}$ was discovered as the anti-pernicious anemia factor in liver.

# ABSORPTION OF VITAMIN $B_{12}$

*active transport* Vitamin $B_{12}$ is absorbed from the gut by two mechanisms: ***active transport***
*and diffusion* involving a specific binding protein (*"**intrinsic factor**"*), and simple diffusion.
The carrier-mediated absorption of vitamin $B_{12}$ is highly efficient and is
important at low doses (e.g., 1-2 $\mu$g) of the vitamin. Diffusion of the
vitamin occurs with low efficiency (~1%) throughout the small intestine and
becomes significant only at higher doses.[4]

*protein-binding* Vitamin $B_{12}$ released in free form by the actions of gastric acidification and/
*in the gut* or peptic digestion is bound to binding proteins secreted by the gastric
mucosa. These include the *"intrinsic factor"* (IF) and the *"R-proteins"*[5].

*intrinsic factor* The ***IF*** is synthesized and secreted, in most animals (including humans),
by the ***gastric parietal cells***[6] in response to ***histamine, gastrin, penta-***
***gastrin***, and the presence of ***food***. A relatively small protein[7], IF binds the
four cobalamins[8] with equivalent affinities. In addition to vitamin $B_{12}$, IF
also binds a ***specific receptor*** in the ileal mucosal brush border. The
binding of a cobalamin appears to have an allosteric effect on the ileal
receptor binding center of IF, causing the protein complex to dimerize and
increasing its binding to the receptor. Formation of the ***IF-vitamin $B_{12}$***
***complex*** protects the vitamin from catabolism by intestinal bacteria. It also
protects IF from hydrolytic attack by pepsin and chymotrypsin. That some
free IF, nevertheless, has been found in the ileum indicates that absorption
may occur for cobalamins synthesized by bacteria of that region of the
small intestine.

---

[4]The passive mechanism is utilized in therapy for pernicious anemia, for which cases are given high doses
(>500 $\mu$g/day) of vitamin $B_{12}$ *per os*.

[5]These vitamin $B_{12}$-binding glycoproteins appear to have no physiological function. They have high
electrophoretic mobility; hence, their name is meant to imply *"rapid"*.

[6]Individuals with loss of gastric parietal cell function may be unable to use dietary vitamin $B_{12}$, as these
cells produce both IF and acid, both of which are required for the enteric absorption of the vitamin. For this
reason, geriatric patients, many of whom are hypoacidic, may be at risk to low vitamin $B_{12}$ status.

[7]The molecular weights of human and porcine IFs vary according to the carbohydrate moiety that is
isolated with particular preparations; values in the ranges of 44-63 kD and 50-59 kD have been reported for IF
from these two sources, respectively.

[8]methylcobalamin, adenosylcobalamin, cyanocobalamin and aquocobalamin

| | |
|---|---|
| *ileal IF-*<br>*receptor* | The ileal *IF-receptor* is a glycoprotein[9] which binds specifically the IF-vitamin B$_{12}$ complex; it binds little, if any, free IF or free vitamin B$_{12}$.  The receptor-binding occurs at neutral pH and depends on the presence of Ca$^{++}$, which forms a stable complex with the IF-vitamin B$_{12}$-receptor.  The receptor is anchored to the brush border membrane[10] and effects the enteric absorption of Vitamin B$_{12}$ through the endocytotic internalization of the receptor-bound complex.  Human patients who lack IF have very low abilities to absorb vitamin B$_{12}$, excreting in the feces 80-100% of oral doses (*vs.* the 30-60% fecal excretion rates of persons with adequate IF). |
| *R proteins* | The physiological role(s) of the *"R proteins"*[11] are only speculative, and the binding of vitamin B$_{12}$ to these glycoproteins[12] may be adventitious.  They are found in humans (not only in the gastric juice and intestinal contents but also several other tissues[13]), and probably only a few other species.   They show structural and immunologic similarities, their differences in electrophoretic mobility being due to differing carbohydrate contents.   Most bind the corrinoids non-specifically; however, the R-proteins of milk and plasma have high affinities for *methylcobalamin*.  Those found in the intestine are not involved in the enteric absorption of vitamin B$_{12}$, as they are normally digested proteolytically in the intestine and, thus, do not compete with IF for the binding of the vitamin[14]. |

---

[9]The human and porcine IF-receptors each consist of two subunits: $\alpha$-subunits of 70 kD and 90 kD, respectively (antigenically related to IF in each species); hydrophobic $\beta$-subunits of 130 kD or 140 kD, respectively. In contrast, the canine IF receptor consists of a single 200 kD unit.

[10]Biophysical studies of the canine IF-receptor have revealed that it mostly (83%) protrudes from the membrane, being only anchored there by ca. 17% of the protein structure.

[11]These proteins are also called *"haptocorrins"*.

[12]They contain sialic acid and fucose.

[13]e.g., plasma, saliva, tears, bile, cerebrospinal fluid, amniotic fluid, leukocytes, erythrocytes and milk

[14]Patients with pancreatic exocrine insufficiency and consequent deficiencies of proteolytic activities in the intestinal lumen can achieve high concentrations of R-proteins. In those conditions, vitamin B$_{12}$ binds primarily to the R-proteins rather than to IF and is, therefore, poorly absorbed. The malabsorption can be corrected by treatment with pancreatic enzymes and, at least partially, with bicarbonate.

# TRANSPORT OF VITAMIN B$_{12}$

specific
transport
proteins

Upon absorption from the intestine, vitamin B$_{12}$ is initially transported in the plasma bound (as the **adenosylcobalamin** and **methylcobalamin**) to highly specific binding proteins called **"transcobalamins" (TCs)**. Transcobalamins are synthesized in several tissues including the intestinal mucosa[15]. One type, **transcobalamin I (TC$_I$)**, is a 60 kD α-glycoprotein. The other, **transcobalamin II (TC$_{II}$)**, is somewhat smaller (38 kD); the chief transport protein of the vitamin, it binds vitamin B$_{12}$ stoichiometrically in a 1:1 molar ratio. A third binding protein, **transcobalamin III (TC$_{III}$)**, has also been described in normal human serum; it is electrophoretically similar to TC$_I$, but antigenically similar to TC$_{II}$. The movement of vitamin B$_{12}$ from the intestinal mucosal cell into the plasma appears to depend on the formation of the TC$_{II}$-vitamin B$_{12}$ complex (the vitamin is shuttled from IF to TC$_{II}$). This complex turns over exceedingly rapidly (its half-life is ca. 6 min.)[16]. Within hours of absorption, however, much of the vitamin originally associated with TC$_{II}$ becomes bound to TC$_I$ and, in humans, to other plasma proteins (**"R-proteins"**)[17]. Whereas deficiency of TC$_I$ does not appear to impair cobalamin metabolism, TC$_{II}$ is clearly necessary for normal cellular maturation of the hematopoietic system[18].

transfer to
"R" proteins
in humans

In humans, most recently absorbed vitamin B$_{12}$ is transferred in the plasma from TC to R-proteins which, therefore, bind most of the circulating vitamin B$_{12}$ in that species. Due to the specificity of the R-proteins for **methylcobalamin**, that vitamer predominates in the circulation of humans[19]. In contrast, this is *not* the case for other species which, lacking R-proteins, transport the vitamin exclusively as the TC-complex. In all species other than the human, the predominant circulating form is **adenosylcobalamin**.

TC-receptor

A membrane-bound receptor protein for TC has been identified in human placenta and rabbit liver. The **TC-receptor** is structurally similar to TC; it is a 50 kD glycoprotein with a single binding-site for the TC-vitamin B$_{12}$ complex. The binding is of high affinity and requires Ca$^{++}$. It is thought

---

[15] Other tissues which appear to synthesize TC are seminal vesicles, liver, fibroblasts, bone marrow and macrophages. The highest concentrations of TC are found in seminal fluid (e.g., vitamin B$_{12}$-binding capacity of ca. 11,550 pg/ml), which contains 10-fold that of the second ranking tissue, plasma.

[16] Human plasma typically contains 500-1400 pmoles TC per liter, with a vitamin B$_{12}$-binding capacity of ca. 800 pg/ml.

[17] Therefore, the transcobalamins belong to a heterogeneous class of proteins called **"R-binders"**.

[18] A rare autosomal recessive deficiency in TC$_{II}$ has been described.

[19] Congenital deficiencies of R-proteins result in low concentrations of vitamin B$_{12}$ in the plasma, but not in detectable losses in function.

that the cellular uptake of vitamin B$_{12}$ involves such TC-receptors mediating the pinocytotic entrance of the vitamin-TC complex to the cell.

*intracellular protein binding*

After its cellular uptake, the TC-receptor complex is degraded in the lysosome to yield the free vitamin, which can be converted to methylcobalamin in the cytosol. Virtually all of the vitamin within the cell is bound to protein, mainly by two vitamin B$_{12}$-dependent enzymes: ***methionine synthetase***[20] in the cytosol and ***methylmalonyl-CoA mutase*** in mitochondria.

*distribution in tissues*

Vitamin B$_{12}$ is stored in very appreciable amounts in the body, mainly in the ***liver*** (ca. 60% of the total body store[21]) and ***muscles*** (ca. 30% of the total). The greatest concentrations of vitamin B$_{12}$ occur in the pituitary gland; kidneys, heart, spleen and brain also contain substantial amounts[22]. The great storage and long biological half-life (350-400 days in humans) of the vitamin provide substantial protection against periods of deprivation[23]. The predominant form in human plasma is ***methylcobalamin*** (60-80% of the total)[24], due to the presence of R-proteins that selectively bind that vitamer. However, the predominant vitamer in the plasma of other species, and in other tissues of all species, is ***adenosylcobalamin*** (in humans, this form accounts for 60-70% of the total vitamin in liver and ca. 50% of that in other tissues). While methylcobalamin is the main form bound by TC$_I$ and TC$_{III}$, both it and adenosylcobalamin are bound in similar amounts by TC$_{II}$. Normal plasma vitamin B$_{12}$ concentrations vary widely among various mammalian species, from only hundreds (humans) to thousands (rabbits) of pmoles per liter.

Cobalamins in normal human plasma:

| cobalamin | range, pmoles/l |
|---|---|
| total cobalamins | 173-545 |
| methylcobalamin | 135-427 |
| adenosylcobalamin | 2- 77 |
| cyanocobalamin | 2- 48 |
| aquocobalamin | 5- 67 |

---

[20] The enzyme is also called *"methyl-FH$_4$ methyltransferase"*.

[21] This amount varies with the intake of the vitamin, but tends to be greater in older subjects. Concentrations approaching 2000 ng/g have been reported in humans; however, a total hepatic reserve of ca. 1.5 mg is typical. Mean total body stores of vitamin B$_{12}$ in humans are in the range of 2-5 mg.

[22] In humans, these organs each contain 20-30 µg of vitamin B$_{12}$.

[23] The low reserve of the human infant (~25 µg) is sufficient to meet physiological needs for about a year.

[24] Methylcobalamin is lost in pernicious anemia patients preferentially to the other forms of the vitamin.

The vitamin $B_{12}$ concentration of human milk varies widely (330-320 pg/ml) and is particularly great (10-fold that of mature milk) in colostrum. Although those products contain TC, most of the vitamin (mainly methyl-cobalamin) is bound to R-proteins, which they also contain in large amounts. In contrast, cow's milk, which does *not* contain R-proteins, typically shows lower concentrations of the vitamin, present in that product mainly as adenosylcobalamin.

## METABOLISM OF VITAMIN $B_{12}$

*activation to coenzyme forms*

Vitamin $B_{12}$ is active in metabolism *only* as derivatives that have a 5'-deoxy-adenosine or methyl group attached covalently to the Co atom (*adenosyl-cobalamin* and *methylcobalamin*, respectively). The conversion of the vitamin to adenosylcobalamin is accomplished by an enzyme system present in many tissues, *vitamin $B_{12}$ coenzyme synthetase*. That system catalyzes the thiol- and reduced flavin-dependent reduction of the cobalt center of the vitamin (to $Co^+$) to form an intermediate[25] which reacts with a deoxyadenosyl moiety derived from ATP. The conversion of the vitamin to methylcobalamin is accomplished by *5-methyl-$FH_4$: homocysteine methyltransferase*, which transfers the single-C unit to vitamin $B_{12}$ as an intermediate step in the biosynthesis of methionine from homocysteine.

*catabolism*

Little, if any, metabolism of the corrinoid ring system is apparent in animals, and vitamin $B_{12}$ excreted as the intact cobalamin. Apparently, only the free cobalamins (not the adenosylated or methylated forms) in the plasma are available for excretion.

*excretion*

Vitamin $B_{12}$ is excreted *via* both renal and biliary routes at the daily rate of 0.1-0.2% of total body reserves (in humans, this constitutes 2-5 $\mu$g/day)[26]. Although it is found in the urine, glomerular filtration of the vitamin is minimal (<0.25 $\mu$g/day in humans), and it is thought that urinary cobal-amin is derived from the tubular epithelial cells and lymph[27]. The biliary excretion of the vitamin is substantial, accounting in humans for the secretion into the intestine of 0.5-5 $\mu$g/day. Most (65-75%) of this amount is reabsorbed in the ileum by IF-mediated active transport. This entero-hepatic circulation constitutes a highly efficient means of conservation with biliary vitamin $B_{12}$ contributing only a small amount to the feces.

---

[25] vitamin $B_{12s}$

[26] This amount, therefore, constitutes the daily requirement for the vitamin.

[27] Urinary excretion of the vitamin after a small oral dose (the *Schilling test*), is used to assess vitamin $B_{12}$ status.

# METABOLIC FUNCTIONS OF VITAMIN B$_{12}$

*coenzyme*
*functions*

Vitamin B$_{12}$ functions in metabolism in two coenzyme forms, ***adenosyl-cobalamin*** and ***methylcobalamin***.  While several vitamin B$_{12}$-dependent metabolic reactions have been identified in microorganisms[28], only *three vitamin B$_{12}$-dependent enzymes have been discovered in animals*: ***methylmalonyl CoA mutase*** and ***leucine mutase*** which each require adenosylcobalamin, and ***methionine synthetase*** which requires methyl-cobalamin).  The reactions catalyzed by the adenosylcobalamin-dependent enzymes each involve intermolecular rearrangements of a C-bound H atom to the neighboring C atom with the adenosylcobalamin C-5' serving as the H-carrier.  This H-transfer is accompanied by the movement of a larger substituent group in the opposite direction (a *"mutase"* reaction).  Methyl-cobalamin, in contrast, is the immediate methyl group donor for the last step of methionine synthesis.  Vitamin B$_{12}$-dependent enzymes play key roles in the metabolism of propionate, amino acids and single carbon.

Metabolic roles of vitamin B$_{12}$ in animals:

| enzyme | metabolic function |
|---|---|
| **adenosylcobalamin** | |
| methylmalonyl CoA mutase | conversion of methylmalonyl CoA to succinyl CoA in the degradation of propionate[a,b] |
| L-*a*-leucine mutase | conversion of L-*a*-leucine to 3-aminoisocapronate as the first step in the synthesis/degradation of the amino acid[c,d] |
| **methylcobalamin** | |
| methionine synthetase | methylation of homocysteine to produce methionine, serving as the methyl group carrier between the donor 5-methyl-FH$_4$ and the acceptor homocysteine[e] |

[a]Propionate, formed from odd-chain fatty acids, is an important energy source for ruminants in which it is produced by rumen microflora.  That the propionic acid pathway is also important in nerve tissue *per se* is suggested by the delayed onset of neurological signs of vitamin B$_{12}$ deficiency effected in animal by dietary supplements of direct (valine and isoleucine) or indirect (methionine) precursors of propionate.
[b]Vitamin B$_{12}$-deficient subjects show methylmalonic aciduria, especially after feeding odd-chain fatty acids.
[c]Vitamin B$_{12}$-deficient subjects show increased circulating levels of 3-aminoisocaproate.
[d]Loss of leucine mutase generally leads to increased 3-aminoisocapronate and decreased leucine, suggesting the main role of the enzyme to be in leucine synthesis.
[e]Vitamin B$_{12}$-deficient subjects show losses of FH$_4$, the key functional form of folate, which accumulates as 5-methyl-FH$_4$ *via* the *"methyl-folate trap"* (see Chapter 16).

---

[28]The following microbial enzymes require *adenosylcobalamin*: glutamate mutase, 2-methylene-glutarate mutase, L-$\beta$-lysine mutase, D-*a*-lysine mutase, D-*a*-ornithine mutase, 1,2-dioldehydratase, glyceroldehydratase, ethanolamine deaminase and ribonucleotide reductase; *methylcobalamin* is also required for the bacterial formation of methane and acetate.

## EXTREMES IN VITAMIN B₁₂ INTAKE

*deficiency*  Vitamin B$_{12}$ deficiency causes ***delay or failure of normal cell division***, particularly in the ***bone marrow*** and ***intestinal mucosa***. Because the biochemical lesion involves arrested synthesis of DNA precursors[29], a reduction in mitotic rate results and abnormally large (cytoplasm-rich) cells are formed. This is called a ***"megaloblastic transformation"***; it is manifest as a characteristic type of anemia in which such enlarged cells are found (***megaloblastic anemia***). ***Neurological abnormalities*** develop in most species[30] with *much later onset* due to the effective storage and conservation of the vitamin. Neurological lesions of vitamin B$_{12}$ deficiency involve diffuse and progressive nerve ***demyelination***, manifest as progressive neuropathy often beginning in the peripheral nerves and progressing eventually to the posterior and lateral columns of the spinal cord. Deficiency of vitamin B$_{12}$ can be produced by several factors; however, inadequate dietary intake is *not* the most common one.

Potential causes of vitamin B$_{12}$ deficiency:

| | |
|---|---|
| *inadequate intake:* | e.g., diet contains only plant-derived, unsupplemented foods |
| *impaired absorption:* | lack of IF<br>pancreatic insufficiency<br>intestinal parasitism<br>drug treatment |

*strict vegetarian diets*  Strict vegetarian diets, containing no meats, fish, animal products (e.g., milk, eggs) or vitamin B$_{12}$ supplements (e.g., multi-vitamin supplements, *"nutritional"* yeasts) contain practically no vitamin B$_{12}$. Therefore, persons consuming such diets typically show very low circulating levels of the vitamin. Nevertheless, clinical signs among such individuals appear to be rare and may not be manifest for many years, though they are more common among their breast-fed infants.

*lack of IF leads to pernicious anemia*  One of the most common causes of vitamin B$_{12}$ deficiency is malabsorption of the vitamin due to ***inadequate production and secretion of IF***. Lack of IF results from ***atrophy of the gastric parietal cells*** which, because they also produce the gastric acid, also results in ***achlorhydria***. Such conditions are caused by atrophy or surgical removal of gastric parietal cells (e.g., ***gastrectomy***), by congenital deficiencies in IF synthesis, and by autoimmune incapacitation of IF. The latter condition, involving the

---

[29]This appears to be due to the failure of ***methionine biosynthesis***, a lack of ***folate coenzymes***, an inadequate synthesis of ***thymidylate*** and, thus, *DNA*.

[30]The neurological lesions, too, appear to result from impaired ***methionine biosynthesis***; however, some investigators dispute this conclusion, proposing that those signs result from the loss of adenosylcobalamin instead.

production of *"blocking antibodies"* that prevent the binding of vitamin B$_{12}$ by IF or of *"binding antibodies"* that bind at the IF receptor-binding site, is characterized by malabsorption of the vitamin ultimately resulting in anemia[31]. It is called *"pernicious anemia"*.

*pancreatic insufficiency*    The loss of pancreatic exocrine function can impair the utilization of vitamin B$_{12}$. For example, about one-half of all human patients with pancreatic insufficiency show abnormally low enteric absorption of the vitamin. This effect can be corrected by pancreatic enzyme replacement therapy using oral pancreas powder or pancreatic proteases. Thus, the lesion appears to involve specifically the loss of proteolytic activity resulting in the failure to digest intestinal R-proteins which, thus, retain vitamin B$_{12}$ bound in the stomach instead of freeing for binding by IF.

*other causes of deficiency*    Other factors that may impair the utilization of vitamin B$_{12}$ include intestinal parasitism (e.g., tapeworms and explosively growing bacterial floras can effectively compete with the host for the vitamin), certain xenobiotic agents (e.g., biguanides[32], alcohol, smoking and N$_2$O[33])[34] and other intestinal defects involving loss of ileal IF-receptors (e.g., sprue, ileitis, etc.).

Signs of vitamin B$_{12}$ deficiency:

| organ system | signs |
|---|---|
| growth | decrease |
| vital organs | hepatic, cardiac and renal steatosis |
| erythrocytes | anemia |
| nervous | peripheral neuropathy |
| fetus | hemorrhage, myopathy, death |

*deficiency syndromes in animals*    Vitamin B$_{12}$ deficiency in animals is characterized most frequently by reductions in rates of *growth* and *feed intake* and impairments in the efficiency of feed utilization. In a few species (e.g., swine) a *mild anemia* develops. In growing chicks and turkey poults, *neurologic signs* may appear. Vitamin B$_{12}$ deficiency has also been related to the etiology of *perosis* in poultry, but this effect seems to be secondary to those of methionine and choline, and related to the availability of labile methyl groups. Also related to *limited methyl group availability* (for the synthesis

---

[31] In humans, megaloblastic anemia may not result for 2-7 years after loss of IF production.

[32] Examples are guanylguanidine, amidinoguanidine and diguanidine, the sulfates of which are used as reagents for the chemical determination of Cu and Ni.

[33] Much of the toxicity of N$_2$O may be due to impaired vitamin B$_{12}$ function. Indeed, it is known that excessive dental use of *"laughing gas"* can lead to neurologic impairment.

[34] The use of oral contraceptive agents (steroids) has been shown to cause a slight drop in plasma vitamin B$_{12}$ concentration; however, no signs of impaired function have been reported.

of phosphatidylcholine) in poultry in increased lipid deposition in the liver, heart and kidneys[35]. Vitamin $B_{12}$ deficiency also causes *embryonic death* in the chicken[36].

*deficiency signs in humans*

Vitamin $B_{12}$ deficiency in humans is characterized by *megaloblastic anemia* and, after prolonged periods, neurological signs including *peripheral neuropathy*, *memory loss* and *dementia*. Abnormalities of lipid metabolism are also observed.

*distinguishing deficiencies of folate and vitamin $B_{12}$*

Some clinical signs (e.g., macrocytic anemia) can result from deficiencies of *either* vitamin $B_{12}$ *or* folate. The only metabolic process that is common to the two vitamins is the methyl group transfer from 5'-methyl $FH_4$ to methylcobalamin for the subsequent methylation of homocysteine to yield methionine and the return of folate to its most important central metabolite, $FH_4$. Thus, deficiencies of either vitamin will reduce the $FH_4$ pool either directly by deprivation of folate or indirectly *via* the *"methylfolate trap"* resulting from deprivation of vitamin $B_{12}$. In either case, the availability of $FH_4$ is reduced and, consequently, its conversion ultimately to 5,10-methylene-$FH_4$ is also reduced. This limits the production of thymidylate and, thus, of DNA, resulting in impaired mitosis which is manifest as macrocytosis and anemia. Similarly, the urinary excretion of the histidine metabolite *formiminoglutamic acid (FIGLU)* is elevated by deficiencies of either folate or vitamin $B_{12}$ as $FH_4$ is required to accept the formimino group, yielding *5'-formimino-$FH_4$*. While supplemental folate can mask the anemia or FIGLU excretion (especially after *histidine loading*) associated with vitamin $B_{12}$ deficiency by maintaining $FH_4$ in spite of the *"methylfolate trap"*, supplemental vitamin $B_{12}$ does not affect the anemia (nor other signs) of folate deficiency. Although such signs as macrocytic anemia, urinary FIGLU and subnormal circulating folate concentrations are, therefore, *not* diagnostic for either vitamin $B_{12}$ or folate deficiencies (these deficiencies *cannot* be distinguished based on these signs), the urinary excretion of *methylmalonic acid (MMA)* can be used for that purpose. *Methylmalonic aciduria* (especially after a meal of odd-chain fatty acids or a load of propionate) occurs *only* in vitamin $B_{12}$ deficiency (*methylmalonyl CoA mutase* requires *adenosylcobalamin*). Therefore, patients with macrocytic anemia, increased urinary FIGLU and low blood folate levels can be diagnosed as being vitamin $B_{12}$-deficient if their urinary MMA levels are elevated, but as being folate-deficient if they are not.

*congenital disorders of vitamin $B_{12}$ metabolism*

Several congenital deficiencies in proteins involved in vitamin $B_{12}$ metabolism, each an autosomal recessive trait, have been reported in humans. Most of these disorders result in signs alleviated by high parenteral doses of the vitamin. The exception is congenital R-protein deficiency; the few

---

[35] For this reason, vitamin $B_{12}$ is known as a *"lipotrope"* for poultry.

[36] Embryos show myopathy of the muscles of the leg, hemorrhage, myocardial hypertrophy and perosis.

documented cases have involved healthy individuals.

Congenital disorders of vitamin B$_{12}$ metabolism:

| condition | missing/deficient factor | signs/symptoms |
|---|---|---|
| methylmalonic aciduria | methylmalonyl CoA mutase | methylmalonic aciduria, homocystein-uria, lethargy, muscle cramps, vomiting, mental retardation |
| lack of Intrinsic Factor | Intrinsic Factor | signs consistent with vitamin B$_{12}$ deficiency |
| Imerslund-Gräsbeck syndrome | IF-receptor | specific malabsorption of vitamin B$_{12}$ |
| lack of transcobalamins | transcobalamins | severe (fatal) megaloblastic anemia appearing early in life |
| lack of R-proteins | R-proteins | no clinical signs |

*hyper-vitaminosis*   Vitamin B$_{12}$ has no appreciable toxicity.  Results of studies with mice indicate that it is ***innocuous*** when administered parenterally in very high doses.  Dietary levels of at least *several hundred* times the nutritional requirements are safe.

# CASE STUDY

*Instructions:*   Review the following case report, paying special attention to the diagnostic indicators upon which the treatment was based.  Then, answer the questions that follow.

*case*   A-six-month old boy was admitted in comatose condition.  He had been born at term, weighing 3 kg, the first child of an apparently healthy 26-year-old ***vegan***[37].  The mother had knowingly eaten no animal products for 8 years and took no supplemental vitamins.  The infant was exclusively breast fed.  He smiled at 1-2 months of age and appeared to be developing normally.  At 4 months, his development began to regress; this was manifest by his loss of head control, decreased vocalization, lethargy and increased irritability.  Physical examination revealed a pale and flaccid infant who was completely unresponsive even to painful stimuli.  His pulse was 136/min, the respirations 22/min and the blood pressure 100 mm Hg by palpation.  His length was 65 cm (50th percentile for age) and the weight 5.6 kg (<3rd percentile, and at the 50th percentile for three months of age).  His head circumference was 41 cm (3rd percentile).  His optic

---

[37] a strict vegetarian

disks[38] were pale. There were scattered ecchymoses[39] over his legs and buttocks. He had increased pigmentation over the dorsa of his hands and the feet, most prominently over the knuckles. He had no head control and a poor grasp. He showed no deep tendon reflexes. His liver edge was palpable 2 cm below the right costal margin.

Laboratory results:

| parameter | patient | normal range |
| --- | --- | --- |
| hemoglobin, g/dl | 5.4 | 10.0-15.0 |
| hematocrit, % | 17 | 36 |
| erythrocytes, $\times 10^6/\mu l$ | 1.63 | 3.9-5.3 |
| white blood cells, $\times 10^3/\mu l$ | 3.8 | 6-17.5 |
| reticulocytes, % | 0.1 | < 1 |
| platelets, $\times 10^3/\mu l$ | 45 | 200-480 |

A peripheral blood smear revealed mild macrocytosis[40], some hypersegmentation of the neutrophils[41]. Bone-marrow aspiration showed frank *megaloblastic changes* in both the myeloid[42] and the erythroid[43] series. Megakaryocytes[44] were decreased in number. The sedimentation rate, urinalysis, spinal-fluid analysis, blood glucose, electrolytes and tests of renal and liver function gave normal results. An electroencephalogram was markedly abnormal, as manifested by minimal background Θ-activity and epileptiform transients in both temporal regions. Analysis of the urine obtained on admission demonstrated markedly elevated excretion of *methylmalonic acid*, *glycine*, *methylcitric acid* and *homocysteine*. Shortly after admission, respiratory distress developed, and 5 mg of *folic acid* was given, followed by transfusion of 10 ml/kg of packed RBCs. Four days later, a repeat bone-marrow examination showed *partial reversal* of the megaloblastic abnormalities.

---

[38] circular area of thinning of the sclera (the fibrous membrane forming the outer envelope of the eye) through which the fibers of the optic nerve pass

[39] purple patches caused by extravasation of blood into the skin, differing from *petechiae* only in size (the latter being very small)

[40] occurrence of unusually large numbers of *macrocytes* (large erythrocytes) in the circulating blood; also called *megalocytosis*, *magalocythemia* and *macrocythemia*

[41] a type of mature white blood cell in the *granulocyte* series

[42] related to *myocytes*

[43] related to *erythrocytes*

[44] an unusually large cell thought to be derived from the primitive mesenchymal tissue that differentiates from hemaotcytoblasts

Other laboratory results:

| parameter | patient | normal range |
|---|---|---|
| serum vitamin B$_{12}$, pg/ml | 20 | 150-1,000 |
| serum folates, ng/ml | 10 | 3-15 |
| serum Fe, $\mu$g/dl | 165 | 65-175 |
| serum Fe-binding capacity, $\mu$/dl | 177 | 250-410 |

*Cyanocobalamin* (1 mg/day) was administered for four days. The patient began to respond to stimuli after the transfusion; however, the response to vitamin B$_{12}$ was *dramatic*. Four days after the initial dose he was alert, smiling, responding to visual stimuli and maintaining his body temperature. As he responded, rhythmical twitching activity in the right hand and arm developed that persisted despite anticonvulsant therapy, despite a concomitant resolution of electroencephalographic abnormalities. The mother showed a completely normal hemogram. Her serum vitamin B$_{12}$ concentration was 160 pg/ml (normal: 150-1,000 pg/ml), but she showed moderate methylmalonic aciduria. Her breast milk contained 75 pg vitamin B$_{12}$/ml (normal: 1-3 ng/ml).

With vitamin B$_{12}$ therapy, the infant's plasma vitamin B$_{12}$ rose to 600 pg/ml and he continued to improve clinically. The abnormal urinary acids and homocystine disappeared by the 10th day; cystathionine persisted until the 20th day. On the 14th day, the Hb was 14.4 g/dl, hematocrit was 41% and the WBC was 5,700/ml. The platelet count had become normal 20 days after admission. The unusual pigment on the extremities had improved considerably 2 weeks after he received the parenteral vitamin B$_{12}$ and disappeared gradually over the next month. The liver was no longer palpable. The twitching of the hands disappeared within a month of therapy. Developmental assessment at 9 months of age revealed him to be functioning at the 5-month age level. A month later, he was sitting and taking steps with support. Head circumference had exhibited catch-up growth and at 44 cm was in the normal range for the first time since admission. His length was 70 cm (10th percentile) and weight 8.4 kg (10th percentile). By this time, the mother's serum vitamin B$_{12}$ had dropped to only 100 pg/ml, and she began taking supplemental vitamin B$_{12}$.

Questions:

i. Which clinical findings suggested that *two* important coenzyme forms of vitamin B$_{12}$ were deficient or defective in this infant? How do the clinical findings relate specifically to each coenzyme?

ii. What findings enable the distinction of vitamin B$_{12}$ deficiency from a possible folic acid-related disorder in this patient?

iii. Offer a reasonable explanation for the fact that the mother, who had avoided vitamin B$_{12}$-containing foods for 8 years prior to her pregnancy, did *not* show overt signs of vitamin B$_{12}$ deficiency.

## Study Questions and Exercises:

i.     Construct a *"decision tree"* for the diagnosis of vitamin $B_{12}$ deficiency in humans or an animal species and, in particular, the distinction of this deficiency from that of folate.

ii.    What key feature of the *chemistry* of vitamin $B_{12}$ relates to its coenzyme functions?

iii.   What parameters might you measure to *assess vitamin $B_{12}$ status* of a human or animal?

iv.    What is the relationship of normal function of the *stomach* and *pancreas* with the utilization of dietary vitamin $B_{12}$?

## Recommended Reading:

Cooper, B.A. and D.S. Rosenblatt. 1987. Inherited defects of vitamin $B_{12}$ metabolism. Ann. Rev. Nutr. 7:291-320.

Ellenbogen, L. and B.A. Cooper. 1991. Vitamin $B_{12}$, Chapter 13 *in* Handbook of Vitamins, 2 ed. (L.J. Machlin, ed.), Marcel Dekker, New York. pp. 491-536.

Flodin, N.W. 1988. Pharmacology of Micronutrients. Alan R. Liss., Inc., New York, pp. 179-188.

Friedrich, W. 1988. Vitamins. Walter de Gruyter, New York. pp. 839-928.

Herbert, V. 1990. Vitamin B-12, Chapter 20 *in* Present Knowledge in Nutrition, 6th ed. (M. Brown, ed.), Int. Life Sci. Inst.-Nutr. Found., Washington, D.C., pp. 170-178.

Herbert, V. 1988. Vitamin B-12: plant sources, requirements, and assay. Am. J. Clin. Nutr. 48:852-858.

Herbert, V. 1987. The 1986 Herman Award Lecture. Nutrition science as a continually unfolding story: the folate and vitamin $B_{12}$ paradigm. Am. J. Clin. Nutr. 46:387-402.

# CHAPTER 18    *QUASI-VITAMINS*

*"Have all the vitamins been discovered? From all indications in the extensive recent and current publications in the scientific literature dealing with the purification and effects of 'unidentified factors', the answer appears to be 'no'. It is from such studies that new vitamins may be recognized and characterized."*    A.F. Wagner and K. Folkers

## Anchoring Concepts:

i.    The designation *"vitamin"* is specific for animal species, stage of development or production, and/or particular conditions of the physical environment and diet.

ii.    Each of the presently recognized vitamins was initially called an *"accessory factor"* or an *"unidentified growth factor"*, and that these terms continue to be used to describe biologically active substances, particularly for species of lower orders.

## Learning Objectives:

i.    To understand that the usual designation of the vitamins has a strong *bias* in favor of those compounds required by higher animals, especially humans.

ii.    To understand that *other substances have been proposed as vitamins*.

iii.    To understand the metabolic functions of *choline* and *carnitine*, which clearly fit the vitamin designation for certain animal species.

iv.    To understand the metabolic functions of *myo-inositol, pyrroloquinoline quinone*, the *ubiquinones, orotic acid* and *bioflavanoids*, and the biological activities of each.

v.    To understand why *p-aminobenzoic acid* and *lipoic acid* are not called vitamins.

vi.    That understanding of the list of vitamins *may not be complete*.

## Vocabulary:

acetylcholine
acetyl transferase
acylcarnitine
p-aminobenzoic acid
arachidonic acid
betaine
betaine aldehyde dehydrogenase
betaine:homocysteine methyltransferase
bioflavonoids
γ-butyrobetaine hydroxylase
Ca$^{++}$ channels
calcisome
carnitine
carnitine acyltransferases I and II
carnitine translocase
chelate
choline dehydrogenase
choline kinase
choline oxidase
choline phosphotransferase
coenzyme Q$_{10}$
cyanogenic glycoside
cytidine diphosphorylcholine
dimethylglycine
eicosanoid
glycerylphosphorylcholine
glycerylphosphorylcholine diesterase
myo-inositol
inositol triphosphate
intestinal dystrophy

labile methyl groups
lecithin
lipoic acid
lipoamide
lysolecithin
lysyl oxidase
orotic acid
perosis
phosphatidylcholine
phosphatidylcholine glyceride choline
   transferase
phosphatidylethanolamine
phosphatidylethanolamine N-
   methyl transferase
phosphatidylinositol
phosphatidylinositol phosphate
phosphatidylinositol diphosphate
phospholipases A$_1$, A$_2$, B and C
phosphorylcholine
phytic acid
pyrroloquinoline quinone
quinoprotein
second messenger
sphingomyelins
stearic acid
trimethylamine
ε-N-trimethyllysine
ubiqinones
vitamin B$_T$

# IS THE LIST OF VITAMINS COMPLETE?

*common*
*features*
*in the*
*recognition*
*of the*
*vitamins*

Reflection upon the ways in which the traditional vitamins were recognized reveals a process of discovery involving both *empirical* and *experimental* phases (see Chapter 2). That is, initial associations between diet and health status were the sources of hypotheses that could be tested in controlled experiments. As is generally true in science, where hypotheses were clearly enunciated and adequate experimental approaches were available, insightful investigators were able to make remarkable progress in identifying these essential nutrients. Those endeavors, of course, also revealed some **"unidentified factors"** not to be new at all[1], some to be identical or otherwise related to each other[2], some to be biologically active but not essential in diets[3], and some to be without basis in fact[4]. The apparently irregular and often confusing array of informal names of the vitamins[5] reveals this history of discovery.

*limitations*
*of traditional*
*designations*
*of vitamins*

The development of the *"Vitamine Theory"* was instrumental in conditioning thought such that the discovery of the vitamins could occur. Indeed, it provided the basis for the evolution of the operating definition that has been used to designate vitamin status for biologically active substances. However, after several decades of learning more and more about the metabolism and biochemical actions of the substances called vitamins, it has become clear that the traditional criteria for that designation[6] are, in several cases[7], inappropriate unless they are used with specific reference to animal species, stage of development, diet or nutritional status, and physical environment. However, because it is often more convenient to consider nutrients by general group without such referents, the designation of vitamin status has become a bit arbitrary as well as anthropocentric in that the traditional designation of the vitamins reflects, to a large extent, the

---

[1] An example is *"vitamin T"* (also called *"termitin"*, *"penicin"*, *"torutilin"*, *"insectine"*, *"hypomycin"*, *"myocoine"* or *"sesame seed factor"*). This extract from yeast, sesame seeds or insects appeared to stimulate the growth of guppies, hamsters, baby pigs, chicks, mice and insects, promoted wound healing in mice, and improved certain human skin lesions. It was found to be a varied mixture containing folate, vitamin $B_{12}$ and amino acids.

[2] For example, vitamins *"M"*, *"$B_c$"*, *"$B_{10}$"*, *"T"* and *"$B_x$"* were found to be various forms of folate.

[3] e.g., the ubiquinones

[4] e.g., pangamic acid (*"vitamin $B_{15}$"*), laetrile (*"vitamin $B_{17}$"*), orotic acid (*"vitamin $B_{13}$"*), *"vitamins $H_3$"* and *"U"*.

[5] See Chapter 2: tables of *"Current and obsolete designations of 'vitamins', 'factors' and other terms"*.

[6] See Chapter 1.

[7] Examples are vitamins D and C, niacin and choline.

nutritional needs of humans and, to a lesser extent, those of domestic animals. For example, although it is now very clear that $1,25\text{-}(OH)_2\text{-}$cholecalciferol is actually a hormone produced endogenously by all species exposed to sunlight, the parent compound cholecalciferol continues to be called "*vitamin D₃*" in recognition of its importance to the health of many people whose minimal sunlight exposure renders them in need of it in their diets.

*vitamin designation should be species-specific*

Nevertheless, it is important to keep in mind that other species may have obligate dietary needs for substances that are biosynthesized by humans and/or higher animals, and that such substances can be considered to be vitamins in the most proper sense of the word. Available evidence indicates this to be true for *at least three substances*, and some reports have suggested this for others. As more is learned, it is certainly possible that **more vitamins** may be discovered!

*quasi-vitamins*

It is useful to recognize the other factors that appear to satisfy the criteria of vitamin status for only a few species or under only certain conditions, and to do so without according them the full status of a vitamin. This is done using the term "*quasi-vitamin*". Thus, the list of quasi-vitamins includes such factors as **choline** (clearly required in the diets of young growing poultry for optimal growth and freedom of leg disorders), **carnitine** (clearly required for growth of certain insects) and **myo-*inositol*** (clearly required for optimal growth of fishes and to prevent intestinal lesions in gerbils). It also includes other factors for which evidence of nutritional essentiality is less compelling (***pyrroloquinoline quinone***, ***ubiquinones***, ***orotic acid***, ***bioflavanoids***, ***p-aminobenzoic acid***, ***lipoic acid***). In addition, the biologically active properties of certain natural products ("***unidentified growth factors***", or "***UGFs***") are worthy of consideration in view of the fact that most of the consensus vitamins were initially recognized as UGFs.

Quasi-vitamins:

| |
|---|
| choline |
| carnitine |
| *myo*-inositol |
| pyrroloquinoline quinone |
| ubiquinones |
| orotic acid |
| bioflavonoids |
| *p*-aminobenzoic acid |
| lipoic acid |

# CHOLINE

*known
metabolite
acts like
vitamin*

The discovery of insulin by **Banting** and **Best** in the mid 1920s, led to studies of the metabolism of depancreatized dogs that showed dietary lecithin (phosphatidylcholine) to be effective in mobilizing the excess lipids in the livers of insulin-deprived animals.  **Best** and **Huntsman** showed that **choline** was the active component of lecithin in mediating this effect.  Choline had been isolated by **Strecker** in 1862, and its structure had been determined by **Bayer** shortly after that.  Yet, it was these latter findings of choline as a **"lipotropic factor"**, that stimulated interest in its nutritional role.

*poultry have
special needs
for choline*

In 1940, **Jukes** showed that choline is required for normal growth and the prevention of the leg disorder called **"perosis"**[8] in turkeys; he found that the amount required to prevent perosis is greater than that required to support normal growth.  Further studies by Jukes and by **Norris'** group at Cornell showed that betaine, the metabolic precursor to choline, was not always effective in preventing choline-responsive perosis in turkeys and chicks. These findings stimulated further interest in the metabolic roles and nutritional needs for choline, as it was clear that its function was more than simply that of a **"lipotrope"**.

*chemical
nature*

Choline is the trivial designation for the compound **2-hydroxy-N,N,N-tri-methylethanaminium** (also, [$\beta$-hydroxyethyl]trimethylammonium).   It is freely soluble in water and ethanol, but insoluble in organic solvents. It is a strong base and decomposes in alkaline solution with the release of trimethylamine.  The prominent feature of its chemical structure is its triplet of methyl groups, which enables it to serve as a methyl donor.

*distribution
in foods*

All natural fats contain some choline; therefore, the vitamin is widely distributed in foods and feedstuffs.  It occurs naturally mostly in the form of **phosphatidylcholine**[9] which, because it is a good emulsifying agent, is used as an ingredient or additive to many processed foods and food supplements[10].  Choline is added (as **choline chloride** and **choline bitartrate**)

---

[8]**Perosis** occurs in rapidly growing heavy-bodied poultry, involving the misalignment of the tibiotarsus and consequent slippage of the Achilles tendon.  This impairs ambulation, and can reduce feeding, consequently, impairing growth.  Perosis can also be caused by dietary deficiencies of **niacin** or **Mn**.

[9]*lecithin*

[10]Some dietary choline (<10%) is present as the **free base** and **sphingomyelins** (phosphatidylcholine analogues containing, instead of a fatty acid, *sphingosine* [2-amino-4-octadecene-1,3-diol] at the glycerol $a$-C).

## Choline

to infant formulas as a means of fortification.  The richest sources in human diets are egg yolk, glandular meats (e.g., liver, kidney, brain), soybean products, wheat germ and peanuts.  The best sources of choline for animal feeding are the germs of cereals, legumes and oil-seed meals (e.g., soybean meal).  Corn is notably low in choline (half the levels found in barley, oats and wheat).  Wheat is rich in the choline-sparing factor *betaine*[11].  Little is known about the bioavailability of choline in foods and feedstuffs.  Naturally occurring choline, as well as the choline salts used as supplements to human diets and animal feeds have *good stability*.

Choline contents of common foods:

| food | choline mg/g | food | choline mg/g |
|---|---|---|---|
| meats | | vegetables | |
| beef brain | 410 | asparagus | 128 |
| beef liver | 630 | cabbage | 46 |
| beef kidney | 333 | carrots | 10 |
| ham | 120 | cauliflower | 78 |
| trout | 84 | lettuce | 18 |
| cereals | | soybeans | 237 |
| barley | 139 | peanuts | 145 |
| oats | 151 | dairy and egg products | |
| rice, polished | 126 | milk | 10 |
| wheat germ | 423 | egg yolk | 1713 |

*absorption*  Choline is released from *phosphatidylcholine* by hydrolysis of the latter in the intestinal lumen.  This is accomplished enzymatically through the action of *phospholipases* produced by the pancreas (*phospholipase $A_2$*, which cleaves the $\beta$-ester bond) and the intestinal mucosa (*phospholipases $A_1$ and B*, both of which cleave the $a$-ester bond to yield *glycerylphosphorylcholine*).  The mucosal enzymes are much less efficient than the pancreatic enzyme.  Therefore, most of the phosphatidylcholine that is ingested is absorbed as *lysolecithin* (deacylated only in the $a$-position) which is re-acylated to yield phosphatidylcholine[12].  The analogous reactions occur with *sphingomyelin* which, unlike phosphatidylcholine, is not degraded in the intestinal lumen, but is taken up intact by the intestinal mucosa.  When free choline or one of its salts are consumed, a large amount (e.g., nearly two-thirds is catabolized by intestinal microorganisms to the end product

---

[11]Therefore, the choline needs of livestock fed diets based on wheat are much lower than those of animals fed diets based on corn.

[12]This reaction involves the *dismutation* of two molecules of lysolecithin to yield one molecule of glycerylphosphorylcholine and one molecule of phosphatidylcholine.

## *Choline*

*trimethylamine*[13] much of which is absorbed and excreted in the urine. The remaining portion is absorbed intact.  Phosphatidylcholine is not subject to such extensive microbial metabolism and, therefore, produces less urinary trimethylamine.

*uptake*   Choline is absorbed in the upper portion of the small intestine by a saturable, *carrier-mediated process* involving a carrier localized in the brush border, and efficient at low luminal concentrations (<4 mM). At high lumenal concentrations, it is also absorbed by *passive diffusion.*

*transport*   Recently absorbed choline is transported into the lymphatic circulation[14] primarily in the form of *phosphatidylcholine* bound to *chylomicra*, which are subject to clearance to the *lipoproteins* that circulate to the peripheral tissues.  Thus, choline is transported to the tissues predominantly as phospholipids associated with the plasma lipoproteins.

Distribution of phospholipids in plasma lipoproteins:

| lipoprotein class | phospholipid content (% total weight) |
|---|---|
| high-density lipoproteins (HDL) | ~30 |
| low-density lipoproteins (LDL) | ~22 |
| very low-density lipoproteins (VLDL) | 10-25 |
| chylomicra | 3-15 |

*tissue distribution*   Choline is present in *all tissues* as an essential component of *phospholipids* in membranes of all types.  It is stored in the greatest concentrations in the essential organs (e.g., *brain*, *liver*, *kidney*) in the forms of *phosphatidylcholine* and *sphingomeylins*.

*biosynthesis*   Most species can synthesize choline, as phosphatidylcholine, by the sequential *methylation of phosphatidylethanolamine*[15] by *phosphatidylethanolamine-N-methyltransferase*.  This activity is actually due to two enzymes: a cell inner membrane enzyme adds the first methyl group; a cell outer membrane enzyme adds the second and third methyl groups. Each enzyme uses *S-adenosylmethionine* as the methyl donor.  The first is rate-limiting to choline synthesis; this activity is low in male rats and absent from

---

[13]The characteristic *"fishy"* odor of this product is identifiable after consumption of a choline supplement.

[14]or the portal circulation in birds, fishes and reptiles

[15]Of the three means of phosphatidylcholine synthesis (methylation of ethanolamine, reaction of cytidine diphosphate, phospholipid base-exchange [e.g., substitution of choline for serine, ethanolamine or inositol in endogenous phospholipids]), only the methylation pathway involves the *de novo* synthesis of choline.

## *Choline*

chicks until ca. 13 weeks of age[16]. The activity is greatest in liver, but is also found in many other tissues. It accounts for the synthesis of 15-40% of the phosphatidylcholine in the liver (most of the balance being derived from the cytidine diphosphate [CDP-choline] pathway).

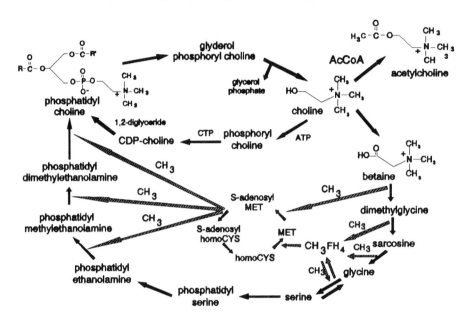

*metabolism*    Choline is released in free form in the tissues by the actions of ***phospholipase C***, which cleaves the circulating form (phosphatidylcholine) to yield a diglyceride and ***phosphorylcholine***. The latter species is converted to free choline by ***alkaline phosphatase***. In addition, peripheral tissues also contain ***phospholipase B*** activity and can, therefore produce ***glycerylphosphorylcholine*** from the circulating form of the vitamin. That product can then be cleaved to yield free choline by ***glycerylphosphorylcholine diesterase***. The brain also contains ***phospholipase D***, which cleaves free choline directly from the circulating form (also yielding glycerylphosphate).

Free choline can be oxidized by the mitochondrial enzyme ***choline dehydrogenase*** to yield ***betaine aldehyde***, which is then converted by the cytosolic enzyme ***betaine aldehyde dehydrogenase*** to ***betaine***[17]. This

---

[16]Due to the developmental deficiency of this methylating enzyme, young chicks require a dietary source of pre-formed choline. Other species require choline only if this methylation pathway is limited by the availability of methyl groups. The feeding of methyl donors (methionine, betaine) spares choline needs.

[17]1-carboxy-N,N,N-trimethylmethanaminium hydroxide inner salt

# *Choline*

dual enzyme system is called *"choline oxidase"*; it is found is several tissues (e.g., liver and kidney), but is notably absent from brain, muscle and blood.  Choline is oxidized to betaine at a rate that is an order of magnitude *greater* than that of its incorporation into phosphorylcholine. *Betaine cannot be reduced back to form choline*, but it can donate its *methyl groups* to *homocysteine* to produce *dimethylglycine* and *methionine (MET)* by the action of the enzyme *betaine:homocysteine methyltransferase*.  Therefore, while the choline oxidase pathway removes free choline from the body, it also serves as a source of labile methyl groups.

Free choline is phosphorylated by the cytosolic enzyme *choline phosphotransferase*[18] using ATP as the phosphate donor.  This step occurs in many tissues and constitutes the first step in the generation of *cytidine diphosphatylcholine* (CDP-choline), which combines with diacylglycerol (by the action of *phosphatidylcholine glyceride transferase*) in the synthesis of phosphatidylcholine.

Only a small fraction of choline is *acetylated*, but that amount provides the important neurotransmitter *acetylcholine*.  This step involves the reaction of choline with *acetyl CoA* and is catalyzed by an enzyme *choline acetyltransferase* localized in cholinergic nerve terminals, as well as in certain other non-nervous tissues (e.g., placenta).  Because brain choline acetyltransferase appears not to be saturated with either substrate, it is likely that the availability of choline (as well as that of acetyl CoA) may determine the rate of synthesis of acetylcholine.

*metabolic functions*

Choline has four basic functions in metabolism:

> i.   As *phosphatidylcholine*, it is a *structural element of biological membranes*
>
> ii.  As *phosphatidylcholine*, it *promotes lipid transport* (is a *"lipotrope"*)
>
> iii. As *acetylcholine*, it is a *neurotransmitter*
>
> iv.  *After conversion to betaine*, it is a *source of labile methyl groups* for transmethylation reactions (e.g., the formation of methionine from homocysteine, or creatine from guanidoacetic acid)

*deficiency*

Choline deficiency can occur in young poultry (e.g., chicks less than *ca.* 13 weeks of age) fed diets low in choline, and in older poultry and other animals fed diets deficient in methyl groups (methionine-deficient diets). Choline deficiency in most animal species is characterized by *depressed growth*, *hepatic steatosis* and *hemorrhagic renal degeneration*.  Poultry also show *perosis*, but this disorder is thought to be a secondary lesion related to impaired lipid transport.

---

[18] *choline kinase*

## *Choline*

Clear cases of choline deficiency have not been reported in humans, but this may only reflect the adequacy of other methyl donors in the types of subjects frequently studied. A recent study wherein healthy adults were fed a diet adequate (but not excessive) in methionine and folacin showed that deprivation of choline produced signs of hepatic dysfunction (increased serum transaminase activities) which were corrected by feeding choline. Further, some evidence supports benefits of choline in the treatment of diseases involving hepatic steatosis and of liver dysfunction associated with total parenteral feeding of low-choline fluids.

Signs of choline deficiency:

| organ system | signs |
|---|---|
| growth | decrease |
| skeletal | perosis |
| vital organs | hepatic steatosis, renal hemorrhage |

*pharmacologic uses*
The intake of choline can affect the concentrations of the neurotransmitter *acetylcholine* in the brain, suggesting that choline-loading may be beneficial to patients with diseases involving deficiencies of cholinergic neurotransmission. Therefore, large doses (multiple-gram quantities) of choline have been used to increase brain choline concentrations above normal levels, thereby stimulating the synthesis of acetylcholine in nerve terminals. Notable success has been achieved with choline therapy[19] for the movement disorder *tardive dyskinesia*, which appears to involve inadequate neurotransmission at striatal cholinergic interneurons[20]. Choline has also been used with some success to diminish *short-term memory losses* associated with *Alzheimer's disease*, a disorder involving deficiency of hippocampal cholinergic neurons. Studies with experimental animal models have shown that choline therapy can improve short-term memory deficits; these findings are supported by several human case reports. Further support comes from the finding that patients treated with anticholinergic drugs develop short-term memory deficits that resemble those of patients with hippocampal lesions. Phosphatidylcholine has been reported to *reduce manic episodes* in patients, suggesting that it can be centrally active; however, such treatment has been found to *exacerbate depression* among tardive dyskinesia patients.

---

[19] Oral choline or phosphatidylcholine are the only effective therapies to date.

[20] *Tardive dyskinesia* is prevalent among patients treated with neuroleptic drugs (drugs affecting the autonomic nervous system) and is characterized by choreoathetotic movements (involuntary movements resembling those of both *chorea*, which are irregular and spasmodic, and those of *athetosis*, which are slow, and writhing) of the face, the extremities and, usually, the trunk.

## Choline

*hyper-*
*vitaminosis*

The toxicity of choline appears to be **very low**.  However, deleterious effects have been reported for the salt choline chloride; these have included growth depression, **impaired utilization of vitamin B$_6$** and **increased mortality**. It is not clear, however, whether the apparent toxicity of that form of the vitamin may actually have been due to the perturbation of acid-base balance caused by the high level of chloride administered with large doses of the salt.  In humans, high doses (e.g., 20 g) have produced **dizziness**, **nausea** and **diarrhea**.

## CARNITINE

*insect growth*
*factor*

In the 1950s, entomologists at the University of Illinois, **Gottfried Fraenkel** and colleagues, found that the successful growth of the yellow mealworm *Tenebrio molitor* in culture required the feeding of a natural substance which they found to be present in milk, yeast and many animal tissues. They purified the growth factor, which they named *"vitamin B$_T$"*, from whey solids and identified it as **carnitine**[21], a known metabolite isolated at the turn of the century from extracts of mammalian muscle.  Although this finding established carnitine as a biologically active substance, the first indication of its metabolic role came a decade later when **Irving Fritz** at the University of Michigan found it to stimulate the *in vitro* oxidation of long-chain fatty acids by subcellular fractions of heart muscle.   Research interest in carnitine has increased dramatically in recent years, stimulated by the finding of **Broquist** and colleagues at Vanderbilt University that carnitine is biosynthesized by mammals from the amino acid lysine, which is limiting in the diets of many third-world populations, and by the description by **Engel** and colleagues of clinical syndromes (of apparently genetic origin) associated with carnitine deficiency.

*chemical*
*nature*

Carnitine is a quaternary amine, $\beta$-hydroxy-$\gamma$-N-trimethylaminobutyrate.

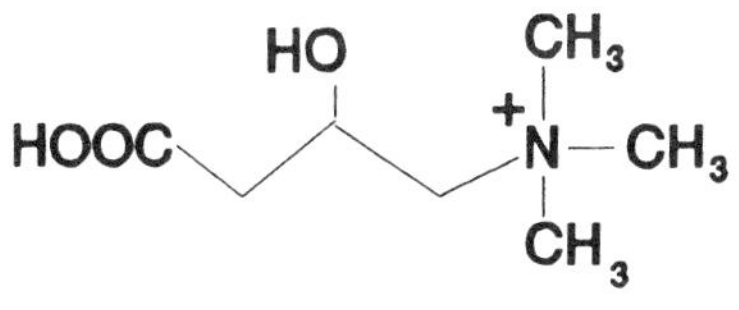

---

[21]Carter, H.E., P.K. Bhattacharyya, K.R. Weidman and G. Fraenkel. 1952. Arch. Biochem. Biophys. 38:405-426.

## Carnitine

*biosynthesis*      Carnitine is synthesized in mammals[22] from the indispensable amino acid
                    *lysine*. The biosynthetic process commences with the enzymatic trimethyl-
                    ation of a peptide-bound lysine residue to form **ε-N-trimethyllysine**, using
                    **S-adenosylmethionine** as the methyl-donor.   The ε-N-trimethyllysine,
                    released as the protein turns over, is converted to **L-carnitine** through a
                    sequence of enzymatic reactions involving two $Fe^{++}$- and ascorbate-
                    dependent hydroxylases and one $NAD^+$-dependent dehydrogenase[23].

The enzymes that catalyze the conversion of ε-N-trimethyllysine to γ-butyrobetaine appear to occur in all tissues.  In contrast, the last enzyme in the
biosynthetic pathway, **γ-butyrobetaine hydroxylase**, is *not* found in human
skeletal muscle or heart, although it is present in other tissues. In human
liver and kidney, it is present as multiple isoenzymes; the activity increases
during development[24], reaching maxima in the mid-teens.   Little direct
evidence is available concerning the quantitative aspects of carnitine
biosynthesis relative to physiological needs in humans.  That healthy adults
can synthesize carnitine at rates sufficient for their needs is indicated by
findings that subjects in southeast Asia, whose cereal-based diets provide

---

[22] Carnitine biosynthesis has been investigated most extensively in the rat; available evidence indicates that the biosynthetic pathways in humans, and probably other mammals, are identical.

[23] That tissue carnitine concentrations are depressed in vitamin $B_6$ deficiency suggests that the vitamin may be required for carnitine biosynthesis. An hypothesis for this effect is that *serine transhydroxymethylase*, a pyridoxal 5'-phosphate-dependent enzyme, has the capacity to cleave 3-hydroxy-6-N-trimethyllysine.

[24] For example, the hepatic γ-butyrobetaine hydroxylase activities of three infants and a 2.5 year old boy were 12% and 30%, respectively, of the mean adult activity.

## *Carnitine*

very little preformed carnitine, show plasma carnitine concentrations[25] comparable to those of subjects in Western nations whose diets tend to have abundant amounts of the factor.  Similarly, attempts to produce carnitine deficiency in experimental animals by restricting carnitine in the diet have proved unsuccessful apparently due to their capacities for the biosynthesis of the factor.  However, because neonates of several species, including humans, have been found to have low tissue carnitine levels when fed low-carnitine diets, it is likely that the total carnitine biosynthetic capacity may be immature in newborns, thus, rendering them dependent on their diets for preformed carnitine[26].

*dietary sources*

The available data concerning the carnitine contents of foods is scant and must be considered suspect due to the use of non-standard analytical methods.  Nevertheless, it is apparent that materials of plant origin tend to be low in carnitine, while those derived from animals tend to be rich in the factor.  Red meats and dairy products are particularly rich sources.

Approximate amounts of total carnitine in selected foods and feedstuffs:

| food | carnitine $\mu$g/100g | feedstuff | carnitine $\mu$g/100g |
|---|---|---|---|
| *plant-derived:* | | | |
| avocado | 1.25 | alfalfa concentrate | 2.00 |
| cabbage | -ª | barley | -ª |
| cauliflower | 0.13 | casein, vit. | 1.5 |
| orange juice | -ª | "  acid-washed | 0.4 |
| peanut | 0.76 | corn | -ª |
| spinach | -ª | wheat | 0.35-1.22 |
| bread | 0.24 | Torula yeast | 1.60-3.29 |
| *animal origin:* | | | |
| beef | 59.8-67.4 | beef liver | 2.6 |
| beef kidney | 1.8 | beef heart | 19.3 |
| chicken | 4.6-9.1 | lamb, muscle | 78.0 |
| cow's milk | 0.53-3.91 | egg | -ª |
| | | | ªnone detected |

source: Mitchell, M. 1978. Am. J. Clin. Nutr. 31:293-306.

*absorption*

Carnitine appears to be absorbed across the gut by an active process dependent on *Na⁺ co-transport*, as well as by a passive, diffusional which may be important for the absorption of large doses of the factor.  The

---

[25]Mean±S.D.: men, 59±12 $\mu$M (n=40); women, 52±12 $\mu$M (n=45).

[26]That the milks of various species contain appreciable amounts of carnitine supports this view.  For example, human milk contains 28-95 nmoles carnitine per ml, and cow's milk contains 190-270 nmoles carnitine per ml.

## *Carnitine*

efficiency of absorption appears to be virtually complete[27]. The uptake of carnitine from the intestinal lumen into the mucosa is rapid, and about one-half of the carnitine taken up is ***acetylated*** in that tissue.

*transport*      Carnitine is released slowly from tissues (e.g., erythrocytes) into the plasma in both the free and acetylated forms, which are found there in simple solution[28]. Carnitine is taken up by peripheral tissues most of which can also synthesize it. Carnitine is located principally in the ***skeletal muscle***, which contains 90% of the total carnitine in the body[29,30].

*excretion*      The turnover of carnitine in muscle is relatively slow[31]; however, it is increased substantially by exercise, which reduces muscle carnitine concentrations[32]. Carnitine is highly conserved by the human kidney, which reabsorbs more than 90% of filtered carnitine, thus, playing a dominant role in the regulation of plasma carnitine concentration. A small amount of carnitine is normally found in the urine, even in subjects with low plasma carnitine concentrations; some of this may come from the renal secretion of carnitine either in free form or as short-chain ***acylcarnitine esters***[33].

---

[27] After a dose of carnitine, a human will typically show < 1% of the dose appearing in the urine and very little appearing in the feces.

[28] Plasma total carnitine concentrations in healthy adults are 30-89 $\mu$M, with men typically showing slightly greater (by ~15%) concentrations than women (see footnote #26).

[29] Carnitine is taken up by peripheral tissues against concentration gradients. The carnitine concentrations of skeletal muscles are typically 70-fold that of plasma; somewhat smaller differences have been reported between other tissues and extracellular fluids.

[30] The carnitine concentrations in healthy adults are are 11-52 nmoles/mg non-collagen protein, with mand and women showing comparable concentrations.

[31] The turnover times for carnitine in human tissues have been estimated to be ~8 days in skeletal muscle and heart, 11.6 hrs. in liver and kidney, and 68 min, in extracellular fluid. Whole-body turnover time has been estimated to be 66 days, indicating significant re-utilization of carnitine among the various tissues in the body.

[32] Exercise appears to produce a preferential mobilization of free carnitine, thus, resulting in an apparent shift towards fatty acid esters of carnitine in the muscle.

[33] Short-chain acyl-CoAs are normally utilized as rapidly as they are generated and little acylcarnitine accumulates. Some conditions, however, lead to the accumulation and, thus, excretion of acylcarnitine: propionic aciduria (propionyl CoA carboxylase deficiency) and methylmalonic aciduria (methylmalonyl CoA mutase deficiency), due to either hereditary abnormalities or dietary deficiencies (of biotin and vitamin $B_{12}$, respectively).

# Carnitine

*metabolic function*   Carnitine functions in the transport of long-chain fatty acids (fatty acyl CoA) from the cytosol into the mitochondrial matrix for oxidation as sources of energy[34]. This transport process, referred to as the *"carnitine transport shuttle"*, is effected by two trans-esterifications involving fatty acyl esters of CoA and carnitine and the action of three mitochondrial enzymes: *carnitine acyltransferases I and II*, and *carnitine translocase*.

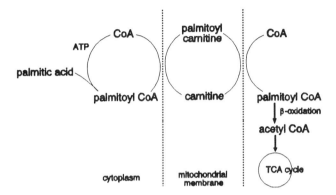

Carnitine acyltransferase I resides on the outer side of the inner mitochondrial membrane, while carnitine acyltransferase II is located on the matrix side and acyl carnitine translocase spans the inner membrane. The acyltransferases catalyze the formation and hydrolysis of fatty acyl carnitine esters[35]. The translocase catalyzes the exchange of carnitine and acyl carnitines (produced by carnitine acyltransferase I) across the membrane. The result of the concert action of these enzymes is that long-chain fatty acids are brought into the mitochondrion by first being esterified to carnitine and transported as fatty acyl carnitine esters, after which carnitine is released and returned to the outer side of the membrane, thus, rendering the free fatty acid available for $\beta$-oxidation within the particle[36].

---

[34] The mitochondrial inner membrane is impermeable to long-chain fatty acids and their CoA-derivatives which are, therefore, dependent on activation as carnitine esters for entry into that organelle.

[35] The carnitine acyltransferases are actually a family of related enzymes. Six carnitine acyltransferases with different but overlapping chain length specificities have been isolated from mitochondria (three from each of the inner and outer sides of the membrane).

[36] It has been suggested that the carnitine transport shuttle may also function in the reverse direction for transporting acetyl groups back to the cytoplasm for fatty acid synthesis. Even if such a *reverse shuttle* were to function, its contribution to fatty acid synthesis would be insignificant in comparison to that of the *citrate shuttle* that transports acetyl CoA to the cytoplasm by the action of a citrate cleavage enzyme.

## *Carnitine*

The activity of the carnitine transport shuttle is typically low at birth but increases dramatically after birth[37]. These increases correspond to the parallel development of fatty acid oxidation in the heart, liver and adipose tissue and suggest that the carnitine transport shuttle is rate-limiting to that process. While the mechanism of the postpartum increase in carnitine transport shuttle activity remains poorly understood, it is clear that one factor influencing it is carnitine status.

*evidence for nutritional essentiality*

It is clear that carnitine is an essential nutrient for some insect species including beetles of the family *Tenebrionidai*[38], the beetle *Oryzaephilus surinamensis* and the fly *Drosophila melanogaster*. It is presumed that carnitine plays the same essential role in the metabolism of fatty acids in insects that it does in mammals, and that their special requirement for the factor as an essential nutrient is due to their inability to synthesize it from endogenous sources. For these species, carnitine clearly *is* a vitamin[39].

Needs for preformed carnitine have also been demonstrated in mammals in certain circumstances in which the biosynthesis of carnitine is impaired by nutritional deprivation of the precursors lysine[40] or methionine[41]. For example, rats fed such diets have been shown to develop mild depressions in tissue carnitine concentrations and to suffer growth depression and fatty liver, both of which are at least partially alleviated by feeding carnitine. Abnormally low circulating carnitine levels have been found in humans with severe ***protein malnutrition***, presumably for the same reasons.

---

[37]For example, the carnitine palmitoyl transferase I activity in rat liver increases nearly five-fold within 24 hrs. of birth, peaking within 2-3 days. Similar increases in the hepatic activities of carnitine acetyl transferase I and carnitine palmitoyl transferase I have been observed in human infants.

[38]a family of mealworms

[39]Although carnitine is an amino acid, because it has no role in protein synthesis it meets the criteria of vitamin status (*"an organic compound that is distinct from fats, carbohydrates and proteins"*, see Chapter 1).

[40]It is estimated that ca. 0.1% of the lysine required by the rat may be consigned to carnitine biosynthesis.

[41]The feeding of a lysine-deficient diet to rats produced a severe depression in growth, but only marginal depressions in the carnitine concentrations of some tissues (e.g., the carnitine concentrations of skeletal muscle and heart were each ca. 70% or normal) and an elevation of the carnitine concentration of the liver. Despite that increase, hepatic steatosis occurred unless L-carnitine was fed. Other experiments have shown that such mild carnitine deficiency produced in lysine-deficient rats can, indeed, reduce palmitic acid oxidation in homogenates of those tissues. Other experiments have shown that rats fed low-protein diets limiting in methionine show reduced growth and develop fatty livers; supplementation of that diet with 0.2% L-carnitine overcame part of the growth depression and markedly reduced the hepatic signs.

## *Carnitine*

Apparent carnitine deficiency in protein-malnourished children:

| group | plasma carnitine µmoles/dl | plasma albumin g/dl |
|---|---|---|
| healthy controls | $9.0\pm0.6$ (8)[b] | $3.5\pm0.1$ (8) |
| undernourished patients | $6.4\pm0.9$ (10) | $2.7\pm0.2$ (5) |
| marasmus patients | $3.7\pm0.5$ (12) | $2.7\pm0.2$ (8) |
| kwashiorkor patients | $2.6\pm0.5$ (13) | $1.7\pm0.1$ (9) |

[a]mean$\pm$S.D. for (n) children

source: Khan and Bamji. 1977. Clin. Chim. Acta 75:163

Low plasma carnitine concentrations, which responded to nutritional therapy have been found in children with schistosomiasis and associated signs of anemia[42] and protein malnutrition (low serum albumin) in the Middle East.  Hypocarnitinemia[43] and tissue carnitine depletion appears to be common in patients with advanced cirrhosis who not only tend to have marginal intakes of carnitine and its precursors, but also have loss of hepatic function including the capacity to synthesize carnitine.  Hemodialysis patients can also be depleted of carnitine[44] due to the loss of carnitine in the dialysate, which greatly exceeds the amount normally lost in the urine (this can be prevented if carnitine is added to the dialysate[45]). Tissue depletion of carnitine has been related to the complications attendant to intermittent hemodialysis:  hyperlipidemia, cardiomyopathy, skeletal muscle asthenia and cramps[46].  Oral carnitine has also been found effective in correcting the hypertriglyceridemia that is frequent in uremic patients undergoing hemodialysis[47].

---

[42]Two steps in the biosynthesis of carnitine require $Fe^{++}$ (the mitochondrial *ε-N-trimethyllysine hydroxylase* and the cytosolic *γ-butyrobetaine hydroxylase*).  Therefore, it is possible that both the Fe deficiency (manifest as anemia) and the protein deficiency (manifest as low serum albumin concentration) of these patients may have reduced their abilities to synthesize carnitine.

[43]$< 55\mu M$

[44]In one study, the muscle carnitine concentrations of 8 patients after hemodialysis was only 10% of that of healthy controls.  It is of interest, however, that not all hemodialysis patients experience carnitine depletion. Some show chronic hypocarnitinemia, whereas others show a return of plasma carnitine concentrations to normal or higher than normal within ca. 6 hrs. after dialysis. The recovery of the latter group is hastened (to ca. 2 hrs.) if each patient is given 3 g D,L-carnitine orally at the end of the dialysis period.

[45]e.g., at a concentration of 65 nmoles/ml

[46]post-dialysis syndrome

[47]Daily oral doses of 2.4 g D,L-carnitine corrected within 14 days the type IV hypertriglyceridemias that six uremic patients undergoing hemodialysis had shown for 6-24 months.

## Carnitine

carnitine in        Carnitine is of special relevance to the nutrition of the **human infant**. For
infant nutrition    the reason that neonates appear to have compromised endogenous carni-
                    tine synthesis[48], their carnitine status is dependent on that of the mother,
                    on the placental transfer of carnitine *in utero*, and on the availability of
                    exogenous sources[49] after birth.  Accordingly, infants fed soya-based
                    formulas (which contain little or no carnitine) have been found to be unable
                    to maintain normal plasma carnitine levels, whereas intravenous administra-
                    tion of L-carnitine allows them to do so.  Pre-term infants can be at special
                    risk in this regard; although their plasma carnitine levels tend to be nearly
                    normal, they can be depleted rapidly during the course of intravenous
                    feeding with solutions which have not been supplemented with carnitine[50].

                    The consequences of suboptimal carnitine status would appear to be great
                    for the infant who, at birth, changes from a pattern of energy metabolism
                    based on glucose as the major fuel to one based on the utilization of
                    fats[51].  Thus, for the newborn, free fatty acids appear to be the preferred
                    metabolic fuels, especially for the heart and skeletal muscle[52], when
                    glucose availability is limited.  Accordingly, carnitine is an important
                    cofactor for neonatal energy metabolism.

                    Carnitine deficiency in human infants has been found to produce several
                    subclinical biochemical changes.  Infants fed soy-based formula diets for
                    as long as two weeks after birth have shown reduced hepatic carnitine
                    concentrations with associated reductions in hepatic fatty acid oxidation
                    and ketogenesis.  Hypertriglyceridemia has also been reported in infants
                    fed soy-based diets not supplemented with carnitine.  However, the long-

---

[48]They have very low hepatic activities of **butyrobetaine hydroxylase**.

[49]Examples are mother's milk, prepared infant formulas and milk replacers. It has been suggested that
natural selection has resulted in mother's milk containing carnitine in proportion to the needs of the infant. In
fact, the greatest concentrations of carnitine in human milk occur during the first 2-3 days of suckling. During
the first three weeks of lactation, the carnitine content of human milk varies from 50-70 nmoles/ml; after that
time, it declines to ca. 35 nmoles/ml by 6-8 weeks. Most milk-based infant formulas contain comparable or
slightly greater amounts of carnitine; however, formulas based on soybean protein or casein and casein
hydrolysate contain little or no carnitine. Lipid emulsions also contain no appreciable carnitine.

[50]One study found the plasma carnitine concentrations of pre-term (gestational age: <36 weeks) infants
to drop from 29 $\mu$M to 13$\mu$M during total parenteral nutrition.

[51]At birth, plasma free fatty acids and $\beta$-hydroxybutyrate concentrations are rapidly elevated due to the
mobilization of fat from adipose tissue. These elevated levels are maintained by the utilization of high-fat diets
such as human milk and many infant formulas which typically contain more than 40% of total calories as lipid.

[52]These tissue depend on the oxidation of fatty acids for more than half of their total energy metabolism.

## Carnitine

term physiological consequences of these reductions are unknown and no clinical symptoms of carnitine deficiency in infants have been described.

*disorders of carnitine metabolism*

Carnitine deficiencies can also result from genetic disorders of carnitine metabolism which affect its tissue utilization. Disorders in which carnitine metabolism is specifically affected are of two types: myopathic and systemic. *Primary muscle carnitine deficiency* is thought to involve defective transport of carnitine into skeletal muscle. Its major clinical feature is mild to severe muscular weakness and, frequently, excessive lipid accumulation in skeletal muscle fibers. *Primary systemic carnitine deficiency* has a much more heterogeneous clinical picture, including such features as multiple episodes of metabolic encephalopathy, cardiomyopathy, hypoglycemia, hypoprothrombinemia, hyperammonemia and hepatic steatosis. The etiology of this syndrome is thought to be heterogenous; carnitine biosynthesis is thought to be normal but, in at least some cases, renal carnitine reabsorption is impaired. Responses to treatment with carnitine supplements have been varied. Carnitine deficiency has also been recognized as a secondary feature of a variety of other genetic disorders, e.g., organic acidurias[53] and Fanconi syndrome[54] in which the urinary loss of total carnitine and, particularly, acylcarnitine esters is elevated. It is thought that, in these abnormal metabolic conditions, carnitine may function to remove excess organic acids. If true, this would be a new physiological role for carnitine.

## myo-INOSITOL

*anti-alopecia factor*

Although *myo-inositol* had been discovered in extracts of animal tissues almost one hundred years earlier, interest in its potential nutritional role was first stimulated in the 1940s when *Wolley* reported it to be a *new vitamin* required for normal growth and for the maintenance of normal hair and skin of the mouse (the *"mouse anti-alopecia factor"*). Subsequently, that original report was questioned on regarding the adequacy of the diet with respect to other known vitamins. Nevertheless, several groups found dietary supplements of *myo*-inositol to stimulate growth of chicks, turkeys, rats and mice, in ways that appeared to depend on such other factors as

---

[53]Examples include isovaleric, glutaric, propionic and methylmalonic acidemias, which result from long- and medium-chain acyl CoA dehydrogenase deficiencies.

[54]*Fanconi syndrome* is a renal disease characterized by the excessive renal excretion of a number of metabolites that are normally reabsorbed (e.g., amino acids).

# myo-*Inositol*

the presence/absence of other sources or antagonists of biotin and folate. Whether these effects were actually responses to a missing nutrient was debated due to the observation by **Needham** that the daily urinary excretion of *myo*-inositol by the rat *exceeds* the amount ingested, which lead to the conclusion the factor was synthesized by that species. However, *myo*-inositol was found to be essential for the growth of most cells in culture. More recently, it has been found that deprivation of inositol can render the hepatic triglyceride accumulation by the rat susceptible to influence by the fatty acid composition of dietary fat, indicating a function of the nature of an essential nutrient. Further, **Hegsted** and colleagues at Harvard found that the female Mongolian gerbil[55] develops intestinal lipodystrophy when depleted of the factor. In fact, that group demonstrated a dietary requirement for *myo*-inositol to prevent that disorder in the gerbil fed a diet containing adequate levels of all other known nutrients.

*chemical nature*

*Myo*-inositol is a water-soluble hydroxylated, cyclic 6-carbon compound (*cis*-1,2,3,5-*trans*-4,6-cyclohexanehexol). It is the only one of the nine possible stereoisomeric forms of cyclohexitol with biological activity.

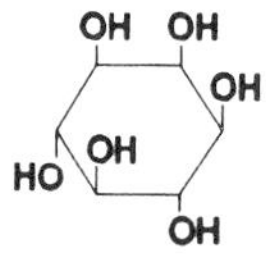

*biosynthesis from glucose*

It appears that most, if not all, mammals can synthesize *myo*-inositol *de novo* ultimately from **glucose**; biosynthetic capacity has been found in the liver, kidney, brain and testis of rats and rabbits, and in the kidney[56] and other tissues in humans. The biosynthesis involves the cyclization of **glucose-6-phosphate** to **inositol-1-phosphate** by **inositol-1-phosphate synthase** followed by a dephosphorylation by **inositol-1-phosphatase**.

*dietary sources*

*Myo*-inositol occurs in foods and feedstuffs in three forms: **free myo-inositol**, **phytic acid**[57], and **inositol-containing phospholipids**. The richest

---

[55] *Meriones unguiculatus*

[56] Renal synthesis of *myo*-inositol has been found to be ca. 4 g/day (~2 g/kidney/day).

[57] inositol hexaphosphate

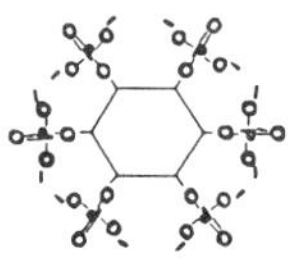

# myo-*Inositol*

Total *myo*-inositol contents of selected foods:

| food | myo-inositol, mg/g | food | myo-inositol, mg/g |
|---|---|---|---|
| vegetables | | fruits | |
| asparagus | 0.29-0.68 | apple | 0.10-0.24 |
| beans, green | 0.55-1.93 | cantaloupe | 3.55 |
| beans, white | 2.83-4.40 | grape | 0.07-0.16 |
| beans, red | 2.49 | grapefruit | 1.17-1.99 |
| broccoli | 0.11-0.30 | orange | 3.07 |
| cabbage | 0.18-0.70 | peach | 0.19-0.58 |
| carrot | 0.52 | pear | 0.46-0.73 |
| cauliflower | 0.15-0.18 | strawberry | 0.13 |
| celery | 0.05 | watermelon | 0.48 |
| okra | 0.28-1.17 | cereals | |
| pea | 1.16-2.35 | rice | 0.15-0.30 |
| potato | 0.97 | wheat | 1.42-11.5 |
| spinach | 0.06-0.25 | meats | |
| squash, yellow | 0.25-0.32 | beef | 0.09-0.37 |
| tomato | 0.34-0.41 | chicken | 0.30-0.39 |
| dairy products and eggs | | lamb | 0.37 |
| milk | 0.04 | pork | 0.14-0.42 |
| ice cream | 0.09 | turkey | 0.08-0.23 |
| cheese | 0.01-0.09 | liver, beef | 0.64 |
| egg, whole | 0.09 | liver, chicken | 1.31 |
| egg yolk | 0.34 | liver, pork | 0.17 |
| nuts | | tuna | 0.11-0.15 |
| almond | 2.78 | trout | 0.11 |
| peanut | 1.33-3.04 | | |

source: Clements and Darnell. Am. J. Clin. Nutr. 33:1954 (1980)

sources of *myo*-inositol are the seeds of plants (e.g., beans, grains and nuts). However, the predominant form occurring in plant materials is phytic acid (which can comprise most of the total P present in materials such as cereal grains[58]). Because most mammals have little or no intestinal phytase activity, phytic acid is poorly utilized as a source of either *myo*-inositol or P[59,60]. In animal products, *myo*-inositol occurs in free form as

---

[58]Of the total phosphorus present, phytic acid-P comprises 48-73% for cereal grains (corn, barley, rye, wheat, rice, sorghum), 48-79% for brans (rice, wheat), 27-41% for legume seeds (soybeans, peas, broad beans), and 40-65% for oil-seed meals (soybean meal, cottonseed meal, rapeseed meal).

[59]The bioavailability of P from most plant sources is relatively good (>50%) for ruminants, which benefit from the phytase activities of their rumen microflora. Non-ruminants, however, lack their own intestinal phytase and generally show much poorer bioavailabilities of plant-P, depending upon the phytase contributions of their intestinal microflora. For pigs and rats, such contributions appear to be significant, giving them moderate abilities (ca. 37% and 44%, respectively) to utilize phytic acid-P. In contrast, the chick, which has a short gut and rapid intestinal transit time and, thus, has only a sparse intestinal microflora, can use little (ca. 8%) phytic acid-P.

# myo-*Inositol*

well as in inositol-containing phospholipids (primarily **phosphatidyl-inositol**)[61]. The richest animal sources are organ meats. Human milk is relatively rich in *myo*-inositol[62] (colostrum: 200-500 mg/l; mature milk: 100-200 mg/l) in comparison to cow's milk (30-80 mg/l).

*Myo*-inositol is a GRAS substance[63], and is added to many prepared infant formulas[64]. It is estimated that typical American diets provide adults with ca. 900 mg *myo*-inositol per day, slightly over half of which is in phospholipid form.

*absorption*

The enteric absorption of **free myo-*inositol*** occurs by **active transport**; the uptake of *myo*-inositol from the gut is virtually complete. The enteric absorption of **phytic acid**, however, depends on the ability to digest that form, and on the amounts of divalent cations in the diet/meal. Most animal species lack intestinal **phytase** activities and are, therefore, dependent on the presence of a gut microflora that produces those enzymes. For species that harbor such microfloral populations (e.g., ruminants and long-gutted non-ruminants), phytate is digestible, thus, constituting a useful dietary source of *myo*-inositol. Dietary cations (particularly $Ca^{++}$) can reduce the utilization of phytate by forming insoluble (and, thus, non-digestible and non-absorbable) phytate chelates. Because a large portion of the total *myo*-inositol in mixed diets typically is in the form of phytic acid, the utilization of *myo*-inositol from high-Ca diets can be less than half of that from

---

[60]Phytic acid can also form a very stable chelation complex with zinc ($Zn^{++}$ is held by the negative charges on adjacent pyrophosphate groups), thus, reducing its nutritional availability. For this reason, the bioavailability of Zn in such plant-derived foods as soybean is very low.

[61]Free *myo*-inositol predominates in brain and kidney, whereas phospholipid-inositol predominates in skeletal muscle, heart, liver and pancreas.

[62]Milk contains a disaccharide form of *myo*-inositol, **6-β-galactinol** (6-o-β-D-galactopyranolsyl-*myo*-inositol), which comprises ca. one-sixth of the non-lipid *myo*-inositol in that material.

[63]It is classified by the U.S. Food and Drug Administration among the substances **'generally recognized as safe'** and, therefore, can be used in the formulation of foods without the demonstrations of safety and efficacy required by the Food, Drug and Cosmetic Act.

[64]e.g., at 0.1%

# myo-*Inositol*

diets containing low to moderate amounts of the mineral[85].    Little information is available concerning the mechanism of absorption of *phospholipid*-**myo-inositol**; it is probable that it is analogous to that of phosphatidylcholine[86].

transport

*Myo*-inositol is transported in the blood predominately in the **free form**[87]. A small but significant amount of **phosphatidylinositol (PI)** is found in association with the circulating lipoproteins.  Free *myo*-inositol appears to be taken up by an **active transport** process in some tissues (kidney, brain) and by **carrier-mediated diffusion** in others (liver).  The active process requires $Na^+$ and energy, and is inhibited by high levels of glucose[88].

metabolism

Free *myo*-inositol is converted to PI within cells either by **de novo synthesis** of the latter by reacting with the liponucleotide **cytidine diphosphate (CDP)-diacylglycerol**[69], or by an exchange with **endogenous PI**[70]. Phosphatidylinositol can, in turn, be sequentially phosphorylated to the mono- (**phosphatidylinositol 4-phosphate, PIP**) and di-phosphate (**phosphatidylinositol 4,5-biphosphate, PIP₂**) forms by membrane kinases[71]. Thus, in tissues, *myo*-inositol is found as the free form, as PI, PIP and $PIP_2$[72].  The *myo*-inositol-containing phospholipids tend to be

---

[85]For the same reason, the bioavailability of Ca is also low for high-phytate diets.  This effect also occurs for the nutritionally important divalent cations $Mn^{++}$ and $Zn^{++}$; the bioavailability of each is reduced by the presence of phytic acid in the diet.

[66]This would involve hydrolysis by pancreatic **phospholipase A** in the intestinal lumen to produce a **lysophosphatidylinositol** which, upon uptake by the enterocyte, would be re-acylated by an **acyltransferase** or hydrolyzed further to yield **glycerylphosphorylinositol**.

[67]The normal circulating concentration of *myo*-inositol in humans is ca. 30 $\mu M$.

[68]Apparently because of this antagonism, untreated diabetics show impaired tissue uptake and impaired urinary excretion of *myo*-inositol.

[69]This step is catalyzed by the microsomal enzyme **CDP-diacylglycerol:inositol phosphatidyltransferase** (also called **PI synthetase**).

[70]This reaction is stimulated by $Mn^{++}$; like phosphatidylinositol synthetase, it is localized in the microsomal fraction of the cell.

[71]These are **ATP:phosphatidylinositol 4-phosphotransferase** and **ATP:phosphatidylinositol-4-phosphate 5-phosphotransferase**, respectively.  They are located on the cytosolic surface of the erythrocyte membrane.

[72]The disaccharide **6-β-galactinol** appears to be a unique mammary metabolite.

# myo-*Inositol*

enriched in ***stearic acid*** (predominately at the 1-position) and ***arachidonic acid*** (predominately at the 2-position) in comparison to the fatty acid compositions of other phospholipids[73]. The greatest concentrations of *myo*-inositol are found in neural and renal tissues.

The turnover of the *myo*-inositol phospholipids is accomplished intracellularly. Phosphatidylinositol phosphates can be catabolized by cellular ***phosphomonoesterases*** (phosphatases) ultimately to yield ***PI***. In the presence of cytidine monophosphate, PI synthetase functions (in the reverse direction) to breakdown that form to yield ***CDP-diacylglycerol*** and ***myo-inositol***. The kidney appears to perform most of the further catabolism of *myo*-inositol, first clearing it from the plasma and converting it to ***glucose*** and, then, oxidizing it to ***$CO_2$*** via the pentose phosphate shunt[74].

*metabolic functions*

The metabolically active form of *myo*-inositol appears to be ***phosphatidylinositol***, which is thought to have several physiologically important roles.

Metabolic functions of *myo*-inositol:

| | |
|---|---|
| *i.* | affecter of the ***structure and function of membranes*** |
| *ii.* | ***source of arachidonic acid*** for the eicosanoid production |
| *iii.* | ***mediator of cellular responses*** to external stimuli |

Phosphatidylinositol has been proposed to be active in the ***regulation of membrane-associated enzymes*** and ***transport processes***[75]. It has been suggested that such effects involve the special membrane-active properties conferred on the phospholipid by its unique fatty acid composition. For example, its polar head group and highly nonpolar fatty acyl chains may facilitate specific electrostatic interactions while providing a hydrophobic microenvironment for enzyme proteins on or in membranes. Such properties may render PI an effective anchor for the hydrophobic attachment of proteins to membranes. Phosphatidylinositol also serves as a source of

---

[73]For example, the *myo*-inositol-containing phospholipids on the plasma membrane from human platelets contain ca. 42 molar % stearic acid and ca. 44 molar % arachidonic acid.

[74]The metabolism of *myo*-inositol appears to be relatively rapid. The rat can oxidize half of an ingested dose in 48 hrs.

[75]For example, phosphatidylinositol has been reported to be an endogenous activator of a microsomal ***$Na^+,K^+$-ATPase***, an essential constituent of ***acetyl CoA carboxylase***, a stimulator of ***tyrosine hydroxylase***, a factor bound to ***alkaline phosphatase*** and ***5'-nucleotidase***, and a membrane-anchor for ***acetylcholinesterase***.

## *myo-Inositol*

releasable *arachidonic acid* for the formation of the *eicosanoids*[76] by the cellular activities of *cyclooxygenase* and/or *lipoxygenase*. Although PI is less abundant in cells than the other phospholipids (phosphatidylcholine, phosphatidylethanolamine and phosphatidylserine), its enrichment in arachidonic acid renders it an effective source of that eicosanoid precursor.

That the metabolism of PI is stimulated in target tissues by stimuli having abilities to produce rapid (e.g., cholinergic or $\alpha$-adrenergic agonists) or medium-term (e.g., mitogens) physiological responses suggests a role as a mediator of such responses. It is thought that this role involves the conversion of the less abundant species, $PIP_2$, to a water-soluble metabolite *inositol-1,4,5-triphosphate (IP₃)*, which serves as a *second messenger* to activate the release of $Ca^{++}$ from intracellular stores[77].

The release of arachidonic acid can be effected in several ways:

> i.   *Direct deacylation of PI by phospholipase A₂* releases arachidonic acid and the lyso(1-acyl)phosphatide
>
> ii.  *Indirect deacylation of PI by phospholipase A₁* produces lyso(2-acyl)phosphatide from which arachidonic acid is released by a *lysophospholipase*
>
> iii. *Direct deacylation of PI by phospholipase C* (phosphodiesterase activity) releases arachidonic acid
>
> iv.  *Phosphorylation of PI by kinases to PIP and PIP₂*, which are hydrolyzed to 1,2-diacylglycerols (by *phosphodiesterase*), then to 2-monoacylglycerol (by *diacylglycerol lipase*), then to arachidonic acid (by *monoacylglycerol lipase*)

The occupancy of a variety of *cell surface receptors* has been shown to effect primary control over the hydrolysis of $PIP_2$ by regulating the activity of *phospholipase C* (phosphodiesterase) on the plasma membrane. Receptor occupancy, thus, activates the hydrolysis of $PIP_2$, which is favored at low intracellular concentrations of $Ca^{++}$, to produce $IP_3$ and, perhaps, other inositol polyphosphates. The $IP_3$ that is produced signals the release of $Ca^{++}$ from discrete organelles called *"calcisomes"*, as well as the entry

---

[76]The eicosanoids include *prostaglandins*, *thromboxanes* and *leukotrienes*. The prostaglandins are hormone-like substances secreted for short-range action on neighboring tissues; they are involved in inflammation, in the regulation of blood pressure, in headaches and in the induction of labor. The functions of the leukotrienes and thromboxanes are less well understood; they are thought to be involved in regulation of blood pressure and in the pathogenesis of some types of disease.

[77]There is some controversy concerning whether other inositol phosphates (e.g., *inositol-1,3,4,5-tetraphosphate [IP₄]*, which is a product of a *3-kinase* acting on IP₃) can also signal $Ca^{++}$ mobilization. Recent evidence suggest that, in at least some cells, $IP_3$ and $IP_4$ may have cooperative roles in $Ca^{++}$-signaling.

# myo-*Inositol*

of $Ca^{++}$ into the cell across the plasma membrane[78]. The former process involves a specific *IP₃-receptor* on the calcisomal membrane; the binding of $IP_3$ to this receptor opens a *$Ca^{++}$ channel* closely associated with the receptor. The latter process is less well understood.

It is thought that the $IP_3$-stimulated entry of $Ca^{++}$ into the cell involves an increase in the permeability to $Ca^{++}$ of the plasma membrane that is signaled by the emptying of the $IP_3$-sensitive intracellular pool. The mechanism whereby the $IP_3$-sensitive pool and the plasma membrane communicate to effect this response is not understood. There is also some evidence to suggest that *1,2-diacylglycerol*, which is formed from the receptor-stimulated metabolism of the *myo*-inositol-containing phospholipids, may also serve a second messenger function in activating *protein kinase C* for the phosphorylation of various proteins important to cell function[79].

*evidence for nutritional essentiality* Although early reports indicated dietary needs for *myo*-inositol to prevent alopecia in rodents, fatty liver in rats and growth retardation in guinea chicks, guinea pigs and hamsters, more recent studies with more complete diets have failed to confirm such needs. Hence, it has been concluded that most, if not all, of those lesions actually involved deficiencies of other nutrients (e.g., biotin, choline and vitamin E). Because *myo*-inositol appears to be synthesized by most, if not all, species, it has been suggested that the observed responses to dietary supplements of *myo*-inositol may have involved favorable effects of the compound to the intestinal microflora. This hypothesis would suggest that the addition of *myo*-inositol to diets would be beneficial when those diets contain marginal amounts of such factors as choline and biotin the gut synthesis of which can be important. Accordingly, it has been shown that supplements of *myo*-inositol reduced hepatic lipid accumulation in rats fed a choline-deficient diet, improved growth in rats fed a diet deficient in several vitamins, and reduced the incidence of fatty liver and improved the growth of chicks fed a biotin-deficient diet containing an antibiotic. Thus, it appears that, under certain conditions, animals can have needs for pre-formed *myo*-inositol. Such conditions are not well defined; but it has been suggested that they include situations in which the intestinal microflora is disturbed[80], the diet contains high levels

# myo-*Inositol*

---

[78]The $Ca^{++}$-mobilizing activity of $IP_3$ is terminated by its dephosphorylation (*via* a 5-phosphatase) to the inactive *inositol-1,4-bisphosphate*, or its phosphorylation (*via* a 3-kinase) to a product of uncertain activity, $IP_4$.

[79]According to this hypothesis, 1,2-diacylglycerol functions with $Ca^{++}$ and phosphatidylserine, both of which are know to be involved in the activation of protein kinase C.

[80]The use of antibiotics that reduce the numbers of microorganisms that normally produce *myo*-inositol as well as other required nutrients.

of fat[81], and the physical environment creates physiological stress.  This kind of need would indicate that *myo*-inositol is a ***conditional nutrient***.

For a few species, however, overt dietary needs for *myo*-inositol have been demonstrated.  These include several ***fishes*** and the ***gerbil***.  Studies with fish have shown dietary deprivation of *myo*-inositol to result in ***anorexia***, ***fin degeneration***, ***edema***, ***anemia***, ***decreased gastric emptying rate***, ***reduced growth*** and ***impaired efficiency of feed utilization***.  Studies with gerbils have shown *myo*-inositol deprivation to result in ***intestinal lipodystrophy***, with associated ***hypocholesterolemia*** and ***reduced survival***.  It is interesting to note that these effects are *only observed in female gerbils*; males appear to have a sufficient testicular synthesis of *myo*-inositol.  For at least these species, *myo*-inositol must be considered a dietary essential.

## *PYRROLOQUINOLINE QUINONE*

*newly discovered co-enzyme*

In the late 1970s, studies of specialized bacteria, the methylotrophs[82], resulted in the discovery of a *new enzyme cofactor **pyrroloquinoline quinone (PQQ)***.  That cofactor was found in several different bacterial oxido-reductases.  Subsequently, PQQ has been identified in several other important enzymes (now collectively called *"quinoproteins"*) in yeasts, plants and animals.  In 1989, ***Killgore*** and colleagues at the University of California, demonstrated beneficial effects of PQQ in preventing skin lesions in mice fed a diet containing low concentrations of that factor.

*chemical nature*

Pyrroloquinoline quinone, sometimes called *"methoxatin"*, is a tricarboxylic acid with a fused heterocylcic (*o*-quinone) ring system[83].  Its C-5 carbonyl group is very reactive toward nucleophiles[84], leading to adduct formation.

---

[81]High-fat diets may increase the needs for *myo*-inositol for lipid transport.

[82]The methylotrophs dissimilate single-carbon compounds, e.g., methane, methanol and methylamine.

[83]4,5-dihydro-4,5-dioxo-1*H*-pyrrolo(2,3-*f*)quinoline-2,7,9-tricarboxylic acid

[84]e.g., amino groups, thiol groups

## Pyrroloquinoline Quinone

*dietary sources*

Little quantitative information is available concerning the distribution of PQQ in foods and feedstuffs. Some reports indicate PQQ to be present in egg yolk, adrenal tissue and many citrus fruits in the range of 500-20,000 ppb and in casein, starch and isolated soy protein in the range of 10-100 ppb.

*metabolic function*

Pyrroloquinoline quinone functions, at least in prokaryotes, as the **redox center** in the quinoprotein enzymes. In the bacterial **quinoproteins**, PQQ is covalently bound to the apoprotein, probably by an amide or ester bond *via* its carboxylic acid group(s). The redox behavior of PQQ involves its ability to form adducts that facilitate both one- and two-electron transfers.

Its function as a cofactor in dehydrogenases appears to involve electron transfers of both types (substrate oxidation by a two-electron transfer to PQQ, followed by single-electron transfer to such acceptors as Cu-containing proteins and cytochromes). Accordingly, two forms of the cofactor, the semiquinone **PQQH·** and the catechol **PQQH₂**, have been found in the bacterial quinoproteins.

The role of PQQ in eukaryotes is less clear. Although several animal quinoproteins have been proposed, more recent investigations with sensitive physical methods have failed to confirm earlier claims of covalent binding of PQQ or derivatives at the active centers of those enzymes. One important enzyme that has been proposed to be a quinoprotein is **lysyl oxidase**, which plays a key role in the cross-linking of collagen and elastin cross-linking[85]. Recent studies indicate that the needs of this and related enzymes for PQQ may not be specific, as other quinones appear to be able to support the catalytic activities of some[86].

*evidence for nutritional essentiality*

**Killgore** and colleagues fed mice for 10 weeks a chemically defined diet that contained <30 ppb PQQ. It was supplemented with vitamins[87] at 5-fold required levels, and special precautions were taken to minimize the

---

[85]by catalyzing the oxidative deamination of peptidyl lysine to peptidyl $\alpha$-aminoadipic-$\delta$-semialdehyde

[86]In fact, the apparent quinone requirement of plasma monoamine oxidase, after which other putative animal quinoproteins have been modeled, has been found to be satisfied by 6-hydroxyDOPA.

[87]thiamin, pyridoxine, vitamin A, vitamin E, vitamin $B_{12}$, folate, vitamin $K_2$ and biotin

# Pyrroloquinoline Quinone

potential for exposure of mice to PQQ from microbial sources[88]. The positive control group was treated in like manner, but was fed the basal diet supplemented with 800 ppb PQQ. The results showed a clear difference in rate of growth in favor of the PQQ-supplemented mice. Further, about one-quarter of the PQQ-deprived animals showed *friable skin*, mild *alopecia* and a *"hunched" posture*. About one-fifth of the PQQ-deprived mice died by 8 weeks of feeding with *aortic aneurysms* or *abdominal hemorrhages*. The most frequent sign, friable skin, was taken to suggest an abnormality of collagen metabolism; subsequent study revealed *increased collagen solubility* (indicating reduced cross-linking) and abnormally *low activities of lysyl oxidase* in PQQ-deprived animals. Attempts to breed PQQ-deprived mice were unsuccessful[89].

Proposed quinoproteins:

| enzyme | organism |
|---|---|
| bacteria | |
| methanol dehydrogenase | methylotrophic bacteria |
| ethanol dehydrogenase | *Pseudomonas aeruginosa* |
| ethanol dehydrogenase° | *Pseudomonas testosteroni* |
| glucose dehydrogenase | many species |
| methylamine dehydrogenase | some methylotrophic bacteria |
| methylamine oxidase | *Arthrobacter* P1 |
| quinate dehydrogenase | several species |
| glycerol dehydrogenase | *Gluconobacter industrius* |
| polyethylene glycol dehydrogenase | *Flavobacterium* sp. |
| polyvinyl alcohol dehydrogenase | *Pseudomonas* sp. |
| yeasts and fungi | |
| amine oxidase | several yeasts and fungi |
| galactose oxidase | several fungi |
| plants | |
| amine oxidase | pea (*Pisum sativum*) |
| lipoxygenase-1 | soybean (*Glycine max*) |
| animals | |
| amine oxidase | cow (serum) |
| dopamine $\beta$-hydroxylase | cow |
| diamine oxidase | pig (kidney) |
| lysyl oxidase | human (placenta) |
| choline dehydrogenase | dog (liver) |
| °a quinohemoprotein | |
| source: Duine and Jongejan, Vit. Horm. 45:223-262, 1989. | |

---

[88]An antibiotic (2% succinyl sulfathiozole) was added to the diet; the major dietary ingredients were autoclaved; drinking water was distilled and ultra-filtered; mice were housed in a laminar flow cage unit with microbiologically filtered air.

[89]Mice fed the low-PQQ diet for 8-9 weeks produced either no litters, or litters in which the pups were immediately cannibalized at birth.

## Pyrroloquinoline Quinone

These results show clear physiologic impairment due to PQQ deprivation; yet, the lack of a clear enzyme cofactor function renders the metabolic significance difficult to assess. Indeed, it has been proposed that PQQ and/or PQQ-derived factors may not function as specific enzyme cofactors at all, acting instead as oxidant radical scavengers. There is still much to be learned about the metabolism, distribution and biochemical functions of PQQ. At present, while it is clear that PQQ and/or related factors can have nutritional significance, available evidence is insufficient to support designating PQQ as a vitamin.

# UBIQUINONES

*mitochondrial respiratory chain component*

The ubiquinones are a group of tetra-substituted 1,4-benzoquinone derivatives with isoprenoid side-chains of variable length. Originally isolated from the unsaponifiable fractions of the hepatic lipids from vitamin A-deficient rats, the principal species of the group (*"ubiquinone[50]"*[90]) was subsequently identified as an essential component (*"coenzyme $Q_{10}$"* or *"CoQ_{10}"*) of the mitochondrial electron transport chains of most prokaryotic and all eukaryotic cells. Over the four decades since that recognition, the term *"coenzyme Q"* has come to be used to describe generally this family of compounds, all of which are synthesized from precursors in the inner mitochondrial membrane[91].

*metabolic function*

The ubiquinones function in *mitochondrial electron transport chains* by passing electrons from *flavoproteins* (e.g., NADH or succinic dehydrogenases) to the *cytochromes* via cytochrome $b_5$. They perform this function by undergoing reversible reduction/oxidation to cycle between the 1,4-quinone (oxidized) and 1,4-dihydroxybenzene (reduced) species.

---

[90]The conventions of nomenclature for the ubiquinone/CoQ group are similar to that of the vitamin K group. For the ubiquinones, the number of side-chain carbons is indicated parenthetically; for the CoQ designation, the number of side-chain isoprenyl units is indicated in subscript.

[91]The isoprenyl side-chain is derived from mevalonate, the ring system from tyrosine, the hydroxyl groups from molecular oxygen and the methyl groups from S-adenosylmethionine.

## Ubiquinones

| | |
|---|---|
| *relationship with tocopherols* | The **6-chromanols** of the CoQ group have remarkably similar structure to the oxidized form of **vitamin E (tocopherylquinone)**, the difference being the two methoxyl groups on the $CoQ_{10}$ ring in place of two methyl groups on the tocopherylquinone ring.  Although $CoQ_{10}$, itself, does not spare vitamin E for preventing the gestation-resorption syndrome in the rat, the oxidized form, that is, the 6-chromanol of hexahydro-$CoQ_4$ has been found to prevent the syndrome in vitamin E-deficient rats and to produce significant reductions (but not full protection) in both the anemia and the myopathy of vitamin E-deficient Rhesus monkeys[92].  Recent studies have shown the administration of $CoQ_{10}$ to protect against myocardial damage mediated by free radical mechanisms (ischemia, drug toxicities). The latter effects appear to related to the antioxidant properties of the ubiquinones[93], suggesting roles for them as physiological antioxidants. |
| *effects of exogenous $CoQ_{10}$* | Important though $CoQ_{10}$ is in oxidative metabolism, it is difficult to consider ubiquinones as important dietary nutrients because their tissue levels appear to be maintained at high levels[94] by biosynthesis from endogenous precursors[95].  Nevertheless, the responses observed experimentally to exogenous $CoQ_{10}$ raise important questions:  Do reduced forms of the ubiquinones actually share some of the functions of vitamin E, or do they merely substitute for the vitamin due to their structural similarities to it?  Do the ubiquinones and vitamin E simply protect each other by virtue of their similar antioxidant properties? |
| | Present information indicates that the redox properties of $CoQ_{10}$ enable it to function both as an essential component of the mitochondrial respiratory chain as well as a fat-soluble antioxidant that protects and, thus, spares $a$-tocopherol in subcellular membranes. Thus, it appears that dietary ubiquinones may be important as potential sources of antioxidant protection, but |

---

[92]In fact, the responses (e.g., increases reticulocyte count, reduced creatinine excretion, reduced dystrophic signs) were more rapid than have been observed for therapy with $a$-tocopherol.

[93]A study which compared the *in vivo* antioxidant effects of dietary sources of $CoQ_{10}$, $a$-tocopherol, $\beta$-carotene and Se in rat tissues showed $CoQ_{10}$ to provide significant protection from lipid peroxidation.  In some tissues (e.g., liver) its effect appeared to be greater than those of the other antioxidant nutrients, while in other tissues it appeared to be somewhat less effective than the others at the dietary levels used (*see* Leibovitz, et al., J. Nutr. 120: 97-104, 1990).

[94]Relatively great concentrations of $CoQ_{10}$ are found in the liver, heart, spleen, kidney, pancreas and adrenals.  The total $CoQ_{10}$ pool size in the human adult is estimated to be 0.5-1.5 g.

[95]The contributions of foods and feedstuffs, many of which are now known to contain appreciable concentrations of ubiquinones, to these high tissue levels are unknown.

## *Ubiquinones*

that they share that role with other antioxidant nutrients[96] several of which are likely to be more potent in this regard. For this reason, and the lack of evidence of specifically impaired physiological function due to deprivation of Coenzyme Q, *these compounds cannot be considered vitamins*.

## *OROTIC ACID*

*intermediate in pyrimidine biosynthesis*  Orotic acid was isolated in the late 1940s from distillers' dried solubles[97] and called, for a while, *"vitamin B$_{13}$"*. A substituted pyrimidine[98], orotic acid is an important intermediate in the biosynthesis of *pyrimidines*.

Orotic acid is biosynthesized from *N-carbamylphosphate* by dehydration (*via* *dihydroorotase*), which is oxidized (*via* *orotate reductase*) to *orotate*. When studies failed to confirm vitamin-like activity, that designation of this normal metabolite was dropped. In fact, orotic acid supplements (0.1%) to the diets of rats have been found to *induce* hepatic steatosis and hepatomegaly, and to *increase* hepatic levels of uracil nucleotides, presumably by increasing the flux through the pyrimidine pathway. In contrast, these adverse effects have not been observed in other species (monkeys, guinea pigs, hamsters, mice or pigs) fed comparable levels of orotic acid. Recent interest in orotic acid has concerned its *hypocholesterolemic effect*, an apparent consequence of its inhibition of hepatic cholesterol synthesis at the level of *3-hydroxy-3-methylglutaryl CoA reductase*. On the basis of present understanding, *orotic acid cannot be considered a vitamin*.

---

[96]e.g., the tocopherols, Se (*via* the Se-dependent glutathione peroxidase), ascorbic acid, and β-carotene.

[97]This feedstuff consists of the dried aqueous residue from the distillation of fermented corn. It is used mainly as a component of mixed diets for poultry, swine and dairy calves. It is rich in several B-vitamins and has been valued as s source of *'unidentified growth factors'*, particularly for growing chicks and turkey poults.

[98]1,2,3,6-tetrahydro-2,6-dioxo-4-pyrimidinecarboxylic acid

## *BIOFLAVONOIDS*

*synergists of vitamin C*

The group of compounds now referred to as the *"bioflavonoids"* was discovered by *Szent-Györgyi* as the factor in lemon juice or red peppers that potentiated the anti-scorbutic activity for the guinea pig of the ascorbic acid contained in those foods. The factor was called by various groups *"citrin"*, *"vitamin P"*[99] and *"vitamin $C_2$"*, but was ultimately found to be a mixture of phenolic derivatives of 2-phenyl-1,4-benzopyrone.

*ubiquitous in plants*

Flavonoids are ubiquitous in foods and feedstuffs of plant origin. More than 800 different flavonoids have been isolated from plants where they comprise the major sources of red, blue and yellow pigments other than the carotenoids. The greatest contributors of flavonoids in human diets[100] are fruits and vegetables[101], fruit juices being the richest sources. The hydroxyl groups of these polyphenols enable them to form glycosidic linkages with sugars. Most flavonoids occur naturally as *glycosides*; these are hydrolyzed prior to absorption by glycosidases of the intestinal microflora. Upon absorption, flavonoids are conjugated as glucuronides or sulfates in the liver, and are degraded to a variety of phenolic compounds that are rapidly excreted.

*physiological effects*

Many inconsistent biological effects of bioflavonoids[102] have been reported. One finding, however, is consistently observed: *some bioflavonoids reduce capillary fragility and/or permeability*. This effect, which would appear to *"spare"* vitamin C, may be due to the ability of flavonoids to *chelate divalent metal cations* (e.g., $Cu^{++}$, $Fe^{++}$), thus, serving *antioxidant functions* by removing those catalysts of lipid peroxidation reactions. Other actions that may have physiological significance

---

[99]The letter P indicated the *"permeability vitamin"*, because it improved capillary permeability.

[100]The average daily intake of flavonoids from a *"typical"* American diet has been estimated to be ~1 g.

[101]Most flavonoids tend to be concentrated in the outer layers of fruit and vegetable tissues (e.g., skin, peel). In general, the flavonoid contents of leafy vegetables are high, whereas those of root vegetables (with the notable exception of onions with colored skins) are low.

[102]Biological activity has been reported for the aglycone flavonoids *quercetin* and *hesperidin*, and for the rhamnoglucosides *rutin* and *naringin*.

## Bioflavonoids

include the inhibition by certain flavonoids of **aldose reductase**[103], **phosphodiesterases**[104] and **o-methyltransferase**[105]. Nevertheless, the reported beneficial clinical responses to bioflavonoids are highly controversial, and no clinical syndromes associated with bioflavonoid deprivation have been reported. It is likely that all of the biological effects attributed to the bioflavonoids may relate to their chelation and antioxidant properties. While those properties may be beneficial under some circumstances, they produce essentially pharmacologic effects rather than *unique* nutritional ones. Therefore, **the bioflavonoids cannot be considered vitamins**.

## *p*-AMINOBENZOIC ACID

*precursor to folate in bacteria*

**p-Aminobenzoic acid** is an essential growth factor for many species of **bacteria**, which use it as a precursor for the biosynthesis of **folate**. Some early studies showed responses of chicks (increased growth) and rats (enhanced lactation) to supplements of *p*-aminobenzoic acid to diets containing marginal concentrations of folate. In fact, for a time *p*-aminobenzoic acid was called *"vitamin B$_x$"*.

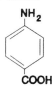

Such responses, however, were shown to be due to the use by the intestinal microflora of *p*-aminobenzoic acid for the synthesis of folate made available to the host either directly in the gut or indirectly *via* the feces. In addition, *p*-aminobenzoic acid can antagonize the bacteriostatic effects of sulfonamide drugs due to its similarities in chemical structure. It has a very high absorbance in the ultraviolet range and is used as a UV-screening agent in sun-blocking creams. Because animals lack the enzymes of the folate synthetic pathway, they cannot convert this precursor to the actual vitamin. Therefore, **p-aminobenzoic acid is not a vitamin**.

---

[103]Aldose reductase converts glucose and galactose to their corresponding polyols which have been implicated in diabetic neuropathy and in the cataracts associated with diabetes and galactosemia.

[104]Phosphodiesterases break down cyclic nucleotides and, thus, affect smooth muscle tone.

[105]*o*-Methyltransferase inactivates epinephrine and norepinephrine.

## LIPOIC ACID

co-enzyme

**Lipoic acid**[106] is an essential cofactor for the **oxidative decarboxylations of α-ketoacids** where, linked to the ε-amino group of a lysine residue of the enzyme **dihydrolipoyl transacetylase**, it is one of several prosthetic groups in a multi-enzyme complex[107]. Thus, as **lipoamide**, it undergoes both reversible acylation/deacylation to transfer acyl groups to CoA and reversible redox ring opening/closing[108], coupling that function with the oxidation of the α-ketoacid. No other metabolic function of lipoic acid has been identified.

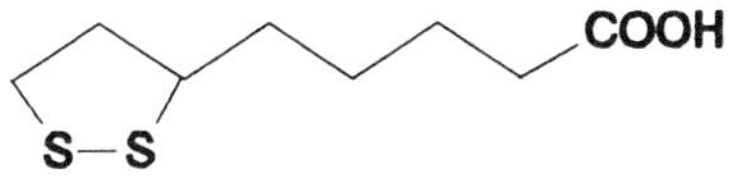

Because only trace amounts of lipoic acid are found in tissues, and because some species of bacteria[109] and protozoa[110] have a clear need for exogenous sources of it, the question arises as to whether diet and/or biosynthesis provides adequate amounts of this metabolically important factor for animals under all circumstances. Available information indicates that animals are fully capable of lipoic acid biosynthesis: no deficiency disorders have been reported and lipoic acid supplements to purified diets of chicks, rats and turkey poults has been without effect. Therefore, **lipoic acid is not considered a vitamin**.

## INEFFECTIVE FACTORS

The term "vitamin" has been used from time to time in association with factors with no apparent metabolic activity that would justify that designation. Further, opportunities afforded by patent law have permitted a substance to be **trade-named** a "vitamin" in the 1940s, a situation bound to mislead the uniformed.

---

[106] 6-thiotic acid

[107] e.g., lactate dehydrogenase complex

[108] interconversion of the disulfide bond with two free sulfhydryls

[109] e.g., *Streptococcus faecalis, Lactobacillus casei*

[110] e.g., *Tetrahymena geleii*

## Ineffective Factors

"vitamin B₁₅"     A substance isolated from apricot kernels and other natural sources was
                  trade-named *"vitamin B₁₅"* and also called *"pangamic acid"* by its discov-
                  erers[111]; it was ***patented*** with a claim of therapeutic efficacy against a
                  wide range of diseases of the skin, respiratory tract, nerves and joints -
                  despite the fact that *no data* were presented in the patent application.
                  Whereas "pangamic acid" was originally described as ***d-gluconodimethyl-***
                  ***amino acetic acid***[112], the term now appears to be used indiscriminately;
                  products also containing ***N,N-diisopropylammonium dichloroacetate***, ***Na***
                  ***gluconolactone***, ***N,N-dimethylglycine***, ***Ca gluconate*** and/or ***glycine*** in
                  various proportions also go by the names "pangamic acid", "pangamate",
                  "aangamik 15" or "vitamin B₁₅". Thus, "vitamin B₁₅" is not a definable
                  chemical entity; in fact, the substance originally called "pangamic acid" has
                  frequently been absent from such preparations. Of the compounds likely
                  to be present, N,N-diisopropylammonium dichloroacetate is known to be
                  hypotensive, hypothermic and potentially toxic and dichloroacetate is a
                  weak mutagen. Despite intermittent popular interest in these prepara-
                  tions[113], the only information that would appear to support positive
                  clinical results come from anecdotal sources and the undocumented
                  claims by vendors of these preparations. ***No substantive data*** appear to
                  have ever been presented to support any beneficial biological effects of the
                  so-called "vitamin B₁₅", and there is no evidence that deprivation of the
                  factor(s) caused any physiological impairment.

gerovital         As its name implies, ***Gerovital*** was promoted as a nutritional substance
                  that alleviated age-related degenerative diseases. Also called *"vitamin H₃"*
                  and *"vitamin GH3"*, it is actually a buffered solution of ***procaine HCl***, the
                  dental anesthetic Novocain[114]. Its health claims are unsubstantiated.

laetrile          Trade-named *"vitamin B₁₇"*, *laetrile* was first isolated from apricot kernels.
                  It is a discrete chemical entity, the ***cyanogenic glysoside***, 1-mandelonitrile-
                  β-glucuronic acid. The term *"laetrile"* is often used interchangeably with the
                  related cyanogenic glycoside *"amygdalin"* that occurs naturally in the seeds
                  of most fruits. These compounds have been *claimed* effective in cancer
                  treatment due either to the cyanide they provide as being selectively toxic
                  to tumor cells, or to the disease itself being a result of an unsatisfied meta-

---

[111]Ernst Krebs, Sr. and Ernst Krebs, Jr. - not to be confused with the great biochemist Sir Hans Krebs.

[112]the ester of *d*-gluconic acid and dimethylglycine

[113]For example, in its March 13, 1978, cover story, *New York Magazine* presented "vitamin B₁₅" as *"a possible cure for everything short of a transit strike."*

[114]Procain hydrochloride, i.e., 4-aminobenzoic acid 2-(diethylamino)ethyl ester hydrochloride.

## Ineffective Factors

bolic need for laetrile.  The contention that either compound provides a source of cyanide ignore the fact that animals, lacking *β-glucosidases*, cannot degrade the mandelonitrile moiety.  In fact, laetrile and amygdalin are each *non-toxic* to animals and humans for that reason.  Apricot kernels and other fruit seeds, however, contain β-glucosidases; if these are liberated (e.g., by crushing) prior to eating such seeds, then cyanide-poisoning can occur[115].   Extensive animal tumor model studies and clinical trials have tested the putative anti-tumor effects of laetrile; these have yielded consistently negative results.

# UNIDENTIFIED GROWTH FACTORS

*present status*   Since the discovery of vitamin $B_{12}$, experimental nutritionists have observed
*of UGFs*          many instances of stimulated growth by the addition of natural materials to purified diets.  Many such responses have been found to involve *interrelationships of known nutrients*[116].    Some have involved *diet palatability* and, thus, the rate of food intake of experimental animals.  Some have resulted in the discovery of *new essential nutrients*, e.g., *selenium*.   Other responses remain to be understood.   For young monogastrics (particularly poultry) several feedstuffs are popularly regarded as having *"UGF activity"*.

Sources of UGF activity for poultry:

| | |
|---|---|
| condensed fish solubles | fish meal |
| dried whey | brewers' dried yeast |
| corn distillers' dried solubles | other fermentation residues |

Elucidating the natures of these UGFs has been complicated by the fact that the growth responses are small and, often, poorly reproducible.  This suggests that other interacting effects of environment, gut microfloral, diet, etc., may be involved.  As has happened in the past, perhaps the *next vitamins* will be discovered through studies of these or other *UGFs*.

---

[115]Normally, cyanide-poisoning is not a problem for animals that eat apricot or peach kernels, as those seeds generally pass intact through the gut.

[116]An example is the enhancement, by the natural chelating activity in corn distiller's dried solubles of, the utilization of zinc by chicks fed a soybean meal-based diet.

## Study Questions and Exercises:

i.  List the *questions* that must be answered in determining the eligibility of a substance for vitamin status.

ii.  For each of the substances discussed in this chapter, list the available information that would *support* its designation as a vitamin, and that which would *refute* such a designation.

iii.  Outline the *general approaches* one would need to take in order to characterize the UGF activity of a natural material such as fish meal for the chick.

iv.  Prepare a *concept map* of the relationships of *micronutrients* and *physiological function*, including the specific relationships of the traditional vitamins, the quasi-vitamins and ineffective factors.

## Recommended Reading:

Choline  Chan, M.M. 1991. Choline, Chapter 14 *in* Handbook of Vitamins, 2nd ed. (L.J. Machlin, ed.), Marcel Dekker, New York, pp. 537-556.

Zeisel, S.H. 1981. Dietary choline: Biochemistry, physiology and pharmacology. Ann. Rev. Nutr. 1:95-121.

Carnitine  Atkins, J. and M.T. Clandinin. 1990. Nutritional significance of factors affecting carnitine dependent transport of fatty acids in neonates: a review. Nutr.Res. 10:117-128.

Borum, P. 1991. Carnitine, Chapter 15 *in* Handbook of Vitamins, 2nd ed. (L.J. Machlin, ed.), Marcel Dekker, New York, pp. 557-563.

Rebouche, C.J. and D.J. Paulson. 1986. Carnitine metabolism and function in humans. Ann. Rev. Nutr. 6:41-66.

myo-*Inositol*  Cody, M.M. 1991. Substances without vitamin status, Chapter 16 *in* Handbook of Vitamins, 2nd ed. (L.J. Machlin, ed.), Marcel Dekker, New York, pp. 567-572.

Holub, B.J. 1987. The cellular forms and functions of the inositol phospholipids and their metabolic derivatives. Nutr. Rev. 45:65-71.

Putney, Jr., J.W., H. Takemura, A.R. Hughes, D.A. Horstman, and O. Thastrup. 1989. How do inositol phosphates regulate calcium signaling? FASEB J. 3:1899-1905.

*Recommended Reading (continued):*

*Pyrroloquinoline quinone*

Duine, J.A., R.A. van de Meer and B.W. Green. 1990. The cofactor pyrroloquinoline quinone. Ann. Rev. Nutr. 10:297-318.

Killgore, J., C. Smidt, L. Duich, N. Romero-Chapman, D. Tinker, K. Reiser, M. Melko, D. Hyde, and R.B. Rucker. 1989. Nutritional importance of pyrroloquinoline quinone. Science 245:850-852.

Smidt, C.R., F.M. Steinberg and R.B. Rucker. 1991. Physiologic importance of pyrroloquinoline quinone. Proc. Soc. Exp. Biol. Med. 197:19-26.

*Ubiquinone*       Olson, R.E., and H. Rudney. 1983. Biosynthesis of Ubiquinone. Vit. Horm. 40:1-43.

*Bioflavonoids*    Cody, M.M. 1991. Substances without vitamin status, Chapter 16 *in* Handbook of Vitamins, 2nd ed. (L.J. Machlin, ed.), Marcel Dekker, New York, pp. 572-575.

# SECTION III

## USING CURRENT KNOWLEDGE OF THE VITAMINS

# CHAPTER 19    *SOURCES OF THE VITAMINS*

*"The intakes of vitamins into the body calculated from standard tables are rarely accurate."*                                                                J. Marks

---

## Anchoring Concepts:

| | |
|---|---|
| *i.* | *Estimates* of vitamin contents of many foods and feedstuffs are available. |
| *ii.* | For some vitamins, only a portion of the total present in certain foods or feedstuffs is *biologically available*. |
| *iii.* | The *total vitamin intake* of an individual is the sum of the amounts of bioavailable vitamins in the various foods, feedstuffs and supplements consumed. |

## Learning Objectives:

| | |
|---|---|
| *i.* | To understand the concept of a *core food*, and to know the core foods for each of the vitamins. |
| *ii.* | To understand the *sources of potential losses* of the vitamins from foods and feedstuffs. |
| *iii.* | To understand which of the vitamins are *most likely* to be in *insufficient supply* in the diets of humans and livestock. |
| *iv.* | To understand the means available for the *supplementation* of individual foods and total diets with vitamins. |

## Vocabulary:

| | |
|---|---|
| bioavailability | nutrient composition tables |
| core foods | vitamin premix |
| National Nutrient Database | |

## VITAMINS IN FOODS AND FEEDSTUFFS

*tabulated*
*vitamin*
*composition*
*data*

Collation of best estimates of the nutrient composition of foods and feedstuffs has been an ongoing activity by several groups in the United States since the turn of the century[1]. Nutrient composition data for foods and feedstuffs are now available in many forms (e.g., books, wall charts, tables and appendices of books, computer tapes and diskettes). However, most compilations derive from a relatively few sources. This is particularly true for the nutrient composition data for foods; almost all current versions are renditions of the *USDA National Nutrient Database*[2] developed through an ongoing program of the U.S. Department of Agriculture. The nutrient composition of feedstuffs has, with few exceptions[3], been developed less systematically and extensively. Data sets presently in the public domain have been compiled largely from original reports in the scientific literature. Therefore, effects of uncontrolled sampling, multiple and often old analytical methods, multiple analysts, unreported analytical precision, unreported sample variance, etc., are likely to be far greater for the nutrient databases for feedstuffs than for those for foods.

Use of any database for estimating vitamin intake is limited for reasons of the *accuracy* and *completeness* of the data. Although the USDA National Nutrient Database is much more complete than most feed tables with respect to data for the vitamins, it is only reasonable complete with respect to *thiamin*, *riboflavin* and *niacin*; data for vitamins D and E are particularly

---

[1] The formal compilation of food composition data was initiated by USDA food chemist W.O. Atwater in 1896. Since that time, developing information on the nutrient composition of foods has been an ongoing program of the USDA. The development of nutrient composition information for feedstuffs started in the US after the turn of the century at several land grant colleges; in recent times those activities have passed largely into the private sector, being in the interest of corporate feed producers to have reliable data for contents in feedstuffs of those nutrients that most directly affect the cost of their formulations (e.g., metabolizable energy, protein, indispensible amino acids, Ca, P, etc.)

[2] These data are available in several forms: <u>Agricultural Handbook No. 8, Composition of Foods: Raw, Processed, Prepared</u>, revised (a series of looseleaf printed publications each dealing with a particular group of foods, e.g., 'Fats and Oils', 'Vegetables and Vegetable Products', 'Baby Foods'); <u>USDA Nutrient Database for Standard Reference</u> (computer tape); <u>USDA Nutrient Database for Standard Reference for Microcomputers</u> (floppy disk, also available in an abbreviated version with only 21 nutrients); <u>USDA Nutrient Database for Individual Food Intake Surveys</u> (computer tape with a recipe-calculation program with the nutrient data set).

[3] The notable exception in the public domain was the program at the University of Maryland which involved the ongoing analysis of feedstuffs commonly used in feeding poultry in the US. That program focused on the macro-nutrients. It was discontinued in the late 1970s; the last version of the data (i.e., *"1979 Maryland Feed Composition Data"*) was published as a supplement in the Proceedings of the Maryland Nutrition Conference in that year. Other widely used feed tables (e.g., Scott, et al. 1982, <u>Nutrition of the Chicken</u>, pp. 482-489) were derived in part from this source.

scant[4]. In addition, accurate and robust[5] analytical methods are available only for *vitamin E, thiamin, riboflavin, niacin* and *pyridoxine*. For the other vitamins, this means that the quality of available analytical data can render them unacceptable for inclusion in the database or be low enough to raise serious questions concerning reliability.

*core foods*
*for vitamins*

**Foods** are the most important sources of vitamins in the daily for diets of humans. However, *the vitamins are unevenly distributed among the various foods* that comprise human diets. Therefore, the evaluation of the degree of vitamin-adequacy of total diets is served by knowing which foods are likely to contribute significantly to the total intake of each particular vitamin, by virtue both of the frequency and the amount of the food consumed as well as the probable concentration of the vitamin in that food. Identifying such *"core foods"* is difficult because both the voluntary intakes of foods by free-living people and the concentrations of vitamins in those foods are extremely difficult to estimate quantitatively with acceptable certainty. Nevertheless, attempts to do that have indicated a manageable number of *"core foods"* for each of the vitamins, e.g., for Americans it has been estimated that 80% of the total intakes of several vitamins are provided by 50-200 foods[6].

*sources of*
*vitamins in*
*feedstuffs*

Several feedstuffs in common use in the formulation of livestock diets contain nutritionally significant concentrations of the vitamins. However, a *"core feedstuffs"* concept (analogous to the *"core food"* concept) for the vitamins is less useful in the practice of animal nutrition than it is in human nutrition because, unlike the ways in which people are fed or chose to feed themselves, the economic considerations in feeding livestock generally dictate the use of a relatively small number of feedstuffs with few (if any) day-to-day changes in diet formulation[7]. In agriculture, the continued use of the same or very similar diets has resulted in the empirical development of the knowledge of the vitamin contents of feedstuffs.

---

[4]Missing data create problems in the estimation of the nutrient contents of diets and of nutrient intakes of individuals and groups. In computer programs for diet analyses, missing data for a the nutrient content of a food used will result in an estimate of the amount of that nutrient present or consumed that may be lower than the actual amount; programs that fail to identify missing data will, therefore, under-represent the uncertainty associated with the estimates they produce.

[5]Accuracy is minimally influenced by such factors as unusual technical skill of the analyst, particular instrumental conditions, etc.

[6]Using data from the 1976 Nationwide Food Consumption Survey and the Continuing Survey of Food Intakes by Individuals, USDA nutritionists have estimated that, on a national basis, Americans obtain 80% of their total intakes of the following vitamins from the following numbers of food: vitamin A, 60; vitamin E, 100; thiamin, 168; riboflavin, 165; niacin, 159; pyridoxine, 175; folate, 129; vitamin $B_{12}$, 58.

[7]For example, starting broiler chicks are typically fed the same diet from hatching to 3 wks. of age, and laying hens in some management systems may be fed the same diet for 20 wks. before its formula is changed.

Adequacy of the USDA National Nutrient Database vitamin contents of foods:

| food | A | D | E | K | C | thiamin | ribo-flavin | niacin | B$_6$ | panto. acid | folate | B$_{12}$ |
|---|---|---|---|---|---|---|---|---|---|---|---|---|
| baby foods | ▪ | | ▪ | □ | ■ | ■ | | ■ | ■ | ▪ | □ | ▪ | ▪ |
| baked foods | | | | | | | | | | | | |
|   breads | □ | | ▪ | □ | | ■ | ■ | ■ | ■ | ▪ | ▪ | □ |
|   sweet goods | ▪ | | ▪ | | | ■ | ■ | ■ | ▪ | ▪ | ▪ | ▪ |
|   cookies/crackers | ▪ | | ▪ | | | ■ | ■ | ■ | ■ | ▪ | ▪ | ▪ |
| beverages | ▪ | | | | ▪ | ▪ | ▪ | ▪ | ▪ | ▪ | ▪ | ▪ |
| breakfast cereals | ▪ | □ | ▪ | □ | ▪ | ▪ | ▪ | ▪ | ▪ | ▪ | ▪ | ▪ |
| candies | ▪ | | □ | | ▪ | □ | ▪ | ▪ | ▪ | ▪ | ▪ | □ |
| cereal grains | | | | | | | | | | | | |
|   whole | ▪ | | ▪ | ▪ | | ■ | ■ | ■ | ■ | ■ | ■ | |
|   flour | | | ▪ | □ | | ■ | ■ | ■ | ■ | ■ | ■ | |
|   pasta | | | □ | □ | | ■ | ■ | ■ | ■ | ■ | ■ | |
| dairy products | ■ | ■ | ▪ | ▪ | ■ | ■ | ■ | ■ | ■ | ■ | ▪ | ■ |
| eggs, egg products | ▪ | ▪ | ▪ | ▪ | □ | ■ | ■ | ■ | ■ | ■ | ▪ | ■ |
| fast foods | ■ | □ | ▪ | □ | ▪ | ■ | ■ | ■ | ▪ | ▪ | □ | ▪ |
| fats and oils | ▪ | ▪ | ▪ | ▪ | | | | | | | | |
| fish, shellfish | | | | | | | | | | | | |
|   raw | ▪ | ▪ | ▪ | □ | | ▪ | ▪ | ▪ | ▪ | ▪ | ▪ | ▪ |
|   cooked | □ | ▪ | ▪ | □ | | □ | □ | □ | □ | ▪ | ▪ | □ |
| fruits | | | | | | | | | | | | |
|   raw | ■ | | □ | ▪ | ■ | ▪ | ▪ | ▪ | ▪ | ▪ | ▪ | |
|   cooked | ▪ | | □ | □ | ▪ | ▪ | ▪ | ▪ | ▪ | ▪ | ▪ | |
|   frozen, canned | ■ | | □ | □ | ▪ | ▪ | □ | ■ | ▪ | ▪ | ▪ | |
| legumes | | | | | | | | | | | | |
|   raw | ▪ | | ■ | ▪ | | ■ | ■ | ■ | ▪ | ■ | ■ | |
|   cooked | □ | | ■ | □ | | ■ | ■ | ■ | ▪ | ■ | ■ | |
| meat | | | | | | | | | | | | |
|   beef | ■ | ▪ | ▪ | ▪ | | ■ | ■ | ■ | ■ | ▪ | ▪ | ■ |
|   lamb | ▪ | ▪ | ▪ | □ | | ■ | ■ | ■ | ▪ | ▪ | ▪ | ■ |
|   pork | ▪ | ▪ | ▪ | □ | | ■ | ■ | ■ | ■ | ▪ | ▪ | ■ |
|   sausage | ▪ | ▪ | □ | □ | ■ | ■ | ■ | ■ | ■ | ▪ | ▪ | ■ |
|   veal | ▪ | ▪ | ▪ | □ | | ■ | ■ | ■ | ■ | ▪ | ■ | ■ |
|   poultry | ▪ | ▪ | ▪ | □ | | ■ | ■ | ■ | ▪ | ▪ | ▪ | ▪ |
| nuts, seeds | ▪ | ▪ | ▪ | □ | ▪ | ▪ | ▪ | ▪ | ▪ | ▪ | □ | |
| snack foods | ▪ | ▪ | ▪ | □ | □ | ▪ | ■ | ■ | ▪ | ▪ | ▪ | □ |
| soups | ■ | | □ | □ | ■ | ■ | ▪ | ■ | ▪ | □ | □ | ▪ |
| vegetables | | | | | | | | | | | | |
|   raw | ■ | | ▪ | ▪ | ■ | ▪ | | ■ | ■ | ▪ | □ | ▪ |
|   cooked | ▪ | | ▪ | □ | ▪ | ▪ | ▪ | ▪ | ▪ | □ | ▪ | |
|   frozen | ■ | | □ | □ | ■ | ■ | ■ | ■ | □ | ▪ | ▪ | |
|   canned | ■ | | □ | □ | ■ | ■ | ■ | ■ | □ | ▪ | ▪ | |

key:

□   *few or no data*
▪   *inadequate data*
■   *substantial data*

source: Beecher, G. and R. Matthews. 1990. Nutrient composition of foods. Chapter 15 *in* <u>Present Knowledge in Nutrition</u>, 6th ed. (M. Brown, ed.), Int. Life Sci. Inst.-Nutr.Found., Wash., DC, pp. 430-439.

Core foods for the traditional vitamins:

| vitamin A | vitamin D | vitamin E | vitamin K |
|---|---|---|---|
| liver | milk* | vegetable oils | broccoli |
| red peppers | margarine* | | lettuce |
| spinach | chicken (skin) | | cauliflower |
| carrots | liver | | cabbage |
| eggs | fatty fish | | Brussels sprouts |
| kale | (e.g., herring) | | turnip greens |
| butter | egg yolk | | liver |
| margarine* | | | spinach |
| milk* | | | asparagus |

| vitamin C | thiamin | riboflavin | niacin |
|---|---|---|---|
| tomatoes | meats | eggs | meats |
| potatoes | potatoes | liver | eggs |
| many other | liver | meats | fish |
|   fruits and | whole grains | some fish | whole grains |
|   vegetables | some fish | asparagus | legumes |
| | legumes | milk | milk |
| | | whole grains | |

| vitamin $B_6$ | biotin | pantothenic acid | folate |
|---|---|---|---|
| meats | liver | liver | tomatoes |
| cabbage | egg yolk | milk | beets |
| potatoes | cauliflower | meats | potatoes |
| liver | kidney | eggs | wheat germ |
| beans | peanuts | fish | cabbage |
| whole grains | soybeans | whole grains | eggs |
| peanuts | wheat germ | legumes | meats |
| soybeans | oatmeal | | spinach |
| some fish | carrots | | asparagus |
| milk | | | liver |
| | | | soybeans |
| vitamin $B_{12}$ | | | whole grains |
| liver | | | milk |
| fish | | | |
| eggs | | | |
| milk | *The high vitamin content is due to fortification. | | |

*vitamin supplements simplify feeds*
As purified sources of the vitamins have become available at low cost, it has become possible to use fewer feedstuffs in less complicated blends to produce diets of high quality that will support efficient and predictable animal performance.  Thus, many feedstuffs formerly valuable as sources of vitamins (e.g., brewers' yeast, dried buttermilk, "green feeds"[8]) are no longer economical to use in intensive animal management systems[9].

---

[8] e.g., fresh cabbage, grass, etc.

[9] This phenomenon is most true in the economically developed parts of the world.  In the developing world, such factors as the shortage of "hard" currency may make purified sources of vitamins too expensive to use in animal diets, thus, making natural sources of the vitamins more valuable.  Under such circumstances, it is prudent to exploit a wide variety of local feedstuffs, food wastes and food by-products in the formulation of animal feeds that are adequate in the vitamins as well as all other known nutrients.

Feedstuffs containing significant amounts of the vitamins:

| vitamin A | vitamin D | vitamin E |
|---|---|---|
| none[a] | none[a] | dehydrated alfalfa meal |
| | | sun-cured alfalfa meal |
| | | wheat germ meal |
| | | unmilled grains |
| | | corn germ meal |
| | | stabilized vegetable oils |

| vitamin K | vitamin C | thiamin |
|---|---|---|
| dehydrated alfalfa meal | none[a,b] | none[a] |
| sun-cured alfalfa meal | | |

| riboflavin | niacin | vitamin $B_6$ |
|---|---|---|
| dried skim milk | barley | sunflower seed meal |
| peanut meal | cottonseed meal | sesame meal |
| brewers' yeast | dried fish solubles | meat and bone meal |
| dried buttermilk | rice bran | |
| dried whey | wheat bran | |
| Torula yeast | corn gluten feed | |
| corn distillers' solubles | fish meals | |
| liver and glandular meal | peanut meal | |
| | rice polishings | |
| | Torula yeast | |
| | corn gluten meal | |
| | corn distillers' solubles | |
| | liver and glandular meal | |
| | sunflower seed meal | |
| | brewers' yeast | |

| biotin | pantothenic acid | folate |
|---|---|---|
| corn germ meal | molasses | dried brewers' grains |
| brewers' yeast | rice polishings | dehydrated alfalfa meal |
| molasses | sunflower seed meal | brewers' yeast |
| Torula yeast | peanut meal | soybean meal |
| hydrolyzed feathers | Torula yeast | Torula yeast |
| safflower meal | liver and glandular meal | meat and bone meal |
| | brewers' yeast | corn distillers' solubles |
| | | sun-cured alfalfa meal |

| vitamin $B_{12}$ | choline | |
|---|---|---|
| dried fish solubles | liver and glandular meal | |
| liver and glandular meal | dried fish solubles | |
| hydrolyzed feathers | soybean meal | |
| fish meals | corn distillers' solubles | |
| crab meal | | |
| dried skim milk | | |
| meat and bone meal | | |
| dried butter milk | | |

[a]Instability of the vitamin in most feedstuffs renders few, if any, predictable sources of appreciable amounts of it.
[b]not required by livestock species.

*vitamins in human diets*    Foods of both plant and animal origin provide vitamins in mixed diets for humans. ***Meats*** and ***meat products*** are generally excellent sources of thiamin, riboflavin, niacin, pyridoxine and vitamin $B_{12}$. ***Liver*** is a very good source of vitamins A, D, E, $B_{12}$, and folacin.   These animal products, however, are generally not good sources of vitamins C or K (the exception being pork liver) or folate.   ***Milk products*** are important sources of vitamins A and C, thiamin, riboflavin[10], pyridoxine and vitamin $B_{12}$. Because milk is widely enriched with irradiated ergosterol (vitamin $D_2$), it is also an important source of vitamin $D$[11]. ***Vegetables*** are generally good sources of vitamins A, K and C, and pyridoxine. ***Grain products*** are generally good sources of thiamin, riboflavin and niacin.

Contributions (%) of various foods to the intakes of vitamins by Americans:

| foods | vit. A | vit. C | thiamin | ribo-flavin | niacin | vit. $B_6$ | vit. $B_{12}$ |
|---|---|---|---|---|---|---|---|
| vegetables | 39.4 | 51.8 | 11.7 | 6.9 | 12.0 | 22.2 | - |
| legumes | - | - | 5.4 | - | 8.2 | 5.4 | - |
| fruits | 8.0 | 39.0 | 4.4 | 2.2 | 2.5 | 8.2 | - |
| grain products | - | - | 41.2 | 22.1 | 27.4 | 10.2 | 1.6 |
| meats | 22.5 | 2.0 | 27.1 | 22.2 | 45.0 | 40.0 | 69.2 |
| milk products | 13.2 | 3.7 | 8.1 | 39.1 | 1.4 | 11.6 | 20.7 |
| eggs | 5.8 | - | 2.0 | 4.9 | - | 2.1 | 8.5 |
| fats and oils | 8.2 | - | - | - | - | - | - |
| other | 2.7 | 3.4 | - | - | 3.3 | - | - |

source:   Sauberlich, et al. 1982. *in* Animal Products in Human Nutrition (D.C. Beitz and R.G. Hansen, eds.), Academic Press, New York, p. 339.

Sources of the vitamins by food group:

| food group | vitamins provided in significant amounts |
|---|---|
| meats, poultry, fish, beans | thiamin, riboflavin, niacin, pyridoxine, pantothenic acid, biotin, vitamin $B_{12}$ |
| milk, milk products | vitamin A, vitamin D, riboflavin, pyridoxine, vitamin $B_{12}$ |
| breads, cereals | thiamin, riboflavin, niacin, pyridoxine, folate, pantothenic acid, biotin |
| fruits, vegetables | vitamin A, vitamin K, ascorbic acid, riboflavin, folate |
| fats, oils | vitamin A, vitamin E |

*vitamins in breast milk formula foods*    The vitamin contents of foods that are intended for use as the main or sole components of diets (e.g., ***human milk, infant formulas, parenteral feeding solutions***) are particularly important determinants of the vitamin status

---

[10]In the U.S., milk products supply an estimated 40% of the required riboflavin.

[11]This practice has practically eliminated rickets in countries that practice it.

of individuals consuming them.  Studies of the vitamin contents of human milk have yielded variable results, particularly for the fat-soluble vitamins. In general, it has been observed that the concentrations of all vitamins *except vitamin B$_{12}$* in human milk tend to increase during lactation.   In comparison to cow's milk, human milk contains *more* of vitamins A, E, C, and niacin, but *less* vitamin K, thiamin, riboflavin and pyridoxine.

Because infant formulas and parenteral feeding solutions are carefully prepared and quality-controlled products, each is formulated largely from purified or partially refined ingredients to contain known amounts of the vitamins.  For parenteral feeding solutions, however, some problems related to vitamin nutrition have occurred.  One problem involved biotin, which was not added to such solutions prior to 1981 in the belief that intestinal synthesis of the vitamin was adequate for all patients except children with inborn metabolic errors or individuals ingesting large amounts of raw egg white.   When it was found that children supported by total parenteral nutrition (TPN) frequently suffered from gastro-intestinal abnormalities which responded to biotin[12], the vitamin was added to TPN solutions[13]. Another problem with parenteral feeding solutions has been the loss of fat-soluble vitamins and riboflavin either by absorption to the plastic bags and tubing most frequently used, or by decomposition upon exposure to light. Such effects can reduce the delivery of vitamins A, D and E to the patient by two-thirds, and to result in the loss of one-third of the riboflavin.

Vitamin contents of human and cow's milk:

| vitamin | human milk | cow's milk |
|---|---|---|
| vitamin A (retinol), mg/l | 0.60 | 0.31 |
| vitamin D$_3$, $\mu$g/l | 0.3 | 0.2 |
| vitamin E, mg/l | 3.5 | 0.9 |
| vitamin K, mg/l | 0.15 | 0.6 |
| ascorbic acid, mg/l | 38 | 20 |
| thiamin, mg/l | 0.16 | 0.40 |
| riboflavin, mg/l | 0.30 | 1.90 |
| niacin, mg/l | 2.3 | 0.8 |
| pyridoxine, mg/l | 0.06 | 0.40 |
| biotin, $\mu$g/l | 7.6 | 20 |
| pantothenic acid, mg/l | 0.26 | 0.36 |
| folate, mg/l | 0.05 | 0.05 |
| vitamin B$_{12}$, $\mu$g/l | <0.1 | 3 |

source:  Porter, J.W.G. Proc. Nutr. Soc. 37:225 (1978).

[12]These cases appeared to have had altered gut microflora secondary to antibiotic treatment.

[13]Although there are no recommended dietary allowances (RDAs) for biotin, it has been suggested that biotin supplements be given to persons being fed parenterally (infants: 30 $\mu$g/kg/day; adults: 5 $\mu$g/kg/day). These levels are consistent with the provisional recommendations (infants: 10 $\mu$g/day; adults: 30-100 $\mu$g/day) of the National Research Council Food Nutrition Board (1989).

*vitamins in animal feeds*

Unlike human diets, formulated diets for livestock generally do not provide adequate amounts of the vitamins unless they are supplemented with either certain vitamin-rich feedstuffs or purified vitamins. In general, the relative vitamin-adequacy of unsupplemented animal feeds depends on the relative complexity (the number of feedstuffs used in the mixture) of the diet. The vitamin contents of simple rations tend to be less than those of complex ones.

Vitamins provided by constituent feedstuffs in two chick starter diets:

| | 1936 diet[a]<br>(complex) | contemporary diet<br>(simple) |
|---|---|---|
| *ingredients, %* | | |
| corn meal | 27.5 | 65.11 |
| oats | 10.0 | |
| wheat bran | 20.0 | |
| wheat middlings | 10.0 | |
| soybean meal, 49% protein | 10.0 | 19.08 |
| meat and bone meal | 10.0 | 4.78 |
| poultry by-product meal | | 7.00 |
| dried whey | 5.0 | |
| dehydrated alfalfa meal | 5.0 | |
| blended fat | | 3.18 |
| limestone | 2.0 | |
| salt | .5 | .25 |
| D,L-methionine, 98% | | .10 |
| trace minerals | +[a] | +[b] |
| vitamins | +[c] | +[d] |
| | | |
| *vitamins provided by feedstuffs, amounts per kg of diet* | | |
| vitamin A, IU | 6000 (400)[f] | 1360 ( 91)[f,g] |
| vitamin E, IU | 27 (270) | 20.5 (205)[g] |
| vitamin K, mg | 0.73 (146) | 0 ( 0)[g] |
| thiamin, mg | 4.7 (261) | 3.1 (172) |
| riboflavin, mg | 5.4 (150) | 2.3 ( 64)[g] |
| niacin, mg | 69.9 (259) | 28.3 (105)[g] |
| pyridoxine, mg | 5.7 (190) | 5.3 (177) |
| biotin, $\mu$g | 208 (139) | 141 ( 94) |
| pantothenic acid, mg | 15.7 (157) | 7.4 ( 74)[g] |
| folate, mg | 0.81 (145) | .32 ( 58) |
| vitamin $B_{12}$, $\mu$g | 6.5 ( 72) | 21.0 (233)[g] |
| choline, mg | 1115 ( 86) | 1395 (107)[g] |

[a]This was a state-of-art diet for starting chicks at Cornell University in 1942.   [b]$MnSO_4$, 125 mg/kg   [c]Provides per kg of diet: ZnO, 66 mg; $MnSO_4$, 220 mg; $Na_2SeO_3$, 220 $\mu$g [d]vit. $D_3$, 790 IU/kg   [e]Provides per kg of diet: vit. A, 4400 IU; vit. $D_3$, 2200 IU; vit. E, 5.5 IU; vit. $K_3$, 2 mg; riboflavin, 4 mg; nicotinic acid, 33 mg; pantothenic acid, 11 mg; vitamin $B_{12}$, 1 $\mu$g; choline, 220 mg   [f]Numbers in parentheses give amounts of each vitamin as a percentage of current (1984) recommendations of the U.S. National Research Council   [g]Included in the vitamin-mineral premix.

For example, complex diets such as those used for feeding poultry or swine in the 1950s[14], would be expected to contain *in constituent feedstuffs* more than an adequate amount of vitamin $B_{12}$, and adequate (or nearly so) amounts of vitamin K, vitamin E, thiamin, riboflavin, niacin, pyridoxine, pantothenic acid, folate and choline. In contrast, the simpler rations (based almost exclusively on corn and soybean meal) that are used today contain lower amounts, if any, of the more costly vitamin-rich feedstuffs previously used. Such simple rations can be expected to contain *in constituent feedstuffs* adequate levels of *only* vitamin E, thiamin, pyridoxine and biotin. The availability of stable, biologically available, and economical vitamins facilitated this change in complexity of animal feeds by replacing with inexpensive mixtures of vitamins the more costly vitamin-rich feedstuffs used previously.

# *DISCREPANCIES BETWEEN PREDICTED AND ACTUAL AMOUNTS OF VITAMINS IN FOODS AND FEEDSTUFFS*

*sources of inaccuracy*

The availability of data for the vitamin contents of foods and feedstuffs can be extremely useful in making judgments concerning the adequacy of food supplies and feedstuff inventories; however, estimates of the nutrient intakes of individuals based upon these data are seldom accurate due to the variety of factors that may alter the nutrient composition of a food or feedstuff before it is actually ingested. The errors associated with such estimates are particularly great for the vitamins.

Sources of error in estimating vitamins in foods and feedstuffs:

| | |
|---|---|
| i. | *analytical errors* in sampling food/feedstuffs and measuring the vitamin |
| ii. | *variation in the actual amount* of the vitamin present |
| iii. | *less than full bioavailability* of the form of the vitamin present |
| iv. | *losses during storage* of the raw food/feedstuff |
| v. | *losses during processing* the food/feedstuff |
| vi. | *losses during cooking* the food |

To accommodate these sources of potential error, most of which operate to inflate estimates of nutrient intake, it has been a common practice to discount by 10-25% the analytical values in the databases. It is likely that such modest discounts may still result in overestimates of intakes of at least some of the vitamins.

---

[14]Those complex diets contained, in addition to a major grain and soybean meal, small amounts of the following: alfalfa meal, corn distillers' dried solubles, fish meal, meat and bone meal.

*analytical*
*errors*

Errors in the sampling of and actual analysis of foods and feedstuffs for vitamins can be an important contributor to the inaccuracy of predicted values. Analytical errors are less likely to be problematic for vitamin E, thiamin, riboflavin, niacin and pyridoxine, for which robust (not prone to analyst-effects) analytical techniques are available.

*natural*
*variation in*
*vitamin*
*contents*

The concentration of vitamins in individual foods and feedstuffs can vary widely. The vitamin contents of materials of animal origin can be affected by the conditions of feeding the source animal, which can be highly variable according to country of origin, season of the year, size of the farm, age at slaughter, the composition of the diets used, etc. For example, the vitamin E contents of poultry meat are greater from chickens fed supplements of the vitamin than from those that are not[15]. For foods and feedstuffs of plant origin, vitamin contents may vary among different cultivars of the same species and according to local agronomic factors and weather conditions that affect growth rate and yield. Different cultivars of corn have been found to vary in vitamin E content three-fold (11-36 IU/kg). For many plants, growing conditions that favor the production of lush vegetation will result in increased concentrations of vitamin E, vitamin K and $\beta$-carotene. For some (e.g., tomatoes), sunlight intensity affects ascorbic acid concentrations. Conditions at harvest can also affect the vitamin content of some crops, e.g., the vitamin E content of fungal infected corn grain can be less than half of that of non-blighted corn. Legumes (e.g., alfalfa, soybeans) contain the enzyme lipoxygenase which, if not inactivated (e.g., by drying) soon after harvest, results in massive destruction of carotenoids and vitamin E. Therefore, plant-derived foods can show a considerable range of concentrations of the vitamins. For example, the ascorbic acid contents of potatoes can vary by more than 6-fold (in the range of 40-260 mg/kg). Values reported for the vitamin contents of wheat vary considerably[16].

Natural variation in the nutritional composition of foods and feedstuffs have generally accommodated by the analysis of multiple representative samples of each material of interest. Nevertheless, most databases include only a single value, the mean of all analyses, and fail to indicate the variance around that mean. The practical necessity of using databases so constructed means that the nutritionist is faced with the dilemma of estimating vitamin intake through the use of data that are likely to be inaccurate but to an uncertain and unascertainable degree. Thus, if an average value of 150 mg/kg is used to represent the ascorbic acid concentration of potatoes, as is frequently the case, then it must be recognized that half of all samples will exceed that value (thus yielding an underestimate) while half

---

[15]A practical example of this comparison is the intensively managed commercial poultry flock fed formulated feeds in the US vs. the small courtyard flock largely subsisting on table scraps, insects and grasses in China and much of the developing world.

[16]Reported variations are: vitamin E, 8.9-fold; thiamin, 7.9-fold; riboflavin, 5.2-fold; niacin, 8.9-fold; pyridoxine, 8.6-fold; pantothenic acid, 2.8-fold; folate, 4.9-fold.

will be less than that value (thus, yielding an overestimate). In constructing databases for use in meal planning or feed formulation, a better way to accommodate such natural variation is to enter into the database values discounted by a multiple of the standard deviation that would yield acceptably low probability of overestimating actual nutrient amounts[17]. That approach, however, requires a fairly extensive body of data from which to generate meaningful estimates of variance. Few, if any sets of food/feedstuff vitamin composition data are that extensive.

*bioavailability*    Apart from considerations of analytical accuracy and natural variation associated with estimates of the vitamin contents of foods and feedstuffs, chemical analyses of vitamin contents may not provide useful information regarding the amounts of vitamin that are biologically available. Many vitamins can be present in foods and feedstuffs in forms that are not readily absorbed by humans or animals. The chemical analyses of such vitamins will yield measures of the total vitamin contents, which will be overestimates of the biologically relevant amounts. The bioavailabilities of *niacin*, *biotin*, *pyridoxine*, *vitamin B^12* and *choline* in certain foods and feedstuffs can be low. Because only the amounts of *biologically available* vitamins in foods and feedstuffs have nutritional relevance, it would be useful to have *in vitro* methods for assessing vitamin bioavailability. Such a method has been developed to measure niacin bioavailability[18]; but for most vitamins bioavailability must be determined *experimentally* using appropriate *animal models*.

Foods and feedstuffs with low vitamin bioavailabilities:

| vitamin | form | food/feedstuff |
|---|---|---|
| vitamin A | pro-vitamins A | corn |
| vitamin E | non-$\alpha$-tocopherols | corn oil, soybean oil |
| ascorbic acid | ascorbinogen | cabbage |
| niacin | niacytin | corn, potatoes, rice, sorghum grain, wheat |
| pyridoxine | pyridoxine 5'-$\beta$-glucoside | corn, rice bran, unpolished rice, peanuts, soybeans, soybean meal, wheat bran, whole wheat |
| biotin | biocytin | barley, fishmeal, oats, sorghum grain, wheat |
| choline | phospholipids | soybean meal |

---

[17]This approach was originated in the 1950s by G.F. Combs, Sr. (the author's father) at the University of Maryland when he developed the Maryland Feed Composition Table. The data included in that table were based on replicate analyses from multiple samples of each feedstuff and were expressed as the **mean-0.9 SD** units. That adjustment was selected to allow a likelihood of overestimating actual nutrient concentration of $P = 0.20$, which level was acceptable in his judgment.

[18]This method, developed by Carpenter, involves the comparison of the amounts of niacin determined chemically before (free niacin) and after (total niacin) alkaline hydrolysis. The free niacin thus determined correlates with the available niacin determined using the growth response of niacin-deficient rats fed a low-TRY diet.

Vitamin bioavailabilities can be affected by extrinsic and intrinsic factors:

> *extrinsic factors:*
> i.    ***concentration*** (effects on solubility and absorption kinetics)
> ii.   ***physical form*** (effects of physical interactions with other food components and/or of coatings, emulsifiers, etc. vitamin supplements)
> iii.  ***food/diet composition*** (effects on intestinal transit time, digestion, vitamin emulsification, vitamin absorption and/or intestinal microflora)
> iv.   ***non-food agonists*** (cholestyramine, alcohol and other drugs that may impair vitamin absorption or metabolism)
> *intrinsic factors:*
> i.    ***age*** (age-related differences in gastro-intestinal function)
> ii.   ***health status*** (effects on gastro-intestinal function)

*storage losses*  The storage of untreated foods can result in considerable losses, particularly of ascorbic acid[19], due to post-harvest enzymatic decomposition. Such losses can vary according to specific techniques of food processing and preservation.

Effects of preservation techniques on vitamin contents of foods:

| technique | main effects | vitamins destroyed[a] |
|---|---|---|
| blanching | partial removal of oxygen | vitamin C (13-60%)[b,c] |
|  | partial heat-inactivation of enzymes | thiamin (2-30%) |
|  |  | riboflavin (5-40%) |
|  |  | carotene (<5%)[c] |
| pasteurization | removal of oxygen[d] | thiamin (10-15%) |
|  | inactivation of enzymes | minor losses (1-5%) of riboflavin, niacin, vit. $B_6$ and pantothenic acid |
| canning | exclusion of oxygen | minor losses[e,f] |
| freezing | inhibition of enzyme activity[g] | vitamin C (ca. 25%) |
| freeze drying | removal of water | very slight losses of most vitamins |
| hot air drying | removal of water | vitamin C (10-15%) thiamin |
| γ-irradiation | inactivation of enzymes | some losses of vitamins C, E and thiamin |

[a]Actual losses are variable, depending on exact conditions of time, temperature, etc.
[b]Loss of vitamin C is due to both oxidation and leeching.
[c]Losses of oxidizable vitamins can be reduced by rapid cooling after blanching.
[d]Vitamin losses are usually small due to the exclusion of oxygen during this process.
[e]Losses in addition to those associated with heat sterilization prior to canning.
[f]e.g., 15% loss of vitamin C after 2 years at 10°C
[g]While enzymatic decomposition is completely inhibited in frozen vegetables, re-activation occurs during thawing such that significant vitamin losses can occur.  This is avoided by rapidly blanching before freezing.

---

[19]The ascorbic acid contents of cold-stored apples and potatoes can drop by two-thirds and one-third, respectively, within 1-2 months.  Those of some green vegetables can drop to 20-78% of original levels after a few days of storage at temperature.

*losses in food*  The milling of grain to produce flour involves the removal of large amounts
*preparation*    of the bran and germ portions of the native product.  Because those
                 portions are typically rich in vitamin E and many of the water-soluble
                 vitamins, highly refined flours[20] are low in these vitamins.

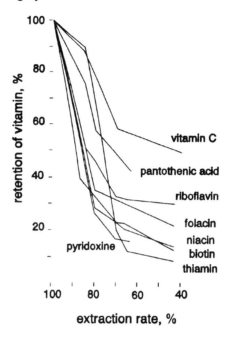

Loss of vitamins in the making of flour.
source:  Moran, T., 1959. Nutr. Abst. Rev. 29:1.

Comparison of typical vitamin contents of whole wheat and white flour:

| vitamin | whole wheat mg/100g | white flour mg/100g |
|---|---|---|
| thiamin | 0.5 | 0.1 |
| riboflavin | 0.15 | 0.05 |
| niacin | 5.0 | 0.9 |
| pyridoxine | 0.45 | 0.17 |

*cooking*   Cooking can introduce further losses of vitamins from native food materials.
*losses*    However, methods used for cooking vary widely between different cultures
            and among different individuals, making vitamin losses associated with
            cooking highly variable.  The washing of vegetables in water prior to
            cooking, can result in the extraction of water-soluble vitamins, particularly
            if they are soaked for long periods of time.  The peeling of vegetables can
            remove vitamins associated with the outer tissues of the vegetable[21].

---

[20] Such flours consist mainly of the starchy endosperm.

[21] For example, the peeling of potatoes can substantially reduce the ascorbic acid content of that food.

Vitamin losses associated with cooking processes are also highly variable, but generally amount to ca. 50% for the less stable vitamins.  The greatest losses are associated with long cooking times under conditions of exposure to air.  Vitamin losses are less when food is cooked rapidly as in a pressure cooker or a microwave oven, or by high temperature stir-frying.  The baking of bread can reduce the thiamin content of flour by ca. 25% without affecting its contents of niacin or riboflavin.

*cumulative losses of vitamins from foods*

The losses of vitamins from foods are ***cumulative***.  Every step in the post-harvest storage, processing and cooking of a food can contribute to the loss of its vitamin contents.  In theory, these losses can be modeled and, thus, predicted.  However, in practice, the variation in the actual conditions of handling foods through each of these steps is so great that the only way to estimate vitamin intakes of people is to analyze the vitamin contents of foods *as they are eaten.*

Vitamin losses from foods can be minimized:

| | |
|---|---|
| *i.* | by ***using fresh food*** instead of stored food; |
| *ii.* | by ***using minimum amounts of water*** in food preparation and cooking; |
| *iii.* | by ***using minimum cooking*** (where necessary, using high temperatures for short periods of time); |
| *iv.* | by ***avoiding the storage of cooked food*** before it is eaten. |

General stabilities of vitamins to food processing and cooking:

| vitamin | conditions that enhance loss |
|---|---|
| vitamin A | highly variable but significant losses during storage and preparation |
| vitamin D | [stable to normal household procedures] |
| vitamin E | frying can result in losses of 70-90%; bleaching of flour destroys 100%; other losses in preparation or baking are small |
| vitamin K | [losses not significant due to synthesis by intestinal microflora] |
| vitamin C | readily lost by oxidation and/or extraction in many steps of food preparation, heat-sterilization, drying and cooking |
| thiamin | readily lost by leaching, by removal of thiamin-rich fractions from native foods (e.g., flour milling) and by heating; losses as great as 75% may occur in meats, and 25-33% in breads |
| riboflavin | readily lost upon exposure to light (90% in milk exposed to sun light for 2 hrs., 30% from milk exposed to room light for 1 day), but very stable when stored in dark; small losses (12-25%) upon heating during cooking |
| niacin | leached during blanching of vegetables ($\leq$40%), but very stable to cooking |
| pyridoxine | leached during food preparation; pasteurization causes losses of 67%; roasting of beef causes losses of ca. 50% |
| biotin | [apparently very stable; limited data] |
| pantothenic acid | losses of 60% by milling of flour and of ca. 30% by cooking of meat; small losses in vegetable preparation |
| folate | [data not available] |
| vitamin $B_{12}$ | only small losses upon irradiation of milk by visible or UV light |

*losses of*        The vitamin contents of feedstuffs and finished feeds[22] are subject to
*vitamins from*    destruction in ways very similar to those of foods. The storage losses that
*feedstuffs and*   can occur in particular feedstuffs are dependent on the conditions of
*finished feeds*   *temperature* and *moisture* during storage; heat and humidity enhance
oxidation reactions of several of the vitamins (vitamins A and E, thiamin,
riboflavin, biotin). Vitamin losses are, therefore, minimized by drying
feedstuffs quickly and storing them dry in weather-proof bins. Where the
drying of a feedstuff is slow[23] or incomplete[24], or where leaky bins are
used for its storage, vitamin losses are greatest.

Most likely limiting vitamins in human and non-ruminant livestock diets:

| humans | livestock |
|---|---|
| vitamin A | vitamin A |
| vitamin E | vitamin E |
| vitamin C | niacin |
| riboflavin | riboflavin |
| folate | pantothenic acid |
| *conditional:* | *conditional:* |
| vitamin D, if house-bound | vitamin D, if raised indoors |
| vitamin $B_{12}$, if strict vegetarian | vitamin K, if raised on slatted or raised-wire floors |
| | vitamin $B_{12}$, if raised on slatted or raised wire floors |
| | choline, chicks only |

Vitamin losses from finished feeds are usually greater than those of individual feedstuffs. Finished feeds are supplemented with essential *trace
elements* some of which ($Cu^{++}$, $Fe^{+++}$) can act as catalytic centers of
oxidation reactions leading to vitamin destruction. Such effects are
particularly important in high-energy feeds (e.g., broiler diets), which
generally contain significant amounts of polyunsaturated fats. It is a
common practice in many countries to compress many of these (and
other) feeds into pellet form[25] by processes involving steam, heat and
pressure. Evidence suggests that *pelleting* can *enhance the bioavailability*
of niacin and biotin, which occur in feedstuffs in bound forms; but it
generally results in the *destruction* of vitamins A, D, E, $K_3$, C and thiamin.

---

[22]complete, blended, ready-to-feed rations

[23]For example, sun-drying enhances the destruction of vitamin E in corn (although sun-curing of cut hay
is essential to provide vitamin D activity).

[24]where moisture is not reduced to less than ca. 15%

[25]There are many reasons for pelleting finished feeds. Pelleting prevents de-mixing of the feed during
handling and transit. It can improve the economy of feed handling due to the associated increase in bulk
density. For the same reason, it can improve the consumption of bulky, low-density feeds. It can also improve
the efficiency of feed utilization by reducing wastage at the feeder. It is thought that the metabolizable energy
values of some feedstuffs may be improved by the steam treatment used in pelleting (e.g., soybean meal with
significant residual anti-tryptic activity). Pelleting also improves the handling of feeds that are very dusty.

## VITAMIN SUPPLEMENTATION

| | |
|---|---|
| *availability of purified vitamins* | All of the vitamins are produced commercially in pure forms.  Most are produced by chemical synthesis, but some are also isolated from natural sources (e.g., the fat-soluble vitamins)[26] and some are produced microbiologically (e.g., thiamin, riboflavin, folate, pyridoxine, biotin, pantothenic acid and vitamin $B_{12}$[27]).  The annual world production of vitamins is estimated to exceed of 20,000 metric tons[28]; purified vitamins are used as additives to foods and feeds, as pharmaceuticals and in cosmetics. |
| *addition of vitamins to foods* | The addition of vitamins to certain foods is a common practice in most countries.  In some cases, vitamins are added to selected, widely used foods (***fortification***[29], e.g., bread[30], milk[31], margarine[31]) for the purpose of ensuring vitamin-adequacy of populations.  In other cases, vitamins are added to restore the vitamin content to that originally present before processing (***re-vitaminization***, e.g., white flour), to increase the amounts of vitamins already present (***enrichment***), or to make foods carriers of vitamins not normally present (***vitaminization***, e.g., many breakfast cereals).  Studies show that the bioavailabilities of purified vitamins added to foods are equivalent, if not better, than those of the vitamins intrinsic to foods. |
| *vitamin supplements for human use* | Many preparations of vitamins are available by prescription and over-the-counter.  A common sight on the shelves of American grocery, drug and health food stores is the wide variety of individual and multi-vitamin supplements that is available.  Many multi-vitamin preparations also contain trace minerals.  The use of vitamin supplements among peoples in developed countries is great enough to make this means a significant contributor to the vitamin nutriture of those populations.  Several surveys have found that about one-half of the U.S. population take oral vitamin supple- |

---

[26] Examples are:  vitamin A from fish liver, vitamin $D_3$ from liver oil or irradiated yeast, vitamin E from soybean or corn oils, and vitamin K from fish meal.

[27] The commercial production of vitamin $B_{12}$ is strictly from microorganisms.

[28] The growth of commercial vitamin production has been steady since the discovery of vitamin $B_{12}$.  For example, in 1950 annual world vitamin production was estimated to be only 1,567 metric tons.

[29] The term *"fortification"* has come to be used to describe *all* types of additions of vitamins to foods.

[30] In the United States, thiamin, riboflavin, niacin and iron are added to white flour.

[31] In most western countries, both vitamin A and vitamin D are added.

ments at least occasionally, and that about one-quarter do so daily[32,33]. The use of vitamin supplements, however, has not resulted in excessive intakes of vitamins among the general American population. With the exception of vitamin C, most Americans receive amounts of vitamin that do not greatly exceed the RDAs. Although vitamin C appears to be consumed in quantities greatly above the RDAs for adults, there is no indication of hazard associated with such intakes.

Prevalence of vitamin supplement use by Americans:

| population | percentage who are daily users | | | | |
|---|---|---|---|---|---|
| | any supplement | multi-type | vit. A | vit. C | vit. E |
| total | 23.2 | 17.4 | 1.2 | 7.6 | 4.1 |
| *gender:* | | | | | |
| men | 19.2 | 14.9 | 1.2 | 6.9 | 3.6 |
| women | 26.8ª | 15.6 | 1.3 | 8.3ª | 4.6ª |
| *race:* | | | | | |
| white | 24.8ª | 18.5ª | 1.3 | 4.5ª | 7.1ª |
| black | 15.9 | 12.2 | 4.5ª | 2.4 | 1.7 |
| hispanic | 18.6 | 14.0 | 5.5 | 3.0 | 3.3ª |
| other | 17.2 | 13.5 | 5.8 | 2.1 | 5.0ª |

ªsignificantly different from rate of lowest percentile group

source: Subar, A.F. and G. Block. 1990. Am. J. Epidemiol. 132:1091-1101.
(1987 National Health Interview Survey data)

Average daily intakes of several vitamins from supplements by Americans:

| vitamin | total population, percentile | | | daily supplement users, percentile | | | |
|---|---|---|---|---|---|---|---|
| | 50th | 75th | 90th | 25th | 50th | 75th | 90th |
| vitamin A, IU | 0 | 2466 | 5000 | 1699 | 5000 | 5000 | 10,010 |
| vitamin D, IU | 0 | 148 | 400 | 136 | 395 | 400 | 400 |
| vitamin E, IU | 0 | 20 | 30 | 12 | 30 | 30 | 230 |
| vitamin C, mg | 0 | 60 | 368 | 39 | 60 | 307 | 629 |
| thiamin/ribo., mg | 0 | .8 | 1.5 | .6 | 1.5 | 1.5 | 7.6 |

source: Subar, A.F. and G. Block. 1990. Am. J. Epidemiol. 132:1091-1101.
(1987 National Health Interview Survey data)

---

[32] The prevalence of daily vitamin supplement use has been estimated at 21.4% (National Health and Examination Survey [NHANES], 1971-74), 22.8% (NHANES-II, 1976-80), 39.9% (FDA, 1983), 36.4% (National Health Interview Survey [NHIS], 1986), and 23.1 (NHIS, 1987).

[33] Whether individuals take vitamin supplements appears to be affected by strong socioeconomic influences. For example, results of the 1987 U.S. National Health Interview Survey indicate that vitamin supplement use was greatest among: individuals who believe that diet affects disease (*vs.* those who do not); non-drinkers and lighter drinkers of alcohol (*vs.* heavy drinkers); former smokers and persons who never smoked (*vs.* current smokers); individuals in the lowest three quartiles of body mass index (kg/m$^2$).

Effects of supplement use on vitamin intakes of Americans:

| vitamin | total population | | supplement users | |
|---|---|---|---|---|
| | mean | % C.V.[*] | mean | % C.V.[*] |
| vitamin A, IU | 7419 | 67 | 8673 | 49 |
| vitamin C, mg | 277 | 110 | 422 | 84 |
| thiamin, mg | 7.5 | 231 | 13.0 | 172 |
| riboflavin, mg | 7.3 | 220 | 12.4 | 168 |
| niacin, mg | 35.4 | 98 | 50.3 | 84 |

[*]coefficient of variation
source:  Bowering, J., A.F. Subar and K.L. Clancy. 1988. Nutr. Res. 8:1073-1077.

*guidelines for use of vitamin supplements*    Healthy individuals can and should obtain adequate amounts of all nutrients including the vitamins from a well-balanced diet based on a variety of foods of good quality.  Such an approach minimizes the risks of deficiencies as well as excesses of all nutrients.  Nevertheless, certain circumstances may warrant the use of vitamin supplements.  These would include:  the use of folate for women who are pregnant or lactating[34]; the use of several vitamins for persons with very low caloric intakes (such that their consumption of total food is insufficient to provide all nutrients); the use of vitamin $B_{12}$ for some vegetarians[35]; the use of a single dose of vitamin K for newborn infants to prevent abnormal bleeding; and the use of certain vitamins for patients with diseases or medications that may interfere with vitamin utilization.  For other persons with varied, balanced diets, the actual benefit of taking vitamin supplements is doubtful.

*vitamin premixes for animal feeding*    The use of purified vitamins as supplements to animal feeds has increased the economy of animal feeding by obviating the need to include relatively expensive vitamin-rich feedstuffs in favor of lower-priced feedstuffs that are lower in vitamin content but provide useful energy and protein.  In modern practice, the addition of vitamins to animal feeds is accomplished by preparing a mixture of the specific vitamins required with a suitable carrier[36] to ensure homogeneous distribution in the feed as it is mixed.  Such a preparation is referred to as *"vitamin premix"* and is handled in much the same way as other feedstuffs in the blending of animal feeds.  Typically, vitamin premixes are formulated to be blended into diets at rates of 0.5-1.0%[37].

---

[34]Pregnant and lactating women may also need supplements of Fe and Ca.

[35]Some vegetarians may also not receive adequate amounts of Ca, Fe and Zn.

[36]Examples are:  soybean meal, finely ground corn or wheat, corn gluten meal, wheat middlings.

[37]The cost of the vitamin premix typically comprises less than 2% of the total cost of most finished feeds. Of that amount, approximately two-thirds of the vitamin cost is accounted by vitamin E, niacin, vitamin A and riboflavin (roughly in that order).

Feedstuffs in turkey starter diets provide insufficient amounts of vitamins:

| vitamin | level from feedstuffs, % NRC requirement | |
|---|---|---|
| | simple feed[a] | complex feed[b] |
| vitamin A | 20 | 40 |
| vitamin E | 130 | 130 |
| thiamin | 170 | 160 |
| riboflavin | 60 | 90 |
| niacin | 30 | 60 |
| vitamin $B_6$ | 130 | 100 |
| pantothenic acid | 90 | 110 |
| biotin | 120 | 140 |
| folate | 50 | 50 |
| vitamin $B_{12}$ | 0 | 74 |
| choline | 90 | 100 |

[a]corn, 40.5%; soybean meal, 51.2%; animal fat, 4%; $CaHPO_4$, 3%; limestone, .8%; salt, .3%; methionine, .15%; trace minerals, .05%
[b]milo, 20.5%; wheat, 20%; soybean meal, 33.9%; poultry meal, 6%; animal fat, 5%; meat & bone meal, 5%; fish meal, 4%; alfalfa meal, 2%; distillers' grains & solubles, 2%; limestone, .7%; $CaHPO_4$, .5%; salt, .3%; methionine, .13%; trace minerals, .05%

source: anonymous, 1989. Vitamin Nutrition for Poultry. Hoffman-La Roche, Inc., Nutley, NJ. pp.13-14.

Premixes generally also contain synthetic antioxidants (e.g., ethoxyquin, BHT) to enhance vitamin stability during storage[38]. In many cases, trace minerals are included in *"vitamin-mineral premixes"* [39]. It is standard practice in the formulation of vitamin premixes to use amounts of vitamins that, when added to the expected amounts intrinsic to the component feedstuffs, will provide a comfortable excess above those levels found experimentally to be required to prevent overt deficiency signs. This is done in view of the many potential causes of increased vitamin needs; due to the low cost of vitamin supplementation, this approach is considered a kind of low-cost[40] *"nutrition insurance"*. It should be remembered, however, that purified vitamins may not always be cheap, particularly in developing countries. Under those circumstances, the appropriate way to assess the value of using vitamin supplements is to compare their market prices to the estimated loss of production realized by not supplementing feeds that can be economically produced using locally available feedstuffs.

---

[38] Studies have shown that the loss of vitamin A from poultry feeds stored at moderate temperatures (ca. 15% in 30 days) was slightly reduced (to ca. 10%) by the addition of any of several synthetic antioxidants. Under conditions of high temperature and high humidity, vitamin A losses from finished feeds can be much greater (e.g., 80-95%). Maximal protection by antioxidants is expected under conditions in which vitamin oxidation is moderate (e.g., short-term feed storage in hot, humid environments).

[39] Due to the presence of mineral catalysts of oxidative reactions, the stabilities of oxidant-sensitive vitamins in compound premixes can be expected to be less than in premixes of the vitamins alone.

[40] Vitamin premixes usually account for only 1-2% of the total cost of feeds for non-ruminant livestock.

Vitamins generally included in vitamin premixes for livestock diets:

| vitamin | poultry | piglets | hogs | calves | cattle |
|---|---|---|---|---|---|
| vitamin A | + | + | + | + | + |
| vitamin D$_3$ | + | + | + | + | + |
| vitamin E | + | + | + | + | +[b] |
| vitamin K | + | + | +[b] | | |
| ascorbic acid | +[a] | + | | + | |
| thiamin | | +[b] | | +[b] | |
| riboflavin | + | + | + | +[b] | |
| niacin | + | + | | | |
| pyridoxine | +[b] | + | +[b] | +[b] | |
| pantothenic acid | + | + | + | +[b] | |
| biotin | +[b] | +[b] | +[b] | | |
| folate | | | | | |
| vitamin B$_{12}$ | + | + | | +[b] | |
| choline | + | + | | | |

[a]added in situations of stress    [b]sometimes added

Examples of vitamin premixes for animal feeds:

| vitamin units/1000 kg diet | practical diet[a] for chicks[c] | semipurified diet[b] for chicks[c] | semipurified diet[b] for rats |
|---|---|---|---|
| vitamin A[g], IU | 8,800,000 | 50,000 | 40,000,000 |
| vitamin D$_3$, IU | 2,200,000 | 4,500,000 | 1,000,000 |
| vitamin E, IU[h] | 5,500 | 50,000 | 50,000 |
| menadione NaHSO$_3$, g | 2.2 | 1.5 | 50 |
| thiamin HCl, g | | 15 | 6 |
| riboflavin, g | 4.4 | 15 | 6 |
| niacin, g | 33 | 50 | 30 |
| pyridoxine HCl, g | | 6 | 7 |
| d-Ca-pantothenate, g | 11 | 20 | 16 |
| biotin, mg | | 0.6 | 0.2 |
| folic acid, g | | 6 | 2 |
| vitamin B$^{12}$, mg | 10 | 20 | 10 |
| choline Cl, g | 220 | 2,000 | +[j] |
| minerals | +[k] | +[l] | +[l] |
| other ingredients | | | |
| antioxidant, g | 125 | 100 | 100 |
| carrier, g | to make weight[m] | to make weight[n] | to make weight[n] |

[a]composed of non-purified natural feedstuffs (e.g., corn, soybean meal, etc.)
[b]composed of purified/partially purified ingredients (e.g., isolated soy protein, casein, sucrose, starch)    [c]from Scott, M., M. Nesheim and R. Young. 1982. Nutrition of the Chicken. 3rd ed. M.L. Scott & Assoc., Ithaca, NY, p. 494    [d]ibid., p. 546    [e]AIN-76 diet, Am. Inst. Nutr.    [f]as all-trans-retinyl palmitate    [g]as all-rac-tocopheryl acetate [h]e.g., ethoxyquin, BHT    [i]e.g., corn meal    [j]added as 0.2% choline bitartrate [k]includes 66 g ZnO, 220 g MnSO$_4$ and 220 mg Na$_2$SeO$_3$    [l]includes CaHPO$_4$·2H$_2$O, CaCO$_3$, KH$_2$PO$_4$, NaHCO$_3$, KHCO$_3$, KCl, NaCl, MnSO$_4$·H$_2$O, FeSO$_4$·7H$_2$O, MgCO$_3$, MgSO$_4$, KIO$_3$, CuO$_4$·5H$_2$O, ZnCO$_3$, CoCl$_2$, NaMoO$_4$·2H$_2$O and/or Na$_2$SeO$_3$ in amounts appropriate for the composition of the particular diet    [m]corn meal    [n]sucrose

## Study Questions and Exercises:

i.        For a core food for any particular vitamin, construct a **flow diagram** showing all of the processes, from the growing of the food to the eating of it by a human, that might reduce the useful amount of that vitamin in the food.

ii.       In consideration of the core foods for the vitamins and your personal food habits, which vitamin(s) might you expect to have the lowest intakes from *your* diet? Which might you expect to be low in the *"typical American diet"*. Which might you expect to be low in vegetarian and low-meat diets?

iii.      Use a **concept map** to show the relationships of *vitamin supplementation of animal feeds* with to the concepts of *chemical stability*, *bioavailability* and *physiological utilization*?

iv.       Prepare a **flow diagram** to show the means by which you might first *evaluate the dietary vitamin status* of a specific population (e.g., in an institutional setting) and then, *improve it*, if necessary.

## Recommended Reading:

Beecher, G.R. and R.H. Matthews. 1990. Nutrient composition of foods, Chapter 51 *in* Present Knowledge in Nutrition (M. Brown, ed.). Int. Life Sci. Inst.-Nutr. Found., Washington, DC. pp. 430-443.

Marks, J. 1968. The Vitamins in Health and Disease - a Modern Reappraisal. J. &. A. Churchill, Ltd., London, pp.158-172.

McDowell, L.R. 1989. Vitamins in Animal Nutrition. Comparative Aspects to Human Nutrition. Academic Press, New York, pp. 422-444.

White, P.L. and D.C. Fletcher (eds.). 1974. Nutrients in Processed Foods: Vitamins, Minerals. Am. Med. Assoc., Publ. Sci. Group, Acton, Mass., 193 pp.

# CHAPTER 20    *ASSESSING VITAMIN STATUS*

*". . . the old idea, that the state of nutrition of a child could be at once established by mere cursory inspection by the doctor, has to be abandoned . . . (such methods) gave us very little information about the occurrence of the milder degrees of deficiency, or of the earlier stages of their development."*
                                                                L.J. Harris

## Anchoring Concepts:

| | |
|---|---|
| *i.* | Detection of sub-optimal vitamin status at early stages (before manifestation of overt deficiency disease) is desirable for the reason that vitamin deficiencies are most easily correctable in their early stages. |
| *ii.* | Vitamin status can be estimated by evaluating diets and food habits, but these methods are not precise. |
| *iii.* | Vitamin status can be determined by measuring the concentrations of vitamins and metabolites, and the activities of vitamin-dependent enzymes in samples of tissues and urine. |
| *iv.* | Sub-optimal status is more probable for some vitamins than for others. |

## Learning Objectives:

| | |
|---|---|
| *i.* | To understand the *requirements of valid methods* for assessing vitamin status. |
| *ii.* | To understand the *methods available* for assessing the vitamin status of humans and animals. |
| *iii.* | To be familiar with available information regarding the *vitamin status of human populations*. |

*Vocabulary:*

anthropometric evaluation          nutrient loading
biochemical evaluation             nutritional assessment
clinical evaluation                sociologic evaluation
dietary evaluation

# GENERAL ASPECTS OF NUTRITIONAL ASSESSMENT

*purposes*     The need to understand and describe the health status of individuals, a basic tenet of medicine, spawned the development of methods to assess nutrition status as appreciation grew for the important relationship of nutrition and health.  The first applications of nutritional assessment were in investigations of feed-related health and production problems of livestock and, later, in examinations of human populations in developing countries.  Activities of the latter type, consisting mainly of organized nutrition surveys, resulted in the first efforts to standardize both the methods employed to collect such data as well as the ways to interpret the results[1].  In recent years, nutritional assessment has also become an essential part of the nutritional care of hospitalized patients, and has become increasingly important as a means of evaluating the impact of public nutrition intervention programs.

Nutritional assessment, in any application, has three general purposes:

| | |
|---|---|
| *i.* | detection of deficiency states |
| *ii.* | evaluation of nutritional qualities of diets, food habits, and/or food supplies |
| *iii.* | prediction of health effects |

*systems of*       Three types of nutritional assessment systems have been employed both
*nutritional*      in population-based studies and in the care of hospitalized patients.
*assessment*

Systems of nutritional assessment:

| | |
|---|---|
| *i.* | ***nutrition surveys*** - cross-sectional evaluations of selected population groups conducted to generate baseline nutritional data, to learn overall nutrition status, and to identify sub-groups at nutritional risk |
| *ii.* | ***nutrition surveillance*** - continuous monitoring of the nutritional status of selected population groups (e.g., "at-risk" groups) for an extended period of time conducted to identify possible causes of malnutrition |
| *iii.* | ***nutrition screening*** - comparison of individuals' parameters of nutritional status with predetermined standards conducted to identify malnourished individuals requiring nutritional intervention |

---

[1]In 1955, the U.S. Government organized the Interdepartmental Committee on Nutrition for National Defense (ICNND) to assist developing countries in assessing the nutritional status of their peoples, identifying problems of malnutrition, and developing practical ways of solving their nutrition-related problems.  The ICNND teams conducted nutrition surveys in 24 countries.  In 1963, the ICNND published the first comprehensive manual (ICNND. 1963. Manual for Nutrition Surveys, 2nd edition, U.S. Government Printing Office, Washington, DC, 327 pp.) in which analytical methods were described and interpretive guidelines were presented.

Systems of nutritional assessment can employ a wide variety of specific methods. In general, however, these methods fall into five categories.

Methods of nutritional assessment:

| | |
|---|---|
| i. | **dietary evaluation** - estimation of nutrient intakes from evaluations of diets, food availability and food habits (using such instruments as food frequency questionnaires, food recall procedures, diet histories, food records) |
| ii. | **anthropometric evaluation** - estimation of nutritional status on the basis of measurements of the physical dimensions and gross composition of an individual's body |
| iii. | **clinical evaluation** - estimation of nutritional status on the basis of recording a medical history and conducting a physical examination to detect signs (observations made by a qualified observer) and symptoms (manifestations reported by the patient) associated with malnutrition |
| iv. | **biochemical methods** - estimation of nutritional status on the basis of measurements of nutrient stores, functional forms, excreted forms and/or metabolic functions |
| v. | **sociologic evaluation** - collection of information on non-nutrient-related variables known to affect or be related to nutritional status (e.g., socio-economic status, food habits and beliefs, food prices and availability, food storage and cooking practices, drinking water quality, immunization records, incidence of low-birth weight infants, breast-feeding and weaning practices, age- and cause-specific mortality rates, birth order, family structure, etc.). |

Typically, nutritional assessment systems employ *many or all* of these types of methods for the complete evaluation of nutritional status. Some of these approaches, however, are more informative than others with respect to specific nutrients and, particularly, to early stages of vitamin deficiencies.

Relevance of assessment methods to the stages of vitamin deficiency:

| | **stage of deficiency** | **most informative methods** |
|---|---|---|
| i. | depletion of vitamin stores | dietary evaluation<br>biochemical methods |
| ii. | cellular metabolic changes | biochemical methods |
| iii. | clinical defects | anthropometric evaluation<br>clinical evaluation<br>biochemical evaluation |
| iv. | morphological changes | anthropometric evaluation<br>clinical evaluation |

## ASSESSMENT OF VITAMIN STATUS

*approaches*        The assessment of vitamin status is best achieved by the application of **biochemical methods**, **clinical evaluation** and, to a lesser extent, **dietary methods**. Anthropometric evaluation can be informative regarding energy and protein status, but yields no information relevant to vitamin status. Clinical evaluation can be effective in the diagnosis of late-stage vitamin deficiencies, that is, those involving physiologic dysfunction and/or morphological changes. However, overt vitamin deficiency syndromes are relatively rare compared to the incidence of sub-optimal vitamin status about which clinical evaluation is informative.  Diets and food habits that are likely to provide insufficient amounts of available vitamins can be identified by dietary evaluation.  However, as discussed in Chapter 19, these methods are almost always imprecise with respect to the vitamins, and the parameters they measure usually have greater inherent variability than those for other nutrients.   The detection of early stage vitamin deficiencies is, therefore, best achieved using the variety of biochemical methods that are available.

*requirements*      Many biochemical parameters of vitamin status can be identified. However,
*of useful*          in order to be useful for the purposes of assessment of vitamin status, a
*biochemical*        parameter must satisfy several requirements.
*methods*

To be useful in assessing vitamin status, a biochemical parameter must:

| | |
|---|---|
| *i.* | **correlate with the rate of vitamin intake**, at least within the nutritionally significant range, and **respond to deprivation of the vitamin** |
| *ii.* | relate to a **meaningful period of time** |
| *iii.* | relate to **normal physiologic function** |
| *iv.* | be measurable in an **accessible specimen** |
| *v.* | be **technically feasible, reproducible and affordable** |
| *vi.* | have an available base of **normative data** |

*available*         The ideal parameter of vitamin status would be a measure of actual meta-
*biochemical*        bolic function of the vitamin.  In some cases this is possible[2]; however, in
*methods for*        most cases, direct measurement of vitamin metabolic function is not
*assessing*          possible due to the absence of a discrete functional parameter[3], to the
*vitamin status*     existence of more than one metabolic function with different sensitivities to

---

[2]Examples include the measurement of prothrombin time to assess vitamin K status, and the measurement of stimulation coefficients of erythrocyte transketolase and glutathione reductase to assess thiamin and riboflavin status, respectively.

[3]For example, vitamin E appears to function as a biological lipid antioxidant; but measuring that function is not possible with any physiological relevance because all of the known products of lipid peroxidation (e.g., malonaldehyde, alkanes) are known to be metabolized.  This makes such measurements difficult to interpret with respect simply to vitamin E status.

vitamin supply[4], to the function of the vitamin in a loosely bound fashion which is unstable to the methods of tissue preparation[5], etc. Therefore, other parameters are useful for assessing vitamin status. These include measurements in accessible tissues or urine of the vitamin, certain metabolites or other enzymes related to the metabolic function of the vitamin.

Accessible tissues for biochemical assessment of vitamin status:

| tissue | relevance |
| --- | --- |
| *blood* | |
| plasma/serum | contain newly absorbed nutrients as well as vitamins being transported to other tissues and, therefore, tend to reflect recent nutrient intake; this effect can be reduced by collecting blood after a fast |
| erythrocytes | with a half life of ca. 120 days, they tend to reflect chronic nutrient status; analyses can be technically difficult |
| leukocytes | have relatively short half-lives and, therefore, can be used to monitor short-term changes in nutrient status; isolation of these cells can present technical difficulties |
| *tissues* | |
| liver, adipose, bone, marrow, muscle | sampling is invasive, requiring research or clinical settings |
| hair, nails | easily collected and stored specimens offer advantages particularly for population studies of trace element status; not useful for assessing vitamin status |

*interpreting results of biochemical tests of vitamin status*

The guidelines originally developed by the ICNND are generally used for the interpretation of the results of biochemical parameters of vitamin status. It is important to note, however, that those interpretive guidelines were originally developed for use in surveys of populations. Their relevance to the assessment of the vitamin status of individuals is not straightforward, due to issues of *intra-individual variation* and *confounding effects* which may be quantitatively more significant for individuals than for populations. For example, intra-individual ("*within-person*") variation is frequently noted in serum analytes. Therefore, a measurement of a single blood sample may not be appropriate for estimating the usual circulating level of the analyte of an individual, even though it may be useful in estimating the mean level of a population. Several factors can confound the interpretation of parameters of vitamin status: those affecting the response parameters directly,

---

[4]For example, pyridoxal phosphate is a cofactor for each of two enzymes involved in the metabolic conversion of tryptophan to niacin: *kynureninase* and a *transaminase*. Although the cofactor is essential for the activity of each enzyme, kynureninase has a much greater affinity for pyridoxal phosphate ($K_m = 10^{-3}$ M) than does the transaminase ($K_m = 10^{-8}$ M). Therefore, under conditions of pyridoxine deprivation, the transaminase activity can be reduced even though kynureninase activity is unaffected.

[5]For example, the metabolically active forms of niacin, NAD(P)H, function as the co-substrates of many redox enzymes. These enzyme-co-substrate complexes are only transiently associated; therefore, dilution of biological specimens results in their dissociation and usually in the oxidation of the co-substrate.

drugs that can increase vitamin needs, seasonal effects related to the physical environment[6] or food availability[7], use of parenteral feeding solutions[8], use of vitamin supplements[9], smoking[10], etc.

Limitations of some biochemical methods of assessing vitamin status:

| vitamin | parameter | limitation |
|---|---|---|
| vitamin A | plasma* retinol | reflects body vitamin A stores *only* at severely depleted or excessive levels; confounding effects of protein and Zn deficiencies and renal dysfunction |
| vitamin D | plasma* alk. P-ase | affected by other disease states |
| vitamin E | plasma* tocopherol | affected by blood lipid transport capacity |
| thiamin | plasma* thiamin | low sensitivity to changes in thiamin intake |
| riboflavin | plasma* riboflavin | low sensitivity to changes in riboflavin intake |
| vitamin $B_6$ | RBC glutam.-pyruv. transaminase | genetic polymorphism |
| folate | RBC folates | also reduced in vitamin $B_{12}$ deficiency |
| | urinary FIGLU[b] | also increased in vitamin $B_{12}$ deficiency |
| vitamin $B_{12}$ | urinary FIGLU[b] | also increased in folate deficiency |

*or serum
[b]formiminoglutamic acid

---

[6]For example, persons living in northern latitudes typically show peak plasma levels of $25(OH)D_3$ around September and low levels around February, with inverse patterns of plasma PTH concentrations, due to the seasonal variation in exposure to solar ultraviolet light.

[7]For example, residents of Finland showed peak plasma ascorbic acid levels in Aug.-Sept. and lowest levels in Nov.-Jan., due to seasonal differences in the availability of vitamin C-rich fruits and vegetables.

[8]Persons supported by total parenteral nutrition (TPN) have frequently been found to be of low status with respect to biotin (due to their abnormal intestinal microflora) and the fat-soluble vitamins (due to absorption by the plastic bags and tubing, and to destruction by UV light used to sterilize TPN solutions).

[9]The NHANESI survey showed that over 51% of Americans over 18 years of age used vitamin/mineral supplements, with 23.1% doing so on a daily basis. Further, the National Ambulatory Medical Care Survey (1981) showed that 1% of office visits to physicians (particularly, general and family practitioners) involved a prescription or recommendation for multi-vitamins. *Multi-vitamins* appear to be the most commonly used supplements, followed by *vitamin C*, calcium, *vitamin E* and *vitamin A*. The use of vitamin supplements have been found to have greater impact than that of vitamin-fortified food on both the mean and coefficient of variation (C.V.) of estimates of vitamin intake in free-living populations.

[10]Smokers have been found to have abnormally low plasma levels of ascorbic acid (with a corresponding increase in dehydroascorbic acid), pyridoxal and pyridoxal phosphate.

Biochemical methods for assessing vitamin status:

| vitamin | functional parameters | tissue levels | urinary excretion |
|---|---|---|---|
| vitamin A | | **serum retinol**[a]<br>change in serum retinol with oral vitamin A dose[b]<br>liver retinyl esters | |
| vitamin D | | **serum 25(OH)$_2$-vitamin D$_3$**[a]<br>serum vitamin D$_3$<br>serum 1,25-(OH)$_2$D$_3$<br>serum alkaline phosphatase | |
| vitamin E | erythrocyte hemolysis | **serum tocopherols**[a]<br>breath alkanes | |
| vitamin K | clotting time<br>**prothrombin time**[a] | | |
| vitamin C | | serum ascorbic acid<br>**leucocyte ascorbic acid**[a] | ascorbic acid<br>ascorbic ac. after load[c] |
| thiamin | **erythrocyte transketolase stimulation**[a] | blood thiamin<br>blood pyruvate | thiamin (thiochrome)<br>thiamin after load[c] |
| niacin | | erythrocyte NAD<br>erythrocyte NAD:NADP ratio | 1-methylnicotinamide<br>1-methyl-6-pyridone-3-carboxamide |
| riboflavin | **erythrocyte glutathione reductase stimulation**[a] | blood riboflavin | riboflavin<br>riboflavin after load[c] |
| vitamin B$_6$ | erythrocyte transaminase | plasma pyridoxal phosphate<br>erythrocyte transaminase stimulation<br>erythrocyte pyridoxal-P<br>plasma pyridoxal | **xanthurenic acid after TRY load**[a,c]<br>quinolinic acid<br>pyridoxine<br>4-pyridoxic acid |
| biotin | | **blood biotin**[a] | biotin |
| pantothenic acid | erythrocyte sulfanilamide acetylase | serum pantothenic acid<br>erythrocyte pantothenic acid<br>**blood pantothenic acid**[a] | pantothenic acid |
| folate | | **serum folates**[a]<br>**erythrocyte folates**[a]<br>leucocyte folates<br>liver folates | **FIGLU**[c] **after HIS load**[a,c]<br>urocanic acid after HIS load[c] |
| vitamin B$_{12}$ | | **serum vitamin B$_{12}$**[a]<br>erythrocyte vitamin B$_{12}$ | FIGLU[d]<br>**methylmalonic acid**[a] |

[a] most useful parameter
[b] relative dose-response test
[c] a single large oral dose
[d] formininoglutamic acid

Interpretive guidelines for assessing vitamin status [part 1]:

| vitamin | parameter | age group | values, by category of status (risk)[a] | | |
|---|---|---|---|---|---|
| | | | deficient (high risk) | low (moderate risk) | acceptable (low risk) |
| vitamin A | plasma[b] retinol, $\mu$g/dl | <5 mo. | <10 | 10-19 | >20 |
| | | .5-17 yrs. | <20 | 20-29 | >30 |
| | | adult | <10 | 10-19 | >20 |
| vitamin D | plasma[b] 25-(OH)-$D_3$[c], ng/ml | all ages | <3 | 3-10 | >10 |
| | plasma[b] alk. P-ase[c], u/ml | infants | >390 | 298-390 | 99-298 |
| | | adults | <40 | 40-56 | 57-99 |
| vitamin E | plasma[b] $\alpha$-tocopherol, mg/dl | all ages | <.35 | .35-.80 | >.80 |
| vitamin K | clotting time, min. | all ages | | >10 | ca. 10 |
| | prothrombin time, min. | | _[d] | _[d] | _[d] |
| vitamin C | plasma[b] ascorbic acid, mg/dl | all ages | <.20 | .20-.30 | >.30 |
| | leucocyte ascorbic acid, mg/dl | all ages | <8 | 8-15 | >15 |
| | whole blood ascorbic ac., mg/dl | all ages | <.30 | .30-.50 | >.50 |
| thiamin | urinary thiamin, $\mu$g/g creat. | 1-3 yrs. | <120 | 120-175 | >175 |
| | | 4-6 yrs. | <85 | 85-120 | >120 |
| | | 7-9 yrs. | <70 | 70-180 | >180 |
| | | 10-12 yrs. | <60 | 60-180 | >180 |
| | | 13-15 yrs. | <50 | 50-150 | >150 |
| | | adults | <27 | 27-65 | >65 |
| | | pregnant | | | |
| | | 2nd trim. | <23 | 23-55 | >55 |
| | | 3rd trim. | <21 | 21-50 | >50 |
| | urinary thiamin, $\mu$g/24 hrs. | adults | <40 | 40-100 | >100 |
| | urinary thiamin, $\mu$g/6 hrs. | adults | <10 | 10-25 | >25 |
| | urinary thiamin after | | | | |
| | thiamin load[e], $\mu$g/4 hrs. | adults | <20 | 20-80 | >80 |
| | erythrocyte transketolase | | | | |
| | stimulation by TPP[f,g], % | adults | >25 | 15-25 | <15 |

[a]from ICNND. 1963. <u>Manual for Nutrition Surveys</u>, 2nd ed., U.S. Gov. Printing Off., Washington, D.C., 327 pp.; Sauberlich, H.E., J.H. Skala and R.P. Dowdy. 1974. <u>Laboratory Tests for the Assessment of Nutritional Status</u>, CRC Press, Cleveland, 136 pp.; and Gibson, R.S. 1990 <u>Principles of Nutritional Assessment</u>, Oxford Univ. Press, New York, 691 pp.    [b]or serum    [c]subject to effects of season and gender    [d]Results vary according to assay conditions; most assays are designed such that normal prothrombin times are 12-13 sec., with greater values indicating suboptimal vitamin K status.    [e]single oral 2 mg dose    [f]thiamin pyrophosphate    [g]the "TPP effect"

Interpretive guidelines for assessing vitamin status [part 2]:

| vitamin | parameter | age group | values, by category of status (risk)[a] deficient (high risk) | low (moderate risk) | acceptable (low risk) |
|---|---|---|---|---|---|
| riboflavin | urinary riboflavin, µg/g creat. | 1-3 yrs. | <150 | 150-500 | >500 |
| | | 4-6 yrs. | <100 | 100-300 | >300 |
| | | 7-9 yrs. | <85 | 85-270 | >270 |
| | | 10-15 yrs. | <70 | 70-200 | >200 |
| | | adults | <27 | 27-80 | >80 |
| | | pregnant | | | |
| | | 2nd trim. | <39 | 39-120 | >120 |
| | | 3rd trim. | <30 | 30-90 | >90 |
| | urinary riboflavin, µg/24 hrs. | adults | <40 | 40-120 | >120 |
| | urinary riboflavin, µg/6 hrs. | adults | <10 | 10-30 | >30 |
| | urinary riboflavin after riboflavin load[b], µg/4 hrs. | adults | <1000 | 1000-1400 | >1400 |
| | erythrocyte riboflavin, µg/d | adults | <10.0 | 10.0-14.9 | >14.9 |
| | erythrocyte glutathione red. stimulation by FAD[c], % | adults | >40 | 20-40 | <20 |
| niacin | urinary N'-methylnicotinamide µg/g creatinine | adults | <.5 | .5-1.6 | >1.6 |
| | | pregnant | | | |
| | | 2nd trim. | <.6 | .6-2.0 | >2.0 |
| | | 3rd trim. | <.8 | .8-2.5 | >2.5 |
| | urinary N'-methylnicotinamide µg/6 hrs. | adults | <.2 | .2-.6 | >.6 |
| | urinary 2-pyridone[d]/N'-methyl nicotinamide ratio | all ages | -[e] | <1.0 | ≥1.0 |
| vitamin B₆ | plasma[i] pyridoxal-P, nM[j] | all ages | -[e] | <60[d] | ≥60[d] |
| | urinary pyridoxine, µg/g creat. | 1-3 yrs. | -[e] | <90[d] | ≥90[d] |
| | | 4-6 yrs. | -[e] | <75[d] | ≥75[d] |
| | | 7-9 yrs. | -[e] | <50[d] | ≥50[d] |
| | | 10-12 yrs. | -[e] | <40[d] | ≥40[d] |
| | | 13-15 yrs. | -[e] | <30[d] | ≥30[d] |
| | | adults | -[e] | <20[d] | ≥20[d] |
| | urin. 4-pyridoxic ac., mg/24 hrs. | adults | <.5[f] | .5-.8[d] | >.8[d] |
| | urinary xanthurenic acid after TRY load[b], mg/24 hrs. | adults | >50[f] | 25-50[d] | <25[d] |
| | urinary 3-OH-kynurenine after TRY load[b], mg/24 hrs. | adults | >50[f] | 25-50[d] | <25[d] |
| | urinary kynurenine after TRY load[b], mg/24 hrs. | adults | >50[f] | 10-50[d] | <10[d] |
| | quinolinic acid after TRY load[b], mg/24 hrs. | adults | >50[f] | 25-50[d] | <25[d] |
| | erythrocyte alanine aminotransferase stimulation by PalP[h], % | adults | -[e] | >25[d] | ≤25[d] |
| | erythrocyte aspartate aminotransferase stimulation by PalP[h], % | adults | -[e] | >50[d] | ≤50[d] |

[a]from ICNND. 1963. Manual for Nutrition Surveys, 2nd ed., U.S. Gov. Printing Off., Washington, D.C., 327 pp.; Sauberlich, H.E., J.H. Skala and R.P. Dowdy. 1974. Laboratory Tests for the Assessment of Nutritional Status, CRC Press, Cleveland, 136 pp.; and Gibson, R.S. 1990 Principles of Nutritional Assessment, Oxford Univ. Press, New York, 691 pp.   [b]single 2 g oral dose  [c]flavin adenine dinucleotide, reduced form, 1-3 µM  [d]N'-methyl-2 pyridone-5-carboxamide   [e]data base is insufficient to support a guideline   [f]These values have only a small data base and, therefore, are considered as tentative.   [g]pyridoxal phosphate

Interpretive guidelines for assessing vitamin status [part 3]:

| vitamin | parameter | age group | values, by category of status (risk)[a] | | |
| --- | --- | --- | --- | --- | --- |
| | | | deficient (high risk) | low (moderate risk) | acceptable (low risk) |
| biotin | urinary biotin, $\mu$g/24 hrs. | adults | $< 10^b$ | $10\text{-}25^b$ | $> 25^b$ |
| | whole blood biotin, ng/ml | adults | $< .4^b$ | $.4\text{-}.8^b$ | $> .8^b$ |
| pantothenic acid | plasma[c] pantothenic acid, $\mu$g/dl | adults | $\_^d$ | $< 6^b$ | $\geq 6^b$ |
| | blood pantothenic acid, $\mu$g/dl | adults | $\_^d$ | $< 80^b$ | $\geq 80^{b,e}$ |
| | urinary pantoth. ac., mg/24 hrs. | adults | $\_^d$ | $< 1^b$ | $\geq 1^{b,f}$ |
| folate | plasma[c] folates, ng/ml | all ages | $< 3$ | $3\text{-}6$ | $> 6$ |
| | erythrocyte folates, ng/ml | all ages | $140$ | $140\text{-}160$ | $> 160$ |
| | leucocyte folates, ng/ml | all ages | $\_^d$ | $< 60$ | $> 60$ |
| | urinary FIGLU[g] after HIS load[h], mg/8 hrs. | adults | $> 50^b$ | $5\text{-}50$ | $< 5^m$ |
| vitamin $B_{12}$ | plasma[c] vitamin $B_{12}$, pg/ml | all ages | $100$ | $100\text{-}150$ | $> 150^n$ |
| | urinary methylmalonic acid after VAL load[k], mg/24 hrs. | adults | $\geq 300$ | $2\text{-}300$ | $\leq 2$ |
| | urinary excretion of a radiolabelled vitamin $B_{12}$ dose after vitamin $B_{12}$ flushing dose[i], % | adults | $< 3$ | $3\text{-}8$ | $> 8$ |

[a]from ICNND. 1963. Manual for Nutrition Surveys, 2nd ed., U.S. Gov. Printing Off., Washington, D.C., 327 pp.; Sauberlich, H.E., J.H. Skala and R.P. Dowdy. 1974. Laboratory Tests for the Assessment of Nutritional Status, CRC Press, Cleveland, 136 pp.; and Gibson, R.S. 1990 Principles of Nutritional Assessment, Oxford Univ. Press, New York, 691 pp.   [b]These values have only a small data base and, therefore, are tentative. [c]or serum   [d]data base is insufficient to support a guideline   [e]Normal values are ca. 100 $\mu$g/dl.   [f]Normal values are 2-4 mg/24 hrs.   [g]formininoglutamic acid   [h]single oral 2-20 mg dose   [i]Normal adults excrete 5-20 mg/8 hrs.   [j]Most healthy persons show 200-900 pg/ml.   [k]single oral 5-10 g dose   [l]This is the Schilling Test; it involves measurement of labelled vitamin $B_{12}$ excreted from a .5-2 $\mu$g tracer dose after a large flushing dose (e.g., 1 mg) given 1 hr. after the tracer.

Estimated vitamin reserves of human adults:

| reserve capacity | vitamins | |
| --- | --- | --- |
| 3-5 years | vitamin $B_{12}$ | |
| 1-2 years | vitamin A | |
| 3-4 months | folate | |
| 2-6 weeks | vitamin D | riboflavin |
| | vitamin E | vitamin $B_6$ |
| | vitamin K | choline |
| | vitamin C | |
| 4-10 days | thiamin | pantothenic acid |
| | biotin | |

## VITAMIN STATUS OF HUMAN POPULATIONS

*national*
*nutrition*
*studies*

Many studies have been conducted, particularly in developing countries where problems of malnutrition are of the most severe proportions, to evaluate the nutritional status of target populations (high-risk sub-groups). In addition, several national studies have been conducted, mostly in the United States, to evaluate the nutritional adequacy of the food supply and/or the nutritional status of the people. These have included efforts to obtain information on most of the high-risk vitamins, e.g., vitamin A, vitamin E, ascorbic acid, thiamin, riboflavin, niacin, pyridoxine and vitamin $B_{12}$.

National surveys of dietary intake and nutritional status in North America:

| survey | description |
|---|---|
| USDA historical data of US food supply | tracking since 1909 of foods available to the American public by disappearance to wholesale and retail markets |
| US Nationwide Food Consumption Surveys | USDA studies conducted at ca. 10-yr. intervals since 1935 of dietary intakes and food use patterns of American households and individuals |
| Ten-State Nutrition Survey | NIH study (1968-1970) of nutritional status of >60,000 individuals in ten US states (CA, KY, LA, ME, MS, SC, TX, WI, NY, WV) selected to include low-income groups |
| Total Diet Study | FDA study of average intakes of certain essential mineral elements (I, Fe, Na, K, Cu, Mn, Zn), pesticides, toxicants, and radionuclides, based on analyses of foods purchased in grocery stores across the U.S. |
| Nutrition Canada | Canadian study conducted in the early 1970s of the nutritional status of >19,000 individuals |
| National Health and Nutrition Examination Surveys | USDA studies conducted to monitor the overall nutritional status of the US population; four studies to date: NHANESI (1971-74), NHANESII (1976-80), Hispanic HANES (HHANES, 1982-84), NHANESIII (began in 1988) |

*apparent*
*increases in*
*vitamins in*
*US food*
*supply*

Historical records of the American food supply would indicate general increases in the amounts of most of the vitamins available for consumption. Whether such increases have been reflected in the actual intakes of the vitamins, or whether they have been distributed democratically across the American population is not indicated by such gross evaluations of the food supply. The results of the 1977-1978 Nationwide Food Consumption Survey indicate that the average consumptions of most of the vitamins were generally adequate, the exception being that of *pyridoxine*, which was low in most age groups. In general, however, it is clear that people with low incomes tend to consume less food, although their food tends to have greater nutritional value per calorie than that consumed by people with greater incomes. While differences in diet quality due to income status appear to be small on average, variation in nutrient intake within groups of individuals appears to be very large.

*On average*, at least, the vitamin intakes of Americans would appear to be generally adequate. However, it is clear that substantial variations occur among individuals in the actual intakes of several vitamins, due to both qualitative and quantitative differences in intake. More recent studies by the USDA have shown that the vitamin intakes of many Americans may not meet the RDAs.

Vitamins available for consumption (per person per day) by Americans:

| vitamin | 1909-13 | 1947-49 | 1967-69 | 1977-79 | 1985 |
|---|---|---|---|---|---|
| vitamin A, IU | 7200 | 8100 | 7300 | 9100 | 9900 |
| vitamin E, mg* | 11.2 | 12.5 | 14.3 | 16.0 | 17.6 |
| vitamin C, mg | 101 | 110 | 98 | 108 | 114 |
| thiamin, mg | 1.6 | 2.0 | 2.0 | 2.1 | 2.2 |
| riboflavin, mg | 1.8 | 2.3 | 2.3 | 2.3 | 2.4 |
| niacin, mg | 19 | 20 | 23 | 25 | 26 |
| vitamin $B_6$, mg | 2.2 | 1.9 | 1.9 | 2.0 | 2.1 |
| vitamin $B_{12}$, $\mu$g | 7.9 | 8.6 | 9.2 | 9.0 | 8.8 |

source: Marston and Raper. Nat. Food Rev. 36:18-23 (1987)
*$a$-tocopherol equivalents

Estimated daily vitamin intakes (% of 1980 RDAs) of Americans (all ages):

| vitamin | vegetarians | non-vegetarians |
|---|---|---|
| vitamin A | 163 | 132 |
| vitamin C | 176 | 147 |
| thiamin | 117 | 113 |
| riboflavin | 136 | 124 |
| niacin* | 114 | 124 |
| vitamin $B_6$ | 76 | 75 |
| vitamin $B_{12}$ | 156 | 176 |

source: 1977-1978 Nationwide Food Consumption Survey; based on 3-day intakes
*pre-formed niacin only

Frequency of low vitamin intakes of American women and children:

| vitamin | % with intakes <100%RDA | | | % with intakes <70%RDA |
|---|---|---|---|---|
| | women | children 1-3 yr | 4-5 yr | women |
| vitamin A | 55 | - | - | 35 |
| vitamin E | 70 | - | - | 40 |
| vitamin C | 45 | - | - | 30 |
| vitamin $B_6$ | 95 | 20 | 55 | 75 |
| folate | 100 | 5 | 60 | 85 |

source: USDA data

*nutritional* The above measures of general nutrient supplies and average nutrient con-
*assessment* sumption are necessary for national food and health policy planning; but
*reveals vitamin* they yield no information useful in addressing questions of nutritional status
*deficiencies* of *individuals* within populations. In order to produce such data, the Ten
State Nutrition Survey, Nutrition Canada and the HANES were conducted.

### The Ten-State Survey:

> Results revealed few severe nutritional deficiencies in its study population. However,
> it showed that people in the lowest groupings by income and education had poorer
> nutrition in virtually every respect than those in higher income/education groups. The
> most frequently observed nutritional problems concerned deficiencies of Fe in all age
> groups (especially among blacks), *vitamin A* (assessed by serum retinol level) among
> teenagers and hispanics of all age groups, and *riboflavin*, particularly among blacks.

### Nutrition Canada:

> Results showed the highest incidence of poor nutritional status among lowest income
> groups, particularly among middle-aged women and older men. Low income groups
> showed the greatest frequencies of low blood levels of *ascorbic acid* and *folates*. Low
> blood *thiamin* levels were observed among teenagers and middle-aged adults. Obesity
> was widespread, especially among middle-aged adults.

### NHANESI:

> Results revealed deficiencies of protein, Ca, *vitamin A* (assessed by serum retinol level)
> and Fe, especially among low income groups and more frequently among blacks than
> whites. Low vitamin A status was found among low income white teenagers, young
> adult women, and teenaged blacks of all income groups.

### NHANESII:

> Results showed low *vitamin A* status in 2-3% of all subjects examined. In addition, it
> revealed low blood *thiamin* levels in 14% of whites and 29% of blacks, low serum
> *riboflavin* levels in 3% of whites and 8% of blacks, and low transferrin saturation in 5-
> 15% of whites and 18-27% of blacks. The apparent consumption of *vitamin $B_6$* was less
> than the 1980 RDAs for 71% of males and 90% of females. The prevalence of low
> serum and erythrocyte *folate* levels was greatest in the 20-44 year age group (women:
> 15% and 13%, respectively; men: 18% and 8%, respectively). The prevalence of low
> plasma *ascorbic acid* level was 3% nationally, but was more common in poor adults,
> with the greatest prevalence (16%) among 55-74 year old black males.

## Study Questions and Exercises:

i.     **List the tests and measurements** that might be useful in assessing the vitamin status of *a)* a food, *b)* a meal, *c)* a national food supply, *d)* an individual, and *e)* a population.

ii.    Devise a **system of biochemical measurements** that could be performed on a 7 ml sample of fresh blood to yield as much information as possible about the vitamin status of the donor. [Assume enzyme activities can be assayed using no more than 50 $\mu$l of plasma or erythrocyte lysate and other biochemical measurements can be made using no more than 500 $\mu$l each.]

iii.   Give an example of a situation wherein a particular biochemical test may be necessary for the **diagnosis** of a vitamin-related disorder detected by clinical examination.  In general, what are the relationships of biochemical tests and clinical examination in the assessment of vitamin status?

iv.    In general terms, discuss the advantages and disadvantages of the various **types of biochemical tests** used in assessing vitamin status (e.g., functional tests, load tests, urinary excretion tests, circulating metabolite tests).

*Recommended Reading:*

Committee on Diet and Health, Food and Nutrition Board, Nat. Res. Coun. Dietary intake and nutritional status: trends and assessment, Chapter 3 *in* 1989. Diet and Health, Implications for Reducing Chronic Disease Risk, Nat. Acad. Press, Washington, D.C., pp. 41-84.

Gary, P.J. and K.M. Koehler. 1990. Problems in interpretation of dietary and biochemical data from population studies. Chapter 49 *in* Present Knowledge in Nutrition, 6th ed. (M. Brown, ed.), Int. Life Sci. Inst.-Nutr. Found., Washington, D.C., pp. 407-414.

Gibson, R.S. 1990. Principles of Nutritional Assessment, Oxford University Press, New York, 691 pp.

Interdepartmental Committee on Nutrition for National Defense. 1963. Manual for Nutrition Surveys, 2nd ed., U.S. Gov. Printing Off., Washington, D.C., 327 pp.

Life Sciences Research Office, FASEB. 1989. Nutrition Monitoring in the United States. DHHS Pub. No. 89-1255, U.S. Gov. Printing Office, Washington, D.C., 158 pp.

Livingston, G.E. (ed.) 1989. Nutritional Status Assessment of the Individual. Food and Nutrition Press, Trumbull, Conn., 479 pp.

Pike, R.L. and M.L. Brown. 1984. Determination of nutrient needs: vitamins, Chapter 24 *in* Nutrition: an Integrated Approach, John Wiley & Sons, New York, pp. 795-831.

Pike, R.L. and M.L. Brown. 1984. Nutrition surveys, Chapter 26 *in* Nutrition: an Integrated Approach, John Wiley & Sons, New York, pp. 832-851.

Sauberlich, H.E., J.H. Skala and R.P. Dowdy. 1974. Laboratory Tests for the Assessment of Nutritional Status, CRC Press, Cleveland, 136 pp.

Swan, P.B. 1983. Food consumption by individuals in the United States:  two major surveys. Ann. Rev. Nutr. 3:413-432.

Woteki, C.E. and M.T. Fanelli-Kuczmarski. 1990. The national nutrition monitoring system. Chapter 50 *in* Present Knowledge in Nutrition, 6th ed. (M. Brown, ed.), Int. Life Sci. Inst.-Nutr. Found., Washington, D.C., pp. 415-429.

Yeatley, E. and C. Johnson. 1987. Nutritional applications of the health and nutrition examination surveys (NANES). Ann. Rev. Nutr. 7:441-463.

# CHAPTER 21    QUANTIFYING VITAMIN NEEDS

*"There is not always agreement on the criteria for deciding when a requirement has been met. If the requirement is considered to be the minimal amount that will maintain normal physiological function and reduce the risk of impairment of health from nutritional inadequacy to essentially zero, we are left with questions such as: 'What is normal physiological function?', 'What is health?', and 'What degree of reserve or stores of the nutrient is adequate?' Differences in judgment on such issues are to be expected. "*

A.E. Harper

## Anchoring Concepts:

*i.* The vitamins have many metabolic role(s) essential to normal physiological function; these roles can be compromised by quantitatively insufficient or temporarilly irregular vitamin intakes.

*ii.* Vitamin needs can be determined by monitoring responses of parameters related to the metabolic functions and/or body reserves of the vitamins.

*iii.* Quantitative information is available concerning the vitamin contents of many common foods and feedstuffs.

## Learning Objectives:

*i.* To understand the concepts of *minimum requirement*, *optimal requirement*, and *allowance* as used with respect to the vitamins.

*ii.* To understand the *methods available* for estimating minimal and optimal vitamin requirements of animals and humans.

*iii.* To understand the basis for establishing *allowances* for the vitamins in human and animal feeding.

*iv.* To be familiar with the *sources of information* concerning vitamin requirements and allowances.

*Vocabulary:*

dietary standards                          optimal requirement
FAO                                        RDAs
margin of safety                           RDIs
minimum requirement                        RNIs
National Research Council                  WHO
nutrient allowance

# DIETARY STANDARDS

*purposes of dietary standards*

The need to formulate healthy diets for both humans and animals has stimulated the translation of current nutrition knowledge into a variety of dietary standards for the intakes of specific nutrients.  As these are typically developed by committees of experts reviewing the pertinent scientific literature, they are frequently referred to as dietary *"recommendations"*.  Formally, they may be called *"Recommended Dietary Allowances (RDAs)"* or *"Recommended Dietary Intakes (RDIs)"*.

*differences between allowances and requirements*

Regardless of the ways they may be named, dietary standards are different than *nutrient requirements*, although they are derived from the latter. Dietary standards are relevant to *populations*; they describe the average amounts of particular nutrients that should satisfy the needs of *almost all* healthy individuals in defined groups.  In contrast, nutrient requirements are relevant to *individuals*; they describe amounts of particular nutrients that satisfy *certain criteria* related to the metabolic activity of those nutrients or to general physiological function.  Because recommended allowances and intakes are designed to satisfy the needs of groups of individuals whose nutrient requirements vary, they, by definition, exceed the average requirement.

# DETERMINING DIETARY STANDARDS FOR THE VITAMINS

*determining nutrient requirements*

The *"nutrient requirement"* is a *theoretical construct* that describes the intake of a particular nutrient that supports a body pool of the nutrient and/or its metabolically active forms adequate to maintain normal physiological function.  In practice, it is generally used in reference to the *lowest* intake that supports normal function, that is, the *"minimum requirement"*. Minimum requirements, while seemingly physiologically relevant, are difficult to define and impossible to measure with any reasonable precision. They can vary according to the criteria by which they are defined.  This problem is illustrated by the widely varying estimates of the vitamin A requirement of the calf that may be derived by different criteria.

Therefore, in order to be relevant to the overall health of the typical individual, estimates of minimum nutrient requirements must be based on responses of obvious physiological importance.  For many nutrients (e.g., the indispensable amino acids) it may, thus, be appropriate to define minimum requirements on the basis of a fairly non-specific parameter such as growth.  For the vitamins, however, it is appropriate to define minimum requirements on the basis of parameters more specifically related to their metabolic functions, such as enzyme activities and tissue concentrations, as these can reflect changes at the earlier stages of vitamin deficiencies. The most useful parameters of vitamin status are those that respond early to deprivation of the vitamin, for those can be used to detect sub-optimal vitamin status at the early and most easily corrected stages.

Estimates of vitamin A requirements of calves based on different criteria:

| criteria | estimated requirement |
|---|---|
| | IU/day |
| prevention of nyctalopia | 20 |
| normal growth | 32 |
| normal serum retinol levels | 40 |
| moderate hepatic retinyl ester reserves | 250 |
| substantial hepatic retinyl ester reserves | 1024 |

source:   Marks, J. 1968. <u>The Vitamins in Health and Disease: a Modern Reappraisal</u>. Churchill, London, p.32.

Quantifying the minimum requirement, even with the use of an appropriate parameter, is not straightforward. It generally requires an experimental approach in which the test animals are fed a basal diet constructed to be deficient in the nutrient of interest but otherwise adequate with respect to all known nutrients, with this diet being supplemented with known amounts of the nutrient of interest. This may necessitate the use of uncommon feedstuffs such that the diet bears little similarity with those used in practice; and it usually means that the test nutrient is provided largely in free form, which may not resemble its form in practical foods and feed-stuffs. Even with these caveats in mind, the level of nutrient intake to be identified as the minimum requirement is not always clear, as the desired value for that parameter is usually a matter of judgement.

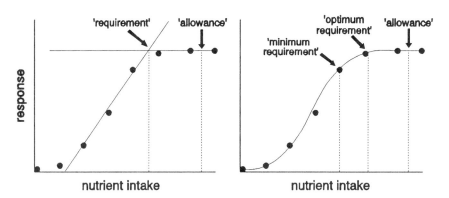

Most responses of specific nutrient-depleted animals to input of the same nutrient appear to be curvilinear; however, in most nutrient requirement experiments both rectilinear and curvilinear models usually fit equally well. For this reason, many investigators have used rectilinear models to impute *"requirements"* (e.g., the x-value of the intercept of the two linear regressions of the observed data in *"broken-line"* regression analyses[1]). Others, however, have used curvilinear models which consider the variations in the experimental population of both the measured response and the nutrient need for maintenance (usually related to body size). From the proposition of curvilinearity, it follows that no value can be properly described as the *"requirement"* of the test populations; nevertheless, the approach can be used to determine the risk of not fully satisfying the nutrient requirement for given proportions of the experimental population. The intake associated with acceptable *risk* of deficiency (a matter of judgment) is frequently called the ***"optimum requirement"*** or level of ***"optimum intake"***.   In public health, such levels are determined on the basis of assumptions regarding putative health risks.  In livestock production, where the cost of feeding accounts for a substantial portion of the total cost of production, *"optimum intakes"* of the more costly nutrients (protein, limiting amino acids, energy) are necessary to optimize economic efficiency.

Potential sources of variation in nutrient requirements:

| | | |
|---|---|---|
| ***physiological determinants*** | | |
| active growth | pregnancy | lactation |
| aging | intra-individual variation | level of physical activity |
| caloric intake | | |
| | | |
| ***hereditary conditions*** | | |
| vitamin-dependent diseases | | |
| | | |
| ***conditions of maldigestion/malabsorption*** | | |
| pancreatitis | gastric resection | endocrine disorders (e.g., |
| hepatobiliary disease | intestinal resection/bypass | diabetes mellitus, hypo- |
| pernicious anemia | regional ileitis | parathyroidism, Addison's |
| radiation injury | kwashiorkor | disease) |
| pellagra | gluten sensitivity | intestinal parasitism (e.g., |
| acute enteritis | enteropathy | hookworm, *Strongyloides*, |
| cystic fibrosis | certain drug treatments | *Giardia lamblia*, *Dibothrio-* |
| | | *cephalus latus*) |
| ***hypermetabolic states*** | | |
| thyrotoxicosis | pyrexial disease | infections |
| | | |
| ***conditions characterized by decreased nutrient utilization*** | | |
| chronic liver disease | chronic renal disease | |
| | | |
| ***conditions involving increased cell turnover*** | | |
| congenital or acquired | sickle cell disease | |
| hemolytic anemias | | |
| | | |
| ***conditions involving increased nutrient loss*** | | |
| extensive burns | bullous dermatoses | enteropathy |
| nephrosis | surgery | hemodialysis |

---

[1]This approach offers the advantage of rendering a *"requirement"* value that is derived mathematically from the observed data; however, that value tends to be in the region of greatest variation in the input-response curve.

*variation in nutrient requirements*

Many factors can affect nutrient requirements, such that those of individuals with the same general characteristics can vary substantially. For most nutrients the requirements of individuals in given populations appear to be normally distributed. For this reason, in the absence of clear information, it is reasonable to assume that the variations in vitamin requirements is similar to those typically observed in biological systems, that is, normally distributed with a coefficients of variation of 10-15%

Physiologically significant drug-vitamin interactions:

| vitamin | drugs |
|---|---|
| vitamin A | spironolactone[a], cholestyramine[b], colestipol[b], phenol-phthalein[c] |
| vitamin D | phenytoin[d], colestipol, phenolphthalein |
| vitamin K | coumarins[e], phenytoin, colestipol, phenolphthalein, cyclosporins[f] |
| thiamin | ethanol |
| niacin | isoniazid[g], phenylbutazone[h] |
| vitamin $B_6$ | isoniazid, penicillamine[i], L-dopa[j], hydralazine[k], ethanol, thiosemicarbazide[l] |
| folate | phenytoin, pyrimethamine[m], methotrexate[n], sodium bicarbonate[o], sulfasalazine[g], cholestyramine, ethanol |
| vitamin $B_{12}$ | p-aminosalicylic acid[g], cholestyramine, biquanides[l], cimetidine[p], neomycin[g], colchicine[q] |

[a]diuretic   [b]bile acid sequestrant   [c]laxative   [d]anti-convulsant   [e]anti-coagulant   [f]immunosuppressants   [g]anti-bacterial   [h]anti-inflammatant   [i]chelating agent, anti-arthritic   [j]anti-cholinergic, anti-parkinsonian   [k]anti-hypertensive   [l]analytical reagent   [m]anti-malarial   [n]anti-neoplastic   [o]antacid   [p]anti-histamine   [q]gout suppressant

*developing vitamin allowances*

Because nutrient *"requirements"*, even for the best cases, are quantitative estimates based on data of uncertain precision derived from a limited number of subjects, those values have only limited practical usefulness. In practice, *"nutrient allowances"* are far more useful. Nutrient allowances, or *"recommended intakes"*, are selected to meet the needs of those individuals with the greatest requirements for those nutrients in given populations, that is, an allowance is set at the right-hand tail of the natural distribution of requirements. An allowance exceeds the *"average"* requirement estimated for a population by an increment sometimes referred to as a *"margin of safety"*. Allowances for vitamins, particularly in livestock feeding, have often been set on the basis of experience; however, rational approaches are available and have been used for establishing *"official"* nutrient allowances for both animals and humans. The latter are generally described in statistical terms relating to the proportion of the target population the requirements of which would be met by the recommended level of intake. For example, WHO and FAO[2] committees have suggested that allowances should be set at 2 standard deviations (SD) above the average requirement for each nutrient, which level covers the needs of 97.5% of the population.

---

[2]*World Health Organization* and *Food and Agricultural Organization*, respectively, of the United Nations

The most common means of deriving nutrient allowances from nutrient requirements is by using the *mean + 2SD conversion algorithm*[3]. This method has yielded satisfactory results, likely in part to the generous estimates of nutrient requirements generally made by expert committees.

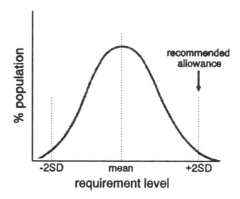

Allowances, therefore, are derived from estimates of requirements (of *"typical"* individuals) made from actual biological data usually from nutritional experiments. Because they are used as standards for populations, allowances are developed with considerations of risk of nutrient deficiency. Therefore, allowances are relevant to *specified populations*, with their characteristic food habits and inherent variations in nutrient requirements. For example, the Recommended Dietary Allowances established by the U.S. National Research Council are implicitly intended to relate to the U.S. population for which they were originally developed to facilitate the wartime planning of food supplies.

Definition of the Recommended Dietary Allowances (RDAs):

> *"Recommended Dietary Allowances (RDAs) are the levels of intake of essential nutrients that, on the basis of scientific knowledge, are judged by the Food and Nutrition Board to be adequate to meet the known nutritional needs of practically all healthy persons."*
>
> Committee on the Tenth Edition of the RDAs, Food and Nutrition, National Research Council, 1989. Recommended Dietary Allowances, 10th ed., National Academy Press, Washington, DC, p. 10.

Considerable confusion surrounds the allowances for the vitamins (and other nutrients) that have been developed by various expert committees. Some questions arise, particularly concerning dietary *"recommendations"* for livestock, because the rationale for such values is frequently not

---

[3] A notable exception is in the setting of allowances for *energy*; these are typically set at the estimated *average requirements* of classes of individuals, for the reason that, unlike other nutrients, both intake and expenditure of energy appear to be regulated such that free-living individuals with free access to food maintain (at least very nearly) energy balance.

presented. A fairly common example is the mistaking, by formulators of animal feeds, of vitamin *"allowances"* to be *"requirements"*; this can lead to vitamin over-fortification of those feeds vitamins. Other questions arise over the publication of differing *"recommendations"* by panels different committees of *"experts"* all of which consider the *same basic data* in their respective reviews of the pertinent literature. This situation results from the paucity of clear and compelling data on nutrient requirements; differences in environmental conditions and food supplies; and the lack of consensus on such issues as criteria for defining requirements, appropriate margins of safety, and whether standards should be based on intakes of food as consumed or as purchased. These considerations make the variable factor of scientific *"judgment"* important in estimating the nature of nutrient requirements. Thus, dietary recommendations are revised periodically[4] as new information becomes available.

History of the NRC Recommended Daily Allowances (RDAs) for vitamins:

| vitamin | 1941 | 1948 | 1957 | 1968 | 1976 | 1980 | 1989 |
|---|---|---|---|---|---|---|---|
| Vitamin A, mg RE | 1000 | 1000 | 1000 | 1000 | 1000 | 1000 | 1000 |
| Vitamin D | | | | 400IU | 400IU | 5$\mu$g | 5$\mu$g |
| Vitamin E, IU | | | | 30 | 15 | 10 | 10 |
| Vitamin K, $\mu$g | | | | | | | 80 |
| Vitamin C, mg | 75 | 75 | 70 | 60 | 45 | 60 | 60 |
| Thiamin, mg | 2.3 | 1.5 | 0.9 | 1.3 | 1.4 | 1.4 | 1.5 |
| Riboflavin, mg | 3.3 | 1.8 | 1.3 | 1.7 | 1.6 | 1.6 | 1.7 |
| Niacin, mg | 23 | 15 | 15 | 17 | 18 | 18 | 19 |
| Vitamin $B_6$, mg | | | | 2.0 | 2.0 | 2.2 | 2.0 |
| Pantothenic Acid | | | | | | | |
| Biotin | | | | | | | |
| Folate, $\mu$g | | | | 400 | 400 | 400 | 200 |
| Vitamin $B_{12}$, $\mu$g | | | | 3.0 | 3.0 | 5.0 | 2.0 |

[males: 25-50 yrs.]

Still other questions about nutrient allowances for humans arise due to the application of those values to purposes for which they were not intended. Although the RDAs were developed originally for use in planning food supplies for *groups* of people[5], they are in fact today used for many other purposes: evaluating the nutritional adequacy of diets; evaluating results of dietary surveys; setting standards for food assistance programs, institutional feeding programs and food and nutrition regulations; developing food and nutrition education programs; formulating new food products and special dietary foods. Many of these uses have fostered criticism of the

---

[4]As available information bases improve, expert committees typically have *reduced* the levels of their recommendations for nutrient allowances. This likely reflects a basically conservative nature of the committee system used for these purposes, whereby the paucity of data tends to be handled by generously estimating quantitative needs.

[5]The RDAs were originated in 1941 for use in planning U.S. food policy during World War II.

RDAs for not dealing with associations of diet and chronic and degenerative diseases, for not including guidelines for appropriate intakes of fat, cholesterol and fiber, and for not providing guidance for food selection and prevention of obesity.  These problems stem from fundamental misunderstandings that, while the RDAs may be used in certain programs to implement sound public health policy, they are not intended to be policy recommendations *per se*.   In fact, RDAs cannot serve as general dietary *guidelines*; by definition, they are reference standards dealing with *nutrients*, while dietary guidelines deal primarily with *foods*.  The RDAs are, in fact, standards upon which sound dietary guidelines are to be based.

*considerations* It should be kept in mind that the RDAs, like other nutrient allowances, are
*implicit to* intended to relate to intakes of nutrients *as part of normal diets*[6] of speci-
*the RDAs* fied populations.  They are intended to be *average daily intakes* based on periods as short as 3 days, for nutrient with fast turnover rates, to several weeks or months, for nutrients with slower turnover rates.

*nutrients and* In one sense, the RDA construct is somewhat archaic in that it fails to
*chronic* pertain to biological functions of nutrients that may be non-specific or non-
*diseases:* traditional in the context of being outside the known functions of nutrients.
*are RDAs* Several such functions have been suggested by fairly recent findings in the
*adequate?* field of Nutritional Epidemiology.  Specifically, evidence is now available for association of several vitamins and other nutrients with risks to such chronic diseases as *cancer*[7] and *cardiovascular diseases*.  Although the mechanisms of these putative nutrient actions remain to be elucidated, they would appear to be *risk-modifiers* of these diseases rather than primary agents in their etiologies.   Nevertheless, findings of such associations have raised questions concerning the concept of the RDA. As it is presently defined, the RDA pertains only to the *specific actions* of nutrients, as in the prevention of specific deficiency diseases, the support of specific coenzyme functions, and the maintenance of tissue reserves of specific metabolites.   Non-specific effects of nutrients, such as those involving interactions with other nutrients and/or non-nutritive factors are simply outside of the current definition of the RDA; the mechanisms for recognizing such needs for nutrients at levels above the RDAs are *dietary guidelines* concerning recommended patterns of food intake.

---

[6]The RDA subcommittee emphasized that the RDAs can typically be met or closely approximated by diets that are based on the consumption of a *variety of foods* from *diverse food groups* that contain *adequate energy*.

[7]Several epidemiological studies have linked intakes of vitamin A-containing foods to reduced risk of cancers of the lung, gastrointestinal tract, bladder, prostate, breast and cervix; there is some question as to whether these effects relate to vitamin A, $\beta$-carotene, other carotenoids or unrelated factors in those foods. Prospective studies have detected links between low plasma $\alpha$-tocopherol levels coupled with low plasma Se to increased risks to cancers of the breast, colon and other sites.  Some studies have linked the consumption of vitamin C-containing foods and, possibly, of vitamin C itself to reduced risk to stomach cancer and, perhaps, cancers of the colon, rectum and lung.  Limited ecologic data from a recent study in China suggest an association of low riboflavin intake with increased risk to esophageal cancer.

## VITAMIN ALLOWANCES FOR HUMANS

*several*
*standards*
*available*

The first nutrient allowances were published 50 years ago by the Food and Nutrition Board of the National Research Council, National Academy of Sciences. Being based on available information, those *"Recommended Dietary Allowances" (RDAs)* have been revised nearly every five years since that time. Since the inception of the publication of RDAs by the U.S. National Research Council, similar dietary standards have been produced by several countries and international organizations. For reasons mentioned above, the various recommendations tend to be similar but not always identical. For example, most are based on food *as consumed*; however, those of West Germany are based on food *as purchased*, making them appear higher than those of other countries.

*the RDAs*

Perhaps the most widely referenced of the dietary standards, and the set that is most comprehensive with respect to the vitamins, are the RDAs produced by the U.S. National Research Council. It is worth noting that the RDAs for the vitamins are still not complete; that is, quantitative recommendations on some (e.g., biotin, pantothenic acid) have not been made due to the lack of a sufficient information base. In 1980, this problem of dealing with nutrients known to be essential for humans but for which insufficient data are available was handled by establishing included *provisional recommendations*; starting with the ninth edition of the RDAs, a table of *"estimated safe and adequate ranges of daily dietary intakes"* was included for such nutrients. In the 1989 publication, vitamin K was removed from that table with the establishment for the first time of RDAs for it; therefore, that edition listed the allowances for only two vitamins (pantothenic acid and biotin) in the provisional category.

*controversy*
*over*
*10th RDAs*

Continuing questions over the means of developing consistent and reliable standards led the tenth RDA Committee to review the scientific basis of the entire RDA table. Their review caused the committee to conclude that the previous allowances for vitamins A and C were high; therefore, they recommended lower RDAs for each in their revision of the 10th RDAs which was to have been published in 1985[8]. It was reported that resistance to this proposal developed within the National Research Council over the earlier recommendation of another NRC committee that intakes of these nutrients be increased as cancer prevention measures. In an unexpected move, the NRC elected not to publish the report of the tenth RDA Committee, instead appointing a five-person panel to prepare the final report. The report of the panel, in which the RDAs for vitamins A and C were *not* changed, was published in 1989 as the tenth RDAs. Discussions of the data upon which the

---

[8]The draft recommendations called for reducing the RDA for vitamin A for adult men and women from 1000 IU RE and 800 IU RE, respectively, to 700 IU RE and 600 IU RE, respectively. Those for vitamin C for adult men and women were recommended to be reduced from 60 mg each to 40 mg for men and 30 mg for women; those for infants were recommended to be reduced from 35 mg to 25 mg.

draft (1985) version of the tenth RDAs were based were published separately by members of the original committee, giving their *recommended dietary intakes* *(RDIs)* for vitamins A, E, K, C, thiamin, riboflavin, niacin, folate and $B_{12}$.

*Canadian* The Committee for the Revision of the Dietary Standard for Canada pro-
*RNIs* duces nutrient standards called *"Recommended Nutrient Intakes"*. The RNIs resemble the RDAs in being defined *"to be adequate to meet the known nutritional needs of practically all healthy persons"*; however, they are somewhat different in quantitative recommendations.

Recommended Vitamin Intakes for Canadians (1983):

| age/condition | vit.A $\mu g^a$ | vit.D $\mu g$ | vit.E $mg^b$ | vit.C $mg$ | folate $\mu g$ | vit.$B_{12}$ $\mu g$ |
|---|---|---|---|---|---|---|
| *Infants:* | | | | | | |
| 0-2 mos. | 400 | 10 | 3 | 20 | 50 | 0.3 |
| 3-5 mos. | 400 | 10 | 3 | 20 | 50 | 0.3 |
| 6-8 mos. | 400 | 10 | 3 | 20 | 50 | 0.3 |
| 9-11 mos. | 400 | 10 | 3 | 20 | 50 | 0.3 |
| *Children:* | | | | | | |
| 1 yr. | 400 | 10 | 3 | 20 | 65 | 0.3 |
| 2-3 yrs. | 400 | 5 | 4 | 20 | 80 | 0.4 |
| 4-6 yrs. | 500 | 5 | 5 | 25 | 90 | 0.5 |
| *Males:* | | | | | | |
| 7-9 yrs. | 700 | 2.5 | 7 | 35 | 125 | 0.8 |
| 10-12 yrs. | 800 | 2.5 | 8 | 40 | 170 | 1.0 |
| 13-15 yrs. | 900 | 2.5 | 9 | 50 | 160 | 1.5 |
| 16-18 yrs. | 1000 | 2.5 | 10 | 55 | 190 | 1.9 |
| 19-24 yrs. | 1000 | 2.5 | 10 | 60 | 210 | 2.0 |
| 25-49 yrs. | 1000 | 2.5 | 9 | 60 | 210 | 2.0 |
| 50-74 yrs. | 1000 | 2.5 | 7 | 60 | 210 | 2.0 |
| 75+ yrs. | 1000 | 2.5 | 6 | 60 | 210 | 2.0 |
| *Females:* | | | | | | |
| 7-9 yrs. | 700 | 2.5 | 6 | 30 | 125 | 0.8 |
| 10-12 yrs. | 800 | 2.5 | 7 | 40 | 170 | 1.0 |
| 13-15 yrs. | 800 | 2.5 | 7 | 45 | 160 | 1.5 |
| 16-18 yrs. | 800 | 2.5 | 7 | 45 | 160 | 1.9 |
| 19-24 yrs. | 800 | 2.5 | 7 | 45 | 165 | 2.0 |
| 25-49 yrs. | 800 | 2.5 | 6 | 45 | 165 | 2.0 |
| 50-74 yrs. | 800 | 2.5 | 6 | 45 | 165 | 2.0 |
| 75+ yrs. | 800 | 2.5 | 5 | 45 | 165 | 2.0 |
| pregnancy (additional) | | | | | | |
| 1st trimester | 100 | 2.5 | 2 | 0 | 305 | 1.0 |
| 2nd trimester | 100 | 2.5 | 2 | 20 | 305 | 1.0 |
| 3rd trimester | 100 | 2.5 | 2 | 20 | 305 | 1.0 |
| lactation (additional) | 400 | 2.5 | 3 | 30 | 120 | 2.0 |

$^a$retinol equivalents    $^b\alpha$-tocopherol equivalents

source: Committee for the Revisions of the Dietary Standard for Canada, Bureau of Nutritional Sciences, Food Directorate, 1983. <u>Recommended Nutrient Intakes for Canadians</u>. Dept. Nat. Health and Welfare, Ottawa, 180 pp.

Recommended Dietary Allowances (RDAs) for vitamins (1989):

| age, (yrs) or condition | vit.A | vit.D | vit.E | vit.K | vit.C | thiamin | ribo-flavin | niacin | vit.B$_6$ | folate | vit.B$_{12}$ |
|---|---|---|---|---|---|---|---|---|---|---|---|
| | µg[a] | µg | mg[b] | µg | mg | mg | mg | mg[c] | mg | µg | µg |
| *Infants:* | | | | | | | | | | | |
| 0-0.5 | 375 | 7.5 | 3 | 5 | 30 | 0.3 | 0.4 | 5 | 0.3 | 25 | 0.3 |
| 0.5-1 | 375 | 10 | 4 | 10 | 35 | 0.4 | 0.5 | 6 | 0.6 | 35 | 0.5 |
| *Children:* | | | | | | | | | | | |
| 1-3 | 400 | 10 | 6 | 15 | 40 | 0.7 | 0.8 | 9 | 1.0 | 50 | 0.7 |
| 4-6 | 500 | 10 | 7 | 20 | 45 | 0.9 | 1.1 | 12 | 1.1 | 75 | 1.0 |
| 7-10 | 700 | 10 | 7 | 30 | 45 | 1.0 | 1.2 | 13 | 1.4 | 100 | 1.4 |
| *Males:* | | | | | | | | | | | |
| 11-14 | 1000 | 10 | 10 | 45 | 50 | 1.3 | 1.5 | 17 | 1.7 | 150 | 2.0 |
| 15-18 | 1000 | 10 | 10 | 65 | 60 | 1.5 | 1.8 | 20 | 2.0 | 200 | 2.0 |
| 19-24 | 1000 | 10 | 10 | 70 | 60 | 1.5 | 1.7 | 19 | 2.0 | 200 | 2.0 |
| 25-50 | 1000 | 5 | 10 | 80 | 60 | 1.5 | 1.7 | 19 | 2.0 | 200 | 2.0 |
| 51+ | 1000 | 5 | 10 | 80 | 60 | 1.2 | 1.4 | 15 | 2.0 | 200 | 2.0 |
| *Females:* | | | | | | | | | | | |
| 11-14 | 800 | 10 | 8 | 45 | 50 | 1.1 | 1.3 | 15 | 1.4 | 150 | 2.0 |
| 15-18 | 800 | 10 | 8 | 55 | 60 | 1.1 | 1.3 | 15 | 1.5 | 180 | 2.0 |
| 19-24 | 800 | 10 | 8 | 60 | 60 | 1.1 | 1.3 | 15 | 1.6 | 180 | 2.0 |
| 25-50 | 800 | 5 | 8 | 65 | 60 | 1.1 | 1.3 | 15 | 1.6 | 180 | 2.0 |
| 51+ | 800 | 5 | 8 | 65 | 60 | 1.0 | 1.2 | 13 | 1.6 | 180 | 2.0 |
| pregnant | 800 | 10 | 10 | 65 | 70 | 1.5 | 1.6 | 17 | 2.2 | 400 | 2.2 |
| lactating 0-6 mos. | 1300 | 10 | 12 | 65 | 95 | 1.6 | 1.8 | 20 | 2.1 | 280 | 2.6 |
| 6-12 mos. | 1200 | 10 | 11 | 65 | 90 | 1.6 | 1.7 | 20 | 2.1 | 280 | 2.6 |

[a]retinol equivalents    [b]α-tocopherol equivalents    [c]niacin equivalents

source:   Subcommittee on the Tenth Edition of the RDAs, Food and Nutrition Board, National Research Council. 1989. Recommended Dietary Allowances, 10 ed., National Academy Press, Washington, DC, 284 pp.

Estimated safe and adequate daily dietary intakes for biotin and pantothenic acid:

| age (yrs.) | biotin µg | pantothenic acid mg |
|---|---|---|
| *Infants:* | | |
| 0-0.5 | 10 | 2 |
| 0.5-1 | 15 | 3 |
| *Children and Adolescents:* | | |
| 1-3 | 20 | 3 |
| 4-6 | 25 | 3-4 |
| 7-10 | 30 | 4-5 |
| 11+ | 30-100 | 4-7 |
| *Adults:* | 30-100 | 4-7 |

source:   Subcommittee on the Tenth Edition of the RDAs, Food and Nutrition Board, National Research Council. 1989. Recommended Dietary Allowances, 10 ed., National Academy Press, Washington, DC, 284 pp.

*International Standards*

The ***Food and Agricultural Organization (FAO)*** and the ***World Health Organization (WHO)*** of the United Nations have established standards for energy, protein, Ca, Fe and 8 of the vitamins. Intended for international use, that is relevant to varied population groups, the FAO/WHO ***"recommended intakes"*** are defined as *"amounts considered sufficient for the maintenance of nearly all people"*. Recently, an FAO/WHO expert group has reviewed available information pertinent to the requirements of humans for vitamin A, Fe, folate and vitamin $B_{12}$. That report provided estimates of averages and variation in the requirements for these nutrients, as well as recommendations for *"safe levels of intake"*[9]. Other dietary standards have been established by many countries; not surprisingly, these show considerable variation.

Recommended intakes of vitamins, FAO/WHO:

| age (yrs.) | vit.A[a] | vit.D[b] | vit.C[b] | thiamin[b] | ribo-flavin[b] | niacin[b] | folate[a] | vit.B$_{12}$[a] |
|---|---|---|---|---|---|---|---|---|
| | $\mu g$[c] | $\mu g$ | mg | mg | mg | mg | $\mu g$ | $\mu g$ |
| *Children:* | | | | | | | | |
| <1 | 350 | 10 | 20 | 0.3 | 0.5 | 5.4 | 6-32 | 0.1 |
| 1-6 | 400 | 10 | 20 | 0.5 | 0.8 | 9.0 | 50 | [0.04][d] |
| 6-10 | 400 | 2.5 | 20 | 0.7 | 1.3 | 14.5 | 102 | [0.04][d] |
| *Male adolescents:* | | | | | | | | |
| 10-12 | 500 | 2.5 | 20 | 0.9 | 1.6 | 17.2 | 102 | [0.04][d] |
| 12-15 | 600 | 2.5 | 30 | 1.0 | 1.7 | 19.1 | 170 | [0.04][d] |
| 15-18 | 600 | 2.5 | 30 | 1.2 | 1.8 | 20.3 | 170 | [0.04][d] |
| *Female adolescents:* | | | | | | | | |
| 10-12 | 500 | 2.5 | 20 | 0.9 | 1.4 | 15.5 | 102 | [0.04][d] |
| 12-15 | 600 | 2.5 | 30 | 1.0 | 1.5 | 16.4 | 170 | [0.04][d] |
| 15-18 | 600 | 2.5 | 30 | 0.9 | 1.4 | 15.2 | 170 | [0.04][d] |
| *Adult men[e]:* | 600 | 2.5 | 30 | 1.2 | 1.8 | 19.8 | 200 | 1.0 |
| *Adult women[e]:* | 500 | 2.5 | 30 | 0.9 | 1.3 | 14.5 | 170 | 1.0 |
| *Pregnant women:* | 600 | 10 | 50 | +0.1 | +0.2 | +2.3 | 340-470 | 1.4 |
| *Lactating women:* | 850 | 10 | 50 | +0.2 | +0.4 | +3.7 | 270 | 1.3 |

[c]retinol equivalents   [d]units per kg body weight   [e]moderately active

sources: [a]Joint FAO/WHO Expert Consultation, 1988. Requirements of Vitamin A, Iron, Folate and Vitamin B$_{12}$. FAO Food and Nutritional Series No. 23, FAO, Rome; and [b]FAO, 1974. Handbook of Human Nutritional Requirements. FAO Nutritional Studies No. 28, FAO, Rome.

---

[9]As the FAO/WHO group used it, the term *"safe level of intake"* (*"the level of intake which, when sustained, will maintain health and appropriate nutrient reserves in almost all health people"*) is synonymous with *"recommended intake"*, which those organizations have used previously to describe the concept that is virtually the same as that indicated by *"nutrient allowance"*. The FAO/WHO group explicitly defined the term to include a consideration of both a *"basal requirement"* and a *"normative storage requirement"*, in that it is used as *"a statement of the level of nutrient intake that is believed to present a very low risk of nutrient depletion in a randomly selected individual"*.

Variations in recommended dietary allowances for vitamins by 30 national or international organizations:

| vitamin | recommended daily allowance[a] | |
| --- | --- | --- |
| | median | range |
| vitamin A, $\mu g$[a] | 800 | 360-1650 |
| vitamin $D_3$, $\mu g$ | 5 | 2.5-20 |
| vitamin E, mg[b] | 10 | 5-50 |
| vitamin K, mg | 140 | 30-3000 |
| vitamin C, mg | 60 | 15-100 |
| thiamin, mg | 1.2 | 0.5-2.2 |
| riboflavin, mg | 1.6 | 0.8-3.2 |
| niacin, mg | 18 | 5.5-22 |
| vitamin $B^6$ | 2 | 1-4 |
| biotion, $\mu g$ | 200 | 100-400 |
| pantothenic acid, mg | 7 | 3-14 |
| folate, mg | 2.1 | 1-20 |
| vitamin $B_{12}$, $\mu g$ | 2 | 1-5 |

[a]for moderately active men    [b]retinol equivalents    [c]$a$-tocopherol equivalents

source: Brubacher, G. 1989. Estimation of daily requirements for vitamins. *in* Elevated Dosages of Vitamins (P. Walter, G. Brubacher and H. Stähelin, eds.), Hans Huber Publ., Toronto, pp. 3-11.

# VITAMIN ALLOWANCES FOR ANIMALS

*public and private information*

The development of livestock production enterprises for the economical production of human food and fiber has superimposed practical needs on the formulation of animal feeds that do not exist in the area of human nutrition. Most notably, this involves access to current information on nutrient requirements and feedstuff nutrient composition. Often, it is the availability of such accurate data that enables commercial animal nutritionists to formulate nutritionally balanced feeds, using computerized linear programming techniques, that maintain cost-competitiveness in a context wherein the cost of feeding can be the largest cost of production[10]. Thus, while recent expansion of understanding in human nutrition has come from discoveries made in public-sponsored research; research in food animal nutrition has, over the past few decades, moved progressively out of the public sector and into the research divisions of agribusinesses with immediate interests in generating such data. The result is that a diminishing proportion of practical animal nutrition data (particularly in the area of amino acid nutrition) remains in the public sector and is, thus, available to the scrutiny of

---

[10]For example, the feed costs for broiler chickens can account for 60-70% of the total cost of producing poultry meat.

Estimated vitamin requirements of domestic and laboratory animals [*part 1*]:

| species | A | D | E | K | C | thiam. | ribo-flavin | niacin | B$_6$ | folate | panto. acid | biotin | B$_{12}$ | choline |
|---|---|---|---|---|---|---|---|---|---|---|---|---|---|---|
| | IU | IU | mg$^a$ | µg$^b$ | mg | mg | mg | mg | mg | mg | mg | µg | µg | g |
| *birds:* | | | | | | | | | | | | | | |
| chickens | | | | | | | | | | | | | | |
| grow. chicks | 1500 | 200 | 10 | .5 | | 1.8 | 3.6 | 27 | 2.5-3 | .55 | 10 | .1-.15 | 3-9 | .5-1.3 |
| laying hens | 4000 | 500 | 5 | .5 | | .8 | 2.2 | 10 | 3 | .25 | 2.2 | .1 | 4 | |
| breeding hens | 4000 | 500 | 10 | .5 | | .8 | 3.8 | 10 | 4.5 | .25 | 10 | .15 | 4 | |
| ducks | | | | | | | | | | | | | | |
| growing | 4000 | 220 | | .4 | | | 4 | 55 | 2.6 | | 11 | | | |
| breeding | 4000 | 500 | | .4 | | | 4 | 40 | 3 | | 11 | | | |
| geese | | | | | | | | | | | | | | |
| growing | 1500 | 200 | | | | | 2.5-4 | 35-55 | | | 15 | | | |
| breeding | 4000 | 200 | | | | | 4 | 20 | | | | | | |
| pheasants | | | | | | | 3.5 | 40-60 | | | 10 | | | 1-1.5 |
| quail | | | | | | | | | | | | | | |
| grow. bobwhite | | | | | | | 3.8 | 30 | | | 13 | | | 1.5 |
| breed. bobwhite | | | | | | | 4 | 20 | | | 15 | | | 1.0 |
| grow. coturnix | 5000 | 1200 | 12 | 1 | | 2 | 4 | 40 | 3 | 1 | 10 | .3 | 3 | 2.0 |
| breed. coturn. | 5000 | 1200 | 25 | 1 | | 2 | 4 | 20 | 3 | 1 | 15 | .15 | 3 | 1.5 |
| turkeys | | | | | | | | | | | | | | |
| grow. poults | 4000 | 900 | 12 | .8-1 | | 2 | 3.6 | 40-70 | 3-4.5 | .7-1 | 9-11 | .1-.2 | 3 | .8-1.9 |
| breed. hens | 4000 | 900 | 25 | 1 | | 2 | 4 | 30 | 4 | 1 | 16 | .15 | 3 | 1.0 |
| *Cats* | 10000 | 1000 | 80 | | | 5 | 5 | 45 | 4 | 1 | 10 | .5 | 20 | 2.0 |
| *Cattle:* | | | | | | | | | | | | | | |
| dry heifers | 2200 | 300 | | | | | | | | | | | | |
| dairy bulls | 2200 | 300 | | | | | | | | | | | | |
| lactating cows | 3200 | 300 | | | | | | | | | | | | |
| beef cattle | 2200 | 300 | | | | | | | | | | | | |
| *Dogs* | 5000 | 275 | 50 | | | 1 | 2.2 | 11.4 | 1 | .18 | 10 | .1 | 22 | 1.25 |
| *Fishes:* | | | | | | | | | | | | | | |
| bream | | | | | | | | | 5-6 | | 30-50 | 1 | | 4.0 |
| carp | 10000 | | 300 | | | | 7 | 28 | 5-6 | | 10-20 | | | |
| catfish | 2000 | 1000 | 30 | | 60 | 1 | 9 | 14 | 3 | 5 | 40 | 1 | 20 | 3.0 |
| coldwater spp. | 2500 | 2400 | 30 | 10 | 100 | 10 | 20 | 150 | 10 | | | | | |
| *Foxes* | 2440 | | | | | 1 | 5.5 | 9.6 | 1.8 | .2 | 7.4 | | | |
| *Goats* | 60$^c$ | 12.9$^c$ | | | | | | | | | | | | |

$^a$α-tocopherol    $^b$menadione    $^c$Unlike almost all of the other values in this table, this requirement is expressed in units (IU) per kg body weight.

sources:
National Research Council, 1984. Nutrient Requirements of Poultry. 8th rev. ed. Nat. Acad. Press, Washington, 71 pp.
*ibid.* 1978. Nutrient Requirements of Cats. rev. ed. Nat. Acad. Press, Washington, 56 pp.
*ibid.* 1978. Nutrient Requirements of Dairy Cattle. 5th rev. ed. Nat. Acad. Press, Washington, 76 pp.
*ibid.* 1984. Nutrient Requirements of Beef Cattle. 6th rev. ed. Nat. Acad. Press, Washington, 90 pp.
*ibid.* 1985. Nutrient Requirements of Dogs. rev. ed. Nat. Acad. Press, Washington, 56 pp.
*ibid.* 1983. Nutrient Requirements of Warmwater Fishes and Shellfishes. rev. ed. Nat. Acad. Press, Washington, 63 pp.
*ibid.* 1981. Nutrient Requirements of Coldwater Fishes. Nat. Acad. Press, Washington, 63 pp.
*ibid.* 1982. Nutrient Requirements of Mink and Foxes. 2nd rev. ed. Nat. Acad. Press, Washington, 72 pp.
*ibid.* 1981. Nutrient Requirements of Goats: Angora, Dairy and Meat Goats in Temperate and Tropical Countries. Nat. Acad. Press, Washington, 91 pp.

Estimated vitamin requirements of domestic and laboratory animals [*part 2*]:

| species | A | D | E | K | C | thiam. | ribo-flavin | niacin | B6 | folate | panto. acid | biotin | B12 | choline |
|---|---|---|---|---|---|---|---|---|---|---|---|---|---|---|
| | IU | IU | mg[a] | μg[b] | g | mg | mg | mg | mg | mg | mg | μg | μg | g |
| *Guinea Pigs* | 23333 | 1000 | 50 | 5 | 200 | 2 | 3 | 10 | 3 | 4 | 20 | .3 | 10 | 1.0 |
| *Hamsters* | 3636 | 2484 | 3 | 4 | | 20 | 15 | 90 | 6 | 2 | 40 | .6 | 20 | 2.0 |
| *Horses:* | | | | | | | | | | | | | | |
| ponies | 25[c] | | | | | | | | | | | | | |
| preg. mares | 50[c] | | | | | | | | | | | | | |
| lact. mares | 55-65[c] | | | | | | | | | | | | | |
| yearlings | 40[c] | | | | | | | | | | | | | |
| 2 yr. olds | 30[c] | | | | | | | | | | | | | |
| *Mice* | 500 | 150 | 20 | 3 | | 5 | 7 | 10 | 1 | .5 | 10 | .2 | 10 | .6 |
| *Mink* | 5930 | | 27 | | | 1.3 | 1.6 | 20 | 1.6 | .5 | 8 | .12 | 32.6 | |
| *Primates*[d] | 15000 | 2000 | 50 | | .1 | | 5 | 50 | 2.5 | .2 | 10 | .1 | | |
| *Rabbits:* | | | | | | | | | | | | | | |
| growing | 580 | | 40 | | | | | 180 | 39 | | | | | 1.2 |
| pregnant | >1160 | | 40 | .2 | | | | | | | | | | |
| lactating | | | 40 | | | | | | | | | | | |
| *Rats* | 4000 | 1000 | 30 | .5 | | 4 | 3 | 20 | 6 | 1 | 8 | | 50 | 1.0 |
| *Sheep:* | | | | | | | | | | | | | | |
| ewes | | | | | | | | | | | | | | |
| early preg. | 26[c] | 5.6[c] | | | | | | | | | | | | |
| late prg./lact. | 35[c] | 5.6[c] | | | | | | | | | | | | |
| rams | 43[c] | 5.6[c] | | | | | | | | | | | | |
| lambs | | | | | | | | | | | | | | |
| early weaned | 35[c] | 6.6[c] | | | | | | | | | | | | |
| finishing | 26[c] | 5.5[c] | | | | | | | | | | | | |
| *Shrimps* | | | | | 10 | | 120 | | | 120 | 120 | | | .6 |
| *Swine:* | | | | | | | | | | | | | | |
| growing | 2200 | 200 | 11 | 2 | | 1.3 | 2.2-3 | 10-22 | 1.5 | .6 | 11-13 | .1 | 22 | .4-1.1 |
| bred gilt/sow | 4000 | 200 | 10 | 2 | | | 3 | 10 | 1 | .6 | 12 | .1 | 15 | 1.25 |
| lact. gilt/sow | 2000 | 200 | 10 | 2 | | | 3 | 10 | 1 | .6 | 12 | .1 | 15 | 1.25 |
| boars | 4000 | 200 | 10 | 2 | | | 3 | 10 | 1 | .6 | 12 | .1 | 15 | 1.25 |

[a] α-tocopherol   [b] menadione   [c] Unlike almost all of the other values in this table, this requirement is expressed in units (IU) per kg body weight.   [d] non-human species

sources:
National Research Council, 1978. Nutrient Requirements of Laboratory Animals. 3rd rev. ed., Nat. Acad. Press, Washington, 96 pp.
*ibid.* 1982. Nutrient Requirements of Mink and Foxes. 2nd rev. ed. Nat. Acad. Press, Washington, 72 pp.
*ibid.* 1978. Nutrient Requirements of Horses. 4th rev. ed. Nat. Acad. Press, Washington, 33 pp.
*ibid.* 1978. Nutrient Requirements of Nonhuman Primates. Nat. Acad. Press, Washington, 83 pp.
*ibid.* 1977. Nutrient Requirements of Rabbits. 2nd rev. ed. Nat. Acad. Press, Washington, 33 pp.
*ibid.* 1975. Nutrient Requirements of Sheep. 5th rev. ed. Nat. Acad. Press, Washington, 72 pp.
*ibid.* 1979. Nutrient Requirements of Swine. 8th rev. ed. Nat. Acad. Press, Washington, 52 pp.

experts.  As a consequence, two type of dietary standards are in use.  The first is the standard developed by review of "open" data available in the scientific literature; the second is the standard developed through "in-house" testing and/or practical experience by animal producers.  Whereas the former are in the public domain, the latter usually are not.

Public information on nutrient allowances is reviewed by expert committees in the U.S., the U.K. and several other countries under programs charged with the responsibility of establishing nutrient recommendations on the basis of the best available data.  Perhaps the most widely used source of such recommendations is the Committee on Animal Nutrition of the U.S. National Research Council.  Through species-based subcommittees of experts, that organization maintains the periodic review of nutrient standards, many of which serve as the bases of recommendations for animal feed formulation throughout the world.  Currently, many gaps remain in knowledge of vitamin requirements.  This is particularly true for ruminant species, for which the substantial ruminal destruction of vitamins appears to be compensated by adequate microbial synthesis, and for several non-ruminant species that are not widely used for commercial purposes.  Therefore, many of the standards for vitamins and other nutrients are imputed from available data on related species; in part for this reason, the "requirements" for some nutrients (e.g., Se) appear to be very similar among many species.

## Study Questions and Exercises:

i.      Prepare a **concept map** illustrating the relationships of the concepts *minimal* and *optimal nutrient requirements* and *nutrient allowances* to the concepts *physiological function* and *health*.

ii.     What *issues* relate to the application of *dietary allowances*, as they are currently defined, to *individuals*?

iii.    What *issues* relate to the consideration of *nutritional status* in such areas as *immune function* or *chronic and degenerative diseases* in the development of *dietary standards*?

## Recommended Reading:

Beaton, G.H. 1985. Nutritional assessment of observed nutrient intake: an interpretation of recent requirement reports. in Advances in Nutritional Research, vol. 7 (H.H. Draper, ed.), Plenum Press, New York, pp. 101-128.

Bieri, J.G. 1987. Are the recommended allowances for dietary antioxidants adequate? Free Radical Biol. Med. 3:193-197.

Harper, A.E. 1990. Dietary standards and guidelines in Present Knowledge in Nutrition, 6th ed. (M.L. Brown, ed.), Int. Life Sci. Inst.-Nutr. Found., Washington, D.C., pp. 491-501.

Harper, A.E. 1987. Evolution of recommended dietary allowances - new directions? Ann. Rev. Nutr. 7:509-537.

Herbert, V. 1987. Recommended dietary intakes (RDI) of folate in humans. Am. J. Clin. Nutr. 45:661-670.

Herbert, V. 1987. Recommended dietary intakes (RDI) of vitamin $B_{12}$ in humans. Am. J. Clin. Nutr. 45:671-678.

Horwitt, M. 1986. Interpretations of requirements for thiamin, riboflavin, niacin-tryptophan, and vitamin E plus comments on balance studies and vitamin $B_6$. Am. J. Clin. Nutr. 44:973-985.

Olson, J.A. 1987. Recommended dietary intakes (RDI) of vitamin K in humans. Am. J. Clin. Nutr. 45:687-692.

Olson, J.A. 1987. Recommended dietary intakes (RDI) of vitamin C in humans. Am. J. Clin. Nutr. 45:693-703.

Olson, J.A. 1987. Recommended dietary intakes (RDI) of vitamin A in humans. Am. J. Clin. Nutr. 45:704-716.

Pike, R.L. and M.L. Brown. 1984. Dietary standards, Chapter 25 in Nutrition: an Integrated Approach, 3rd ed., John Wiley & Sons, New York, pp. 813-831.

Roe, D.A. 1978. Factors affecting nutritional requirements, Chapter 2 in Drug-Induced Nutritional Deficiencies, AVI Publ. Co., Westport, Conn., pp. 70-91.

Southgate, D.A.T., G. Cannon, B.A. Rolls, M.J. Gibney and M.I. Gurr. 1990. Editorial. Dietary recommendations: how do we move forward? Br. J. Nutr. 64:301-305.

Subcommittee on the Tenth Edition of the RDAs, Food and Nutrition Board, National Research Council. 1989. Recommended Dietary Allowances, National Academy Press, Washington, D.C., 284 pp.

# CHAPTER 22     VITAMIN SAFETY

*"Nutriment is both food and poison. The dosage makes it either poison or remedy."*

T. B. von Hohenheim

---

## Anchoring Concepts:

i.     Vitamins are typically used in human feeding, in animal diets and in treating certain clinical conditions at levels in excess of their requirements.

ii.     Several of the vitamins, most notably vitamins A and D, can produce adverse physiological effects when consumed in excessive amounts.

## Learning Objectives:

i.     To understand the concept of *upper safe use level* as used with respect to the vitamins.

ii.     To understand the *margins of safety* above their respective requirements for intakes each of the vitamins.

iii.     To understand the *factors affecting vitamin toxicities*.

iv.     To understand the *signs/symptoms* of vitamin toxicities in humans and animals.

## Vocabulary:

| | |
|---|---|
| hypervitaminosis | safe use level |
| margin of safety | toxic threshold |
| range of safe intake | |

# USES OF VITAMINS ABOVE REQUIRED LEVELS

*typical uses*
*exceed*
*requirements*

Most normal diets that include varieties of foods intake can be expected to provide supplies of the vitamins that meet those levels required to prevent clinical signs of deficiencies. In addition, most *intentional* uses of vitamins are designed to exceed those *requirements* of most individuals. Indeed, that is the principle by which vitamin *allowances* are set. Thus, the formulation of diets, the planning of meals, the vitamin-fortification of foods, and the designing of vitamin supplements are all done to provide vitamins at levels contributing to total intakes that exceed the requirements of most individuals by some *"margins of safety"*. This approach minimizes the probability of producing vitamin deficiencies in populations.

*clinical*
*conditions*
*requiring*
*elevated doses*
*of vitamins*

Some clinical conditions *require* the use of vitamin supplements at levels greater than those normally used to accommodate the usual *"margins of safety"*. These include ***specific vitamin deficiency disorders***[1] and certain rare ***inherited metabolic defects***[2]. In such cases, vitamins are prescribed at doses that far exceed requirement levels; at such pharmacologic doses, many effects may not involve physiological vitamin functions.

*other*
*putative*
*benefits of*
*elevated doses*
*of vitamins*

Elevated doses of vitamins are also frequently prescribed by physicians or are taken as over-the-counter supplements by affected individuals in the treatment of certain other pathological states including neurological pains, psychosis, alopecia, anemia, asthenia, premenstrual tension, carpal tunnel syndrome, and prevention of the common cold. Although the efficacies of vitamin supplementation in most of these conditions remain untested in double-blind clinical trials, vitamin prophylaxis and/or therapy for at least some conditions is perceived as effective by many people in the medical community as well as in the general public. For certain groups, such as athletes, this view supports the widespread use of oral vitamin supplements at dosages greater than 50-100 times RDAs[3].

---

[1] The most commonly encountered vitamin deficiency disorders, particularly in the developing world, are xerophthalmia, rickets, scurvy, beri beri, pellagra, and disorders related to excessive alcohol consumption (polyneuritis, encephalopathy). Of these, the prophylaxis and treatment of xerophthalmia with large doses of vitamin A (100,000 IU for children under 1 yr., and 200,000 IU for others) administered semi-annually has been questioned, as side effects (mild nausea, vomiting, headaches) have been reported in 1-4% of recipients.

[2] Examples are vitamin $B_6$-responsive ***cystathionase deficiency***, vitamin $B_{12}$-responsive ***transcobalamin II deficiency***, and biotin-responsive ***biotinidase deficiency***. Other examples are listed on p. 115.

[3] Several studies have shown that athletes and their coaches generally believe that athletes require higher levels of vitamins than do none-athletes. This attitude appears to affect their behavior, as athletes use vitamin (and mineral) supplements with greater frequencies than the general population. One study found that 84% of international Olympic competitors used vitamin-supplements. Despite this widespread belief, it remains unclear whether any of the vitamins at levels of intake greater than RDAs can affect athletic performance.

# HAZARDS OF EXCESSIVE VITAMIN INTAKES

*non-linear risk responses to vitamin dosage*

The risks of adverse effects (*toxicity*) of the vitamins, like those of any other potentially toxic compounds, are functions of dosage level. In general, the risk-dosage function is curvilinear, indicating a *"toxic threshold"* for vitamin dosage at some level *greater than the requirement* for that vitamin. Thus, a dosage increment exists between the level required to prevent deficiency and that sufficient to produce toxicity. That increment, the *"range of safe intake"*, is bounded on the low-dosage side by the *allowance*, and on the high-dosage side by the *upper safe limit*, each of which is set based on similar considerations of risk to adverse effects within the population.

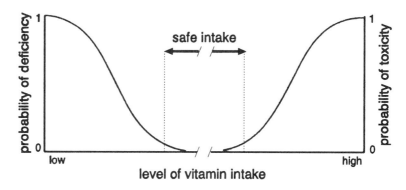

*factors affecting vitamin toxicity*

Several factors can affect the toxicity of any vitamin. These include the *route of exposure*, the *dose regimen* (number of doses and intervals between doses), the general *health of the subject*, and potential effects of *food and drugs*. For example, parenteral routes of vitamin administration may increase the toxic potential of high vitamin doses, as the normal routes of controlled absorption and hepatic first-pass metabolism may be circumvented. Large single doses of the water-soluble vitamins are rarely toxic, as they are generally rapidly excreted, thus, minimally affecting tissue reserves; however, repeated multiple doses of these compounds can produce adverse effects. In contrast, single large doses of the fat-soluble vitamins can produce large tissue stores that can steadily release toxic amounts of the vitamin thereafter. Some disease states, such as those involving malabsorption, can reduce the potential for vitamin toxicity; however, most increase that potential by compromising the subject's ability to metabolize and excrete the vitamin[4], or by rendering the subject particularly susceptible to the hypervitaminosis[5]. Foods and some drugs can reduce the absorption of certain vitamins, thus, reducing their toxicities.

---

[4] For example, persons with liver damage (e.g., alcoholic cirrhosis, viral hepatitis) have increased plasma levels of free (unbound) retinol and a higher incidence of adverse reactions to large doses of vitamin A.

[5] For example, patients with nephrocalcinosis are particularly susceptible to hypervitaminosis D.

## SIGNS OF HYPERVITAMINOSES

*vitamin A*    The potential for vitamin A intoxication is greater than those for other hypervitaminoses, as its *range of safe intakes is relatively small.* For humans, intakes as low as 25 times the RDA are thought to be potentially intoxicating, although actual cases of hypervitaminosis A have been very rare[6] at chronic doses less than ca. 9000 $\mu$g RE per day. The consumption of 25,000-50,000 IU/day for periods of several months has been associated with multiple adverse effects, and intakes by pregnant women of ca. 25,000 IU/day have been associated with birth defects. Infants appear to be especially susceptible to hypervitaminosis A signs of which have been reported in individuals consuming 2100 IU/100 kcal (3-8 times RDAs). Acute hypervitaminosis A can occur in adults after ingestion of $\geq$500,000 IU (100 times RDA). In animals, chronic intakes of 100-1000 times requirement levels have produced clear intoxication, and some adverse effects have been reported at intakes as low as 10 times RDA. Ruminants appear to tolerate high intakes of vitamin A better than non-ruminants, apparently due to substantial destruction of the vitamin by the rumen microflora. The most frequently observed signs are loss of appetite, loss of weight or reduced growth, skeletal malformations, spontaneous fractures and internal hemorrhages; most signs of hypervitaminosis A can be reversed by discontinuing excess exposure to the vitamin.

*vitamin D*    Because they are stored in adipose tissue, vitamins $D_2$ and $D_3$ have relatively high potentials for producing systemic toxicity after single overdoses. Intakes as low as 50 times RDAs have been reported to be toxic to humans. Children appear to be particularly sensitive to the hypervitaminosis; cases of toxicity have been reported resulting from the use of large doses of the vitamin for prophylaxis or treatment of rickets. Studies with animals indicate that vitamin $D_3$ is 10-20 times more toxic than vitamin $D_2$[7], apparently because it is more readily metabolized than the latter vitamer to 25-OH-D, which is thought to produce the lesions that characterize hypervitaminosis D. Those lesions (hypercalcemia, calcinosis) suggest that hypervitaminosis D involves extremes of the normal physiologic functions of Ca-homeostasis for which vitamin D is essential. Accordingly, hypervitaminosis D can be exacerbated by high intakes of Ca and P, and reduced by intakes of low Ca levels or of Ca-chelating agents.

---

[6]According to Bendrich (Am. J. Clin. Nutr. 49:358,1989), fewer than 10 cases per year were reported in 1976-1987. Several of those occurred in persons with concurrent hepatic damage due to drug exposure, viral hepatitis or protein-energy malnutrition.

[7]That is, vitamin $D_3$ can produce effects comparable to vitamin $D_2$ at doses of 5-10% of the latter.

| | |
|---|---|
| *vitamin E* | The toxic potential of vitamin E is very low; intakes of 100+ times typical allowance levels are tolerated without adverse reactions by all species tested. Substantial clinical experience has shown that daily intakes of up to 2 g. for several years or as much as 3.5 g. for several months have produced few or no ill effects in healthy people. Studies with animals indicate that excessive dosages of tocopherols exert most, if not all, of their adverse effects by antagonizing the utilization of the other fat-soluble vitamins, probably at the level of their common micelle-dependent absorption. The scant data available indicate that vitamin E is safe for most animals at dietary levels up to 100 times their typical dietary allowances. |
| *vitamin K* | The toxic potential of the naturally occurring forms of vitamin K are negligible. Phylloquinone exhibits no adverse effects when administered to animals in massive doses by any route; the menaquinones are similarly thought to have little, if any, toxicity. The synthetic vitamer menadione, when administered parenterally, can produce fatal anemia, hyperbilirubinemia and severe jaundice; however, its toxic threshold appears to be at least 1000 times allowance levels. The horse appears to be particularly vulnerable to menadione toxicity. Parenteral doses of 2-8 mg/kg have been found to be lethal in that species; whereas, the parenteral $LD_{50}$[8] values for most other species are an order of magnitude greater than that. |
| *vitamin C* | The only adverse effects of large dosages of vitamin C that have been consistently observed in humans are gastrointestinal disturbances and diarrhea occurring at levels of intake nearly 20-80 times RDAs. Such intakes have been shown to produce slight increases in urinary oxalic acid excretion; however, it is not clear whether such low-magnitude effects, which are still within normal variation, are associated with increased risks of forming urinary calculi. Dietary vitamin C concentrations 100-1000 times allowance levels appear safe for most species. |
| *thiamin* | The toxic potential of thiamin appears to be low, particularly when it is administered orally. Parenteral doses of the vitamin at 100-200 times RDAs have been reported to cause intoxication in humans, characterized by headache, convulsions, muscular weakness, paralysis, cardiac arrhythmia and allergic reactions. The few animal studies to date indicate that thiamin HCl, administered parenterally at dosages of 1000 times allowance levels, can suppress the respiratory center of the brain, producing dyspnea, cyanosis and epileptiform convulsions. |
| *riboflavin* | High oral dosages of riboflavin are very safe, probably due to the relatively poor absorption of the vitamin at high levels. No adverse effects in humans have been reported. Studies with animals indicate that dosages as great as 100 times allowance levels have negligible risks of toxicity. |

---

[8]The $LD_{50}$ value is a useful parameter indicative of the degree of toxicity of a compound. It is defined as the lethal dose for 50% of a reference population, and is calculated from experimental dose-survival data using the probit analysis.

niacin                In humans, high dosages (2-4 g/day) of *nicotinic acid* can cause vasodila-
                      tion, itching, nausea, vomiting, headaches and, less frequently, skin
                      lesions; whereas, *nicotinamide* only rarely produces these reactions. The
                      latter form of the vitamin, therefore, is recommended for medical use.
                      Many patients have taken daily oral doses of 200 mg to 10 g nicotinamide
                      for periods of years with only occasional side effects at the larger dosages
                      (skin rashes, hyperpigmentation, reduced glucose tolerance in diabetics,
                      some liver dysfunction). Nicotinamide dosages of 50-100 times RDAs have
                      not been associated with these effects and, therefore, can be considered
                      safe for most people. Available information on the tolerances of animals
                      for niacin is scant but suggests that daily doses greater than 350-500 mg
                      nicotinic acid equivalents per kg body weight can be toxic.

vitamin $B_6$         Daily dosages as great as 500 mg vitamin $B_6$ have been used for humans
                      (treatment of premenstrual tension in women) for periods of several
                      months without significant adverse effects[9]; however, larger dosages (500
                      mg to 6 g per day) have produced reversible neuropathies after chronic
                      use. It would appear, therefore, that levels as great as 100 times RDAs can
                      be used safely for most people. Substantial information concerning the
                      safety of large doses of vitamin $B_6$ in animals are available for only the dog
                      and the rat. That information indicates that dosages less than 1000 times
                      allowance levels are safe for those species and, by inference, for other
                      animal species.

pantothenic           Pantothenic acid is generally regarded as being *non-toxic*. No ill effects
acid                  have been reported for any species given the vitamin orally; although
                      parenteral administration of very large amounts (e.g., 1 g per kg body
                      weight) of the Ca-salt have been shown to be lethal to rats[10]. A very few
                      reports indicate diarrhea occurring in humans consuming 10-20 g of the
                      vitamin per day. Thus, it appears that pantothenic acid is safe for humans
                      at dosages of *at least* 100 times RDAs; for animals, dosages as great as
                      1000 times allowance levels can be considered safe.

biotin                Biotin is generally regarded as being *non-toxic*. Adverse effects of large
                      dosages of biotin have not been reported in humans or animals given the
                      vitamin orally. Limited data suggests that biotin is safe for most people at
                      dosages of as great as 500 times RDAs and for animals at probably more
                      than 1000 times allowance levels.

---

[9] A transient dependency condition was reported.

[10] Ten times that level, i.e., 10 g/kg body weight, produced no adverse effects on rats.

*folate*  Folate is generally regarded as being *non-toxic*. Adverse reactions to large dosages of it have not been observed in animals. Other than a few cases of apparent allergic reactions, the only proposed adverse effect in humans (interference with the enteric absorption of Zn) is not supported with adequate data. Dosages of 400 mg folate per day for several months have been tolerated without side effects in humans, indicating that levels at least as great as 2000 times RDAs are safe. Because no adverse effects of folate in animals have ever been reported, it would appear that similarly wide ranges of intakes are also safe for animals.

*vitamin B$_{12}$*  Vitamin B$_{12}$ is generally regarded as being *non-toxic*[11]. A few cases of apparent allergic reactions have been reported in humans; otherwise no adverse reactions have been reported for humans or animals given high levels of the vitamin. Upper safe limits of vitamin B$_{12}$ use are, therefore, highly speculative; it appears that dosages at least as great as 1000 times RDAs/allowances are safe for humans and animals.

## SAFE INTAKES OF VITAMINS

*ranges of safe intakes of the vitamins*  The vitamins fall into four categories of relative toxicity. The first category includes those vitamins with the *greatest potentials for producing adverse reactions* at levels of exposure above typical allowances: **vitamin A** and **vitamin D**. The second category includes only one vitamin, which has moderate potentials for toxicity: *niacin*. The third category includes the vitamins with low toxic potentials: **vitamin E, vitamin C, thiamin, riboflavin** and **vitamin B$_6$**. The last category include the vitamins with *negligible toxicities*: **vitamin K, pantothenic acid, biotin, folate** and **vitamin B$_{12}$**. In circumstances of vitamin use at levels appreciably greater than the standard allowances (RDAs for humans, or recommended use levels for animals), prudence dictates giving special consideration to those vitamins with greatest potentials for toxicity (those in the first two or three categories). In practice, it may only be necessary to consider the most potentially toxic vitamins of the first category (vitamins A and D).

---

[11]Indeed, low toxicity would be predicted for this vitamin on the basis of its poor absorption.

Signs and symptoms of vitamin toxicities in humans:

| vitamin | children | adults |
|---|---|---|
| vitamin A | *acute toxicity:*<br>anorexia, bulging frontanelles, lethargy, high intracranial fluid pressure, irritability, nausea, vomiting<br><br>*chronic toxicity:*<br>alopecia, anorexia, bone pain, bulging frontanelles, cheilitis, craniotabes, hepatomegaly, hyperostosis, photophobia, premature epiphyseal closure, pruritus, skin desquamation, insomnia, erythema | *acute toxicity:*<br>abdominal pain, anorexia, blurred vision, lethargy, headache, hypercalcemia, irritability, muscular weakness, nausea, vomiting, peripheral neuritis, skin desquamation<br>*chronic toxicity:*<br>alopecia, anorexia, ataxia, bone pain, cheilitis, conjunctivitis, diarrhea, diplopia, dry mucous membranes, dysuria, edema, high CSF pressure, fever, headache, hepatomegaly, hyperostosis, irritability, lethargy, menstrual abnormalities, muscular pain and weakness, nausea, vomiting, polydypsia, pruritus, skin desquamation, erythema, splenomegaly, weight loss |
| vitamin D | anorexia, diarrhea, hypercalcemia, irritability, lassitude, muscular weakness, neurological abnormalities, polydypsia, polyuria, poor weight gain, renal impairment | anorexia, bone demineralization, constipation, hypercalcemia, muscular weakness and pain, nausea, vomiting, polyuria, renal calculi |
| vitamin E | *no adverse effects reported* | mild gastrointestinal distress, some nausea, coagulopathies in patients receiving anti-convulsants |
| vitamin K[a] | *no adverse effects reported* | *no adverse effects reported* |
| vitamin C | *no adverse effects reported* | gastrointestinal distress, diarrhea, oxaluria |
| thiamin[b] | *no adverse effects reported* | headache, muscular weakness, paralysis, cardiac arrhythmia, convulsions, allergic reactions |
| riboflavin | *no adverse effects reported* | *no adverse effects reported* |
| niacin | *no adverse effects reported* | blood vessel dilation, itching skin, headache, liver damage, jaundice, cardiac arrhythmia, anorexia |
| vitamin $B_6$ | *no adverse effects reported* | neuropathy, skin lesions |
| pantothenic acid | *no adverse effects reported* | diarrhea[c] |
| biotin | *no adverse effects reported* | *no adverse effects reported* |
| folate | *no adverse effects reported* | allergic reactions[c] |
| vitamin $B_{12}$ | *no adverse effects reported* | allergic reactions[c] |

[a]Adverse effects observed only for *menadione*; phylloquinone and the menaquinones appear to have negligible toxicities.
[b]Adverse effects have been observed only when the vitamin was administered *parenterally*; none have been observed when it has been given orally.
[c]This sign has been observed in only a few cases.

Signs of vitamin toxicities in animals [part 1]:

| vitamin | sign | species |
|---|---|---|
| vitamin A | alopecia | rat, mouse |
| | anorexia | cat, cattle, chicken, turkey |
| | cartilage abnormalities | rabbit |
| | convulsions | monkey |
| | elevated heart rate | cattle |
| | fetal malformations | hamster, monkey, mouse, rat |
| | hepatomegaly | rat |
| | gingivitis | cat |
| | irritability | cat |
| | lethargy | cat, monkey |
| | reduced CSF pressure | cattle, goat, pig |
| | reduced growth | chicken, pig, turkey |
| | skeletal abnormalities | cat, cattle, chicken, dog, duck, mouse, pig, rabbit, rat, turkey |
| vitamin D[a] | anorexia | cattle, chicken, fox, pig, rat |
| | bone abnormalities | pig, sheep |
| | cardiovascular calcinosis | cattle, dog, fox, horse, monkey, mouse, pig, rat, sheep, rabbit |
| | renal calcinosis | cattle, chicken, dog, fox, horse, monkey, mouse, pig, rat, sheep, turkey |
| | cardiac dysfunction | cattle, pig |
| | hypercalcemia | cattle, chicken, dog, fox, horse, monkey, mouse, pig, rat, sheep, trout |
| | hyperphosphatemia | horse, pig |
| | hypertension | dog |
| | myopathy | fox, pig |
| | reduced growth, weight loss | catfish, chicken, horse, mouse, pig, rat |
| | lethality | cattle[c] |
| vitamin E | atherosclerotic lesions | rabbit |
| | bone demineralization | chicken, rat |
| | cardiomegaly | rat |
| | hepatomegaly | chicken |
| | hyperalbuminemia | rat |
| | hypertriglyceridemia | rat |
| | hypocholesterolemia | rat |
| | impaired muscular function | chicken |
| | increased hepatic vitamin A | chicken, rat |
| | increased prothrombin time | chicken |
| | reduced adrenal weight | rat |
| | reduced growth | chicken |
| | increased hematocrit | rat |
| | reticulocytosis | chicken |
| | splenomegaly | rat |
| vitamin K[c] | anemia[c] | dog |
| | renal failure[c] | horse |
| | lethality | chicken[c,d], mouse[c,d], rat[c] |

[a]*Vitamin D$_3$ is much more toxic than vitamin D$_2$.*
[b]Only *menadione* produces adverse effects; phylloquinone and the menaquinones have negligible toxicities.
[c]These effects observed after *parenteral administration* of the vitamin.
[d]These effects observed after *oral administration* of the vitamin.

Signs of vitamin toxicities in animals [part 2]:

| vitamin | sign | species |
|---|---|---|
| vitamin C | anemia | mink |
| | bone demineralization | guinea pig |
| | decreased circulating thyroid hormone | rat |
| | liver congestion | guinea pig |
| | oxaluria | rat |
| thiamin | respiratory distress[a] | rat |
| | cyanosis[a] | rat |
| | epileptiform convulsions[a] | rat |
| riboflavin | *no adverse effects reported for oral doses* | |
| | lethality[b] | rat |
| niacin | impaired growth | chicken (embryo) |
| | developmental abnormalities | chicken (embryo), mouse (fetus) |
| | liver damage | mouse |
| | mucocutaneous lesions | chicken |
| | myocardial damage | mouse |
| | decreased weight gain[c] | chicken |
| | lethality | chicken (embryo)[b], mouse[b,d] |
| vitamin B$_6$ | anorexia | dog |
| | ataxia | dog, rat |
| | convulsions | rat |
| | lassitude | dog |
| | muscular weakness | dog |
| | neurologic impairment | dog |
| | vomiting | dog |
| | lethality[d] | mouse, rat |
| pantothenic acid | *no adverse effects reported for oral doses* | |
| | lethality[d] | rat |
| biotin | *no adverse effects reported for oral doses* | |
| | irregular estrus[a] | rat |
| | fetal resorption[a] | rat |
| folate | *no adverse effects reported for oral doses* | |
| | epileptiform convulsions[a] | rat |
| | renal hypertrophy[a] | rat |
| vitamin B$_{12}$ | *no adverse effects reported for oral doses* | |
| | irregular estrus[a] | rat |
| | fetal resorption[a] | rat |
| | reduced fetal weights[a] | rat |

[a]These signs have only been observed when the vitamin was *administered parenterally*.
[b]Lethality has been reported for *parenterally administered* doses of the vitamin.
[c]*Nicotinamide* is more toxic than *nicotinic acid*.
[d]Lethality has been reported for *orally administered* doses of the vitamin.

Recommended upper safe intakes of the vitamins:

| vitamin | humans (x RDA[a]) | animals (x allowance[b]) |
|---|---|---|
| *high potential for toxicity:* | | |
| vitamin A | 20 (5[c],10[d]) | 10[e]-30[f] |
| vitamin D | 20[g] (10[c]) | 10-20[g] |
| *moderate potential for toxicity:* | | |
| niacin[h] | 50 | 50-100 |
| *low potential for toxicity:* | | |
| vitamin E | 100 | 100 |
| vitamin C | 50-100 | 100-1000 |
| thiamin | 100 | 500 |
| riboflavin | 100 | 100-500 |
| vitamin B$_6$ | 100 | 100-1000 |
| *insignificant potential for toxicity:* | | |
| vitamin K[i] | 500 | 1000 |
| pantothenic acid | 100-500 | 1000 |
| biotin | 500 | 1000 |
| folate | 1000 | 1000 |
| vitamin B$_{12}$ | 1000 | 1000 |

[a]based on the 10th RDAs (National Research Council, 1989); *see* p. 484.
[b]based on the Estimated Vitamin Requirements of Domestic and Laboratory Animals (from National Research Council reports); *see* pp. 487-488.
[c]for infants and young children
[d]for pregnant women
[e]for non-ruminant species
[f]for ruminant species
[g]Vitamin D$^3$ is more toxic than vitamin D$_2$.
[h]Nicotinamide is more toxic than nicotinic acid.
[i]Only menadione has significant (low) toxicity.

## Study Questions and Exercises:

i.      Prepare a **concept map** illustrating the relationships of the concepts *minimal* and *optimal nutrient requirements* and *nutrient allowances* to the concepts *physiological function* and *health*.

ii.     What **issues** relate to the application of *dietary allowances*, as they are currently defined, to *individuals*?

iii.    What **issues** relate to the consideration of *nutritional status* in such areas as *immune function* or *chronic and degenerative diseases* in the development of *dietary standards*?

## Recommended Reading:

Baurenfeind, J.C. 1980. The Safe Use of Vitamin A. Rep. Int. Vit. A Consultative Group, Nutrition Foundation, Washington, D.C., 44 pp.

Bendrich, A. and L. Langseth. 1989. Safety of vitamin A. Am. J. Clin. Nutr. 49:358-371.

Bell, E.F. 1989. Upper limit of vitamin E in infant formulas. J. Nutr. 119:1829-1831.

Flodin, N.W. 1988. Pharmacology of Micronutrients, vol. 20 Current Topics in Nutrition and Disease. Alan R. Liss, New York, pp. 3-243.

Hathcock, J.N. 1990. Evaluation of vitamin A toxicity. Am. J. Clin. Nutr. 52:183-202.

Hathcock, J.N. 1989. High nutrient intakes - the toxicologist's view. J. Nutr. 119:1779-1784.

McCormick, D.B. 1989. Water-soluble vitamins: bases for suggested upper limits in infant formulas. J. Nutr. 119:1818-1819.

Olson, J.A. 1989. Upper limits of vitamin A in infant formulas, with some comments on vitamin K. J. Nutr. 119:1820-1824.

Subcommittee on Vitamin Tolerance, Committee on Animal Nutrition, National Research Council. 1987. Vitamin Tolerance in Animals. National Academy Press, Washington, D.C., 96 pp.

Walter, P., G. Brubacher and H. Stähelin. 1989. Elevated Dosages of Vitamins: Benefits and Hazards. Hans Huber Publishers, Toronto, 245 pp.

# APPENDICES

# APPENDIX A: *ORIGINAL REPORTS FOR CASE STUDIES*

Chapter 5    *case 1*
McLaren, D.S., E. Ahirajian, M. Tchalian and G. Koury. 1965. Xeroph-thalmia in Jordan. Am. J. Clin. Nutr. 17: 117-130.

*case 2*
Wechsler, H.L. 1979. Vitamin A deficiency following small-bowel bypass surgery for obesity. Arch. Dermatol. 115: 73-75.

*case 3*
Sauberlich, H.E., R.E. Hodges, D.L. Wallace, H. Kolder, J.E. Canham, H. Hood, N. Racia, Jr. and L.K. Lowry. 1974. Vitamin A metabolism and requirements in the human studied with the use of labeled retinol. Vit. Horm. 32: 251-275.

Chapter 6    Marx, S.J., A.M. Spiegel, E.M. Brown, D.G. Gardner, R.W. Downs, Jr., M. Attie, A.J. Hamstra and H.F. DeLuca. 1978. J. Clin. Endocrinol. Metab. 47:1303-1310.

Chapter 7    *case 1*
Boxer, L.A., J.M. Oliver, S.P. Spielberg, J.M. Allen and J.D. Schulman. 1979. Protection of Granulocytes by vitamin E in glutathione synthetase deficiency. N. Eng. J. Med. 301:901-905.

*case 2*
Harding, A.E., S. Matthews, S. Jones, C.J.K. Ellis, I.W. Booth and D.P.R. Muller. 1985. N. Eng. J. Med. 313:32-35.

Chapter 8    *case 1*
Colvin, B.T. and M.J. Lloyd. 1977. Severe coagulation defect due to a dietary deficiency of vitamin K. J. Clin. Pathol. 30: 1147-1148.

*case 2*
Corrigan, J. and F.I. Marcus. 1974. Coagulopathy associated with vitamin E ingestion. J. Am. Med. Assoc. 230:1300-1301.

Chapter 9    *case 1*
Hodges, R.E., J. Hood, J.E. Canham, H.E. Sauberlich and E.M. Baker. 1971. Clinical manifestations of ascorbic acid deficiency in man. Am. J. Clin. Nutr. 24:432-443.

*case 2*
Dewhurst, K. 1954. A case of scurvy simulating a gastric neoplasm. Br. Med. J. 2:1148-1150.

Chapter 10    *case 1*
Burwell, C.S. and L. Dexter. 1947. Beriberi heart disease. Trans. Assoc. Am. Physiol. 60:59-64.

*case 2*
Blass, J.P. and G.E. Gibson. 1977. Abnormality of a thiamin-requiring enzyme in patients with Wernicke-Korsakoff syndrome. New Eng. J. Med. 297:1367-1370.

Chapter 11    Dutta, P., M. Gee, R.S. Rivlin and J. Pinto. 1988. Riboflavin deficiency and glutathione metabolism in rats: possible mechanisms underlying altered responses to hemolytic stimuli. J. Nutr. 118:1149-1157.

Chapter 12    Vannucchi, H. and F.S. Moreno. 1989. Interaction of niacin and zinc metabolism in patients with alcoholic pellagra. Am. J. Clin. Nutr. 50:364-369.

Chapter 13    *case 1*
Barber, G.W. and G.L. Spaeth. 1969. The successful treatment of homocystinuria with pyridoxine. J. Pediatr. 75:463-478.

*case 2*
Schaumberg, H., J. Kaplan, A. Windebank, N. Vick, S. Rasmus, D. Pleasure and M.J. Brown. 1983. Sensory neuropathy from pyridoxine abuse. New Eng. J. Med. 309:445-448.

Chapter 14    Mock, D.M., A.A. DeLorimer, W.M. Liebman, L. Sweetman and H. Baker. 1981. Biotin deficiency: an unusual complication of parenteral alimentation. New Eng. J. Med. 304:820-823.

Chapter 15    Lacroix, B., E. Didier and J.F. Grenier. 1988. Role of pantothenic and ascorbic acid in wound healing processes: *in vitro* study on fibroblasts. Int. J. Vit. Nutr. Res. 58:407-413.

Chapter 16    Freeman, J.M., J.D. Finkelstein and S.H. Mudd. 1975. Folate-responsive homocystinuria and schizophrenia. A defect in methylation due to deficient 5,10-methylenetetrahydrofolic acid reductase activity. New Eng. J. Med. 292:491-496.

Chapter 17    Higginbottom, M.C., L. Sweetman and W.L. Nyhan. 1978. A syndrome of methylmalonic aciduria, homocystinuria, megaloblastic anemia and neurological abnormalities of a vitamin $B_{12}$-deficient breast-fed infant of a strict vegetarian. New Eng. J. Med. 299: 317-323.

Original research reports:

*Acta Vitaminonologica et Enzymologica*, Acta Vitaminological et Enzymologica, Milan
*American Journal of Clinical Nutrition*, American Society for Clinical Nutrition, Rockville, Md.
*Annals of Nutrition and Metabolism*, Karger, Basel
*British Journal of Nutrition*, Nutrition Society, Cambridge
*Drug-Nutrient Interactions*, Alan R. Liss, Inc., New York
*Ernährungsforschung*, Academie-Verlag, Berlin
*International Journal for Vitamin and Nutrition Research*, H. Huber Publishers, Berne
*Journal of Biological Chemistry*, American Society of Biological Chemists, Rockville, Md.
*Journal of Clinical Biochemistry and Nutrition*, Institute of Applied Biochemistry, Tokyo
*Journal of Lipid Research*, Lipid Research, Inc., Bethesda, Md.
*Journal of Nutrition*, American Institute of Nutrition, Rockville, Md.
*Journal of Nutritional Biochemistry*, Butterworth Publishers, Stoneham, Mass.
*Journal of Nutritional Science and Vitaminology*, Society of Nutrition and Food Science and the Vitamin Society of Japan, Tokyo
*Lipids*, American Oil Chemists' Society, Champaign, Ill.
*Nutrition Research*, Pergamon Press, New York
*Proceedings of the Nutrition Society*, Nutrition Society, Cambridge

Reviews:

*Annual Review of Biochemistry*, Annual Reviews, Inc., Palo Alto, Ca.
*Annual Review of Nutrition*, Annual Reviews, Inc., Palo Alto, Ca.
*Nutrition Abstracts and Reviews*, Aberdeen University Press, Aberdeen, Scotland
*Nutrition Reviews*, International Life Sciences Institute - Nutrition Foundation, Washington, DC
*Vitamins and Hormones*, Academic Press, San Diego

# Index